The SAGES Manual of Pediatric Minimally Invasive Surgery

Danielle S. Walsh • Todd A. Ponsky
Nicholas E. Bruns
Editors

The SAGES Manual of Pediatric Minimally Invasive Surgery

Springer

Editors
Danielle S. Walsh, MD, FACS, FAAP
Associate Professor of Surgery
Division of Pediatric Surgery
East Carolina University
Brody School of Medicine
Greenville, NC, USA

Nicholas E. Bruns, MD
Research Fellow
Division of Pediatric Surgery
Akron Children's Hospital
Akron, OH, USA

Resident in General Surgery
Cleveland Clinic,
Cleveland, OH, USA

Todd A. Ponsky, MD, FACS
Associate Professor of Surgery and Pediatrics
Northeast Ohio Medical College
Division of Pediatric Surgery
Akron Children's Hospital
Akron, OH, USA

ISBN 978-3-319-43640-1 ISBN 978-3-319-43642-5 (eBook)
DOI 10.1007/978-3-319-43642-5

Library of Congress Control Number: 2016959450

Printed on acid-free paper

This Springer imprint is published by Springer Nature
The registered company is Springer International Publishing AG
The registered company address is: Gewerbestrasse 11, 6330 Cham, Switzerland

Preface

...find though she be but little, she is fierce.—Shakespeare

More than once pediatric surgeons have heard general surgeons comment on their "fear" of caring for pediatric surgical patients. The diminutive size of the patient can intimidate, but those of us flourishing in the pediatric world recognize a well-kept secret—infants and children are fierce in their desire to live, handling the surgical insults that would cause many adults to give out, with determination of sometimes Olympic proportions. While they tolerate large incisions for invasive procedures with aplomb, showing their scars as badges of courage on the playground, we believe our kids deserve to reap the same benefits from minimally invasive techniques that the adult population embraces. This book was developed to help current and future surgeons in advancing their comfort in approaching children with laparoscopy, thoracoscopy, and endoscopy.

The mission of the Society of American Gastrointestinal and Endoscopic Surgeons (SAGES) is to improve patient care through education, research, innovation, and leadership, principally in gastrointestinal endoscopic surgery. The pediatric surgery community within SAGES has been grateful that the leadership of SAGES has recognized the need to apply this mission to not only the adult general surgical population but to all patients, including our youngest and smallest. It is with this in mind that these authors set out to educate *ALL* surgeons, not just pediatric specialists, in the applications of minimally invasive surgery to children through this textbook.

The focus of this text is on the technical knowhow of these minimally invasive techniques. There are larger resources for detailed information on pathophysiology and others reviewing each and every alternative technique for managing a particular disorder. However, this publication is for providing a safe way of technically approaching a particular problem utilizing percutaneous or per-orifice methods in a concise compendium. It is appropriate for the trained professional looking for a refresher on a less commonly performed intervention, an adult MIS surgeon with a pediatric emergency unable to be transferred, or a surgical student or resident in need of critical teaching points for understanding.

This coeditor team greatly appreciates the support we have received from SAGES and Springer in making this endeavor come to fruition. We applaud the authors, colleagues, staff, families, and patients who contributed to this book through either time, effort, patience, or use of their surgical journey to build the knowledge and content within these pages. It is our hope that many a student of surgery will benefit from the herein pearls of wisdom as they endeavor to improve the care of a pediatric surgical patient.

Greenville, NC, USA — Danielle S. Walsh
Akron, OH, USA — Todd A. Ponsky
Akron, OH, USA — Nicholas E. Bruns

Contents

Contributors

Mohammad Ali Abbass Pediatric Surgery, Cleveland Clinic Foundation, Cleveland, OH, USA

Sophia Abdulhai General Surgery, East Carolina University, Greenville, NC, USA

Ruchi Amin General Surgery, East Carolina University, Greenville, NC, USA

Kelly Arps Emory University School of Medicine, Atlanta, GA, USA

Wesley Barnes General Surgery, Beaumont Health System, Royal Oak, MI, USA

Lilly Ann Bayouth General Surgery, East Carolina University, Greenville, NC, USA

Nicholas E. Bruns Pediatric Surgery, Akron Children's Hospital, Akron, OH, USA

General Surgery, Cleveland Clinic, Cleveland, OH, USA

Cathy A. Burnweit Nicklaus Children's Hospital, Miami, FL, USA

Juan L. Calisto Pediatric General and Thoracic Surgery, University of Pittsburgh Medical Center, Pittsburgh, PA, USA

Julietta Chang Digestive Diseases Institute, Cleveland Clinic Foundation, Cleveland, OH, USA

Richard Cheek General Surgery, Allegheny General Hospital, Pittsburgh, PA, USA

Curtis J. Clark Urology, Akron Children's Hospital/ Northeast Ohio Medical University, Akron, OH, USA

Brian T. Craig Monroe Carell Jr. Children's Hospital at Vanderbilt, Nashville, TN, USA

Domenic Craner Pediatric General Surgery, Akron Children's Hospital, Akron, OH, USA

Barrett P. Cromeens General Surgery, East Carolina University, Greenville, NC, USA

Anthony L. DeRoss Pediatric Surgery, Cleveland Clinic Children's, Surgery, Cleveland Clinic Lerner College of Medicine of Case Western Reserve University, Cleveland, OH, USA

Diana L. Diesen Pediatric Surgery, Department of Surgery, Southwestern Medical, Children's Health Dallas, Dallas, TX, USA

Robert Michael Dorman Pediatric Surgery, Women and Children's Hospital of Buffalo, Buffalo, NY, USA

Ibrahim Abd el-shafy Pediatric Surgery, Cohen Children's Medical Center, Queens, NY, USA

Meagan Elizabeth Evangelista Pediatric Surgery, East Carolina University, Greenville, NC, USA

Gavin A. Falk Nicklaus Children's Hospital, Miami, FL, USA

Aaron P. Garrison Pediatric Surgery, Akron Children's Hospital, Akron, OH, USA

James D. Geiger Pediatric Surgery, Mott Children's Hospital, University of Michigan, Ann Arbor, MI, USA

Sarah Gilmore University of Alabama School of Medicine in Birmingham, Birmingham, AL, USA

Ian C. Glenn Pediatric Surgery, Akron Children's Hospital, Akron, OH, USA

Joshua Glenn Pediatric Surgery, Mercer University School of Medicine/The Medical Center – Navicent Health, Macon, GA, USA

Michael J. Goretsky Pediatric Surgery, Carolinas HealthCare System, Charlotte, NC, USA

Moriah M. Hagopian General Surgery, University of Texas Southwestern Medical Center, Dallas, TX, USA

Angela M. Hanna Pediatric Surgery, Swedish Medical Center, Seattle, WA, USA

Carroll M. Harmon Pediatric Surgery, Women and Children's Hospital of Buffalo, Buffalo, NY, USA

Celeste Hollands Surgery, University of South Alabama, Mobile, AL, USA

Anne-Sophie Holler Pediatric Surgery, University Medicine, Johannes Gutenberg University Mainz, Mainz, Germany

Zachary Hothem General Surgery, Beaumont Health System, Royal Oak, MI, USA

Sarah T. Hua Pediatric Surgery, Monroe Carell Jr. Children's Hospital at Vanderbilt, Nashville, TN, USA

Gretchen Purcell Jackson Monroe Carell Jr. Children's Hospital at Vanderbilt, Nashville, TN, USA

Kevin N. Johnson Pediatric Innovation, Pediatric Surgery, Mott Children's Hospital, University of Michigan, Ann Arbor, MI, USA

Folashade Adebisi Jose Pediatric Gastroenterology, East Carolina University, Greenville, NC, USA

Timothy D. Kane Surgery and Pediatrics, Children's National Medical Center, George Washington University School of Medicine, Washington, DC, USA

Harveen K. Lamba Pediatric Surgery, Akron Children's Hospital, Akron, OH, USA

Alessandra Landmann General Surgery, University of Oklahoma Health Sciences Center, Oklahoma City, OK, USA

Christine M. Leeper Surgery, University of Pittsburgh Medical Center, Pittsburgh, PA, USA

Thom E. Lobe Regeneveda, The Beverly Hills Institute of Cellular Therapy, Chicago, IL, USA

Shannon W. Longshore Surgery, East Carolina University, Greenville, NC, USA

Jose Alberto Lopez General Surgery, Swedish Medical Center, Seattle, WA, USA

Jeffrey Lukish Johns Hopkins University, Baltimore, MD, USA

Cristina Mamolea General Surgery, Cleveland Clinic Foundation, Cleveland, OH, USA

Colin A. Martin University of Alabama at Birmingham, Birmingham, AL, USA

Laura Y. Martin Surgery, Johns Hopkins Hospital, Baltimore, MD, USA

Mark O. McCollum Pediatric Surgery, Akron Children's Hospital, Akron, OH, USA

J. Hunter Mehaffey General Surgery, University of Virginia Medical Center, Charlottesville, VA, USA

Go Miyano Pediatric Surgery, Shizuoka Children's Hospital, Shizuoka, Japan

Azmath Mohammed General Surgery, Beaumont Health System, Royal Oak, MI, USA

Kevin P. Mollen Children's Hospital of Pittsburgh of UPMC, Pittsburgh, PA, USA

Oliver J. Muensterer Pediatric Surgery, University Medicine Mainz, Mainz, Germany

Heather R. Nolan General Surgery, Mercer University School of Medicine/The Medical Center – Navicent Health, Macon, GA, USA

Nathan Novotny Pediatric Surgery, Beaumont Health System, Oakland University William Beaumont School of Medicine, Royal Oak, MI, USA

Dominic Papandria Pediatric General and Thoracic Surgery, Children's Hospital of Pittsburgh of UPMC, University of Pittsburgh School of Medicine, Pittsburgh, PA, USA

Neel Parekh Urology, Akron Children's Hospital/Northeast Ohio Medical University, Akron, OH, USA

Shawn D. St. Peter Surgery, Children's Mercy Hospital, Kansas City, MO, USA

Hans G. Pohl Urology and Pediatrics, Children's National Medical Center, Washington, DC, USA

Todd A. Ponsky Surgery and Pediatrics, Pediatric Surgery, Akron Children's Hospital, Akron, OH, USA

Ashwini S. Poola Surgery, Children's Mercy Hospital, Kansas City, MO, USA

José M. Prince Pediatric Surgery, Cohen Children's Medical Center of Northwell Health/Hofstra Northwell School of Medicine, New Hyde Park, NY, USA

Priya Rajdev General Surgery, Emory University, Atlanta, GA, USA

Eric J. Rellinger Pediatric Surgery, Monroe Carell Jr. Children's Hospital at Vanderbilt, Nashville, TN, USA

Robert L. Ricca Surgery, Naval Medical Center Portsmouth/ Uniformed Services University, Portsmouth, VA, USA

J. Eli Robins Surgery, East Carolina University, Greenville, NC, USA

David Rodeberg Pediatric Surgery, East Carolina University, Greenville, NC, USA

Armando Rosales Nicklaus Children's Hospital, Miami, FL, USA

Steven S. Rothenberg Pediatric Surgery, Rocky Mountain Hospital for Children, Denver, CO, USA

Melody R. Saeman Surgery, University of Texas Southwestern, Dallas, TX, USA

Lauren Salesi School of Medicine, University of Pittsburgh, Pittsburgh, PA, USA

Avraham Schlager Pediatric Surgery, Akron Children's Hospital, Akron, OH, USA

Stefan Scholz Pediatric General and Thoracic Surgery, Children's Hospital of Pittsburgh of UPMC, School of Medicine, University of Pittsburgh, Pittsburgh, PA, USA

Federico G. Seifarth Pediatric Surgery, Kalispell Regional Healthcare, Kalispell, MT, USA

Bethany J. Slater Rocky Mountain Hospital for Children, Denver, CO, USA

Oliver Soldes Pediatric Surgery, Akron Children's Hospital, Akron, OH, USA

Andrew T. Strong General Surgery, Cleveland Clinic Foundation, Cleveland, OH, USA

Brandon VanderWel General Surgery, Swedish Medical Center, Seattle, WA, USA

John H.T. Waldhausen Division Chief Pediatric General and Thoracic Surgery, Seattle Children's Hospital, Seattle, WA, USA

William Taylor Walsh General Surgery, South Pointe Hospital, Warrensville Heights, OH, USA

Danielle S. Walsh Pediatric Surgery, East Carolina University, Greenville, NC, USA

Craig A. Wengler Surgery, Mercer University School of Medicine/The Medical Center – Navicent Health, Macon, GA, USA

Simon K. Wright Minimally Invasive Head and Neck Surgery, ENT Clinic of Iowa, West Des Moines, IA, USA

Charlotte Wu Urology, Yale–New Haven Hospital, Yale University School of Medicine, New Haven, CT, USA

Jingliang Yan General Surgery, Cleveland Clinic Foundation, Cleveland, CT, USA

Jeh B. Yung General Surgery, Cleveland Clinic Foundation, Cleveland, OH, USA

Jeh B. Yung Pediatric Surgery, Kalispell Regional Healthcare, Kalispell, MT, USA

David C. van der Zee Pediatric Surgery, University Medical Center Utrecht, Wilhelmina Children's Hospital, Utrecht, The Netherlands

1. Physiologic Considerations for Minimally Invasive Surgery in Infants and Children

Brian T. Craig and Gretchen Purcell Jackson

Introduction

Laparoscopy and thoracoscopy have gained widespread acceptance in the surgical approach to infants and children. Minimally invasive procedures are routinely performed and often considered the standard of care for common pediatric operations, such as appendectomy, pyloromyotomy, and fundoplication. Many pediatric surgeons employ laparoscopy or thoracoscopy for advanced procedures including operations for duodenal atresia, malrotation, anorectal malformations, Hirschsprung's disease, congenital diaphragmatic hernia, and tracheoesophageal fistula [1, 2]. Additionally, there are case reports of minimally invasive pancreatectomy, hepatectomy, and resections for neuroblastoma and Wilms tumor in children. The general trend in pediatric surgical practice has been increased adoption of minimally invasive approaches.

Safe application of minimally invasive surgery in pediatric patients necessitates a thorough understanding of the physiologic effects of carbon dioxide (CO_2) insufflation in this population. Regardless of the operation being performed, two main effects produce the physiological consequences of insufflation: (1) increased intra-abdominal or intrathoracic pressure and (2) CO_2 absorption through the visceral and parietal peritoneum (Fig. 1.1). One series reported a 7 % rate of needing to stop insufflation either transiently or permanently for children undergoing laparoscopy [3, 4]. Patients who had insufflation-related incidents and needed the procedure halted were younger with lower immediate preoperative body temperature, and the operations were longer and had higher

D.S. Walsh et al. (eds.), *The SAGES Manual of Pediatric Minimally Invasive Surgery*, DOI 10.1007/978-3-319-43642-5_1

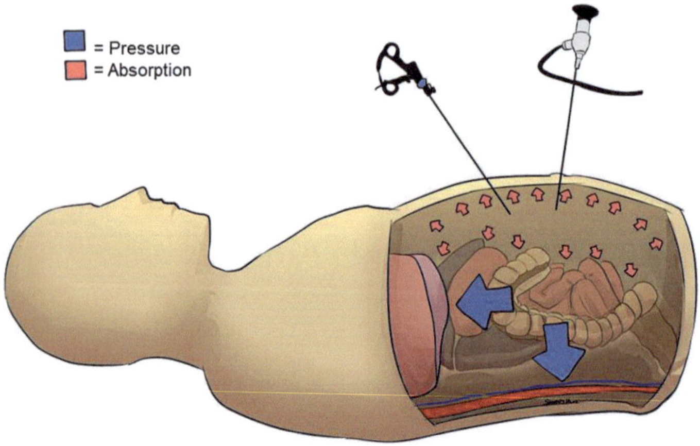

Fig. 1.1. Two major stimuli produce the observed physiologic changes during abdominal insufflation for laparoscopy: (1) increased intra-abdominal pressure (*blue arrows*), which impedes full lung expansion and can decrease flow through the aorta and vascular system, and (2) enhanced CO_2 absorption (*red arrows*) by the visceral and parietal peritoneum, which increases the necessary minute ventilation to maintain acid-base balance. Figure courtesy of Sarah Hua.

insufflation pressures. Therefore, during minimally invasive operations, pediatric surgeons and anesthesiologists frequently contend with acute physiologic changes from abdominal or thoracic insufflation that may significantly change the course of the procedure. They should anticipate such changes and be prepared to manage them.

This chapter describes the effects of abdominal and thoracic insufflation on the cardiovascular, pulmonary, metabolic, and immune/inflammatory systems, with a special emphasis on neonates and infants, as these patients differ significantly from adults and older children both anatomically and physiologically. General principles for preoperative preparation and postoperative care are addressed. Physiologic sequelae of abdominal insufflation are discussed in context of the organ systems affected.

Preoperative Evaluation

As with any pediatric or neonatal operation, general fitness for a planned minimally invasive operation is of paramount importance. Appropriate history related to nutritional status and growth should be obtained for every patient, and any symptoms or signs that could suggest cardiac or pulmonary impairment must be elicited. Anesthetic management plans need to be carefully formulated, especially in neonatal cases with extended procedures, reverse Trendelenburg positioning, and higher insufflation pressures [5]. General endotracheal anesthesia remains the standard for pediatric laparoscopic and thoracoscopic operations to allow the anesthesiologist to contend with the physiologic effects of hypercarbia and increased intra-abdominal or intrathoracic pressures [2].

Several specific comorbidities warrant special consideration in preoperative planning. Minimally invasive procedures are increasingly being performed in infants with congenital heart disease. These patients may be more susceptible to changes in preload due to impaired venous return or changes in systemic resistance associated with increased intra-abdominal pressure [6]. Laparoscopic and thoracoscopic operations can be done safely in these patients in experienced centers with dedicated pediatric cardiac anesthesia teams [6–8].

Underlying pulmonary disease is another important comorbidity to consider before undertaking a minimally invasive procedure in a child. Excretion of excess CO_2 that is absorbed through the visceral and parietal peritoneum is a primary concern of the anesthesiologist managing the infant undergoing laparoscopic or thoracoscopic surgery. Increasing minute ventilation is the primary tool used to remove excess CO_2. Any pulmonary condition that may limit the ability to increase minute ventilation or impair gas exchange could rapidly lead to a respiratory acidosis. If laparoscopy is to be undertaken in a patient with baseline pulmonary dysfunction, intensive postoperative monitoring should be utilized to limit risks of hypoventilation from retained hypercarbia. A related problem is portal hypertension, which has been shown to accelerate absorption of CO_2 to a level twice that of the already increased absorption displayed in children [9]. Similar to the patient with pulmonary disease, patients with portal hypertension should be managed with increased vigilance to limit the negative effects of hypercarbia in the postoperative period.

Physiologic Effects of Pneumoperitoneum by System

Cardiovascular System

Several studies have examined the cardiovascular effects of pneumoperitoneum in children. Direct measurement of flow in the thoracic aorta by transesophageal echocardiography (TEE) in healthy 6- to 30-month-old infants and children undergoing laparoscopic assisted orchiopexy for undescended testicles with a maximum insufflation pressure of 10 mmHg showed significantly decreased flow, decreased stroke volume, and increased systemic resistance. However, these changes resolved completely after desufflation of the abdominal cavity. Significant changes in mean arterial pressure (MAP) or end-tidal CO_2 were not observed during these relatively short procedures, nor were any clinically important sequelae [10]. In another study of healthy 2- to 6-year-old children undergoing laparoscopic inguinal herniorrhaphy, an initial insufflation to an abdominal pressure of 12 mmHg decreased cardiac index (CI) as measured by TEE [11]. Interestingly, CI returned to baseline with a decrease in insufflation pressure to 6 mmHg and did not decrease with a subsequent increase in abdominal pressure to 12 mmHg, suggesting an adaptation to the change in afterload induced by abdominal insufflation. A recent study exposed neonatal and adolescent piglets to 180 min of abdominal insufflation, which caused a decrease in CI and MAP that persisted well into the recovery period after insufflation ended. This effect was more pronounced in the neonates [12]. The extended response to the pressure stimulus suggests a need for vigilant monitoring in the postoperative period to ensure that hypotension does not ensue. Prolonged exposure to higher insufflation pressures (>8–10 mmHg) may also induce capillary microcirculatory changes and impair venous return [1]. In contrast, a study using low-pressure insufflation no greater than 5 mmHg combined with reverse Trendelenburg positioning in children ages 6 to 36 months undergoing laparoscopic fundoplication actually increased CI, heart rate, and MAP [13].

In summary, in the otherwise healthy infant or child, abdominal insufflation pressures of 12 mmHg or less for short- to medium-length procedures may cause changes in CI, MAP, or systemic resistance when specifically measured but rarely (3.2 % of cases) produce clinically significant effects requiring intervention [4]. The location of monitoring may not affect the accuracy of blood pressure measurements. In a piglet model, no difference was found between measured carotid and femoral arterial blood pressures with up to 24 mmHg abdominal insufflation, a level nearly twice that of the highest commonly used clinically [14].

Pulmonary System

The pulmonary effects of pneumoperitoneum in pediatric patients are the result of anatomic and physiologic differences between adults and children. The alveolar surface area to body surface area ratio in infants and children is smaller than that of adults. Therefore, children have a significantly higher minute ventilation and oxygen consumption (up to twice that of an adult) *even at baseline* to maintain $PaCO_2$ in the normal range [1]. In patients younger than 1 year of age, the space-occupying effects of abdominal insufflation lead to increased peak inspiratory pressure, reduced tidal volume, and decreased compliance [15]. These changes in turn produce decreased functional residual capacity (FRC), increased pulmonary vascular resistance, and increased shunt fraction, which in combination with the increased CO_2 absorption can lead to hypercarbia if the minute ventilation is not increased concomitantly [15].

Hypercapnia is a significant concern in minimally invasive surgery, especially in children with underlying pulmonary disease. In one series of laparoscopic and thoracoscopic procedures performed in neonates (i.e., <1 month of age), hypercapnia >45 mmHg was reported in 2.3 % of cases [4]. The degree of hypercapnia depends on insufflation pressure and duration of pneumoperitoneum. In piglet models, $PaCO_2$ has been shown to increase 25 % with stepwise increases in insufflation pressure with associated increases in mortality from CO_2 embolism [16]. In a study of low-pressure (i.e., maximum 5 mmHg) insufflation for fundoplication, CO_2 rose 28 % on average when patients up to 3 years of age were exposed for more than an hour [17]. Careful monitoring for hypercapnia is warranted for all pediatric minimally invasive procedures, and laparoscopic insufflation pressures should be limited, with a maximum recommended pressure of 12 mmHg for neonates [15].

An important consideration for respiratory monitoring is that a gradient will develop between the $PaCO_2$ and the end-tidal CO_2 after abdominal insufflation because of an increased CO_2 and diminished functional residual volume. This gradient has been documented to increase significantly in adults during the first 60 min of insufflation for laparoscopic colorectal surgery but to stabilize or decrease thereafter [18]. In young children with cyanotic congenital heart disease undergoing laparoscopic fundoplication, the gradient increased by a factor of nearly 2.5 soon after initial insufflation of the abdomen [19]. This gradient was shown to be as high as 8 mmHg in one study of laparoscopic fundoplication in children without underlying cardiac or respiratory disease; as in other studies, the gradient decreased with longer insufflation stimulus [20]. Measuring CO_2 elimination has also been used to monitor this process. End-tidal CO_2 increases disproportionately for younger patients compared to older children with the same insufflation pressures and duration, and it remains elevated even after the conclusion of the procedure [15]. For these reasons, postoperative monitoring of respiratory rate is critical to safely performing laparoscopy in infants and neonates.

Another potential problem in infants undergoing laparoscopy is hypoxemia. In neonates and infants, there is a close relationship between functional residual capacity (FRC) and airway closing pressure. When FRC decreases in response to the increased intra-abdominal pressure, airway closure will exacerbate right-to-left intrapulmonary shunt and can lead to hypoxemia [5].

Inflammatory/Immune System

In children, data from a study of procedures for acute abdominal pain suggested that laparoscopic compared to open operations did not result in differences in major inflammatory mediators such as cortisol and IL-6 [21]. However, several subsequent studies have demonstrated a lesser degree of increase in inflammatory mediators including IL-6, CRP, TNF-α, and cortisol with laparoscopy compared to open approach for a variety of operations [22–25]. Cellular responses are also affected by laparoscopy, in a manner similar to the cytokine responses. Both macrophages and neutrophils are recruited to the peritoneal cavity with insufflation, though the numbers are lower with CO_2 insufflation compared to air [26].

Other

Compared with adults, children have a greater body surface area to volume ratio [27] and thus are at increased risk for hypothermia. During minimally invasive surgical procedures in infants and children, hypothermia is reported to occur in 1.8 % of cases [4]. Temperature monitoring is especially important in newborns. Dry CO_2 insufflation on continuous flow of 5–8 L/min will lead to massive evaporative losses relative to body size, and the accompanying heat loss can approach 40 % of a neonate's metabolic power capacity, despite their higher-per-kilogram power capacity compared to adults [3]. Additionally, gas leaks around port sites in a neonate can result in a much greater loss of insufflation gas, thereby requiring higher flow rates and potentially exacerbating hypothermia if non-humidified CO_2 is used.

Reversible anuria during laparoscopy is a consistent observation in the literature, occurring in 88 % of neonates and 14 % in older children. Up to one-third of older children will experience oliguria [28]. Interestingly, these decreases in urine output are not responsive to volume challenge and do not reflect decreases in renal blood flow. Thus, intraoperative fluid resuscitation during laparoscopic procedures should not be governed by urine output alone.

Finally, potential catastrophic events can occur during laparoscopy, and some of these severe complications may be more likely in children. Venous air embolism due to cannulation and insufflation of a patent umbilical vein has been reported in several instances and has sometimes led to cardiac arrest [1]. CO_2 pneumothorax is another rare complication that has been reported in children. In one case, it was discovered at the end of the procedure when the infant did not resume spontaneous respirations with reversal of anesthesia, although the child eventually recovered with no reported long-term effects [29].

Thoracoscopic Surgery Considerations

Many of the major pediatric thoracic operations have been performed thoracoscopically, including resection for congenital pulmonary airway malformation, repair of congenital diaphragmatic hernia, and repair of esophageal atresia with and without concomitant tracheoesophageal fistula [1]. Thoracoscopy is routinely employed in pediatric surgical practice for other procedures such as decortication, sympathectomy, and lung biopsies or resections. A knowledge of the physiology of minimally invasive chest procedures is essential for their safe application.

Two potential effects of thoracoscopic surgery merit consideration. First, single-lung ventilation produces ventilation/ perfusion (V/Q) mismatch, which is most pronounced in neonates. Several factors make neonates particularly susceptible to V/Q mismatch: a narrower window between FRC and residual volume, a compliant chest wall, a lateral decubitus positioning, and a neuromuscular blockade [5]. The end result is hypoxia.

Second, there is a widely held belief that CO_2 absorption is greater during thoracoscopy compared to laparoscopy, which could lead to metabolic acidosis, as reported during congenital diaphragmatic hernia repair [1]. In support of this hypothesis, end-tidal CO_2 has been shown to increase significantly after chest insufflation and persist after desufflation, and these changes are greater in younger patients and larger than those observed during laparoscopy [30]. The data on these two responses are far from conclusive, and more work is needed to identify specific situations that will produce clinically important changes in CO_2 level and acid-base status.

Postoperative Care

The most important consideration in the postoperative care of children undergoing minimally invasive procedures is respiratory monitoring in the first several hours after abdominal desufflation, when residual hypercarbia may be present and the potential for hypoventilation persists. This risk is especially important in neonates, infants, and young children, and we recommend these patients be monitored with continuous pulse oximetry for at least the first several hours after laparoscopy. Further work will be needed to accurately determine if a predefined, mandatory length of stay in the anesthesia recovery area or in a monitored hospital unit is necessary to prevent life-threatening hypoventilation.

Summary

- Laparoscopy is physiologically safe and effective approach in pediatric patients of all ages and for many pediatric abdominal surgical procedures.
- Increased intra-abdominal pressure leading to impaired pulmonary mechanics and increased CO_2 absorption are the two primary stimuli that lead to the array of physiologic sequelae during and after laparoscopy.
- Cardiac index, mean arterial pressure, and aortic blood flow decrease during abdominal insufflation but rarely with important clinical consequences.
- Increased minute ventilation must be achieved during minimally invasive surgery, especially in neonates, to prevent hypercarbia and subsequent acidosis.
- Reversible anuria and oliguria occur with laparoscopy, and this effect is more pronounced in younger patients.
- Increases in inflammatory mediators and cellular responses are decreased during laparoscopic compared to open operations in children.
- Vigilant postoperative monitoring for neonates should be employed as CO_2 retention may persist after abdominal desufflation.

References

1. Lacher M, Kuebler JF, Dingemann J, Ure BM. Minimal invasive surgery in the newborn: current status and evidence. Semin Pediatr Surg. 2014;23(5):249–56.
2. Ponsky TA, Rothenberg SS. Minimally invasive surgery in infants less than 5 kg: experience of 649 cases. Surg Endosc. 2008;22(10):2214–9.
3. Blinman T, Ponsky T. Pediatric minimally invasive surgery: laparoscopy and thoracoscopy in infants and children. Pediatrics. 2012;130(3):539–49.
4. Kalfa N, Allal H, Raux O, et al. Multicentric assessment of the safety of neonatal video surgery. Surg Endosc. 2007;21(2):303–8.
5. Means LJ, Green MC, Bilal R. Anesthesia for minimally invasive surgery. Semin Pediatr Surg. 2004;13(3):181–7.
6. Watkins SC, Morrow SE, McNew BS, Donahue BS. Perioperative management of infants undergoing fundoplication and gastrostomy after stage I palliation of hypoplastic left heart syndrome. Pediatr Cardiol. 2012;95:204–11.
7. Slater B, Rangel S, Ramamoorthy C, Abrajano C, Albanese CT. Outcomes after laparoscopic surgery in neonates with hypoplastic heart left heart syndrome. J Pediatr Surg. 2007;42(6):1118–21.
8. Cribbs RK, Heiss KF, Clabby ML, Wulkan ML. Gastric fundoplication is effective in promoting weight gain in children with severe congenital heart defects. J Pediatr Surg. 2008;43(2):283–9.
9. Bozkurt P, Kaya G, Yeker Y, et al. Arterial carbon dioxide markedly increases during diagnostic laparoscopy in portal hypertensive children. Anesth Analg. 2002;95(5):1236–40.
10. Gueugniaud PY, Abisseror M, Moussa M, et al. The hemodynamic effects of pneumoperitoneum during laparoscopic surgery in healthy infants: assessment by continuous esophageal aortic blood flow echo Doppler. Anesth Analg. 1998;86(2):290–3.
11. Sakka SG, Huettemann E, Petrat G, et al. Transoesophageal echocardiographic assessment of haemodynamic changes during laparoscopic herniorrhaphy in small children. Br J Anaesth. 2000;84:330–4.
12. Metzelder ML, Kuebler JF, Huber D, et al. Cardiovascular responses to prolonged carbon dioxide pneumoperitoneum in neonatal versus adolescent pigs. Surg Endosc. 2010;24(3):670–4.
13. De Waal EEC, Kalkman CJ. Haemodynamic changes during low-pressure carbon dioxide pneumoperitoneum in young children. Paediatr Anaesth. 2003;13(1):18–25.
14. Aksakal D, Hückstädt T, Richter S, et al. Comparison of femoral and carotid blood pressure during laparoscopy in piglets. J Pediatr Surg. 2012;47(9):1688–93.
15. Bannister CF, Brosius KK, Wulkan M. The effect of insufflation pressure on pulmonary mechanics in infants during laparoscopic surgical procedures. Paediatr Anaesth. 2003;13(9):785–9.
16. Beebe DS, Zhu S, Kumar MVS, et al. The effect of insufflation pressure on CO(2) pneumoperitoneum and embolism in piglets. Anesth Analg. 2002;94(5):1182–7.
17. McHoney M, Corizia L, Eaton S, et al. Carbon dioxide elimination during laparoscopy in children is age dependent. J Pediatr Surg. 2003;38(1):105–10.

18. Tanaka T, Satoh K, Torii Y, Suzuki M, Furutani H, Harioka T. Arterial to end-tidal carbon dioxide tension difference during laparoscopic colorectal surgery. Masui. 2006;55(8):988–91.
19. Wulkan ML, Vasudevan SA. Is end-tidal CO_2 an accurate measure of arterial CO_2 during laparoscopic procedures in children and neonates with cyanotic congenital heart disease? J Pediatr Surg. 2001;36(8):1234–6.
20. Sanders JC, Gerstein N. Arterial to endtidal carbon dioxide gradient during pediatric laparoscopic fundoplication. Paediatr Anaesth. 2008;18(11):1096–101.
21. Bozkurt P, Kaya G, Altintas F, et al. Systemic stress response during operations for acute abdominal pain performed via laparoscopy or laparotomy in children. Anaesthesia. 2000;55(1):5–9.
22. Ure BM, Niewold TA, Bax NMA, et al. Peritoneal, systemic, and distant organ inflammatory responses are reduced by a laparoscopic approach and carbon dioxide vs air. Surg Endosc. 2002;16(5):836–42.
23. Wang L, Qin W, Tian F, et al. Cytokine responses following laparoscopic or open pyeloplasty in children. Surg Endosc. 2009;23(3):544–9.
24. Montalto AS, Bitto A, Irrera N, et al. CO_2 pneumoperitoneum impact on early liver and lung cytokine expression in a rat model of abdominal sepsis. Surg Endosc. 2012; 26(4):984–9.
25. Papparella A, Noviello C, Romano M, et al. Local and systemic impact of pneumoperitoneum on prepubertal rats. Pediatr Surg Int. 2007;23(5):453–7.
26. Moehrlen U, Ziegler U, Boneberg E, et al. Impact of carbon dioxide versus air pneumoperitoneum on peritoneal cell migration and cell fate. Surg Endosc. 2006;20(10): 1607–13.
27. Berdan EA, Segura BJ, Saltzman DA. Physiology of the newborn. In: Holcomb GW, Murphy JP, Ostlie DJ, editors. Ashcraft's pediatric surgery. 6th ed. Elsevier Saunders; 2014:3–18.
28. Gómez Dammeier BH, Karanik E, Glüer S, et al. Anuria during pneumoperitoneum in infants and children: a prospective study. J Pediatr Surg. 2005;40(9):1454–8.
29. Lew YS, Thambi Dorai CR, Phyu PT. A case of supercarbia following pneumoperitoneum in an infant. Paediatr Anaesth. 2005;15(4):346–9.
30. Bishay M, Giacomello L, Retrosi G, Thyoka M, Garriboli M, Brierley J, Harding L, Scuplak S, Cross KM, Curry JI, Kiely EM, De Coppi P, Eaton S, Pierro A. Hypercapnia and acidosis during open and thoracoscopic repair of congenital diaphragmatic hernia and esophageal atresia: results of a pilot randomized controlled trial. Ann Surg. 2013;258(6):895–900.

2. Pediatric Laparoscopic and Thoracoscopic Instrumentation

Sarah Gilmore and Colin A. Martin

Early Experience

Pediatric minimally invasive surgery (MIS) has lagged behind its adult counterpart. In 1973, a report in the Journal of Pediatric Surgery by Gans and Berci described 16 early laparoscopic pediatric cases [1]. These early advances were possible in part by the Hopkins rod-lens optical system (Fig. 2.1). However, widespread adoption of pediatric laparoscopy was initially met with criticism. The first adult laparoscopic cholecystectomy was performed in 1985 [2] and was widely regarded as experimental and dangerous. There has been no single procedure that has propelled the advance of MIS in pediatric patients the way laparoscopic cholecystectomies did with adult MIS. Training modules for teaching laparoscopic cholecystectomy to adult surgeons were not well suited for teaching the advanced skills required for pediatric surgery [3]. This procedure was not considered standard of care in pediatrics until many years later. However, great strides have been made within the last 20 years. Today, it is common practice for neonates to undergo minimally invasive surgery. A study conducted by Rothenberg et al. over a 51-month period with 183 infants weighing 1.3–5.0 kg who underwent 195 procedures using minimally invasive techniques "demonstrates that advanced endosurgical techniques in infants is safe, effective, and associated with the same benefit as that seen in older patients" [4].

D.S. Walsh et al. (eds.), *The SAGES Manual of Pediatric Minimally Invasive Surgery*, DOI 10.1007/978-3-319-43642-5_2

June 28, 1966 H. H. HOPKINS **3,257,902**

OPTICAL SYSTEM HAVING CYLINDRICAL ROD-LIKE LENSES

Filed July 14, 1960 4 Sheets-Sheet 1

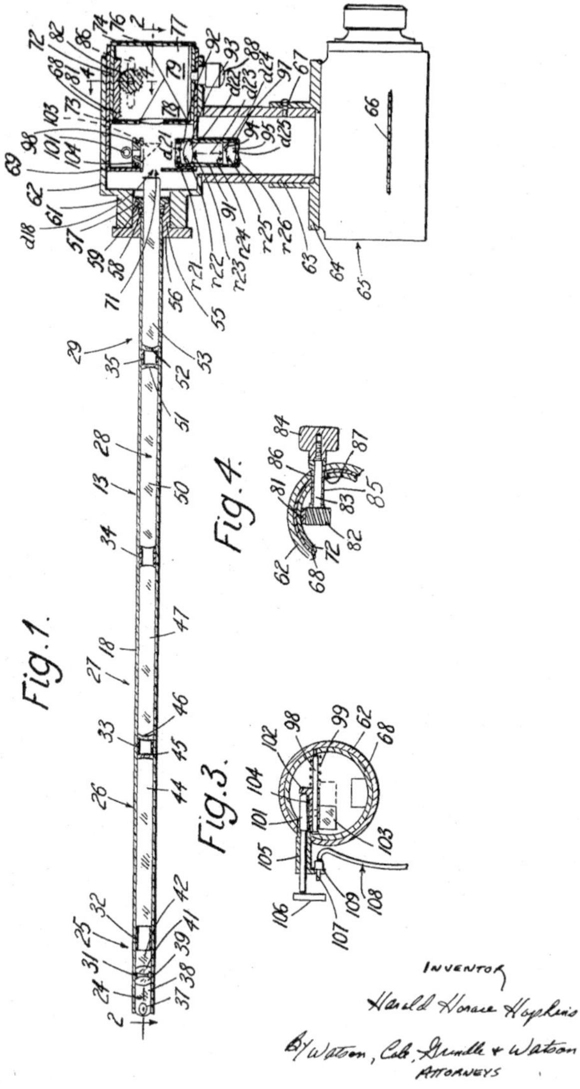

Fig. 2.1. Hopkins rod-lens optical system.

Challenges and Hurdles

The delay in the development of minimally invasive pediatric surgery can be attributed to many factors. There have been many financial constraints. Equipping hospitals with adequate pediatric laparoscopic operating room equipment and staff training is costly [3]. Initial operative times were longer with MIS approaches, also increasing costs [5]. Furthermore, with pediatric open surgery compared to adult, the cosmesis and length of stay are generally better thus requiring an even greater final margin from the MIS approach [6].

In addition to the financial hurdles, a new skill set is needed which includes depth perception, tactile sensation, and operative choreography [3]. New methods of teaching are required for the intricate details of minimally invasive surgery. Surgical instruments that were used for adult surgeries were too large and hazardous when used in infants and children (Fig. 2.2) [7]. Once the surgical instruments decreased in size and safe endoscopic techniques were discovered, pediatric surgeons were more apt to apply thoracoscopy and laparoscopy to neonates.

Trocar Selection

Types and Sizes

There are several commercially available trocar types including the MiniSite system by Covidien, the 3-mm minilaparoscopy set from Storz, the Aesculap Reusable Trocar System, and the Passport trocars from Stryker. The important tenants are safe insertion and ease of instrument exchange. Some trocars, like the MiniSite system, are inserted with a spring-loaded, blunt stylet (Fig. 2.3) or contain a metal conical tipped trocar like the Storz system. Each patient and case is unique; the trocar location and selection are specific to the size of the patient, the instruments being used, and the discretion of the surgeon [8]. Trocar sizes have been a challenge from the onset of minimally invasive surgery in pediatrics. The decrease from 5- and 10-mm instrumentation to 2- and 3-mm instrumentation has greatly aided surgeons in the complicated procedures of their smaller patients. Procedures became feasible in the littlest of children. In general, incisions and trocars are between 2 and 4 mm for neonates. Incisions less than 2 mm heal well without visible scarring. With trocars smaller than 4 mm, a red catheter sleeve can be fit around the outside of

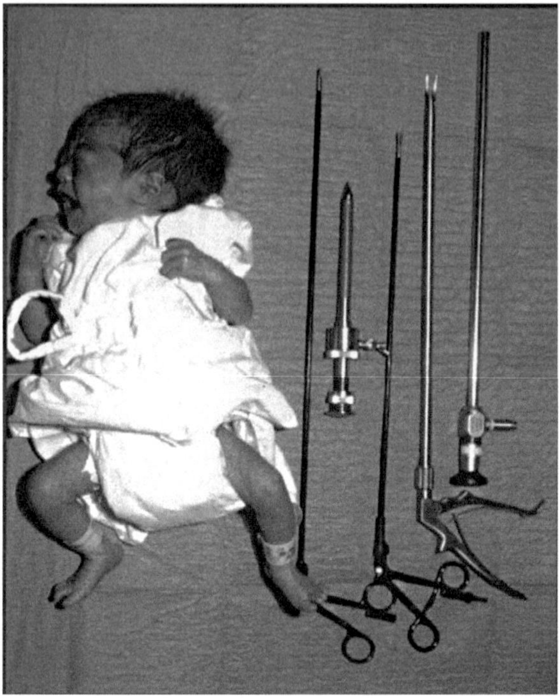

Fig. 2.2. Originally designed adult laparoscopic instruments were too large and hazardous for pediatric surgical use. From Georgeson K. Minimally invasive surgery in neonates. Semin Neonatol. 2003 Jun;8(3):243–8. Reprinted with permission from Elsevier Limited.

the trocar to help stabilize the trocar. The catheter sleeve can then be sutured to the skin thus allowing the trocar mobility without slippage [7]. An example is the two-piece sealing cap that fits at the end of the cannula of Aesculap trocars to preserve the pneumoperitoneum and prevent inadvertent removal when sutured to the abdominal wall. For the more traditional system, the Storz system contains silicone leaflet valves to maintain pneumoperitoneum.

Trocar Complications

The most common injuries from trocars include bleeding, hernias, bowel injuries, and bladder injuries [9]. The abdominal wall of neonates is relatively thin which allows for slippage of the trocars when instruments

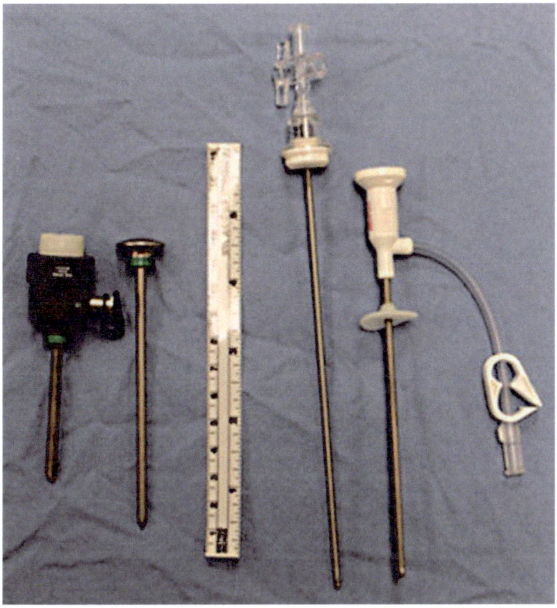

Fig. 2.3. The MiniSite system is inserted with a spring-loaded, blunt stylet. From Krpata, D.M. and T.A. Ponsky, Needlescopic surgery: what's in the toolbox? Surg Endosc, 2013. 27(3): p. 1040–4. Reprinted with permission from Springer.

are placed through them [10]. Trocar instability can cause a gamut of complications, including air leakage, loss of vision, instrument clashing, and others [11]. Rothenberg reports a specific complication directly related to the laparoscopic approach during one of his procedures: the "injury was a bladder wall injury secondary to the replacement of a 3 mm trocar in the suprapubic position after it had slipped out. The injury was extraperitoneal and was managed by Foley catheter drainage for 5 days" [10]. Jayaram et al. describe an efficient way to prevent complications from trocar instability with the use of a 16- or 18-Fr Foley catheter sleeve over the trocar, in which the sleeve is then fixed to the skin with a stitch [11]. In addition, major vascular injury can occur with trocar insertion including iliac, caval, and umbilical vein injury [12].

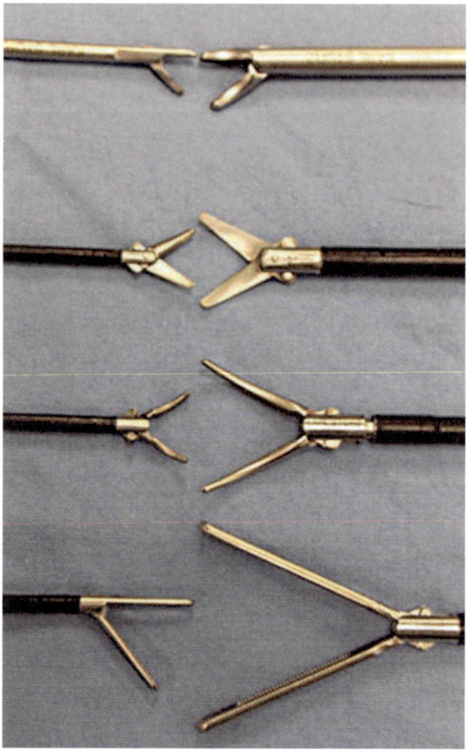

Fig. 2.4. Comparison between 3- and 5-mm instruments. From Krpata, D.M. and T.A. Ponsky, Needlescopic surgery: what's in the toolbox? Surg Endosc, 2013. 27(3): p. 1040–4. Reprinted with permission from Springer.

Laparoscopic Instruments

Smaller and more versatile instruments have greatly expanded the laparoscopic capabilities in neonates. Figure 2.4 demonstrates the comparison between 3- and 5-mm instruments. A reliable and versatile set of reusable instruments for pediatric laparoscopy is essential for success. The 3-mm minilaparoscopy system by Storz has a set with 36-cm-long instruments that include graspers, dissectors, scissors, cautery, suction, and needle holders for intracorporeal suturing (Fig. 2.5). The major advantage of this set is that it is the only 3-mm set that offers a 36-cm length which is helpful for pediatric patients with thicker abdominal walls. In addition Storz offers this set in 20- and 30-cm lengths. Other brands include

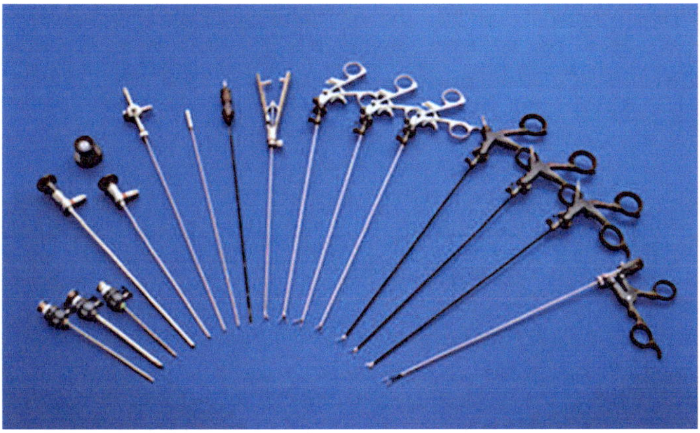

Fig. 2.5. The 3-mm minilaparoscopy system by Storz. From Krpata, D.M. and T.A. Ponsky, Needlescopic surgery: what's in the toolbox? Surg Endosc, 2013. 27(3): p. 1040–4. Reprinted with permission from Springer.

Stryker which offers 3-mm instruments and Sovereign® mini-instruments (Aesculap, Center Valley, PA) which makes 3.5-mm instruments. Finally the MiniSite™ system makes 2-mm instruments that can be used directly through the abdominal wall or through a specially designed part [13].

Insufflation Pressure and Physiology

Respiratory parameters are affected due to the insufflation pressures, the CO_2 absorption, and the position of the patient. Pediatric patients have a higher oxygen consumption, minute ventilation, and airway resistance than adults. Pediatric patients have a lower functional residual capacity (FRC) (10 % of total lung capacity) and high closing volume compared with adults [14]. The low FRC causes a ventilation-perfusion mismatch and alveolar dead space that is further exaggerated during laparoscopic surgery. During laparoscopic surgery, the diaphragm is displaced upward due to the insufflation force, resulting in a reduction of the lung volume and creating a ventilation-perfusion mismatch. Stiffening of the chest wall due to abdominal distention and impaired diaphragmatic motion also restricts lung expansion. Gas exchange is affected more severely in infants than adults due to these physiologic reasons [15]. There is a linear correlation with the changes in respiratory function and the intraperitoneal pressure. Due to the stepwise design of the study performed by Bannister et al., they discovered that significant pulmonary changes occur at a pressure of 10 mmHg and greater [16].

Carbon Dioxide

Carbon dioxide (CO_2) insufflation in the pediatric population can result in hypercarbia secondary to CO_2 absorption, changes in respiratory function, and cardiac output and acidosis [17]. Hypercarbia and increased intra-abdominal pressures can cause increased intracranial pressures and cerebral hemorrhage. Cardiovascular parameters are also affected during laparoscopic surgery. At baseline, infants and neonates have a relatively higher cardiac index and oxygen consumption than adults. The mean arterial pressure is lower, and the central venous pressure is comparable [18]. Cardiac output decreases when intra-abdominal pressure exceeds 20 mmHg and when blood flow to the heart is obstructed via compression of the inferior vena cava from cardiac compression to reduction in end-diastolic volume, respectively. Increased intra-abdominal pressures above 10 mmHg can compromise venous return due to compression of the inferior vena cava thus causing hypotension [19]. Systemic vascular resistance is increased due to compression of the aorta and increase in splanchnic arteriolar vasoconstriction from an increased intra-abdominal pressure [16]. Neonates are especially sensitive to absorption of CO_2, causing hypercapnia and hypoxia, and can develop respiratory acidosis.

Physiology

The main physiological changes upon insufflation are an increase in end-tidal CO_2 and an elevation in peak airway pressures which can be compensated for with slight hyperventilation. Intraoperative minute ventilation should be increased to maintain normocapnia [20], and care should be taken to monitor the neonates that are at risk postoperatively of not being able to maintain increased respiratory rate to blow off the remaining CO_2 [7]. Patients should be monitored with electrocardiogram, pulse oximeter, and end-tidal CO_2 monitor, because at pressure 12–14 mmHg, liver and kidney perfusion is decreased. The insufflation pressure should be set at the lowest possible pressure giving the best possible exposure without causing harm [20].

Thoracoscopy

The very first entirely thoracoscopic repair of a tracheoesophageal fistula was done in 1999, and it described a repair of pure esophageal atresia in a 3.4-kg 8-month-old infant [21]. Since then there have been numerous successfully performed thoracoscopic esophageal atresia repairs since the operation is easier on the patient, requires less dissection than open repair, and provides better visualization of the field. Thoracoscopic procedures require main stem intubation of the opposite lung to provide single-lung ventilation and low-flow, low CO_2 to help collapse the lung on the involved side. Single-lung ventilation is required because double-lumen tubes are not available in sizes small enough to accommodate the airway of a neonate. Insufflation with CO_2 into the pleural space can also help create a larger intrathoracic working space and improve exposure and visualization by pushing the diaphragm down. CO_2 may cause less pulmonary compromise during the operation when compared to standard mechanical retraction [10].

Since bilateral lung expansion is critically important in neonates due to their cylindrical chest, recumbent position, and small airways, thoracoscopy is beneficial over thoracotomy. The lack of a large incision improves pulmonary compliance in the early postoperative period and avoids the child becoming one of the 30 % of patients who develop scoliosis after thoracotomies [7]. Plus, laparoscopic surgery preserves postoperative pulmonary function better than open surgeries [20]. The proper insertion techniques are important due to the potential advantages of the development of less adhesions and scar tissue, less postoperative pain, less disruption of anatomy and function, and better cosmesis [10].

Insertion Techniques

In pediatric patients, the largest trocar is usually inserted through the umbilicus for cosmetic reasons and to use the existing small umbilical hernia. However many neonates have retained umbilical stumps; thus the access is made through an umbilical fold below the umbilicus. Access can be made through the open technique or with a Veress needle. Iwanaka et al. noted in his study that the most common nonspecific complication is related to the introduction of either the Veress or the first trocar [22]. He states that they always use open technique around the umbilicus for the first trocar in order to avoid trocar-related nonspecific complications in the patients, as it minimizes inadvertent major vascular injury. Conversely, Georgeson states that he has used the Veress needle access technique in over 2000 neonatal and pediatric laparoscopic procedures without significant injury. The preference and comfort level of the individual surgeon often dictates whether the open technique or the Veress needle technique is used [7].

Single-Port/Single-Incision Techniques

Reduced port surgery (RPS) aims at performing surgeries with the fewest ports possible. The attractive features about RPS are the minimal scarring and fewer incisions. The main incision for instrumentation, access, and extraction is usually in the umbilicus. Due to the pediatric population size, the usual umbilical incision has limitations in function and use. There are different options to enlarge the incision, each with its own drawbacks. Hizuru et al. describe the umbilical Benz incision that is an inverted Y shape in order to enlarge the opening for surgical instrumentation, extractions, and access [23]. Their reasoning is that the Benz incision creates three skin flaps and preserves the natural shape of the umbilicus while providing a larger orifice. Other alternative incisions are the longitudinal incision, the circumumbilical incision, the zigzag skin incision, and the omega-shaped incision. The conventional longitudinal incision has to extend beyond the umbilicus ring in order to provide enough space to work with but at the cost of visible scarring. The zigzag incision and omega-shaped incision require larger umbilici in order to prevent the incision from extending beyond the umbilicus thus creating visible scarring [23]. In addition to the function and use, the main concerns are the complications of the incision sites: ischemia, wound infections and abscesses, and postoperative scarring.

Robotic Pediatric Experience

A three-dimensional vision in endoscopic surgery is achieved with a robotic surgical system called the da Vinci robot system, a device that weighs 567 kg and is 6-feet tall originally designed for adults. The best available evidence for pediatric robotic assisted surgery is currently Oxford Centre for Evidence-Based Medicine Level 3, relating only to fundoplication and pyeloplasty [24]. Even though there has been an increase in the number of studies reporting RAS in infants and children, there is no currently an up-to-date quality assessment for the different types of procedures. There is a need for more comprehensive data indicating proven patient benefits or significant cost-effectiveness for robotically assisted surgery [24]. Robotically assisted surgeries are helpful in complex procedures that require dissection of delicate, vulnerable, anatomic structures. Currently due to the longer operating times, higher costs, and lack of clinical advantage, robotic surgery is not a general alternative to conventional, minimally invasive surgery [25].

The robotic approach makes the surgery easier, but the sizes of the scopes create the largest barrier for its use in small children [20]. The advantages of robotic surgery include the magnified three-dimensional view and increased depth perception, 6–7 degrees of freedom of movement of the instruments (standard laparoscopic instruments are only capable of 5 degrees of freedom), tremor reduction and greater surgeon comfort, and motion scaling from the surgeon's hand to the instrument tip [26]. The internal articulation of the instruments is especially important in thoracic cavity due to the narrow confines of the cavity and stress that occurs on the intercostal spaces with standard thoracoscopy instruments [27]. The disadvantages and concerns of robotic surgery include high-cost, additional training required for the entire operating room, limited operative space, large size of the camera and instrument ports, loss of tactile sensation, increased operative time for set up/docking and undocking, and potential barrier created between the patient and anesthesia team [28, 29].

One area of success using the robot in pediatric patients is in the field of urology, especially the robot-assisted laparoscopic pyeloplasty. In a multi-institutional cohort by Avery et al., there was a 91 % success rate and an 11 % complication rate among 60 robotic pyeloplasties compared with modern series of open pyeloplasty success rates ranging from 70 to 96 % and complication rates ranging from 0 to 24 % [28]. Bansal et al. concluded in his open cohort comparison that infant robot-assisted laparoscopic pyeloplasty was more feasible and efficacious with shorter operative time, hospital stay, and narcotic utilization than open pyeloplasty [29].

A retrospective review by Meehan looked at 47 procedures of 45 patients of less than 10 kg who underwent various general robot-assisted surgical procedures. All of the procedures were performed with the three-arm da Vinci Standard surgical robot with additional nonrobotic accessory ports used when necessary. They concluded that the biggest limitation is one of space. For children 3 kg and greater, the robot mobility inside the abdomen is very good. For children 4 kg and greater, the robot mobility inside the thoracic cavity is very good. However at sizes below 3 kg for the abdomen and 4 kg for the thoracic cavity, space becomes an issue [8]. While robotic surgery is safe and effective in the pediatric population, robotic technology needs to continue to downsize in order to truly become advantageous for the neonatal population.

Summary

- Pediatric minimally invasive surgery (MIS) has lagged behind its adult counterpart.
- The delay of MIS can be mainly contributed to financial constraints, training limitations, and size of instruments compared with size of the patient.
- Trocar selection and size hold extreme consequences on the outcomes of surgery.
- The pediatric population is more sensitive to insufflation pressures due to their physiology than adults.
- Thoracoscopy is beneficial over thoracotomy due to the lack of large thoracic wall incision which can decrease pulmonary compliance in the early postoperative period and because of the 30 % of patients who develop scoliosis after thoracotomies.
- Reduced port surgery (RPS), aiming for minimal scarring and fewer incisions, has become increasingly popular in the pediatric population.
- Robotic assisted surgery makes pediatric surgery easier, but the sizes of the scopes create the largest barrier for its use in small children.

References

1. Gans SL, Berci G. Peritoneoscopy in infants and children. J Pediatr Surg. 1973; 8(3):399–405.
2. Muhe E. Long-term follow-up after laparoscopic cholecystectomy. Endoscopy. 1992;24(9):754–8.
3. Georgeson KE, Owings E. Advances in minimally invasive surgery in children. Am J Surg. 2000;180(5):362–4.
4. Rothenberg SS, Chang JH, Bealer JF. Experience with minimally invasive surgery in infants. Am J Surg. 1998;176(6):654–8.
5. Luks FI, et al. Cost-effectiveness of laparoscopy in children. Arch Pediatr Adolesc Med. 1999;153(9):965–8.
6. Esposito C, et al. Pediatric laparoscopic splenectomy: are there real advantages in comparison with the traditional open approach? Pediatr Surg Int. 1997;12(7):509–10.
7. Georgeson K. Minimally invasive surgery in neonates. Semin Neonatol. 2003;8(3): 243–8.
8. Meehan JJ. Robotic surgery in small children: is there room for this? J Laparoendosc Adv Surg Tech A. 2009;19(5):707–12.

9. Chen MK, Schropp KP, Lobe TE. Complications of minimal-access surgery in children. J Pediatr Surg. 1996;31(8):1161–5.
10. Georgeson KE, Robertson DJ. Minimally invasive surgery in the neonate: review of current evidence. Semin Perinatol. 2004;28(3):212–20.
11. Jayaram H, Chandrasekharam VV. A simple technique of trocar fixation during pediatric laparoscopy with Foley catheter sleeve. Indian J Surg. 2013;75(4):319–20.
12. Guloglu R, et al. Major retroperitoneal vascular injuries during laparoscopic cholecystectomy and appendectomy. J Laparoendosc Adv Surg Tech A. 2004;14(2):73–6.
13. Krpata DM, Ponsky TA. Needlescopic surgery: what's in the toolbox? Surg Endosc. 2013;27(3):1040–4.
14. van Vonderen JJ, et al. Measuring physiological changes during the transition to life after birth. Neonatology. 2014;105(3):230–42.
15. Bozkurt P, et al. The cardiorespiratory effects of laparoscopic procedures in infants. Anaesthesia. 1999;54(9):831–4.
16. Bannister CF, Brosius KK, Wulkan M. The effect of insufflation pressure on pulmonary mechanics in infants during laparoscopic surgical procedures. Paediatr Anaesth. 2003;13(9):785–9.
17. Maharjan SK, Shrestha BR. Do we have to hyperventilate during laparoscopic surgery? Kathmandu Univ Med J (KUMJ). 2007;5(3):307–11.
18. Ure BM, et al. Physiological responses to endoscopic surgery in children. Semin Pediatr Surg. 2007;16(4):217–23.
19. Gueugniaud PY, et al. The hemodynamic effects of pneumoperitoneum during laparoscopic surgery in healthy infants: assessment by continuous esophageal aortic blood flow echo-Doppler. Anesth Analg. 1998;86(2):290–3.
20. Neudecker J, et al. The European Association for Endoscopic Surgery clinical practice guideline on the pneumoperitoneum for laparoscopic surgery. Surg Endosc. 2002;16(7):1121–43
21. Rothenberg SS. Experience with thoracoscopic tracheal surgery in infants and children. J Laparoendosc Adv Surg Tech A. 2009;19(5):671–4.
22. Iwanaka T, et al. Complications of laparoscopic surgery in neonates and small infants. J Pediatr Surg. 2004;39(12):1838–41.
23. Amano H, et al. The umbilical Benz incision for reduced port surgery in pediatric patients. JSLS. 2015;19(1):e2014 00238.
24. Friedmacher F, Till H. Robotic-assisted procedures in pediatric surgery: a critical appraisal of the current best evidence in comparison to conventional minimally invasive surgery. J Laparoendosc Adv Surg Tech A. 2015;25(11):936–43.
25. van Haasteren G, Levine S, Hayes W. Pediatric robotic surgery: early assessment. Pediatrics. 2009;124(6):1642–9.
26. Woo R, et al. Robot-assisted pediatric surgery. Am J Surg. 2004;188(4A Suppl):27S–37.
27. Ballouhey Q, et al. Assessment of paediatric thoracic robotic surgery. Interact Cardiovasc Thorac Surg. 2015;20(3):300–3.
28. Avery DI, et al. Robot-assisted laparoscopic pyeloplasty: multi-institutional experience in infants. J Pediatr Urol. 2015;11(3):139 e1–5.
29. Bansal D, et al. Infant robotic pyeloplasty: comparison with an open cohort. J Pediatr Urol. 2014;10(2):380–5.

3. Pediatric Endoscopic Instrumentation

Timothy D. Kane, Folashade Adebisi Jose, Danielle S. Walsh, and Nicholas E. Bruns

Introduction

The indications for the use of endoscopic equipment for pediatric surgical conditions primarily involve those that relate gastrointestinal endoscopy and airway endoscopy, including tracheoscopy and bronchoscopy. The instrumentation for pediatric endoscopy routinely utilized by pediatric surgeons includes a broad spectrum of both flexible and rigid endoscopic tools. The main interventions for pediatric upper intestinal endoscopy are for diagnostic purposes, to perform removal of foreign bodies (esophageal and gastric), to treat esophageal strictures, and to perform endoscopic retrograde pancreatography (ERCP) for pancreaticobiliary disease. The indications for the use of pediatric colonoscopy include evaluation of radiographic abnormalities, diarrhea, bleeding, abdominal pain, and abnormal growth patterns. Both diagnostic and therapeutic procedures can be performed endoscopically. The most common indications for airway endoscopy are foreign body removal, removal of airway secretions, and diagnostic purposes (e.g., assessment of/for tracheoesophageal fistula, tracheomalacia, or result following aortopexy).

Upper Endoscopy

Upper endoscopy is commonly performed for a variety of diagnostic and therapeutic purposes. Pediatric surgeons are more likely to be asked to perform therapeutic endoscopic procedures, such as retrieval of a foreign body

D.S. Walsh et al. (eds.), *The SAGES Manual of Pediatric Minimally Invasive Surgery*, DOI 10.1007/978-3-319-43642-5_3

or dilation of the esophagus, than for strictly diagnostic indications. A small number of pediatric surgeons now pursue training in more advanced endoscopic procedures, such as ERCP. Dilation of esophageal strictures is covered in detail in Chap. 19 of this text. This chapter will focus on upper endoscopy for foreign bodies and ERCP.

Esophageal Foreign Body Removal

Preoperative Evaluation

Depending on the age of the patient, there may be a history of foreign body ingestion. This may be accompanied by chest pain, excessive salivation, dysphagia, cough, or respiratory distress. Chest or abdominal radiographs may identify a foreign body if it is radiopaque (Fig. 3.1).

Surgical Indications

The presence of foreign body in the esophagus on imaging is an indication for retrieval. A child with a convincing history of ingestion of a radiolucent object is also an indication. As well, foreign bodies in the esophagus, stomach, or distal intestine require urgent removal if they have potential to cause damage such as batteries or multiple magnets [1].

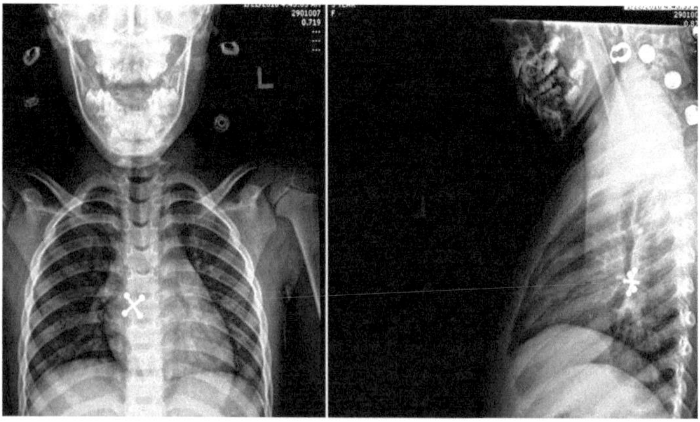

Fig. 3.1. Chest X-ray showing radiopaque foreign body in the upper esophagus in the region of the cricopharyngeus muscle.

Special Considerations

Foreign body removal from the airway is almost always performed with rigid endoscopic tools due to improved grasping ability. Esophageal or gastric foreign bodies may be removed using either rigid or flexible endoscopic tools. Larger children or adolescents may require flexible endoscopy for distal esophageal or gastric foreign bodies due to the length restrictions of rigid instruments.

The usual locations of esophageal foreign bodies, depending upon the child's age, requiring extraction are near the cricopharyngeal sphincter (over 90 %), distal esophagus, or at prior anastomotic sites [2].

Technique

The patient is positioned supine with a shoulder roll. General anesthesia is typically used, and a bite block is placed. Rigid endoscopic equipment appropriate for size/age or flexible endoscopic equipment is required. Among flexible endoscopes, the Olympus GIF 180 (9.3 mm OD) or GIF XP 160 (4.9 mm OD) (Olympus America, Center Valley, PA) are used depending on the size of the patient (Figs. 3.2 and 3.3). Optical grasping forceps (Fig. 3.4) or flexible graspers, snares, or basket should be available (Fig. 3.5).

- For rigid endoscopy, the scope is inserted posteriorly until the esophageal lumen is visualized.

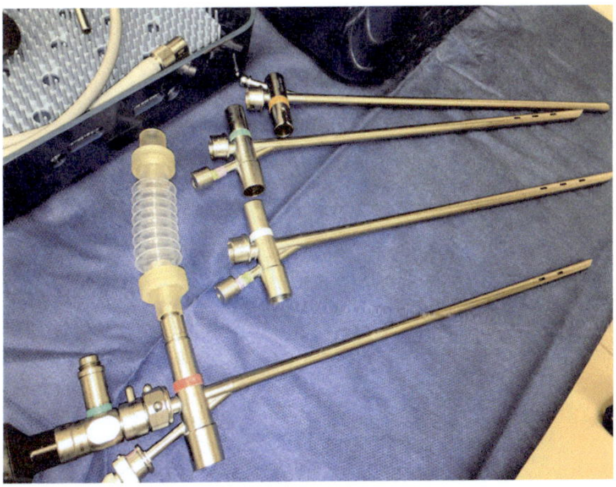

Fig. 3.2. Rigid endoscope.

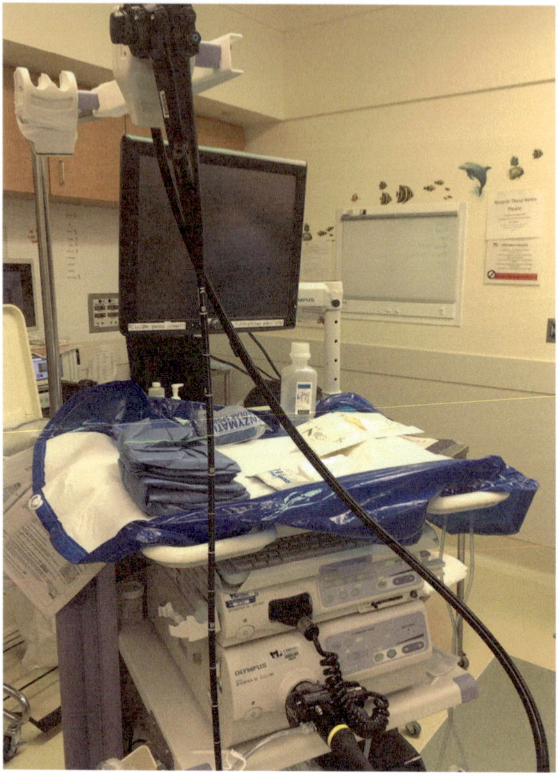

Fig. 3.3. Flexible endoscope.

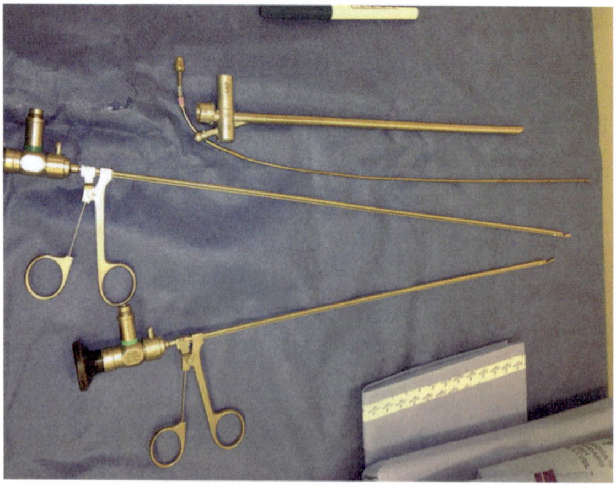

Fig. 3.4. Optical grasping forceps.

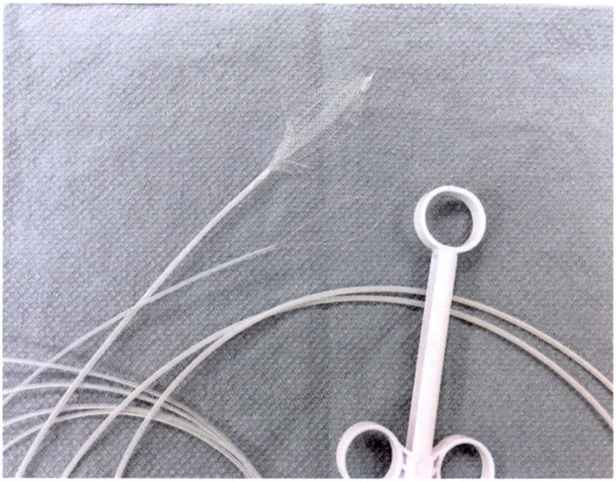

Fig. 3.5. Snare and basket for flexible endoscopy.

- Once the foreign body is visualized, the telescope is exchanged for optical grasping forceps.
- The object is grasped, and the entire scope and grasper is removed in a single motion.
- The optical grasper is exchanged for the visualizing scope and reintroduced to inspect the mucosa for trauma or injury. For flexible endoscopy, there is no need for instrument exchange. Objects may be removed by introducing grasping forceps, snare, or basket through the working channel of the scope. Similarly, when the object is grasped, the scope and grasping device are removed in a single motion.

Pearls/Pitfalls

- It is essential to have all of the necessary equipment prepared and sorted out prior to starting the procedure since instrument or scope exchange is frequently necessary. Any delay in this exchange process can lead to loss of visualization of the object.
- With esophageal foreign body removal using rigid scopes, it is sometimes helpful to attach the insufflation tubing of a sigmoidoscope (Fig. 3.6) to the esophagoscope to inflate air to distend the esophageal lumen and prevent the walls from collapsing in to obscure the view.

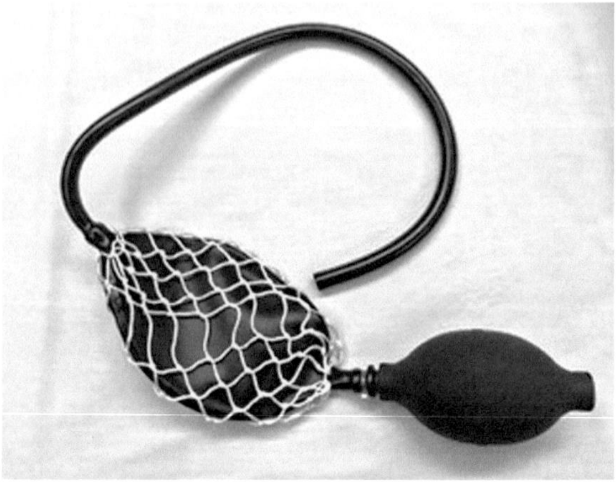

Fig. 3.6. Insufflation tubing (from rigid sigmoidoscopy scope).

- After grasping the object, one must pull the scope and grasper out simultaneously otherwise the object will be knocked off back into the esophagus by the scope if only the grasper is pulled out.

Postoperative Care

Esophageal foreign bodies can be removed by either rigid or flexible endoscopy with good results and minimal complications. It has been shown that if one approach is unsuccessful, then the alternative approach may be utilized with success [2].

Majority of patients may be discharged from the postanesthesia recovery unit. Exceptions to this include patients with perforation or significant erosion, ongoing respiratory symptoms, or comorbidities.

The overall rate of complications after endoscopic esophageal foreign body removal is low (1–2 %) and may include esophageal perforation, mucosal erosion, mediastinitis, pneumothorax, and pulmonary edema [2].

Endoscopic Retrograde Cholangiopancreatography (ERCP)

Preoperative Evaluation

Commonly, there is a diagnosis of choledocholithiasis, cholangitis, pancreatitis, or right upper-quadrant cystic mass. These diagnoses may be supported by jaundice and right upper-quadrant or epigastric pain on physical exam.

Laboratory evaluation may reveal elevated liver function tests such as hyperbilirubinemia or transaminitis, elevated amylase/lipase, or leukocytosis on complete blood count. A metabolic panel may show electrolyte disturbances.

Right upper-quadrant ultrasound, plain abdominal films (may show gallstones), abdominal computed tomography (common bile duct dilation), and/or magnetic resonance cholangiopancreatography (MRCP) may be useful in the workup of jaundice [3].

Surgical Indications

Surgical indications for ERCP include common bile duct (CBD) obstruction with dilation, CBD stones (before or after cholecystectomy), resolved gallstone pancreatitis with persistent CBD dilation, equivocal MRCP findings requiring definition of pancreaticobiliary anatomy, and internal drainage of biliary tree or pancreatic duct [4].

Special Considerations

The indications for ERCP are similar to those utilized for adult patients although smaller patient size conditions need to be considered. The smallest side-viewing duodenoscope for ERCP has an outer diameter (OD) of 7.3 mm. It is possible to use this therapeutic endoscope in infants as small as 10 kg. ERCP should not be performed in the setting of active pancreatitis. For difficult cases, if the endoscopist is not a surgeon, then surgical backup should be available.

The relevant anatomy includes the duodenum, ampulla of Vater, common bile duct, and the pancreatic ducts of Wirsung and Santorini. It is important to consider the possibility of pancreatic divisum.

Surgical Technique

The patient is placed in supine position. Instruments that are required include a side-viewing endoscope (Fig. 3.7), cannulating catheter, guide wire, sphincterotome, biliary stents (Fig. 3.8), and electrocautery attachment.

- For diagnostic purposes, ERCP is performed by cannulating the ampulla of Vater and injecting contrast into the orifice of the pancreatic and common bile ducts. Diagnosis of a choledochal cyst is seen in Fig. 3.9.
- For stone removal/retrieval, the ampulla is cannulated, and then a sphincterotomy is performed to open the ampulla.
- Either balloon extraction and/or flushing of the CBD are performed to remove stones.

Pearls/Pitfalls

- Smaller patients are more challenging with respect to cannulating the ampulla and performing sphincterotomy.

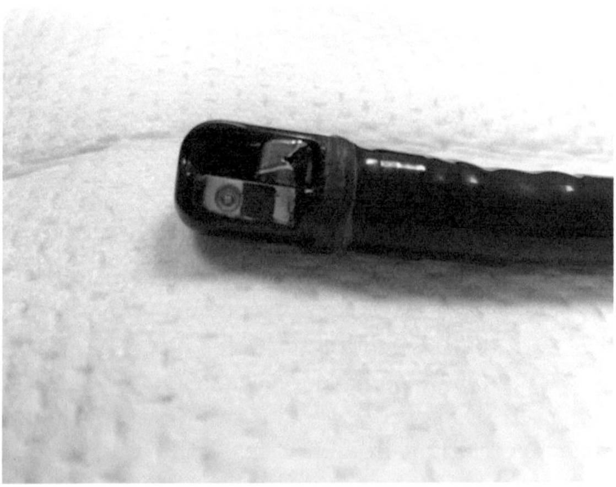

Fig. 3.7. Flexible endoscope for ERCP with side-viewing end.

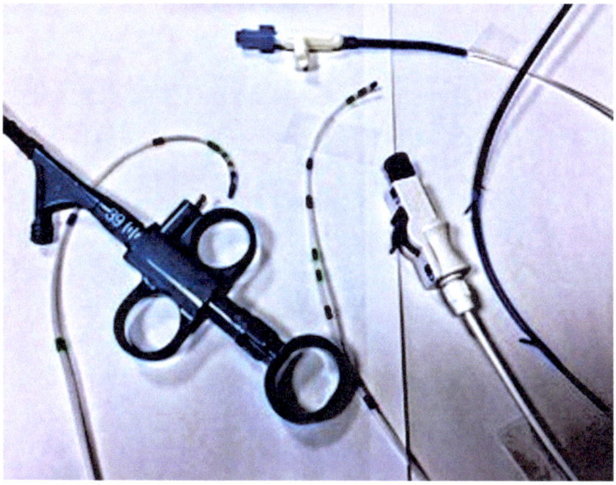

Fig. 3.8. Cannulation catheter, sphincterotome, and stent.

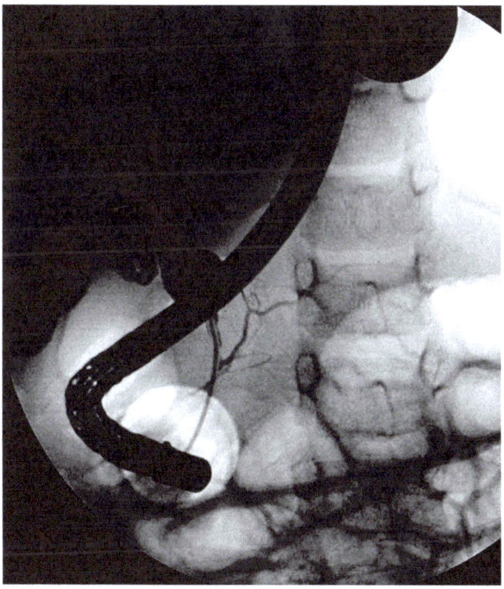

Fig. 3.9. ERCP with cholangiogram demonstrating type I choledochal cyst.

Postoperative Care

The postprocedural management after ERCP is dictated by the disease process that was the indication for ERCP.

The results of ERCP in children are generally good with limited complications. In an experienced center, bile duct cannulation success as well as therapeutic duct clearance success rates are high [5, 6]. Complications after ERCP include pancreatitis (3–8 %), post-sphincterotomy bleed (rare), duodenal perforation (rare), and bile duct perforation (rare) [5, 6].

Lower Endoscopy

Introduction

The indications for the use of pediatric colonoscopy most commonly include diarrhea, bleeding per rectum or bloody stools, abdominal pain with abnormal growth patterns, or constitutional symptoms. Lower endoscopy can also be utilized to investigate abnormalities suspected on barium enema, small bowel follow through or computed tomography. Colonoscopy can also be performed for therapeutic reasons such as retrieval of foreign body, polypectomy, vascular ablations, and decompression of toxic megacolon.

While anal diseases that felt isolated to the anorectal area can be assessed by rigid sigmoidoscopy or anoscopy alone, a thorough colonoscopy can avoid multiple sedated procedures and need for bowel preparation in children. Since both anoscopy and sigmoidoscopy require less technical skills than colonoscopy, they are touched on only briefly here. Rigid sigmoidoscopy can be performed with either the pediatric-sized (11–15 mm diameter) or adult-sized (19–23 mm diameter) scope sets, and these scopes are accompanied by a fiberoptic light source and hand-insufflation bulb and tube for wall distension. The lubricated scope with introducer is inserted posterosuperiorly in the patient in a lithotomy position until resistance is met. After removal of the introducer, the trap door can be closed to permit insufflation, and the walls of the rectum and anus are inspected on withdrawal. A variety of anoscopes, including disposable models, are available, though in smaller infants, a nasal speculum and pediatric gynecologic speculum can permit adequate visualization. When anal intervention is needed, anoscopes with openings along 1/3–1/2 of their diameter can prove useful. The remainder of this section will focus on flexible colonoscopy.

Preoperative Evaluation

A period of fasting and a bowel preparation regimen is necessary as colonoscopy is accomplished successfully only if the colon is free of fecal debris. Many bowel preparation regimens are available for colonic cleansing, such as nonabsorbable polyethylene glycol-electrolyte lavage solution (PEG-ELS), which is not approved for children younger than 6 months as it causes osmotic diarrhea [7]. Magnesium citrate, bisacodyl, and oral sodium phosphate can also be used for bowel cleansing. To be effective, a large volume of solution must be ingested over a relatively short period of time.

Technique

- Sedation is utilized with most pediatrics patients to minimize discomfort and provide amnesia for the procedure. Most pediatric colonoscopists have replaced general anesthesia with intravenous sedation for this procedure.
- Colonoscopy is traditionally performed in the left lateral decubitus position with the knees bent. Rotation of the patient from the left lateral position to a supine or lateral decubitus position may facilitate scope advancement from the hepatic flexure into the ascending colon.
- Instruments: Pediatric colonoscopes have variable insertion tube lengths (1330–1700 mm), shaft diameters (9.8–11.8 mm), and channel size (2.8–3.8 mm). The colonoscope has varying degrees of flexibility throughout the length of the insertion tube [7]. Additional instrumentation, including a biopsy forcep, polypectomy snare, basket, and flexible graspers can be inserted in the channel for procedures.
- The colonoscope is inserted into the anus and advanced into the rectum. There are various landmarks seen during the procedure; the most prominent landmark in the rectum is the fixed "valves of Houston." The anal canal is about 2–3 cm long, followed by is an abrupt decrease resistance with continuous advancement of the scope. The instrument should be advanced past these valves using the dials for tip deflection under direct vision.
- Advancing the scope through the sigmoid colon is smooth and coordinated. It involves torquing the instrument along its shaft with the right hand and using the left hand to control the tip deflection. Intermittent backward and forward motions are usually needed to

telescope the colon onto the instrument. As the tip of the instrument reaches a bend, the combination of dial and torque is used to rotate the tip around the bend into the lumen. Withdrawal of the instrument will often straighten the loop and allow advancement to the next bend. No anatomic landmark is obvious between the sigmoid and descending colon, but the descending colon is smaller in diameter.

- Transverse colon is characterized by the triangular-shaped haustral folds. The scope is advance to the hepatic flexure which is identified by the bluish discoloration of the outer wall caused by approximation of the liver. The cecum can be identified by the triangular-shaped fold and the appendiceal orifice. The ileocecal valve (ICV) is identified on the lateral surface of the prominent ileal fold as a slight irregularity of the valve contour. The ICV is intubated in pediatric colonoscopy especially in the evaluation of inflammatory bowel disease.
- Avoid forming loops, but when loops are formed, reduce them as quickly as possible. Use little air as possible while maintaining adequate visualization. Pull back and telescope the bowel onto the colonoscopy when possible.
- Additional techniques of air insufflation and suction, rotation or torquing of the insertion tube, external pressure applied to the abdomen, and changing position of the patient can assist in navigation throughout the procedure.
- Biopsies are obtained from the terminal ileum and also throughout the colon for histology via biopsy forcep. Polyps are cauterized using polypectomy snares hooked to an energy source.

Pearls/Pitfalls

- It is essential that the patient has complete bowel preparation for clear visualization of the mucosa.
- Always advance the colonoscopy under direct observation.
- Avoidance and reduction of endoscopic looping and minimizing air insufflation will help reduce post colonoscopy bloating and abdominal pain.
- Complications can arise from sedation during colonoscopy, and the proceduralist should be attentive to the patient's hemodynamics.

Postoperative Care

Bleeding after colonoscopy is minimal, and this may follow mucosal biopsy or polypectomy. Bleeding following polypectomy is uncommon in children but may occur in 0.26–2.5 % depending on the series [8, 9]. Bleeding following diagnostic procedure has been reported in 0.1–0.6 % in adult [10] and is most likely rare in children.

Perforation is the most serious complication in children usually related to polypectomy and managed with surgical intervention. The risk of perforation is increased with active colitis, strictures, diverticulitis, adhesions from prior surgery, and large polyps. The risk varies from 0.06 to 0.3 % [8, 11]. Silent or small perforation of the rectum or sigmoid colon can be managed conservatively. Larger perforations may require abdominal exploration and/or repair. Other rare complications include infection due to a contaminated scope, gas explosion, or sedation-related morbidity or mortality.

Airway Endoscopy

Bronchoscopy is a valuable tool for the pediatric surgeon as it has utility in both diagnosis and therapeutic intervention. As such, there are dedicated chapters for various aspects of airway manipulation throughout this text, including Chap. 5 on Tracheobronchial Disorders and Chap. 8 on Aortopexy. However, it is worth mentioning that pediatric surgeons facile in airway endoscopy find it a valuable tool for patient care. Airway foreign bodies can be both confirmed and extracted, even in the presence of normal chest radiographs. Tracheo-esophageal fistulas can be diagnosed and localized to facilitate repair. The degree of tracheomalacia present can be evaluated in the spontaneously breathing infant. Vascular compression of the trachea can be evaluated pre- and post-aortopexy to confirm adequacy of the procedure [12, 13].

The sizes of rigid bronchoscopes, approximate ages for use, and sizes of flexible bronchoscopes with corresponding endotracheal tubes for accommodation are listed in Table 3.1.

Table 3.1. Bronchoscopy equipment sizes.

Rigid scope size	Inner diameter (mm)	Outer diameter (mm)	Patient age	Flexible scope size	ET tube for scope
2.5	3.5	4.2	Premature infant	2.2	2.5
3.0	4.3	5.0	Newborn infant	2.8	3.0
3.5	5.0	5.7	1–6 months	2.8	3.0
3.7	5.7	6.4	6 months–1 year	2.8	3.5
4.0	6.0	6.7	1–2 years	3.6	4.0
5.0	7.1	7.8	3–4 years	3.6	4.5
6.0	7.5	8.2	5–7 years	3.6 or 5.0	5.0
6.5	8.5	9.2	8+ years	5.0	6.5+

Pearls/Pitfalls

- All equipment should be prepared before beginning airway endoscopy as instrument/scope exchange will be required.
- A bag valve mask should be used to elevate oxygen saturations before introduction of the equipment.
- The optical forceps are longer than the bronchoscopic sheath to allow for extension into smaller bronchial segments.

Postoperative Care

Airway foreign body retrieval is generally quite successful with rare complications [7]. Complications include bronchospasm, laryngeal edema, pneumonia, need for prolonged mechanical ventilation, tracheoesophageal fistula, granulation tissue formation, and bronchial stenosis.

Summary

- Pediatric endoscopic equipment involves a combination of rigid and flexible endoscopic tools for safe and effective performance of endoscopic procedures such as foreign body removal from the airway and gastrointestinal tract.

- Diagnostic maneuvers in the airway are predominantly performed using rigid endoscopy by pediatric surgeons, although, both rigid and flexible endoscopes are utilized in the gastrointestinal tract.
- More advanced procedures such as airway or esophageal dilation or endoscopic retrograde pancreatography (ERCP) are performed for diagnostic or therapeutic purposes.
- For colonoscopy, avoidance and reduction of endoscopic looping and minimizing air insufflation will help reduce post colonoscopy bloating and abdominal pain.

References

1. ASGE Standards of Practice Committee, Lightdale JR, Acosta R, et al. Modifications in endoscopic practice for pediatric patients. Gastrointest Endosc. 2014;79:699–710. doi:10.1016/j.gie.2013.08.014.
2. Russell R, Lucas A, Johnson J, et al. Extraction of esophageal foreign bodies in children: rigid versus flexible endoscopy. Pediatr Surg Int. 2014;30:417–22. doi:10.1007/s00383-014-3481-2.
3. Egbert ND, Bloom DA, Dillman JR. Magnetic resonance imaging of the pediatric pancreaticobiliary system. Magn Reson Imaging Clin N Am. 2013;21:681–96. doi:10.1016/j.mric.2013.04.009.
4. Troendle DM, Barth BA. Pediatric considerations in endoscopic retrograde cholangiopancreatography. Gastrointest Endosc Clin N Am. 2016;26:119–36. doi:10.1016/j.giec.2015.08.004.
5. Giefer MJ, Kozarek RA. Technical outcomes and complications of pediatric ERCP. Surg Endosc. 2015;29:3543–50. doi:10.1007/s00464-015-4105-1.
6. Otto AK, Neal MD, Slivka AN, Kane TD. An appraisal of endoscopic retrograde cholangiopancreatography (ERCP) for pancreaticobiliary disease in children: our institutional experience in 231 cases. Surg Endosc. 2011;25:2536–40. doi:10.1007/s00464-011-1582-8.
7. Dahshan A, Lin CH, Peters J, Thomas R, Tolia V. A randomized, prospective study to evaluate the efficacy and acceptance of three bowel preparations for colonoscopy in children. Pediatric bowel preparations for colonoscopy in children. Am J Gastroenterol. 1999;94:3497–501.
8. Sieg A, Hachmoeller-Eisenbach U, Eisenbach T. Prospective evaluation of complications in outpatient GI endoscopy: a survey among German gastroenterologists. Gastrointest Endosc. 2001;53:620–7.
9. Nelson DB, McQuaid KR, Bond JH, et al. Procedural success and complications of large-scale screening colonoscopy. Gastrointest Endosc. 2002;55:307–14. doi:10.1067/mge.2002.121883.
10. Ko CW, Dominitz JA. Complications of colonoscopy: magnitude and management. Gastrointest Endosc Clin N Am. 2010;20:659–71. doi:10.1016/j.giec.2010.07.005.

11. Korman LY, Overholt BF, Box T, Winker CK. Perforation during colonoscopy in endoscopic ambulatory surgical centers. Gastrointest Endosc. 2003;58:554–7.
12. Kane TD, Nadler EP, Potoka DA. Thoracoscopic aortopexy for vascular compression of the trachea: approach from the right. J Laparoendosc Adv Surg Tech. 2008;18:313–6. doi:10.1089/lap.2007.0032.
13. Abdel-Rahman U, Ahrens P, Fieguth HG, et al. Surgical treatment of tracheomalacia by bronchoscopic monitored aortopexy in infants and children. Ann Thorac Surg. 2002;74:315–9.

4. Minimally Invasive Approaches to the Pediatric Thyroid and Parathyroid

Thom E. Lobe, Simon K. Wright, and Go Miyano

Introduction

Epidemiology

Thyroid and parathyroid hormones play a crucial role as a regulator of growth, of nervous system myelination, of metabolism, and of organ functions. Disorders affecting the thyroid gland represent the most common endocrinopathies in children. The etiology and clinical presentation of thyroid and parathyroid disorders in children and adolescents substantially differ from that in adults. Thus, pediatric medical care requires an appreciation of distinct characteristics of these function and dysfunction in childhood and adolescence [1–4].

Pathophysiology

Although the need for thyroid and parathyroid surgery is less common in children, there are a number of conditions that may justify surgical intervention, including malignancy, functional disorder, and nodular disease [5, 6]. Furthermore, this is a population in which a minimally invasive technique is particularly appealing, and many of these patients are eligible for this approach [7]. For example, because youthful patients with differentiated thyroid cancer are more likely to require reoperation than their adult counterparts, the preservation of tissue planes afforded by the reduced dissection may be anticipated to facilitate subsequent surgical encounters [8].

D.S. Walsh et al. (eds.), *The SAGES Manual of Pediatric Minimally Invasive Surgery*, DOI 10.1007/978-3-319-43642-5_4

Preoperative Evaluation

History/Surgical Indications

The first published patient series involving minimally invasive video-assisted thyroid/parathyroid surgery for adults was reported by Miccoli et al. [9]. Although this report confined its use to a select patient cohort, indications for the procedure have expanded widely over the past two decades: in low- to intermediate-risk differentiated cancer, cytologically undermined nodules, and small volume benign disease [10].

Exam/Imaging

Thyroid and parathyroid hormonal profile, neck ultrasound evaluation, and fine needle aspiration are considered depending on the patient's pathology. In cases of hyperparathyroidism, at least two preoperative studies are generally performed; computed tomography scan and a Sestamibi scan are best to help locate the adenoma.

Labs

Preoperative thyroid and parathyroid hormone levels are drawn before making the incision. Rapid thyroxin and parathormone levels are performed perioperatively after removal of the suspected lesion to confirm that the abnormally functioning gland has accurately been removed.

Technique

Special Consideration

Since the beginning of the 1990s, minimally invasive endoscopic techniques have been applied for surgery in natural body cavities such as the thorax and abdomen of children, and the pediatric surgeon had to be trained to work in limited spaces. The head and neck represent an anatomic region that, while not a natural body cavity, is well suited to minimally invasive procedures performed after creating an artificial space.

The past two decades has seen a tremendous transformation in the way in which thyroid surgery is accomplished. In 1996 Gagner published the first case of subtotal resection of the parathyroids via a cervical endoscopic approach in a 37-year-old man [11]. In 1997 Huscher et al. reported their first endoscopic right thyroid lobectomy for a 4-mm adenoma [12], and a year later Yeung reported three endoscopic parathyroidectomies and five endoscopic hemithyroidectomies [13], which were carried out without any complications.

After having performed the authors' first total thyroidectomy using a robotic-assisted bilateral transaxillary endoscopic approach, over the past a decade, the authors have developed a totally endoscopic minimal access approach to head and neck lesions and reviewed their experience [14, 15].

Instruments

Much change has been technologically driven, with the advent of advanced energy devices such as the ultrasonic dissector, the availability of robust nerve monitoring, and the judicious application of high-resolution endoscopy [16–18]. Moreover, with the improvement in technical skills in endoscopic surgery and the development of thinner and shorter instruments, new spaces have become accessible to endoscopic surgery. With the aid of CO_2 pneumodissection, virtual spaces, such as the retroperitoneum, can be turned into real spaces allowing for easy endoscopic surgery in these areas.

Positioning

In the operating room, patient is placed supine on the table and is administered a general anesthesia, and the neck is slightly extended and displaced forward in a sniffing position. The arms are extended anterior at the shoulder and the elbows are bent at right angles, then are suspended from an ether screen or other form of horizontal bar from which to suspend the arms.

Access and Exposure

Three incisions are made in the axilla of the affected side or in both axillae in the case of a total thyroidectomy, and all the incisions are made just posterior to the anterior axillary line. The largest incision is in the center of the axilla for a 10–12 mm trocar, and other two smaller incisions, each ~5 mm, are made for the 5 mm instrument trocars. The trocars are secured with sutures so that they do not dislodge during the procedure. To create the initial space, the surgeon first inserts the index finger of the dominant hand, and by advancing it and sweeping it from side to side creates an initial working space just anterior to the pectoralis fascia; this dissection is carried out medially and cephalad until it is big enough to accommodate trocar placement.

Under 10 mmHg CO_2 insufflation, a 10-mm telescope is inserted, a dissector is inserted through one of the 5-mm cannula, and L-hook electrocautery or the Harmonic Scalpel is inserted through the other. The authors do not use 2-mm instruments as they are not rigid enough to lift up the thyroid, and as the procedure is bloodless, no suction probe or gauze pads are needed. Suction in such a small working space would certainly cause collapse of the working space and hinder further surgery.

Neck Dissection

The dissection can proceed and the space between the subcutaneous fascia and platysma muscle just anterior to the pectoralis fascia can be enlarged to the level of the clavicle cephalad and the sternocleidomastoid muscle medially. Depending on the size and location of the lesion, dissection then continues either underneath or between the two heads of the sternocleidomastoid muscle, medially toward the strap muscles. The junction of the sternocleidomastoid and omohyoid muscles serves as a useful landmark. Dissection continues deeper, dividing the strap muscles as required until the thyroid gland itself is observed. The parathyroid glands are carefully identified. One must remain fully aware of the position of the recurrent laryngeal nerve throughout the case. After the polar vessels are divided, attention is turned to the hilar structures. The vessels are carefully dissected from the hilum and displaced posteriorly, taking care to identify the recurrent laryngeal nerve and parathyroid glands. Once the hilar structures are free and allowed to fall posteriorly, the intact lobe is then dissected from the trachea using an ultrasonic device; when further dissection might risk injury to the nerve, it is preferred to leave a small bit of thyroid tissue adherent to the nerve. One of the dissecting instruments is removed from either of the trocars. Once the intact lobe is extracted, a Petite® wound drain (Vitalcor, Westmont, IL, USA) is placed in the bed of thyroid. This is typically removed the morning after surgery.

For the case of total thyroidectomy, two surgeons work simultaneously toward the midline, one from each axilla performing the procedure described above.

Pearls/Pitfalls

Although the authors initially thought that the robot-assisted approach might be useful, it has since been abandoned for these cases as it seemed simpler and perfectly adequate to perform the procedure without the additional time and expense. There is a learning curve of about 10 cases, after which the surgeon has clearer concept of the anatomic relationships and can perform the procedure more quickly.

Postoperative Care

Outcomes/Complications

In the past 10 years, 4 series of pediatric minimally invasive thyroid surgery have been reported from each different center, and were reviewed [13, 19–21]. These results are summarized in Table 4.1.

Summary

- One of the major limitations inhibiting the use of minimally invasive surgery for thyroid and parathyroid among pediatric patients is the lack of evidence that it can produce results comparable to a conventional thyroidectomy/parathyroidectomy in the treatment of these patients where malignant diseases are relatively much more frequent with respect to adult patients.
- The safety of minimally invasive surgery for thyroid/parathyroid has been already highlighted in several adult studies comparing different endoscopic procedures with the standard open thyroidectomy.
- In this experience the rate of transient and permanent recurrent laryngeal nerve palsy and hypo-PTH was similar to that reported in other series. More interestingly, there were no differences in terms of complications between patients treated with minimally invasive approach and those treated with conventional approach [22, 23].

Table 4.1. The series of minimally invasive approach for thyroid in children.

Author/Year (Ref)	*n*	Pathology	Procedure	Approach from-	Age (y)	Volume	Op-t (min)	Complications
Napoli/2014 (16)	34	Multinodular goiter ($n=5$)	Total thyroidectomy	Suprasternal notch	15	15.8 mm[a]	40	Hypo-PTH ($n=14$: 41 %)[b]
		Toxic goiter ($n=4$)						Vocal cord palsy ($n=2$: 5.9 %)
		Papillary carcinoma ($n=19$)						
		Medullary carcinoma ($n=6$)						
Glynn/2014 (15)	6	Multiple endocrine neoplasia 2 ($n=6$)	Total thyroidectomy	Suprasternal notch	5.3	NA	93	Hematoma ($n=1$: 17 %)
Seybt/2011 (14)	19	Papillary cancer ($n=5$)	Total thyroidectomy ($n=11$)	Suprasternal notch[c]	15.4	NA	NA	Vocal cord palsy ($n=1$: 4.3 %)
		Follicular cancer ($n=3$)	Hemithyroidectomy ($n=12$)					Hypocalcemia ($n=2$: 8.7 %)
		Medullary cancer ($n=1$)						
		Grave's disease ($n=4$)						
		Multinodular goiter ($n=3$)						
		(Completion thyroidectomy; $n=3$)						

Lobe/2011 (13)	31	Hyperparathyroidism ($n=2$)	Hemithyroidectomy ($n=2$)	Transaxillary	12.7 (Avg)	29.0 g (Avg)	197 (Avg)	Hypocalcemia ($n=3$: 9.7 %)
		Adenoma ($n=2$)	Total thyroidectomy ($n=29$)					Neuroplaxia ($n=3$: 9.7 %)
		Grave's disease ($n=27$)	(Robot-assisted; $n=3$)					Hematoma ($n=1$: 3.2 %)
								Pneumothorax ($n=1$: 3.2 %)
								Laryngeal tear ($n=1$: 3.2 %)

PTH parathyroid hormone, *Op-t* operating time, *NA* not available, *Avg* average
[a]Size of nodule
[b]Including two permanent hypo-PTH
[c]Including 16 cases of non-endoscopic minimally invasive approach

- The long-term trend and effects of minimally invasive surgery for pediatric thyroid and parathyroid remain to be seen, and more data in children and adolescence is expected to be accumulated.

References

1. Larsen PR, Davis TF, Hay ID. The thyroid gland. In: Wilson JD, Foster DW, Kronenberg HM, Larsen PR, editors. Williams textbook of endocrinology. Philadelphia: Saunders; 1998. p. 389–515.
2. Bettendorf M. Thyroid disorders in children from birth to adolescence. Eur J Nucl Med Mol Imaging. 2002;29:439–46.
3. Alagaratnam S, Kuzawinski TR. Aetiology, diagnosis and surgical treatment of primary hyperparathyroidism in children: New trends. Horm Res Pediatr. 2015. [Equb ahead of print].
4. Durkin ET, Nichol PF, Lund DP, et al. What is the optimal treatment for children with primary hyperparathyroidism? J Pediatr Surg. 2010;45:1142–6.
5. Bargren AE, Meyer-Rochow GY, Delbridge LW, et al. Outcomes of surgically managed pediatric thyroid cancer. J Surg Res. 2009;156:70–73.
6. Raval MV, Browne M, Chin AC, et al. Total thyroidectomy for benign disease in the pediatric patient – feasible and safe. J Pediatr Surg. 2009;44:1529–33.
7. Spinelli C, Donatini G, Berti P, et al. Minimally invasive video-assisted thyroidectomy in pediatric patients. J Pediatr Surg. 2008;43:1259–61.
8. Thompson GB, Hay ID. Current strategies for surgical management and adjuvant treatment of childhood papillary thyroid carcinoma. World J Surg. 2004;28:1187–98.
9. Miccoli P, Berti P, Conte M, et al. Minimally invasive surgery for thyroid small nodules: preliminally report. J Endocrinol Invest. 1999;22:849–51.
10. Minuto MN, Berti P, Miccoli M, et al. Minimally invasive video-assisted thyroidectomy: an analysis of results and a revision of indications. Surg Endosc. 2012;26:818–22.
11. Gagner M. Endoscopic subtotal parathyroidectomy in patients with primary hyperthyroidism. Br J Surg. 1996;83:875.
12. Huscher CS, Chiodini S, Napolitano C, et al. Endoscopic right thyroid lobectomy. Surg Endosc. 1997;11:877.
13. Yeung GH. Endoscopic surgery of the neck: a new frontier. Surg Laparosc Endosc. 1998;8:227–32.
14. Miyano G, Lobe TE, Wright SK. Bilateral transaxillary endoscopic total thyroidectomy. J Pediatr Surg. 2008;43:299–303.
15. Lobe TE, Wright SK. The transaxillary, totally endoscopic approach for head and neck endocrine surgery in children. J Laparoendosc Adv Surg Tech A. 2011;21: 97–101.
16. Defechereux T, Rinken F, Maweja S, et al. Evaluation of the ultrasonic dissector in thyroid surgery. A prospective randomized study. Acta Chir Gerg. 2003;103:274–77.

17. Randolph GW. Surgical anatomy of the recurrent laryngeal nerve. In: Randolph, editor. Surgery of the thyroid and parathyroid glands. Philadelphia: Saunders; 2003. p. 300–342.
18. Sebag F, Palazzo FF, Harding J, et al. Endoscopic lateral and approach thyroid lobectomy: safe evolution from endoscopic parathyroidectomy. World J Surg. 2006;30:802–5.
19. Seybt MW, Terris DJ. Minimally invasive thyroid surgery in children. Ann Otol Rhinol Laryngol. 2011;120:215–9.
20. Glynn RW, Cashman EC, Doody J, et al. Prophylactic total thyroidectomy using the minimally invasive video-assisted approach in children with multiple endocrine neoplasia type 2. Head Neck. 2014;36:768–71.
21. Napoli LD, Spinelli C, Ambrosini CE, et al. Minimally invasive video-assisted thyroidectomy versus conventional thyroidectomy in pediatric patients. Eur J Pediatr Surg. 2014;24:398–402.
22. Lombardi CP, Raffaelli M, Princi P, et al. Safety of video-assisted thyroidectomy versus conventional surgery. Head Neck. 2005;27:58–64.
23. Miccoli P, Pinchera A, Materazzi G, et al. Surgical treatment of low and intermediate-risk papillary thyroid cancer with minimally invasive video-assisted thyroidectomy. J Clin Endocrinol Metab. 2009;94:1618–22.

5. Bronchoscopy and Tracheobronchial Disorders

Ian C. Glenn, Domenic Craner, and Oliver Soldes

Introduction

The endoluminal examination of the tracheobronchial tree and therapeutic airway interventions is made possible by the technique of bronchoscopy. This chapter reviews the types of bronchoscopy, techniques, and disorders commonly managed with these techniques. Bronchoscopy is generally divided into rigid and flexible bronchoscopies, which are complementary techniques. Pediatric surgeons who care for diseases of the tracheobronchial tree should be familiar with both techniques. They should also be familiar with direct laryngoscopy, which is performed at the time of introduction of the rigid bronchoscope and is a prerequisite for any airway interventions.

Tracheobronchial Disorders Commonly Managed with Bronchoscopy

Foreign Body Aspiration

Foreign body aspiration most commonly occurs between the ages of 6 months and 2 years of age with the most commonly aspirated items being food particles, such as nuts and seeds. This represents a true emergency due to the possibility of partial or complete airway obstruction. Aspiration of a foreign body has an overall mortality rate of approximately 1 %. Approximately 20 % of aspirated foreign bodies are located in the upper airway, while around 80 % of objects are found in the main stem or lobar bronchus.

D.S. Walsh et al. (eds.), *The SAGES Manual of Pediatric Minimally Invasive Surgery*, DOI 10.1007/978-3-319-43642-5_5

Tracheoesophageal Fistula and Esophageal Fistula

It is believed that tracheoesophageal fistula and esophageal atresia occur due to a defect in the process of septation of the foregut into the trachea and esophagus, with or without a residual communication between the two. Congenital tracheoesophageal fistula has an overall incidence of approximately 1 in 4000 live births. It is often also associated with other abnormalities such as cardiac, gastrointestinal, and other elements of the VACTERL association (vertebral, anorectal, cardiac, tracheoesophageal, renal, and limb anomalies).

While most tracheoesophageal fistulas in children are congenital, there is also an acquired form. Acquired tracheoesophageal fistulas can be caused by prolonged intubation, localized infection, malignancy, trauma, and following ingestion of a caustic substance, disk batteries, or other foreign bodies.

Tracheal Atresia and Tracheal Stenosis

Tracheal atresia and stenosis are rare disorders involving the portion of the trachea inferior to the larynx. They are often associated with other anomalies in distinct patterns. Tracheal atresia is a failure of development leading to complete or partial absence of the trachea, with high lethality. It is often accompanied by a fistula between the esophagus and distal trachea or bronchus, which may rarely permit survival with surgical intervention, if a sufficient fistula is present at birth. The patient presents with severe respiratory distress and hypoxia immediately after birth. They are unable to be intubated and readily ventilated, and the cry is absent.

Tracheal stenosis is a segmental, funnel-shaped, or diffuse long narrowing of the trachea. Short segmental stenosis may have reasonably good outcomes. The prognosis for long segment stenosis is poor.

Tracheomalacia

Tracheomalacia is a dynamic functional narrowing of the tracheal lumen that is caused by collapse of the airway during expiration due to an inadequacy of the cartilaginous rings of the trachea. It may be misdiagnosed as bronchial asthma, respiratory tract infection, or an aspirated foreign body. Congenital tracheomalacia is the result of congenital hypoplasia of the tracheal cartilages. The acquired form can be associated with long-term intubation of premature newborns, severe tracheobronchitis, surgical tracheal procedures (tracheostomy), and compression due to tumors, abscess, or cysts. Although often underdiagnosed, tracheomalacia has an incidence of at least 1 in 2100 live births. Bronchomalacia is a similar cartilaginous deficiency of the bronchus, which impairs exhalation from the effected segment of the lung and may lead to lobar hyperinflation and congenital lobar emphysema.

Laryngotracheoesophageal Clefts

Laryngotracheoesophageal cleft is a congenital malformation that leads to a residual congenital communication between the esophagus and the laryngotracheal complex. It presents with varying degrees of aspiration, respiratory distress, pneumonia, feeding difficulties, increased secretions, wheezing, and stridor. It may be limited to the larynx (laryngeal cleft) or extended into the trachea (laryngotracheoesophageal cleft) as far as the carina. It results from a failure of fusion of the posterior cricoid cartilage and improper formation of the septum separating the tracheal and esophageal lumens. It is estimated that the incidence of laryngeal cleft is between 1 in 10,000 to 1 in 20,000 live births, occurring more commonly in boys than in girls. There is often an association with other malformations such as Opitz-Frias syndrome, Pallister-Hall syndrome, DiGeorge syndrome, and CHARGE (coloboma, heart defects, atresia of choanae, retardation of growth/development, genitourinary disorders, and ear defects) syndrome. Laryngotracheal cleft may be part of VACTERL association. Laryngotracheal clefts are classified based on the degree of downward extension of the cleft.

Bronchial Carcinoid

Bronchial carcinoid tumors are neuroendocrine tumors that most often occur within the central bronchi. Bronchial carcinoids produce endoluminal obstruction with atelectasis, pneumonia, wheezing, cough, and sometimes bleeding with hemoptysis. Most are low-grade “typical” carcinoids that are well-differentiated, slow-growing tumors that rarely metastasize. “Atypical” carcinoids are more aggressive intermediate-grade tumors with a greater tendency for local extension and metastases. In addition, they may secrete vasoactive substances that include 5-hydroxytryptamine (5-HT), 5-hydroxytryptophan (5-HTP), and many others that can lead to the classic carcinoid syndrome. Carcinoid syndrome more often occurs with large tumors and in the presence of liver metastases. Carcinoid syndrome consists of vasomotor flushing, episodic hypotension, and diarrhea. This syndrome is rarely seen in children. Carcinoids may also secrete adrenocorticotropic hormone (ACTH), producing Cushing's syndrome. Bronchial carcinoids are the most common primary pulmonary neoplasm of childhood. They account for roughly 80 % of primary malignant lung tumors in children. However, overall, they only represent roughly 1–2 % of all lung tumors. The estimated incidence of bronchial carcinoid tumors in children is approximately 3–5 cases per million per year.

Preoperative Evaluation

Preoperative evaluation of the patient is essential in determining a working diagnosis of tracheobronchial disease and planning for subsequent bronchoscopy.

History

The patient's history is the most important initial element in the evaluation of tracheobronchial disorders. Children with suspected tracheobronchial disease often present with chronic cough, wheezing, stridor, increased secretions, feeding difficulties, hoarseness, respiratory distress, and rarely, hemoptysis. Specifically, children with tracheoesophageal fistula and esophageal atresia will often present with a history of coughing, choking, and cyanosis following feeds, which is caused by aspiration of feeds. Excessive drooling and secretions may also be present. Recurrent or unrecognized tracheoesophageal fistulas, laryngotracheal clefts, and unrecognized airway foreign bodies may present with a history of chronic or recurrent pneumonias. Parents or caregivers of children with foreign body aspiration often report having witnessed the child putting food or object in their mouth and choking on it. Bronchial carcinoid often presents with a history of post-obstructive pneumonia, persistent cough, and hemoptysis.

Exam

A thorough physical exam is essential in the diagnosis of tracheobronchial disease. Auscultation of the chest is imperative. Unequal or decreased sounds, wheezing, stridor, and vocal changes can be indicative of disease. It is important to calm the child for the examination to allow for ideal auscultation and to prevent exacerbation of respiratory distress. A confirmatory test for the diagnosis of esophageal atresia with or without tracheoesophageal fistula is an inability to pass an orogastric or nasogastric tube down the esophagus.

Laboratory Evaluation

In most instances of tracheobronchial disease, blood tests will not be useful unless the patient is in acute respiratory distress. In such cases, blood gasses are useful in determining the degree of respiratory dysfunction that the patient is experiencing, and in managing ventilation. However, pulse oximetry is more rapidly and easily applied in urgent situations and is generally employed first. In the case of bronchial carcinoid, blood serotonin and urine 5-hydroxyindoleacetic acid (5-HIAA) may be elevated.

Imaging

Plain X-rays are an important imaging tool for diagnosis. Posteroanterior (PA) and lateral chest films are commonly obtained. The chest X-ray will demonstrate pulmonary infiltrates, atelectasis, or hyperinflation of the lung due to air trapping. Bilateral decubitus chest X-rays may also be helpful in localizing aspirated objects or bronchial masses causing air trapping (Fig. 5.1) and in the diagnosis of pleural effusions. If not included in the chest X-rays, neck films, often part of a "foreign body series", may be necessary in order to help identify foreign bodies in the proximal airway. Unfortunately, the most commonly aspirated items are radiolucent. Thus, imaging studies should not be used to rule out the presence of a foreign body as radiolucent objects (food, nuts, etc.) can present with a normal chest X-ray with or without focal hyperinflation, infiltrate, or atelectasis. In the case of congenital esophageal atresia, a dilated upper pouch can occasionally be seen on plain chest radiography.

Chest CT scans can be useful in the diagnosis of bronchial masses or foreign bodies, stenosis and intrinsic obstructions, or masses causing extrinsic compression of the airway.

Fluoroscopy with contrast imaging of the esophagus can also be useful in the diagnosis of congenital, recurrent, and acquired tracheoesophageal fistula.

Other Tests

Bronchoscopy itself is the most definitive technique in diagnosis of anatomic disorders of the airways. Other tests outside of those already discussed are infrequently useful in the diagnosis of pediatric surgical tracheobronchial disease.

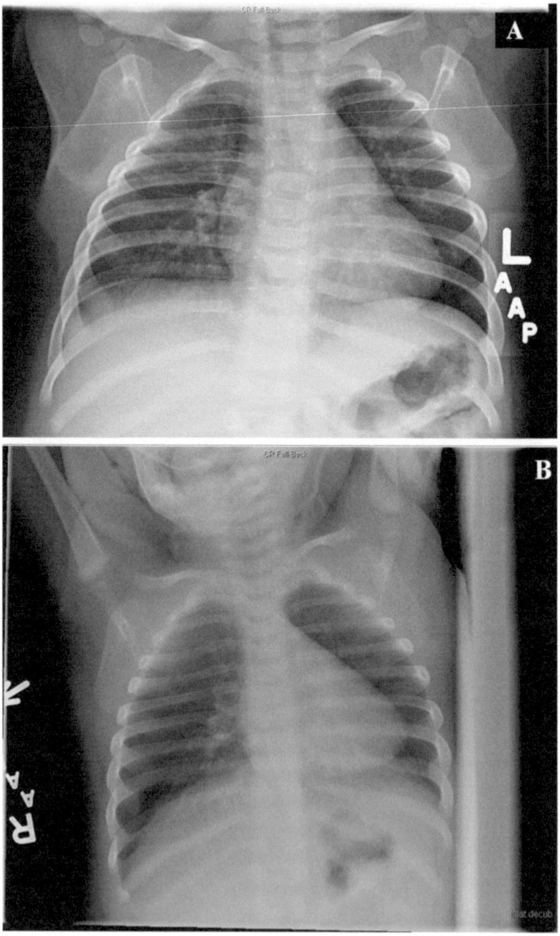

Fig. 5.1. Images of a 9-month-old female who presented with concern for foreign body aspiration. Air trapping on the left side (**a**) is noted on the decubitus films (**b, c**). Note the normal posteroanterior images; emphasize the importance of obtaining decubitus films.

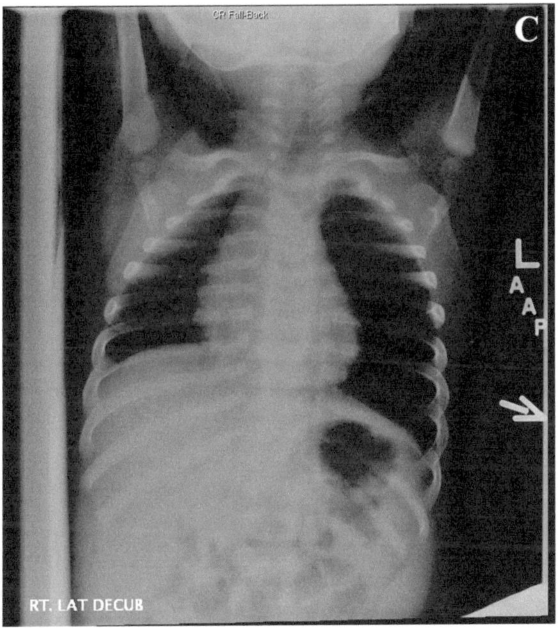

Fig. 5.1. (continued).

Surgical Indications

Rigid and flexible bronchoscopies are indicated for examination of the airway in cases of suspected endoluminal diseases of the trachea and bronchi, airway foreign bodies, stenosis, fistula to the airway, obstructions, and hemorrhage. It is simultaneously a diagnostic and a therapeutic technique, useful for the treatment of endoluminal diseases. It permits clearance and collection of secretions (and blood), biopsy of tissue, removal of foreign bodies, dilation of strictures, destruction of endoluminal lesions, and treatment of some recurrent fistulas. Flexible bronchoscopy may be used to guide selective intubation of a main stem bronchus.

Technique

Bronchoscopy is divided into rigid and flexible types of bronchoscopy, which are complementary techniques.

Special Considerations

1. Children requiring rigid bronchoscopy, especially for acute foreign body removal, usually require general anesthesia in order to tolerate the procedure and permit safe and effective examination. Flexible bronchoscopy may be performed under moderate sedation with topical airway anesthesia. Consultation with the anesthesiologist is required preoperatively when deciding to perform the procedure with or without spontaneous respiration (paralysis).
2. Rigid bronchoscopy requires direct laryngoscopy to visualize the glottic opening and introduce the bronchoscope. Flexible endoscopy may be performed through a laryngeal mask airway, endotracheal tube, tracheostomy, or orally through a bite block. Additionally, a nasal approach may be adopted with the flexible endoscope inserted via the naris.
3. Flexible bronchoscopy permits more distal examination of the airways, due to the smaller size and flexibility of the endoscope (Fig. 5.2). Subsequently, these pediatric bronchoscopes may be too small to have a working channel or have a small diameter channel that permits suctioning but limits instrumentation (graspers, biopsy forceps). The small size of the pediatric flexible bronchoscope may also limit image quality.

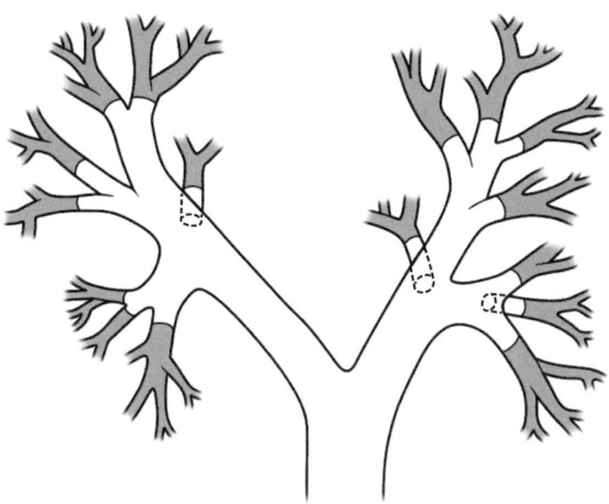

Fig. 5.2. The tracheobronchial tree. The gray portions represent the areas which are beyond the limits of visualization by rigid bronchoscopy. A flexible bronchoscope is required to evaluate these areas. The figure is oriented to represent the anatomy as it is encountered via rigid bronchoscopy.

4. Although both flexible and rigid pediatric bronchoscopies may be both diagnostic and therapeutic techniques, rigid bronchoscopy is more often used therapeutically in pediatrics. Most foreign bodies are removed with rigid bronchoscopy.
5. Patients with bleeding in the airway should undergo rigid over flexible bronchoscopy due to its improved ability to achieve hemostasis and definitively secure the airway.
6. Cervical instability and maxillofacial trauma or anomalies may make rigid endoscopy difficult or hazardous due to the need to extend the neck to allow a straight pathway for introduction of the rigid scope. In patients with head and neck trauma, flexible is preferred over rigid bronchoscopy. This is because the head and neck do not have to be manipulated as dramatically to insert the flexible bronchoscope. Similarly, in patients who are already intubated, flexible bronchoscopy is also preferred as the airway is already secured and the flexible scope may be inserted via the endotracheal tube. Patients with respiratory failure and significant ventilator support may not tolerate extubation and ventilation via the bronchoscope.

Anatomy

There are many important anatomic differences in the airways of adults and children which must be remembered when dealing with tracheobronchial disease. In children, several factors may make intubation of the airway more difficult. The jaw is smaller, the tongue is relatively larger, the epiglottis is larger, and the larynx is more anterior. The occiput is also relatively larger, causing neck flexion. The trachea is shorter and narrower, with the narrowest area in the subglottis.

In terms of physiology, the pediatric airway has a higher resistance to gas flow due to the smaller radius and cross-sectional area. For the same reason, the pediatric airway is more prone to obstruction by foreign bodies and secretions. Due to a relatively lower functional residual capacity and relatively higher rate of oxygen consumption, pediatric patients (and infants in particular) are less tolerant of apnea than adults

Positioning

Proper setup of the operating room table and equipment facilitates performance of bronchoscopy (Fig. 5.3). For rigid bronchoscopy, the

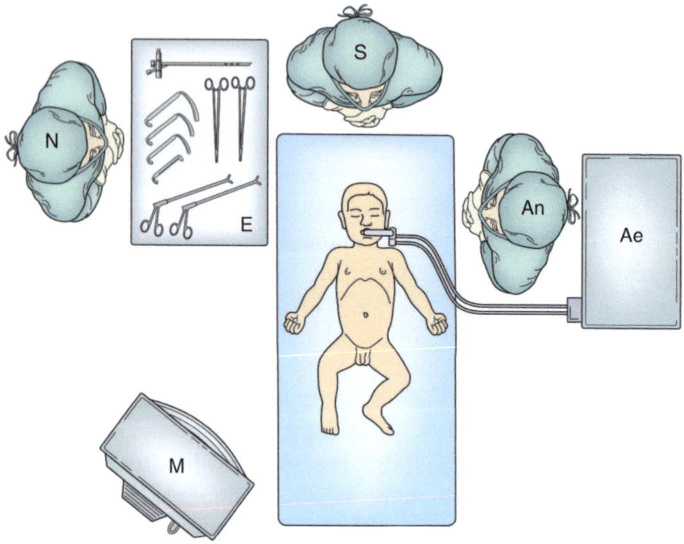

Fig. 5.3. Orientation of personnel and equipment during rigid bronchoscopy. (S) surgeon, (An) anesthesiologist, (Ae) anesthesia equipment, (N) assistant, (M) video monitor, (E) endoscopy equipment and instruments (light source, suction, bronchoscope, etc.).

surgeon sits at the head of the bed, and the video monitor is placed at the foot. The anesthesia provider and anesthesia machine are situated to the left of the head of the bed. The instruments and the surgical assistant are to the right of the head of the bed.

The patient is placed in the supine position and a shoulder roll is placed to compensate for the large occiput and to straighten the airway. The cervical spine and the head are extended into the "sniffing position." Eye protection should always be applied to the patient prior to commencing bronchoscopy. The index finger and thumb of the surgeon's nondominant hand not only support the rigid scope but serve to protect the patient's teeth and lips. The head is positioned such that it can be easily turned to the side during the procedure.

Children undergoing flexible bronchoscopy are generally sedated or anesthetized. They may be placed in the semi-recumbent or supine position. The surgeon stands at the head or to the side of the table with the monitor opposite him/her. The anesthesia provider and his/her equipment are to the side, cephalad to the surgeon, or at the foot.

Instruments

The basic requirements for rigid bronchoscopy are a light source, a rod-lens telescope, and the bronchoscope (Fig. 5.4). There are multiple styles and manufacturers of bronchoscopes, rod-lenses, and light sources, which are integrated with video equipment. Among telescopes, the Hopkins rod-lens style is the most popular. Telescopes have angles from 0° to 120°, and newer rigid telescopes have flexible tips allowing greater ranges of visualization up to 180°. A bite block, or similar device, may be used to protect the lips and teeth, as well as the endoscope.

The standard pediatric flexible bronchoscope (Fig. 5.5) has a diameter of 3.4 to 3.6 mm with a 1.2 mm working channel. Diameters as small as 1.8 mm are available, although these scopes lack a working channel. The adult flexible bronchoscope has a diameter up to 6.3 mm (Table 5.1). A bite block should always be employed if the flexible bronchoscope is used transorally but not via the endotracheal tube.

Most endoscopy suites and operating rooms are equipped with video equipment allowing the bronchoscope image to be projected onto large viewing screens and recorded.

Suction for clearance of oropharyngeal secretions is important to the management of any airway. The suction is connected to the working

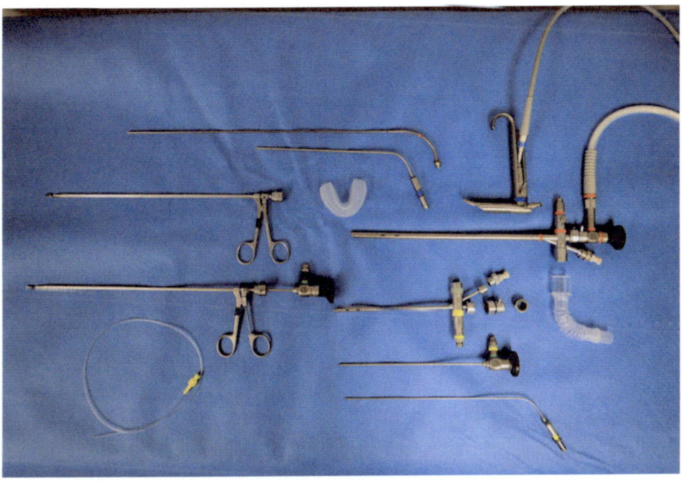

Fig. 5.4. Commonly used rigid bronchoscopy instruments.

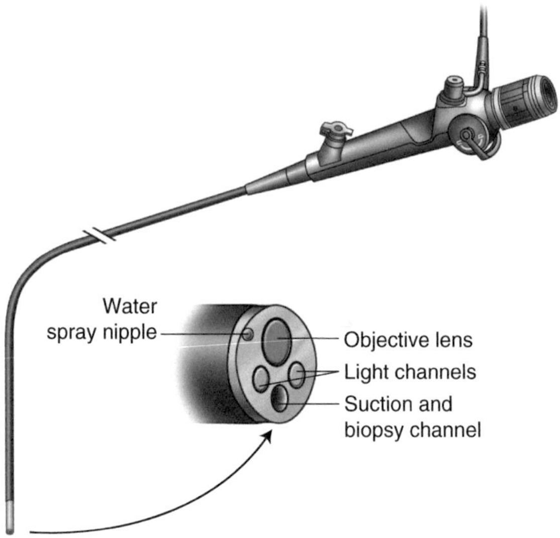

Fig. 5.5. Flexible endoscope with identification of key components.

Table 5.1. Appropriate endotracheal tube (ETT) size for patient age ranges, in addition to compatible flexible bronchoscope sizes for introduction via the ETT.

Age (years)	ETT diameter (mm)	Bronchoscope size (mm)
Preterm	2.0–3.0	2.2
0–2	3.5–4.5	2.2, 2.8
2–4	4.5–5.5	2.8, 3.8
4–8	5.5–6.5	2.8, 3.8, 4.9
8–18	6.5–8.0	2.8, 3.8, 4.9, 5.5

Data from Koumbourlis [5]

channel of the flexible bronchoscope or to a suction catheter or hand-held suction tip that may be passed into the rigid bronchoscope.

Magill forceps should be available at any time when the airway is manipulated. Foreign bodies located in the mouth or oropharynx may potentially be retrieved via this instrument, without the need for bronchoscopy. Additionally, the Magill forceps may be helpful when a foreign body has been brought to the level of the pharynx via the bronchoscope.

Biopsy or grasping forceps may be used in either flexible or rigid bronchoscopy. Of note, the pediatric bronchoscope working channel cannot accommodate standard biopsy forceps and requires special biopsy forceps designed for such scopes.

Snares and baskets, most of which are adapted from urologic surgery for the retrieval of urinary tract calculi, and a vascular balloon catheter may be used via the flexible bronchoscope working channel for retrieval of foreign bodies. Foreign bodies also may be retrieved using a Fogarty-type balloon catheter with a rigid bronchoscope. The balloon is passed beyond the foreign object and inflated. Gentle traction is placed on the balloon in order to move or dislodge the body. At this point, the object is definitively retrieved using one of the above instruments. The use of a magnet to retrieve ferromagnetic foreign bodies is also described.

Both injectable epinephrine and epinephrine-soaked pledgets may be implemented in cases of bleeding within the airway. The epinephrine may be injected via both types of bronchoscope through the use of special catheters. The pledgets may be used via the rigid bronchoscope to hold manual pressure on bleeding sources.

Cryotherapy is used for cryoablation of airway lesions in the field of otolaryngology. However, it may be used for freezing organic foreign bodies, which have a high water content, thus making them easier to manipulate and remove.

Similarly, the laser (Nd:YAG, CO_2, argon, and KTP are common types) may be used to ablate granulation tissue and hemangiomas. However, it can be used to free a foreign body of granulation tissue and also to score the surface of a smooth object, facilitating retrieval.

Both metal (self-expanding and balloon expandable) and silastic stents are available and amenable to placement in the pediatric airway of larger children via the rigid bronchoscope.

Steps

Flexible Bronchoscopy

Flexible bronchoscopy, especially in younger patients, is typically performed with general anesthesia with spontaneous respirations and intubation with a laryngeal mask airway (LMA) or endotracheal tube. The patient is positioned supine. After induction of anesthesia, topical 1 % lidocaine is applied to the larynx, vocal cords, and trachea. A special adapter is attached to the endotracheal tube or laryngeal mask airway to allow for simultaneous ventilation and bronchoscopy. The practitioner stands at the head of the bed with the patient in the supine position, holding the scope housing and controls in the left hand. The thumb is used to operate the control wheel and the index finger to control suction. The flexible portion of the scope is held in the right hand. The scope is introduced into the endotracheal tube or LMA and is advanced until it is in the subglottic space.

Flexible bronchoscopy may also be performed under sedation with topical anesthesia applied to the nose, pharynx, and larynx. The patient is positioned semi-recumbent. After induction of sedation with spontaneous respiration, topical 1 % lidocaine is applied to the nose or pharynx. The scope is introduced via a bite block in the mouth or via the nares. The scope tip is deflected inferiorly, and the scope is advanced to a position just superior to the glottis. When advancing past the tongue base, the patient may be prompted to stick out the tongue, or alternatively, the tongue may be retracted by grasping the tongue with a dry gauze. In scopes with a working channel, local anesthetic is sprayed onto the vocal folds to reduce the risk of laryngospasm. The scope is advanced into the subglottic space, and further local anesthetic is applied into the trachea. The position of the tracheal rings is noted to ensure accurate maintenance of anatomic relations.

Biopsies may be performed with larger scopes with a working channel. The area of interest should be maintained in view while the biopsy forceps are introduced.

Most bleeding related to bronchoscopy will stop spontaneously, but the forceps may be used to apply manual pressure. Additionally, epinephrine may be applied topically or injected.

Rigid Bronchoscopy

Patients undergoing rigid bronchoscopy require general anesthesia with spontaneous or spontaneous-assisted ventilation via a ventilating bronchoscope. Spontaneous ventilation is recommended in cases of foreign body aspiration. A rigid 0° telescope is placed into the bronchoscope, and image quality is verified. After induction of anesthesia, a transverse shoulder roll is placed, and topical 1 % lidocaine is applied to the larynx, vocal cords, and trachea by the anesthetist. The patient is positioned in the "sniffing position" with the head and neck extended (Fig. 5.6). A Miller (straight blade) laryngoscope is held in the left hand, elevated forward, and used to elevate the epiglottis, taking care to protect

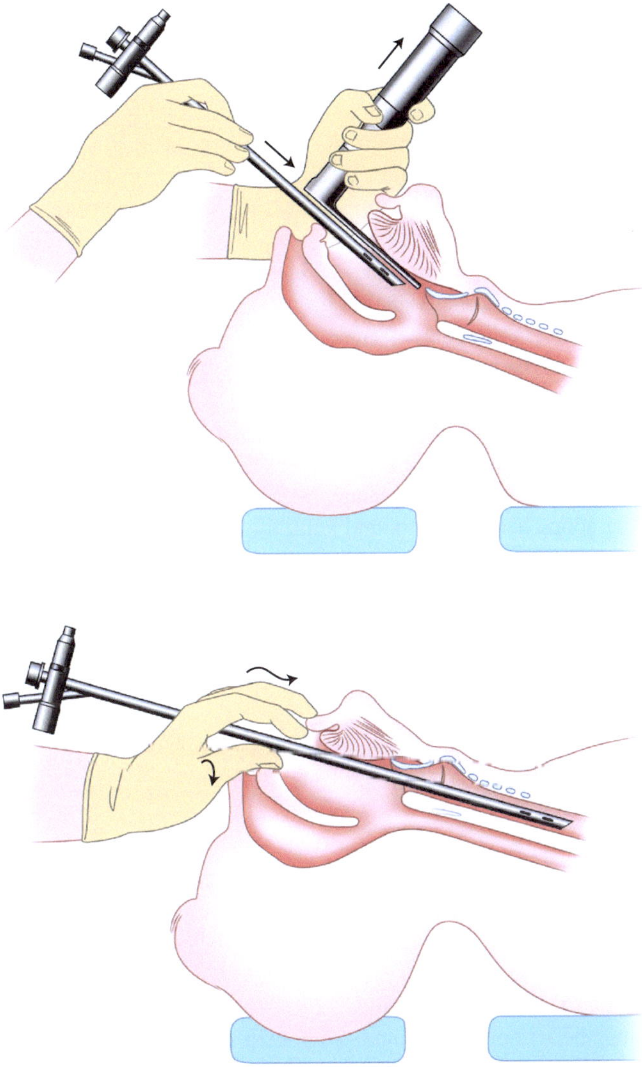

Fig. 5.6. Proper insertion of the rigid bronchoscope using the laryngoscope. The body of the scope is supported and the teeth protected using the left hand, while the right hand is used to advance and guide the tip of the bronchoscope.

the teeth and pharyngeal mucosa. The bronchoscope is introduced along the right side of the laryngoscope and advanced toward the glottic opening. The scope is rotated 90°, allowing the beveled edge of the scope to more easily traverse the vocal cords and advanced into the trachea. The scope is rotated to the neutral position and the laryngoscope removed. The surgeon supports the bronchoscope with the thumb and fingers of the left hand to protect the teeth and lips. Care must be taken to avoid injuring the tracheobronchial mucosa with the pointed beveled edge of the bronchoscope. The anesthesia circuit is attached to the ventilating port. The scope is advanced down the trachea to the level of the carina. The scope is intermittently removed from the bronchoscope sheath to clean the lens, suction, and insert instruments (i.e., optical peanut grasper). A long hand-held suction tip is used to aspirate secretions.

In order to examine the left main stem bronchus and left lobar bronchi, the end of the bronchoscope is rotated to the left and the patient's head rotated to the right. To examine the right side, this maneuver is reversed. Small alligator graspers, biopsy forceps, or urologic snares may be introduced alongside the bronchoscope via the working channel if the bronchoscope is of sufficient size. When the procedure is complete, the scope is withdrawn, and ventilation performed via a mask or the patient may be intubated, until anesthesia is reversed.

If rigid bronchoscopy is being formed for the purpose of removing a foreign body, it is often easier to remove the foreign body, forceps, bronchoscope, and telescope as one unit, particularly for larger foreign bodies.

Special Topics: Endoscopic Repair of Recurrent Tracheoesophageal Fistula

The overall recurrence rate for TEF has been reported as high as 10 %. While the standard for repair of recurrence has been operative, there has been a trend toward endoscopic repair of recurrent TEF via the rigid bronchoscope. Recurrence is typically suspected clinically, and endoscopy may be both diagnostic and therapeutic. A summary of some of the repair techniques is detailed below.

Using the technique detailed previously, the rigid bronchoscope is inserted into the trachea to the level of the suspected TEF. A Fogarty catheter or flexible soft guidewire is inserted into the suspected fistula to confirm its recurrence. A flexible esophagoscope may be concurrently inserted into the esophagus to further confirm the fistula. Alternatively, or additionally, methylene blue may be instilled into the trachea or esophagus. The presence of the dye in the other hollow viscus confirms the fistulous connection.

After the fistula is localized, the epithelial lining of the fistula tract is removed to aid in scar formation. The tissue may be mechanically abraded with a cytology brush or suction catheter tip. It may also be destroyed via electrocautery, applied via Bugbee or ball-type electrode, or application of trichloroacetic acid.

To further aid in closure of the TEF, the tract may be injected and filled with fibrin glue or similar tissue adhesive. After the glue is allowed to dry, excess adhesive is removed and instruments are removed.

Pearls/Pitfalls

- The necessary personnel and equipment for endotracheal intubation, surgical airway placement, and tube thoracostomy should be available at all times when performing either type of bronchoscopy. Topical 1 % lidocaine solution, bronchodilators, suction, and anti-fog solution should be routinely available.
- Rigid bronchoscopes, rod-lenses, graspers, suctions, and assorted accessories are available in a wide variety of sizes. Successful rigid endoscopy is greatly facilitated when all the matching components are preassembled to verify their compatibility prior to starting the procedure. The surgeon should verify the suitability of the equipment personally.
- Care should be taken when manipulating foreign bodies such that they are not forced more deeply into the tracheobronchial system.
- Routine prophylactic antibiotics are not indicated for rigid or flexible bronchoscopy. Prophylactic antibiotics are also indicated in patients at risk for infective endocarditis and in whom an incision in the respiratory mucosa is made.

Postoperative Care

Outcomes

Foreign bodies in the airway are able to be endoscopically removed or naturally eliminated in well over 95 % of cases. One study cited a 2 % rate of need for surgical foreign body extraction via thoracotomy with bronchotomy.

Approximately 10 % of patients who undergo bronchoscopic repair of recurrent tracheoesophageal fistula will have an additional recurrence.

These are amenable to repeat bronchoscopic repair, but open repair may also be elected.

Complications

The serious complication rate of both types of bronchoscopy is less than 0.1 %. Hemorrhage, injury to the airway, and laryngospasm or bronchospasm may occur. Pneumothorax may occur secondary to scope trauma, biopsy, or positive pressure ventilation. Tube thoracostomy supplies should be readily available in the event of development of pneumothorax. Chest X-ray is routinely performed at many centers following rigid bronchoscopy, especially following interventional or difficult procedures.

Damage to the teeth, gums, lips, and tongue are the most common minor complications of bronchoscopy and are more likely to occur with rigid bronchoscopy. These injuries can be prevented by taking special care, particularly when removing or inserting the bronchoscope, as well as by using a shield for the teeth and gums. The eyelids should be closed with adhesive tape to prevent corneal abrasions.

Hemorrhage secondary to bronchoscope trauma may initially be controlled with gentle pressure applied via the scope itself or an instrument. Injection of epinephrine and application of epinephrine-soaked pledgets may be necessary for more persistent bleeding.

Laryngeal or tracheal edema may occur secondary to irritation from instrumentation or (aspirated) foreign body reaction. The risk for this can be reduced by ensuring that bronchoscope size is matched for patient size and can be improved with corticosteroid administration. Some authors recommend administration of IV corticosteroids prior to removal of the rigid bronchoscope.

Summary

- Flexible and rigid bronchoscopy can be used for both diagnostic and therapeutic purposes in the pediatric population.
- Recurrent tracheoesophageal fistula may be amenable to endoscopic repair, thus avoiding open surgery.
- Airway foreign bodies are an emergency, and rigid bronchoscopy is usually performed to remove the foreign body with very high rates of success.

Suggested Reading

1. Grainger J, Hartley B. Bronchoscopy. In: Operative pediatric surgery. 7th ed. CRC Press; 2013.
2. Holcomb III GW, Murphy JD, Ostlie DJ. Foreign bodies. In: Ashcraft's pediatric surgery. 6th ed. Philadelphia, Saunders; 2014.
3. Colt H, Murgu S. Rigid bronchoscopy for removal of a foreign body lodged in the right lower lobe bronchus. In: Bronchoscopy and central airway disorders: a patient-centered approach. 1st ed. Philadelphia, Saunders; 2012.
4. Najmaldin A, Rothenberg S, Crabbe D, et al. Rigid endoscopy of the airway, foreign bodies in the airway. In: Operative endoscopy and endoscopic surgery in infants and children. 1st ed. Hodder Education; 2005.
5. Koumbourlis AC. Flexible fibre-optic bronchoscopy in the intensive-care unit. In: Priftis KN, Anthracopoulos MB, Eber E, Koumbourlis AC, Wood RE, editors. Paediatric bronchoscopy. vol 38. Prog Respir Res. Basel: Karger; 2010. p. 54–63.

6. Thoracoscopic Thymectomy

Christine M. Leeper and Stefan Scholz

Anatomy

The thymus is located in the superior mediastinum, overlying (from anterior to posterior) the innominate vein, the innominate artery, the left common carotid artery, and the trachea (Fig. 6.1). Inferiorly, it overlaps the superior aspect of the pericardial sac, and superiorly, it extends into the neck beneath the upper anterior ribs and approaches the inferior thyroid. Its arterial blood supply originates from the internal thoracic arteries; its veins drain into the brachiocephalic and internal thoracic veins [1].

Physiology

The thymus is the site for generation of mature thymic-derived lymphocytes (T cells) from lymphoid stem cells. During their development, T cells acquire antigen receptors in preparation for responding to antigenic challenges later in life. Once mature and functional, T cells leave the thymus and circulate in the blood and through secondary lymphoid tissues. The thymus develops at the eighth week of gestation and increases in size through fetal development and childhood. The process of thymic involution begins after puberty with size progressively decreasing over time.

Non-thymomatous Myasthenia Gravis

Myasthenia gravis (MG) is an autoimmune condition caused by the formation of antibodies against acetylcholine receptors at neuromuscular junctions. Characteristic symptoms include weakness of skeletal

D.S. Walsh et al. (eds.), *The SAGES Manual of Pediatric Minimally Invasive Surgery*, DOI 10.1007/978-3-319-43642-5_6

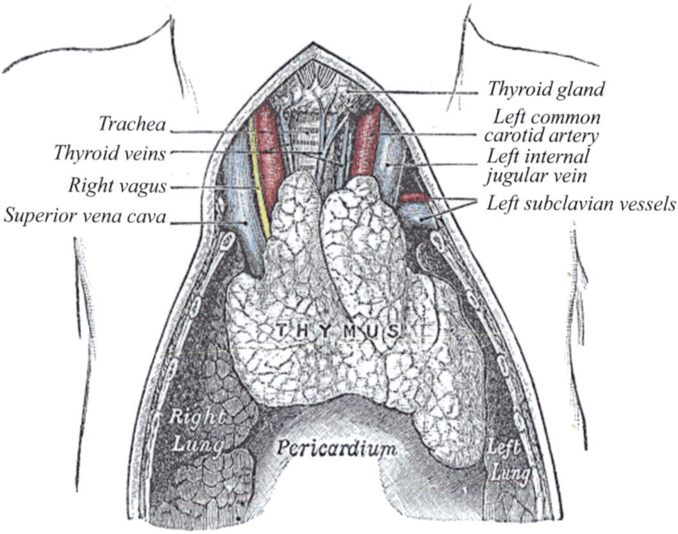

Fig. 6.1. The large thymus gland during childhood. Henry Gray (1918) Anatomy of the Human Body, Bartleby.com: Gray's Anatomy, Plate 1178.

muscles that increases with activity and improves with rest. The Osserman classification of myasthenia gravis (Table 6.1) is a commonly used tool to grade the severity of MG symptoms according to the distribution of affected muscles, which ranges from ocular muscles only in milder disease to generalized body weakness and even respiratory compromise during periods of crisis [2]. Medical management is the primary therapy for MG and may include pyridostigmine bromide (an acetylcholinesterase inhibitor), immunosuppression with corticosteroids, nonsteroid immunosuppressants like cyclosporine, azathioprine and mycophenolate mofetil, immunoglobulin, and plasmapheresis in severe cases of myasthenic crisis. MG in children is rare, with an incidence of about 1.1 per million [3]. It is more prevalent in black children and adolescents, with typical age of diagnosis around 10–12-year-olds (peripubertal) [4].

Alfred Blalock first described the benefits of thymectomy in adult patients with MG in 1939 [5], which has been confirmed by numerous adult studies. Thymectomy is currently the recommended therapy for all patients aged from puberty to 60 with generalized MG [6]. The benefits of thymectomy in this population may include symptom reduction, decreased need for medication, and increased rates of medication-free

Table 6.1. Osserman classification of myasthenia gravis.

Group I	Ocular myasthenia
Group IIA	Mild, generalized symptoms (including bulbar)
Group IIB	Moderate, generalized symptoms
Group III	Acute, fulminating symptoms

remission for patients with MG. Enrolling a pediatric cohort for quality prospective trials is prohibitive due to the rare incidence of MG in children; many studies, therefore, tend to be small and retrospective in nature. Despite this limitation, there is sufficient evidence to suggest that thymectomy has a role in the pediatric MG population as well [7–11]. Current indications for thymectomy in patients with MG include failure of medical management or presence of a thymic mass. In a review of 479 pediatric patients who underwent thymectomy across 50 studies, 68 % saw symptomatic improvement, and 39 % were in medication-free remission at the time of follow-up [12].

The recommendations in children regarding timing of operation are complicated by the role of the thymus in development of the immune system. For that reason, surgical intervention is often delayed until the onset of puberty, if possible. However, for younger patients who are not responding to medical management and otherwise face-prolonged immunosuppression, thymectomy is an acceptable alternative. The literature demonstrates that children of all ages have undergone thymectomy safely and many enjoy symptom improvement without adverse outcome [12].

Traditionally, thymectomy has been performed via an open approach using a median sternotomy or cervical collar incision. Thoracoscopic thymectomy was first described in an adult population in 1995 [13] and in a pediatric population in 2000 [14, 15]. As in adults, VATS thymectomy in pediatric patients does not cause any increased mortality or operative complication and does permit a comparably adequate resection. Importantly, thoracoscopy offers the advantages of improved cosmesis, reduced narcotic and oxygen requirements, decreased incidence of wound infection and pneumonia, and shorter hospital length of stay, all of which contribute to decreased overall cost [8, 12, 16–18]. This decrease in the morbidity of thymectomy may permit resection in patients at an earlier stage of disease, as there is some evidence to suggest that surgical intervention early in the disease course may result in superior symptom control and remission rates [9, 19, 20].

Both left- and right-sided thoracoscopic approaches have been described. Some advocate a right-sided approach because it allows (1) ready identification of the innominate using the vena cava as a landmark, (2) easier maneuverability of instruments in the larger right pleural cavity, and (3) greater ease for right-handed surgeons to dissect the thymus from inferior to superior [21, 22]. Others advocate a left-sided approach because it permits (1) avoidance of the vena cava and (2) easier dissection of the thymus around the left pericardiophrenic angle and aortopulmonary window with good visualization of the left phrenic nerve [23, 24]. Neither approach is clearly superior, and the laterality therefore should be selected based on patient factors and surgeon experience. Robotic-assisted thymectomy has also been described with early success and long-term outcomes pending [25–28]. A robotic approach may offer distinct advantages for minimally invasive thymectomy due to its 3D, high-definition vision system and its wristed instruments that bend and rotate allowing careful dissection in difficult access spaces such as the thoracic inlet and the neck [29].

A unilateral operative approach to thymectomy is widely accepted for its comparable safety and clinical outcomes [30–32]; however, care must be taken during dissection of the contralateral thymus. In particular, the contralateral phrenic nerve should be identified and dissected meticulously along with adjacent large vessels and vital structures that are at risk of injury. Further, when thymectomy is performed for MG, some advocate for the removal of all anterior pericardial fat, as this may occasionally contain ectopic thymic tissue [33]. While this has the potential to be a challenging dissection, pericardial fat tends to be more prominent in older adults as compared to pediatric patients; children typically have little if any pericardial fat tissue to resect.

Other Indications for Thymectomy

Thymoma

Thymomas are neoplasms arising from thymic epithelial cells that are very rarely found in children. The incidence in children is very low; there are approximately 50 cases reported in the literature, with 62 % of cases reported in males and 7 (15 %) presenting with MG. Many patients were asymptomatic, though some experienced dysphagia or dyspnea due to mass effect and compression of nearby structures. All thymomas have the potential for malignant degeneration, and the current recommendation is complete surgical resection plus chemoradiation depending on staging [34]. The International Thymic Malignancy Interest Group (ITMIG) has published recommendations to guide minimally invasive resection of thymic malignancies, namely, (1) a resection that includes the thymoma, thymus, and mediastinal fat; (2) dissection and visualization of the innominate vein and both phrenic nerves; (3) an access incision that is large enough to prevent specimen disruption, which should be removed in a bag and examined after removal for completeness of resection; and (4) conversion to open surgery if oncologic principles are compromised or violated [35].

Thymic Cysts

Thymic cysts are thin-walled structures diagnosed histologically by the presence of thymic tissue in the cyst wall. They can be found anywhere along the anatomic course of embryologic descent of the thymus from the third pharyngeal pouch. On occasion thymic cysts may completely replace normal thymic tissue [36]. Surgical resection is the primary treatment; depending on the location of the cyst (substernal versus cervical), this may necessitate a thoracoscopic- or robotic-assisted approach [37].

Operative Technique

The procedure is performed under general anesthesia with endotracheal intubation. A double-lumen tube may be utilized to assist with ipsilateral lung collapse but is not necessary. The patient is positioned at 30–45° from horizontal using a roll under the back and lateral chest with the ipsilateral right arm raised above the head (Fig. 6.2). All pressure points should be padded appropriately and the endotracheal tube position confirmed after patient positioning is complete. The surgeon and assistant stand together on the side selected for the approach facing a monitor that is placed above the patient's contralateral shoulder. Three 5-mm ports are placed inferior to the axilla: one in the fourth intercostal space of the anterior axillary line (camera), one in the second-third intercostal space of the midaxillary line (instrument), and one in the fifth-sixth intercostal space of the midaxillary line (instrument). Care should be taken to avoid violating mammary tissue (Fig. 6.3). Equipment may include a 30° telescope, tissue-grasping

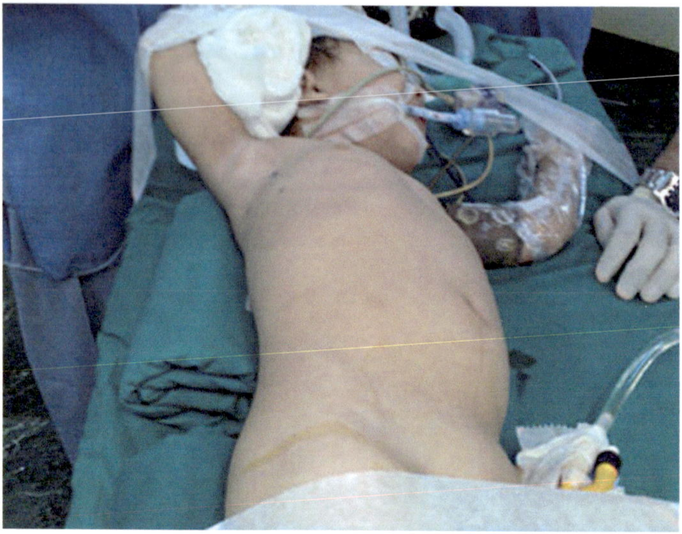

Fig. 6.2. Position of patient [38]. Reprinted with permission from Springer.

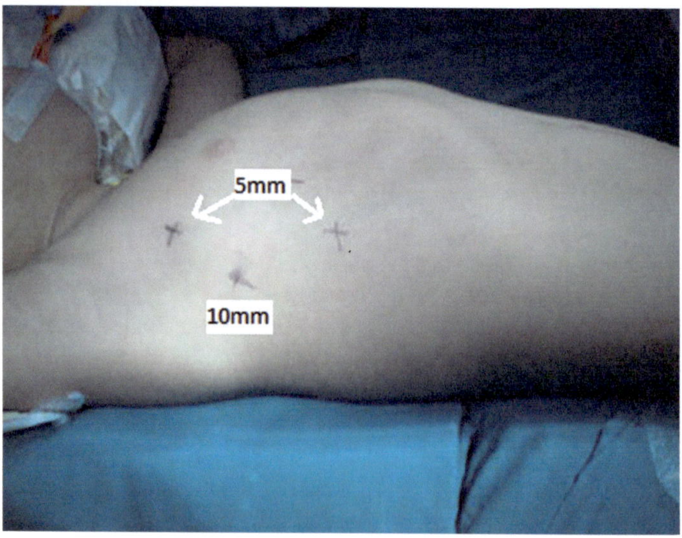

Fig. 6.3. Port positions for thymectomy. We start with three 5-mm ports, and the center port can be upsized to 10 mm or utility incision as needed to extract the specimen [38]. Reprinted with permission from Springer.

forceps, endoscopic scissors or hook cautery, LigaSure™ (Covidien, Mansfield, MA) or energy device, endoscopic clips, endokittner, and specimen retrieval bag.

Insufflation is achieved with CO_2 to a pressure of 6–10 mmHg. Dissection begins at the inferior margin of the thymus, superior to the heart, and anterior to the phrenic nerve. Caution should be taken using energy devices in close proximity to the phrenic nerve, as heat spread and resulting injury may occur. Using a combination of blunt and sharp dissection parallel to the phrenic nerve and posterior to the thymic gland, the thymus is lifted away from the surface of the heart and great vessels. Anteriorly, the mediastinal pleura is incised, and the thymus is dissected free from its retrosternal attachments (Fig. 6.4). The dissection is carried inferiorly to superiorly, elevating the gland and ultimately exposing the vasculature. The thymic branches off the internal thoracic artery (thyro-cervical trunk) originate cephalic and lateral to the gland, while the thymic vein branches drain posteriorly to the innominate vein. Blood vessels should be isolated and divided between clips or cauterized with a LigaSure™ energy device depending on surgeon preference. Next, the thymus is bluntly dissected from its contralateral pleural attachments

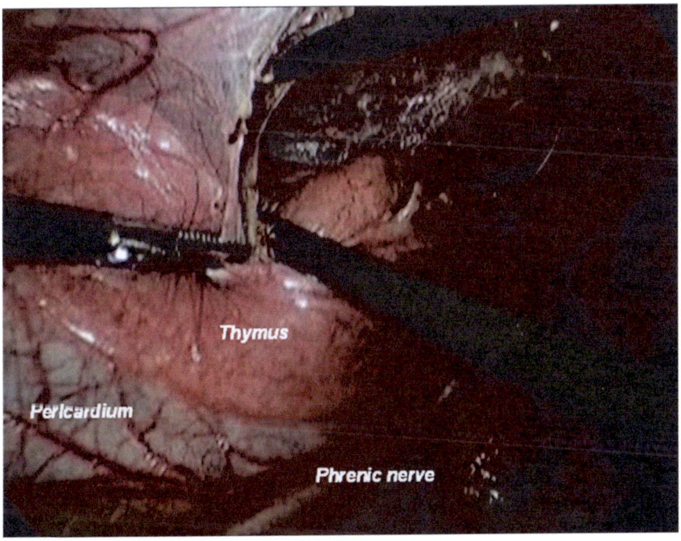

Fig. 6.4. Thymus view from the left. The mediastinal pleura is divided to gain access to the plane between thymus and anterior chest wall. Care is taken not to injure the phrenic nerve.

taking care to avoid injury to the phrenic nerve. This allows the entire gland to be flipped superiorly to allow careful dissection off the innominate vein, freeing the thymic tissue from the great vessels. The remaining attachments in the cervical area, which may include tissue that joins the thymus and inferior thyroid, are separated; this may be assisted by inferior retraction of the superior horns of the thymus (Fig. 6.5).

Once the entire gland has been dissected free, the middle port may be exchanged for a 10-mm port or extended for creation of a small utility incision to permit the introduction of an endoscopic specimen bag. The thymus is placed in the specimen bag before removal to prevent seeding of the tract and allow intact removal of the thymus. The gland may be examined on the back table to assess grossly for adequacy of the resection and is then sent to pathology for microscopic analysis. The mediastinum should then be inspected for residual thymic tissue and to ensure hemostasis. The utility incision (former 10-mm port site) should be closed in two layers, while the 5-mm ports require only skin closure. Gas evacuation from the chest can be facilitated by asking the anesthesiologist to perform Valsalva maneuvers during removal of the last 5-mm port. The same effect can be achieved

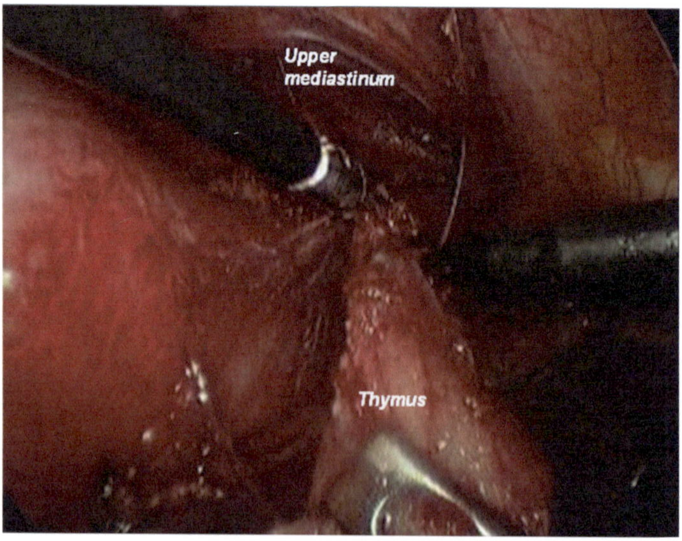

Fig. 6.5. The most difficult part of the operation is dissection of the thymus in the lower neck to assure that no thymic tissue is left behind. Here, the large inferior thymic vein is encountered, which drains directly into the innominate vein.

using a small suction catheter to evacuate the remaining CO_2. A drain or chest tube is not required under most circumstances. The patient is then extubated in the operating room and taken to the Post Anesthesia Care Unit (PACU) for observation.

Postoperative Considerations

From the PACU, the patient is then admitted to a surgical floor bed to recover. Overnight observation is indicated in patients with MG, as very rarely they can develop MG crisis resulting in oropharyngeal and respiratory muscle weakness in the early postoperative period. This may cause upper airway obstruction, respiratory failure requiring intubation and ventilator support, or dysphagia with aspiration. Preoperative medications, including pyridostigmine and corticosteroids, should be resumed immediately. Patients without MG can be discharged home the day of surgery if they recover appropriately. Routine postoperative chest radiograph is not performed. Patients may have some residual pneumothorax if the gas is incompletely evacuated; a chest tube may be placed in the event of respiratory or hemodynamic compromise, but more often this can be safely observed. Pulmonary toilet, early ambulation, and adequate pain control are a priority during the recovery period. Oral pain medications are used for the first few days after surgery. Diet is advanced as tolerated. Patients are usually discharged home 24–48 h after the surgery.

Summary

- The thymus is a large organ in children located in the superior mediastinum and the site for T-cell generation.
- Indications for thymectomy include thymic cyst or thymoma and myasthenia gravis.
- Minimally invasive approaches are ideal for thymectomy and offer decreased morbidity with a much shorter hospital stay in comparison to sternotomy.
- Left or right-sided thoracoscopic or robotic approaches are employed and are equally effective.
- Key surgical steps include preservation of the phrenic nerves, complete resection of all thymic tissue, preferably in toto, for patients with myasthenia gravis, and safe ligation of the inferior thymic vein.

References

1. Kipps T. The organization and structure of lymphoid tissues. In: Lichtman M, editor. Williams hematology. 8th ed. New York: The McGraw-Hill Companies; 2010.
2. Osserman K. Myasthenia gravis. New York: Grune & Stratton; 1958.
3. Gadient P, Bolton J, Puri V. Juvenile myasthenia gravis: three case reports and a literature review. J Child Neurol. 2009;24(5):584–90.
4. Andrews PI, Massey JM, Howard Jr JF, Sanders DB. Race, sex, and puberty influence onset, severity, and outcome in juvenile myasthenia gravis. Neurology. 1994;44(7):1208–14.
5. Blalock A. The treatment of myasthenia gravis by removal of the thymus gland: preliminary report. JAMA. 1941;117(18):1529–33.
6. Drachman DB. Myasthenia gravis. N Engl J Med. 1994;330(25):1797–810.
7. Liew WK, Kang PB. Update on juvenile myasthenia gravis. Curr Opin Pediatr. 2013;25(6):694–700.
8. Christison-Lagay E, Dharia B, Vajsar J, Kim PC. Efficacy and safety of thoracoscopic thymectomy in the treatment of juvenile myasthenia gravis. Pediatr Surg Int. 2013;29(6):583–6.
9. Youssef S. Thymectomy for myasthenia gravis in children. J Pediatr Surg. 1983;18(5):537–41.
10. Molinaro F, Garzi A, Cerchia E, Angotti R, Di Maggio G, Valla JS, et al. Thoracoscopic thymectomy in children: our preliminary experience. J Laparoendosc Adv Surg Tech A. 2013;23(6):556–9.
11. Castro D, Derisavifard S, Anderson M, Greene M, Iannaccone S. Juvenile myasthenia gravis: a twenty-year experience. J Clin Neuromuscul Dis. 2013;14(3):95–102.
12. Tracy MM, McRae W, Millichap JG. Graded response to thymectomy in children with myasthenia gravis. J Child Neurol. 2009;24(4):454–9.
13. Yim AP, Kay RL, Ho JK. Video-assisted thoracoscopic thymectomy for myasthenia gravis. Chest. 1995;108(5):1440–3.
14. Kogut KA, Bufo AJ, Rothenberg SS, Lobe TE. Thoracoscopic thymectomy for myasthenia gravis in children. J Pediatr Surg. 2000;35(11):1576–7.
15. Kolski H, Vajsar J, Kim PC. Thoracoscopic thymectomy in juvenile myasthenia gravis. J Pediatr Surg. 2000;35(5):768–70.
16. Wagner AJ, Cortes RA, Strober J, Grethel EJ, Clifton MS, Harrison MR, et al. Long-term follow-up after thymectomy for myasthenia gravis: thoracoscopic vs open. J Pediatr Surg. 2006;41(1):50–4; discussion 4.
17. Ozkan B, Demir A, Kapdagli M, Sungur Z, Duman S, Cimenoglu B, et al. Results of videothoracoscopic thymectomy in children: an analysis of 40 patientsdagger. Interact Cardiovasc Thorac Surg. 2015;21(3):292–5.
18. Seguier-Lipszyc E, Bonnard A, Evrard P, Garel C, De Ribier A, Aigrain Y, et al. Left thoracoscopic thymectomy in children. Surg Endosc. 2005;19(1):140–2.
19. Lakhoo K, Fonseca JD, Rodda J, Davies MRQ. Thymectomy in black children with juvenile myasthenia gravis. Pediatr Surg Int. 1997;12(2/3):113–5.

20. Seybold ME. Thymectomy in childhood myasthenia gravis. Ann N Y Acad Sci. 1998;841:731–41.
21. Yim AP, Izzat MB, Lee TW, Wan S. Video-assisted thoracoscopic thymectomy. Ann Thoracic Cardiovasc Surg. 1999;5(1):18–20.
22. Ng CS, Wan IY, Yim AP. Video-assisted thoracic surgery thymectomy: the better approach. Ann Thorac Surg. 2010;89(6):S2135–41.
23. Goldstein SD, Culbertson NT, Garrett D, Salazar JH, Van Arendonk K, McIltrot K, et al. Thymectomy for myasthenia gravis in children: a comparison of open and thoracoscopic approaches. J Pediatr Surg. 2015;50(1):92–7.
24. Mineo TC, Pompeo E, Lerut TE, Bernardi G, Coosemans W, Nofroni I. Thoracoscopic thymectomy in autoimmune myasthenia: results of left-sided approach. Ann Thorac Surg. 2000;69(5):1537–41.
25. Rea F, Marulli G, Bortolotti L, Feltracco P, Zuin A, Sartori F. Experience with the "da Vinci" robotic system for thymectomy in patients with myasthenia gravis: report of 33 cases. Ann Thorac Surg. 2006;81(2):455–9.
26. Goldstein SD, Yang SC. Assessment of robotic thymectomy using the Myasthenia Gravis Foundation of America Guidelines. Ann Thorac Surg. 2010;89(4):1080–5. discussion 5-6.
27. Marulli G, Schiavon M, Perissinotto E, Bugana A, Di Chiara F, Rebusso A, et al. Surgical and neurologic outcomes after robotic thymectomy in 100 consecutive patients with myasthenia gravis. J Thorac Cardiovasc Surg. 2013;145(3):730–5. discussion 5-6.
28. Augustin F, Schmid T, Sieb M, Lucciarini P, Bodner J. Video-assisted thoracoscopic surgery versus robotic-assisted thoracoscopic surgery thymectomy. Ann Thorac Surg. 2008;85(2):S768–71.
29. Hartwich J, Tyagi S, Margaron F, Oitcica C, Teasley J, Lanning D. Robot-assisted thoracoscopic thymectomy for treating myasthenia gravis in children. J Laparoendosc Adv Surg Tech A. 2012;22(9):925–9.
30. Liu Z, Yang J, Lin L, Huang J, Jiang G. Unilateral video-assisted thoracoscopic extended thymectomy offers long-term outcomes equivalent to that of the bilateral approach in the treatment of non-thymomatous myasthenia gravis. Interact Cardiovasc Thorac Surg. 2015;21(5):610–5.
31. Ye B, Tantai JC, Ge XX, Li W, Feng J, Cheng M, et al. Surgical techniques for early-stage thymoma: video-assisted thoracoscopic thymectomy versus transsternal thymectomy. J Thorac Cardiovasc Surg. 2014;147(5):1599–603.
32. Maniscalco P, Tamburini N, Quarantotto F, Grossi W, Garelli E, Cavallesco G. Long-term outcome for early stage thymoma: comparison between thoracoscopic and open approaches. Thorac Cardiovasc Surg. 2015;63(3):201–5.
33. Hubka M, Wood D. Primary tumors of the thymus. In: Cameron JL, Cameron AM, editors. Current surgical therapy. 11th ed. Philadelphia: Elsevier; 2014.
34. Fonseca AL, Ozgediz DE, Christison-Lagay ER, Detterbeck FC, Caty MG. Pediatric thymomas: report of two cases and comprehensive review of the literature. Pediatr Surg Int. 2014;30(3):275–86.

35. Toker A, Sonett J, Zielinski M, Rea F, Tomulescu V, Detterbeck FC. Standard terms, definitions, and policies for minimally invasive resection of thymoma. J Thorac Oncol. 2011;6(7 Suppl 3):S1739–42.
36. Cigliano B, Baltogiannis N, De Marco M, Faviou E, Antoniou D, De Luca U, et al. Cervical thymic cysts. Pediatr Surg Int. 2007;23(12):1219–25.
37. Ballouhey Q, Villemagne T, Cros J, Vacquerie V, Berenguer D, Braik K, et al. Assessment of paediatric thoracic robotic surgery. Interact Cardiovasc Thorac Surg. 2015;20(3):300–3.
38. Parikh K, Vaidya A, Jain R. Preliminary results of VATS thymectomy for pediatric myasthenia gravis. Pediatr Surg Int. 2011;27(6):595–8.

7. Thoracoscopic Ligation of the Patent Ductus Arteriosus

Laura Y. Martin and Jeffrey Lukish

Introduction

Patent ductus arteriosus (PDA) is a persistence of the fetal communication between the left pulmonary artery and descending aorta. It is one of the most common congenital heart defects, representing 5–10 % of all congenital heart disease [1, 2]. During fetal development, non-aerated, fluid-filled lungs result in high pulmonary vascular resistance. The ductus arteriosus is necessary for pulmonary bypass from the pulmonary artery to the descending aorta to reduce the afterload on the right ventricle [1, 2]. Patency is maintained by low oxygen concentration and serum prostaglandins. After birth, the lungs begin to aerate and receive more blood flow, oxygen concentration increases, and levels of prostaglandins fall. In response, the ductus arteriosus rapidly constricts, leading to intimal remodeling and closure [1, 2]. In healthy, term infants, this closure typically occurs within 72 h [1, 2]. Patent ductus arteriosus is defined as a delay or failure of this spontaneous closure and can be associated with significant morbidity and mortality.

Epidemiology

PDA is one of the most common congenital heart defects, with an incidence in healthy term infants of 1 in 2000, representing 5–10 % of all congenital heart disease in term infants [1, 2]. With improved diagnostic modalities, this incidence has climbed in recent years and may be as high as 1 in 500 if clinically silent cases are considered [3]. The risk of PDA is inversely proportional to birth weight and gestational age.

D.S. Walsh et al. (eds.), *The SAGES Manual of Pediatric Minimally Invasive Surgery*, DOI 10.1007/978-3-319-43642-5_7

The incidence in preterm infants under 28 weeks of gestational age approaches 70 % and climbs to 80 % at 24–25 weeks' gestation [4]. Low birth weight infants are also at elevated risk, with PDA found in 80 % of infants weighing less than 1200 g at birth [1]. For unknown reasons, the incidence is twice as high in females as in males [1–4]. In rare cases, PDA may be triggered by certain intrauterine events, such as exposure to rubella [1].

Although the majority of cases are sporadic, with the strongest identifiable risk factors being birth weight and gestational age, genetic factors may play a role in a minority of cases. There is an increased incidence observed in association with several known genetic syndromes, as well as an increased risk among siblings [2]. Several genes have been implicated in prolonged patency; however, they are incompletely characterized, and investigation is ongoing. Twin studies suggest there is also genetic familial predisposition for prolonged patency, suggesting heritability for those infants requiring indomethacin therapy and/or surgical ligation [5].

Patent ductus arteriosus is generally defined as failure of closure of the ductus arteriosus by 72 h after birth [1, 2]. However, many PDAs close spontaneously, and it is difficult to determine a timeline of clinical significance and intervention. In infants above 30 weeks' gestation, 98 % of PDAs will close by the first week of life [5]. The highest risk for PDA patency is prematurity. In infants under 24 weeks, the rate of spontaneous closure falls to 8 % by day 4, and only 13 % are closed by 1 week [5]. Due to the high rate of morbidity and mortality, early intervention may be required in severe cases. However, with improvements in critical care, many preterm and low-birth-weight infants avoid intervention in the first year of life. In these infants, the majority of defects are closed upon re-evaluation at 1 year of age.

Pathophysiology

The clinical sequelae of PDA are related to the size and flow dynamics of the vessel and its subsequent effects on the heart. Increased left heart pressures resulting from biventricular circulation result in a left to right shunt. The size of the defect determines the degree of the shunt. The majority of early clinical morbidities are related to either pulmonary hypoperfusion or systemic hypoperfusion [1, 2, 6]. Hypoperfusion of the pulmonary vasculature results in pulmonary edema and may contribute to respiratory failure. Low systemic diastolic pressures may result in acidosis and systemic hypoperfusion, with an increased incidence of renal dysfunction, necrotizing enterocolitis (NEC), and intraventricular hemorrhage (IVH) and prerenal azotemia [1–3]. PDA is also associated with poor neurological outcomes independent of IVH [7].

Long-term sequelae of PDA are largely based on early studies of severe disease in the absence of medical or operative intervention. In persistently patent moderate or large defects, increased work of the left ventricle may lead to hypertrophy and ultimately failure [1, 2]. Persistently elevated pulmonary pressures due to long standing pressure and volume overload can result in irreversible lung disease and pulmonary hypertension [2, 8, 9]. Increased workload of the right ventricle to overcome elevated pulmonary pressures can result in hypertrophy of the right ventricle [2, 8–10]. In large PDAs, this may result in a reversal of flow in the ductus, with shunting of unoxygenated blood from the right ventricle into the systemic circulation, known as Eisenmenger's syndrome [8–10]. Ultimately, persistent volume overload and increased work of the right ventricle may progress to right heart failure [2, 8–10]. With improved diagnostic capabilities and the availability of medical and invasive treatment, these sequelae are rarely seen in contemporary practice.

Initial Evaluation

Clinical Presentation

With increased critical care and diagnostic capabilities, clinically significant PDAs are most commonly discovered in the neonatal period. Early clinical signs and symptoms are dependent on the size of the ductus, which may range from small and asymptomatic to large with significant left to right shunt. Clinical diagnosis typically relies on a high index of suspicion and the presence of one or more clinical signs.

In the first 24 h, neonates with clinically significant PDA typically have decreased blood pressure, due to delayed myocardial adaptation to changes in preload [6]. As the myocardium adapts, subsequent clinical signs may include bounding pulses, wide pulse pressures, and a characteristic murmur [1, 2, 6].

Increased shunt fraction can result in signs of pulmonary overload on physical exam, as well as respiratory distress, apneic episodes, and failure to wean from the ventilator. Diastolic hypotension and unexplained metabolic acidosis may also be observed [1, 2]. Persistent systemic hypotension may result in low end organ perfusion with increased risk of severe clinical presentations such as NEC, renal failure, and IVH [1, 2, 4]. Severe cases can present with early congestive heart failure [2]. Milder presentations often include poor feeding, failure to thrive, tachypnea, and diaphoresis [1, 2, 4].

Imaging

Upon clinical suspicion of PDA, echocardiogram is crucial to confirm the diagnosis, quantify the severity of the defect, and rule out other cardiac comorbidities that require a patent ductus for maintenance of systemic blood flow. Critical echocardiogram findings suggestive of a hemodynamically significant shunt include an absolute ductal diameter greater than 1.5 mm or a ratio of left atrial diameter to aortic diameter greater than or equal to 1.4, pulsatile low flow velocity in the descending aorta, or end diastolic flow velocity in the left pulmonary artery >0.20 m/s [1, 2, 4–6]. The echocardiogram findings must be considered in the context of individual symptoms, risk factors, and comorbidities.

Chest X-ray is largely used as a means to evaluate volume status of the lungs in response to the PDA and treatment measures. It may be normal or may demonstrate increased pulmonary vascular markings due to fluid overload [1, 2]. Cardiomegaly may also be noted in severe cases [1, 2]. In severe cases with prolonged hypotension, head ultrasound must be considered to rule out intraventricular hemorrhage, and abdominal imaging may be necessarily dependent on symptomatic presentation.

Management

There is no consensus regarding what constitutes a hemodynamically significant defect, nor do we fully understand the timeline of pathophysiological morbidity and when this may become irreversible. The data regarding morbidity and mortality are highly variable depending upon the size of the defect, delay to closure, type and timing of medical or surgical intervention, as well as risk factors and comorbidities of the patient population involved. There remain no clear guidelines for timing and indications for medical or surgical treatment. Increasing concerns regarding risks associated with pharmacological and surgical treatments have resulted in a shift toward a more conservative approach in hemodynamically stable infants with minimal risk factors.

Nonsurgical Management

Non-pharmacological Management

Non-pharmacological management is considered by many to be the best approach in infants who are stable enough from a respiratory and hemodynamic standpoint to tolerate a trial waiting period for spontaneous closure [1, 5, 6]. This includes careful fluid management with the use of mild fluid restriction and diuretics to avoid fluid overload and prevent lung injury, while maintaining adequate volume to maintain diastolic pressures and end organ perfusion [1, 4–6]. Ventilator adjustments to lower inspiratory time and elevate PEEP may increase pulmonary vascular resistance and encourage closure [5, 6]. The benefit to this approach is avoidance of unnecessary pharmacological exposure. Drawbacks include delay of alternative treatment options such as prostaglandin inhibitors and concern for diminished efficacy [1, 4].

Pharmacological Management

The mainstay of medical therapy is the administration of prostaglandin inhibitors to encourage remodeling and closure of the PDA [1, 2, 4–6]. Initial studies advocated prophylactic use of prostaglandin inhibitors, which have been shown to reduce the incidence of symptomatic PDA, needed for surgical ligation, IVH, and NEC [4, 5]. However, some studies suggest negative short-term pulmonary outcomes as well as possible increased frequency of bronchopulmonary dysplasia within the first year of life. These concerns, as well as the known effects on mesenteric, cerebral, and renal circulation, have led to the use of a more targeted approach, with intervention only for hemodynamically significant defects, as suggested by symptoms or echocardiogram [4–6].

In patients with PDAs unresponsive to medical management, timing of intervention continues to be debated. In individuals who are relatively asymptomatic without comorbidities, closure may be delayed. Typically, closure of asymptomatic PDAs is recommended by 2 years of age to minimize the risk of bacterial endocarditis and pulmonary hypertension. This is often achieved by transarterial occlusion in adults and larger infants [4, 5].

Transarterial Occlusion

Transarterial occlusion is the standard approach for PDA closure in adults and term infants that has failed medical therapy, with high rates of success [4, 5, 11, 12]. With the advent of new closure devices, this procedure has been increasingly applied to smaller infants. Recent small series in high volume centers report positive outcomes and low rates of complications in preterm and very low-birth-weight babies [11, 12]. Long-term outcomes have yet to be determined, but likely parallel those seen after surgical closure and may provide the most minimally invasive option in the future.

Surgical Management

Review of the literature reveals no significant difference between medical and surgical intervention with regard to success rates or mortality. Therefore timing of intervention and indications for surgical ligation are highly debated.

Early surgical ligation is generally indicated in infants who fail to stabilize from a respiratory and hemodynamic standpoint in spite of medical measures, with persistent ventilator or pressor requirements [1, 4–6, 13–15]. In these patients, surgical duct closure has been shown to facilitate extubation in infants with left ventricular overload and decrease the incidence of sequelae associated with hypoperfusion [4, 5, 15]. Surgical closure should particularly be considered in premature infants with hemodynamically significant defects, as they are less likely to respond to medical therapy and less likely to tolerate prolonged instability associated with delay of definitive treatment.

Early ligation should also be considered for clinically significant defects in patients with comorbid conditions contraindicating NSAID administration, such as necrotizing enterocolitis, acute renal failure, intraventricular hemorrhage, or other evidence of bleeding in the pulmonary or GI tract [4–6, 13–16].

Surgical ligation is generally well-tolerated and may improve lung compliance and extubation [4]. Some studies suggest higher risks of neurosensory impairment, bronchopulmonary dysplasia, and retinopathy of prematurity, but this is confounded by the fact that surgical intervention is more common in premature infants, infants with more severe disease, and is often attempted after more prolonged exposure to the PDA following attempted medical management [1, 4–7, 15, 16].

Surgical Approach

Open and thoracoscopic repair of PDA are well tolerated, with a high rate of success and low rates of morbidity and mortality [13–23]. Video-assisted thoracic surgery has the advantage of improved exposure, with excellent visualization to minimize risk of injury. However, the disadvantage of this approach is the inability to achieve immediate hemostasis. Thoracoscopic repair is associated with decreased operative time, shorter incision, earlier extubation, and decreased hospital and ICU stay compared to thoracotomy. Additionally, it avoids the risk of long term musculoskeletal sequelae that have been observed in association with long thoracotomy incisions [17–19].

Video-Assisted Thoracoscopic Repair

T-PDA initially reported by Laborde et al. in 1993 [20] has become an accepted treatment option at many centers [17–19, 21–24]. Although the initial reports recommended open repair via thoracotomy for infants <1500 g, many now advocate T-PDA in even the smallest of infants. In fact, recent literature provides evidence of safe thoracoscopic repair in very low- and extremely low-birth-weight premature infants while avoiding the negative effects of thoracotomy [22–24].

T-PDA Technique

After induction of general anesthesia, the infant is placed in the right lateral decubitus position. Three incisions are placed along the fifth intercostal space at the site of an intended thoracotomy incision should an open procedure become necessary.

The initial 3-mm incision is made in the left fifth intercostal space in the posterior axillary line. Following placement of a 3-mm port, thoracoscopy is performed. During this phase of the operation, low-volume carbon dioxide insufflation is utilized (pressure set at 6 mm of mercury and flow rate of 0.5 l/min). A second 3-mm incision is made in the left fifth intercostal space in the midaxillary line. Via this site, a 3-mm fan retractor (Karl Storz GmbH and Company, Munich, Germany) that was previously modified using a plastic towel drape (Towel Drape, Medical Concepts Development, St. Paul, Minn) is inserted without a port under direct visualization (Fig. 7.1). Following deployment of the retractor and lung retraction, insufflation is discon-

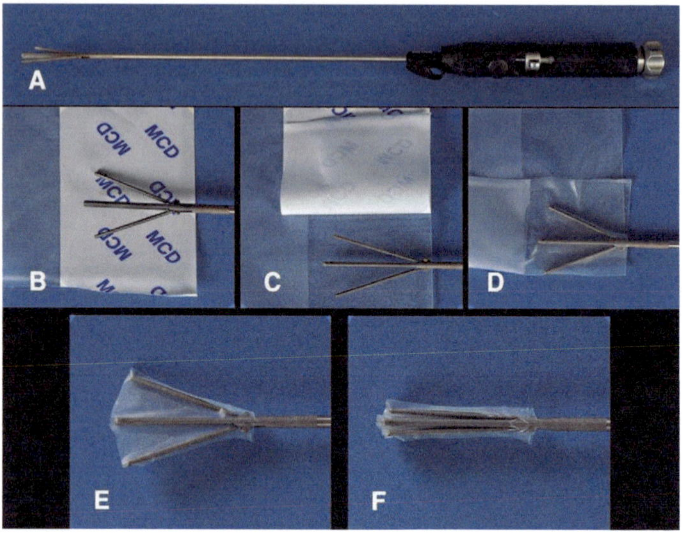

Fig. 7.1. The modification of the 3-mm retractor (Karl Storz GmbH and Company, Germany). (**a**) The 3-mm Storz fan retractor. (**b**) The retractor is placed on the plastic towel drape (Towel Drape, Medical Concepts Development, St. Paul, Minn) in the expanded open position. (**c**) The plastic is allowed to stick to the arms of the retractor. (**d**) The plastic is folded around the arms of the retractor. (**e**) The excess plastic is trimmed. (**f**) The retractor is opened and closed to ensure proper function and plastic adherence. Reprinted from Lukish J. Video-assisted thoracoscopic ligation of a patent ductus arteriosus in a very low-birth-weight infant using a novel retractor. J Pediatr Surg 2009; 44: 1047–50. Published by Elsevier Inc.

tinued. With gentle retraction of the right mid- and apical lung, the aortic arch, descending aorta, left subclavian artery, and PDA should be clearly visualized. The recurrent laryngeal nerve should be identified as it crosses over the medial aspect of the ductus. A final 5-mm incision is made posteriorly in the fifth intercostal space approximately 1 cm below the inferior tip of the scapula. A 3-mm curved dissector is used to begin dissection medial to the descending aorta just below the presumptive PDA/aortic junction (Fig. 7.2). The junction is further defined by the dissection of the PDA inferiorly and superiorly. Care should be taken to avoid unnecessary traction on the recurrent laryngeal nerve. Gentle dissection continues along the superior and inferior edges of the PDA, freeing it from surrounding tissue and carefully defining the ductus until it has been exposed nearly

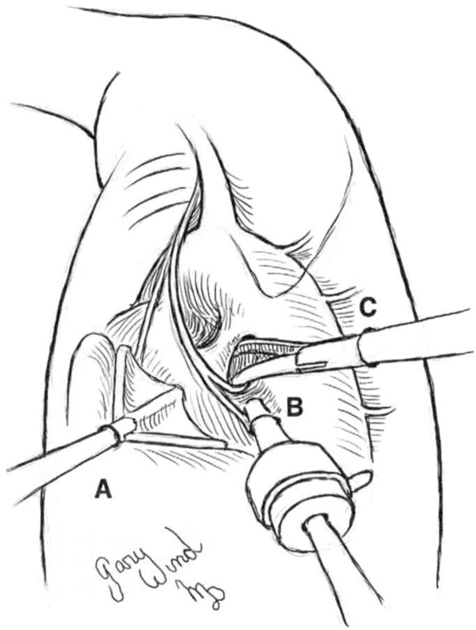

Fig. 7.2. Incision and instrument placement for VATS PDA ligation in VLBW infants. (**a**) Midaxillary line, fifth intercostal space, site for retractor, no port used. (**b**) The posterior axillary line, fifth intercostal space, and site for port placement, camera, and insufflation. (**c**) The posterior site for dissector and clip applier, no port used (original artwork courtesy of Gary Wind, MD, FACS). Reprinted from Lukish J. Video-assisted thoracoscopic ligation of a patent ductus arteriosus in a very low-birth-weight infant using a novel retractor. J Pediatr Surg 2009; 44: 1047–50. Published by Elsevier Inc.

circumferentially. Dissection proceeds toward the PA until a small segment is clearly defined for optimal placement of two clips. It is the practice of the authors to perform a test occlusion prior to clipping the duct, while monitoring pre-ductal and post-ductal oxygen saturations, as well as observing the lung to look for any changes in perfusion.

Following test occlusion, the clip applier (Weck Horizon, Teleflex Medical, Limerick, PA) is inserted through the posterior 5-mm working port, and two medium metal clips are applied near the PDA junction with the aorta (Fig. 7.3). The area is inspected for optimal clip placement and hemostasis, and the thoracic cavity is examined once again to rule out any evidence of lung injury. The incisions are then closed in the standard fashion. Prior to closure of the last incision, positive inspiratory

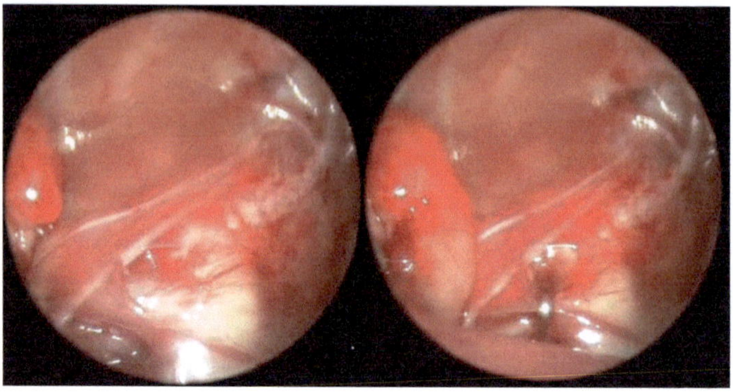

Fig. 7.3. Intraoperative thoracoscopic photo of exposure achieved using the modified retractor. Clip is in place with ligation of PDA. Note that the lung can be assessed through the plastic drape.

pressure is applied to fully inflate the lung to facilitate evacuation of the pneumothorax. The authors do not routinely place thoracostomy tubes in the absence of suspected lung injury.

Postoperative Management

Postoperatively, a chest radiograph should be performed to rule out pneumothorax, and an echocardiogram should be confirmed to confirm occlusion of flow [21–24]. Close hemodynamic monitoring is crucial in the postoperative period, due to the abrupt hemodynamic changes associated with surgical ligation. Following ligation, there is an increase in diastolic arterial pressure and associated increase in MAP compared to preoperative levels [16]. However, there is commonly a transient decrease in systolic arterial pressure, likely associated with delayed left ventricular adaptation to the abrupt increase in afterload [16]. Postoperative MAP frequently fails to rise to normal levels in the immediate postoperative period. Some studies suggest a transient decrease in postoperative cerebral perfusion, further highlighting the need to maintain adequate MAPs [16]. Some studies also suggest increased oxygenation index following ligation [16]. The risk of post-ligation cardiorespiratory decompensation likely depends on the size of the defect, the time of closure, and the gestational age of the infant. Careful titration of fluids and vasopressors must be employed to maintain adequate perfusion while avoiding pulmonary fluid overload.

Complications

The rate of intraoperative mortality is exceedingly low, with the overall rate reported to be <1 %. There are no intraoperative deaths reported in recent literature of thoracoscopic PDA repair, and two reported during open repair. Intraoperative hemorrhage is also uncommon, with rates estimated between 0.5 and 1 % and even lower in recent series [17–19, 22–24]. Injury to surrounding structures, such as the pulmonary artery and descending aorta, is exceedingly rare, usually resulting in death [25–27].

More common complications include injury to the recurrent laryngeal nerve, which are reported to range between 0.5 and 6 %, with no significant difference noted between VATS and open approaches [17–19, 21, 23]. Over half of these are transient injuries with return of function [18, 19]. Rates of pneumothorax are between 0.5 and 6 %, and rates of chylothorax are estimated between 0.5 and 3 %, with no difference between minimally invasive and open repair [17–19, 21, 23]. Reported incidence of residual flow in the duct ranges between 0.5 % and 6 % [17–19, 21, 23], with a trend toward higher incidence in open repair that reaches statistical significance in some studies [17]. In contemporary series, conversion from thoracoscopic to open repair is between 0.5 and 4 %, with the most common cause reported to be poor exposure due to inability to retract the lung safely. Missed concurrent abnormalities are reported in less than 1 % of cases, with the most common abnormality being coarctation of the aorta [21, 23].

In the Johns Hopkins University series of 25 T-PDA ligations in very low-birth-weight infants, there have been no intraoperative deaths, 1 conversion to open procedure, 1 recurrent laryngeal nerve injury, and no other immediate morbidity.

Postoperative mortality approaches 15 % in some series, with the greatest risk factors being prematurity and low birth weight [14, 18, 23]. Sepsis is the leading cause of in-hospital death, frequently with associated necrotizing enterocolitis. Other causes are chronic respiratory disease and multisystem organ failure [14, 18, 23]. In our series we have had 3 deaths postoperatively all from sepsis related to NEC.

Conclusions

Thoracoscopic PDA ligation offers many of the advantages of a minimally invasive surgical approach that have been previously reported as well as a potential reduction in post thoracotomy scoliosis by avoiding rib spreading, muscular division, and minimization of the risk of nerve injury or rupture of intercostal ligaments. T-PDA ligation is effective and can be safely performed in very low-birth-weight infants. Exposure and magnification of important anatomic landmarks are superior compared to open techniques. This factor results in shorter operative time. In addition to the enhanced cosmesis, this minimally invasive approach may reduce postoperative pain, pulmonary morbidity, and the future incidence of chest wall and spine deformities in children.

Summary

- Patent ductus arteriosus is a persistence of the fetal communication between the left pulmonary artery and descending aorta. In term infants, the incidence of PDA is 1 in 2000 and represents 5–10 % of all congenital heart anomalies.
- The incidence of PDA is significantly higher in preterm and low-birth-weight babies, approaching 80 % in some populations.
- Presentation is highly variable depending on the size of the ductus. Small defects may produce no symptoms, moderate defects may result in systemic hypotension and pulmonary overload due to left to right shunt, and the most severe of defects can result in systemic hypotension or early cardiorespiratory failure.
- Diagnosis relies on high suspicion in the context of abnormal clinical or imaging findings such as hypotension, acidosis, respiratory distress, feeding intolerance, apneic episodes, or failure to thrive. The diagnosis is confirmed on echocardiogram, which is also critical to quantify the severity of the defect and rule out other cardiac comorbidities.
- Many PDAs spontaneously close by 1 year. The rate of spontaneous closure is significantly lower in large defects and in preterm and low-birth-weight babies.
- Persistent PDA is associated with increased long term morbidity and mortality related to the sequelae of persistent left to right shunt, thus the goal of management is to achieve closure of the defect prior to these negative sequelae.
- The type and timing of intervention are determined on an individual basis with consideration of symptoms, severity of defect, comorbidities, and other factors.
- Noninvasive treatments of PDA include mild fluid restriction, ventilator management, and prostaglandin administration in an attempt to achieve spontaneous closure

- Transarterial occlusion is the standard approach for PDA closure in infants and adults who have failed medical therapy.
- Surgical ligation is reserved for infants with severe defects who fail to stabilize from a respiratory and hemodynamic standpoint in spite of medical measures. It should also be considered in patients with comorbid conditions contraindicating prostaglandin administration.
- Both video-assisted thoracoscopic and open repair have high rates of success. There is no difference in perioperative mortality, recurrence, or complications. VATS repair is associated with decreased operative time, improved cosmesis, and decreased postoperative pain when compared to thoracotomy. Additionally, there may be a decreased incidence of pulmonary morbidity and chest wall or spine deformities.
- Long-term complications have been reported following medical and invasive and noninvasive intervention and include increased risk of bronchopulmonary dysplasia, as well affects on mesenteric, renal, and cerebral perfusion. Long-term outcomes are still under investigation.
- Both invasive and noninvasive repair of PDA are associated with a high rate of positive outcomes, low morbidity, and significant symptomatic improvement.

References

1. Dice J, Bhatia J. Patent ductus arteriosus: an overview. J Petiatr Phrmacol Ther. 2007;12:138–46.
2. Schneider D. The patent ductus arteriosus in term infants, children, and adults. Semin Perinatol. 2011;36:146–53.
3. Lloyd TR, Beekman III RH. Clinically silent patent ductus arteriosus. Am Heart J. 1994;127:1664–5. Letter.
4. Heuchan AM, Clyman RI. Managing the patent ductus arteriosus: current treatment options. Arch Dis Child Fetal Neonatal Ed. 2014;99:431–6.
5. Mitra S, Ronnestad A, Holmstrom H. Management of patent ductus arteriosus in preterm infants- where do we stand? Congenit Heart Dis. 2013;8:500–12.
6. Jain A, Shah P. Diagnosis, evaluation, and management of patent ductus arteriosus in preterm neonates. JAMA Pediatr. 2015;169(9):863–72.
7. Weisz DE, McNamara PJ. Patent ductus arteriosus ligation and adverse outcomes: causality or bias? J Clin Neonatol. 2014;3(2):67–75.
8. Kriege EV, Learly PJ, Opotowsky AR. Pulmonary hypertension in congenital heart disease: beyond Eisenmenger syndrome. Cardiol Clin. 2015;33(4):599–609.
9. Schneider DJ, Moore JQ. Congenital heart disease for the adult cardiologist. Circulation. 2006;114:1873–82.

10. Waddell TK, Bennett L, Kennedy R, et al. Heart-lung or lung transplantation for Eisenmenger syndrome. J Heart Lung Transplant. 2002;21:731–7.
11. Francis E, Singhi AK, Lakshmivenkateshaiah S, et al. Transcatheter occlusion of patent ductus arteriosus in pre-term infants. J Am Coll Cardiol Intv. 2010;3(5):550–5.
12. Baruteau AE, Hascoet S, Baruteau J, et al. Transcatheter closure of patent ductus arteriosus: past present and future. Arch Cardiovasc Dis. 2014;107(2):122–32.
13. Weinberg JG, Evans FJ, Burns KM, et al. Surgical ligation of patent ductus arteriosus in premature infants: trends and practice variation. Cardiol Young. 2015; Sep 23 [Epub ahead of print].
14. Lee LC, Tillett A, Tulloh R, et al. Outcome following patent ductus arteriosus ligation in premature infants: a retrospective cohort analysis. BMC Pediatr. 2006;11:6–15.
15. Tashiro J, Perez EA, Sola JE. Reduced hospital mortality with surgical ligation of patent ductus arteriosus in premature, extremely low birth weight infants: a propensity score-matched outcome study. Ann Surg. 2015; Mar 27 [Epub ahead of print].
16. Teixeria LS, Shivananda SP, Stephens D, et al. Postoperative cardiorespiratory instability following ligation of the preterm ductus arteriosus is related to early need for intervention. J Perinatol. 2008;28:803–10.
17. Chen H, Weng G, Chen Z, et al. Comparison of posterolateral thoracotomy and video-assisted thoracoscopic clipping for the treatment of patent ductus arteriosus in neonates and infants. Pediatr Cardiol. 2011;32:386–90.
18. Stankowski T, Aboul-Hassan SS, Marczak J, Cichon R. Is thoracoscopic patent ductus arteriosus closure superior to conventional surgery? Interact Cardiovasc Thorac Surg. 2015;21:532–8.
19. Vanamo K, Berg E, Kokki H, et al. Video-assisted thoracoscopic versus open surgery for persistent ductus arteriosus. J Pediatr Surg. 2006;41:1226–9.
20. Laborde F, Noirhomme R, Karam J, et al. A new video-assisted thoracoscopic surgical technique for interruption of patent ductus arteriosus in infants and children. J Thorac Cardiovasc Surg. 1993;105:278–80.
21. Nezafati MH, Soltani G, Vedadian A. Video-assisted ductal closure with new modifications: minimally invasive, maximally effective, 1300 cases. Ann Thorac Surg. 2007;84:1343–8.
22. Slater B, Rothenberg S. Thoracoscopic management of patent ductus arteriosus and vascular rings in infants and children. J Laparoendosc Adv Surg Tech. 2015;25:1–4.
23. Hines MH, Raines KH, Payne RM. Video-assisted ductal ligation in premature infants. Ann Thorac Surg. 2003;76:1417–20.
24. Lukish J. Video-assisted thoracoscopic ligation of a patent ductus arteriosus in a very low-birth-weight infant using a novel retractor. J Pediatr Surg. 2009;44:1047–50.
25. Fuller SJ, Gruber PJ. Patent Ductus Arteriosus. Fundamentals of pediatric surgery; 2011. p. 283–8.
26. Grunenfelder J, Bartram U, Van Praagh R, et al. The large window ductus: a surgical trap. Ann Thorac Surg. 1998;65(6):1790–1.
27. Tefera E, Bermudez-Canete, van Doorn C. Inadvertent ligation of the left pulmonary artery during intended ductal ligation. BMC Res Notes. 2015;8:511.

8. Thoracoscopic Aortopexy

Azmath Mohammed and Nathan Novotny

Introduction

Tracheomalacia is a disorder associated with localized or generalized weakening of the tracheal wall. This results in a dynamic narrowing of the trachea's lumen when intrathoracic pressure exceeds intraluminal pressure, i.e., during coughing, crying, or Valsalva maneuver. Management of severe TM is challenging for clinicians, and aggressive surgical therapy is almost always indicated. Aortopexy is now considered the best approach for severe TM and can be performed as open or thoracoscopic approach [1–3].

Epidemiology

Tracheomalacia is a rare disorder that is almost always confined to infancy and early childhood [4]. It is the most common congenital anomaly of the trachea. The true incidence of the congenital form is unknown [5]. However, based on a recent 7-year retrospective study, estimated incidence of primary airway malacia is 1 in every 2100–2600 newborns [6]. The vast majority are of mild to moderate severity and will never need surgical intervention. There has been an increasing trend in incidence which is likely reflective of increased suspicion by clinicians and also increase in survival of premature infants.

There is evidence that there are a number of undiagnosed cases in children in which they are diagnosed late in life or not at all. There is also an overlap of symptoms compared to other common pulmonary diseases which makes diagnosis difficult. Mild to moderate TM can be self-limiting, and most infants can outgrow the disorder by 2 years of

D.S. Walsh et al. (eds.), *The SAGES Manual of Pediatric Minimally Invasive Surgery*, DOI 10.1007/978-3-319-43642-5_8

age [6]. However, severe cases are associated with mortality rates as high as 80 % with nonoperative management.

TM is also frequently associated with tracheoesophageal atresia (TEA) and tracheoesophageal fistula (TEF). The development of both the trachea and esophagus share the common embryonic foregut [7]. Early histological studies of tracheas with TEF have shown high incidence of deficient cartilage along with increase in length of muscle in the membranous part of the tracheal ring. Acute postoperative respiratory distress after correction of TEA/TEF is likely due to TM. It requires a high index of suspicion, and clinicians need to recognize it early to manage impending respiratory distress [8].

Pathophysiology

The trachea is a relatively rigid structure supported by cartilaginous rings. In normal physiology, the tracheal diameter is dynamic in that it dilates with inspiration and narrows with expiration. However, weakening of the rings leads to a much more significant difference in the luminal diameter during high intrathoracic pressures such as during forced expiration, coughing, crying, or Valsalva maneuver. Involvement of the disease may occur at an isolated segment of trachea, the entire trachea, or even extend into the mainstem bronchi (tracheobronchomalacia) [2, 9].

Although TM can be classified in many ways, the most common classification divides the process into congenital (primary) and acquired disease (secondary). Congenital disease is primarily found in premature infants. Their tracheobronchial cartilage is not fully developed, either from early delivery or lack of maturity in utero despite normal gestation. There are also a number of diseases that lead to inadequate development of the cartilaginous matrix. Ehlers-Danlos syndrome, dyschondroplasia, and polychondritis are examples of inherent abnormalities in the collagen fibers leading to weakening of the trachea. Several genetic syndromes like Trisomy 9, Trisomy 21, and VATER anomaly have been associated with TM as well.

Acquired processes are much more common than the former congenital diseases. Prolonged intubation especially in premature infants is associated with higher risk of TM. Tracheostomy sites and even the cuffed portion of the tube can weaken the tracheal rings. Mechanical friction, pressure necrosis, and infections have been implicated as mechanisms.

External compression of the trachea from space occupying lesions can cause either intermittent or, if severe, persistent obstruction.

Congenital vascular abnormalities like the abnormal branch of the innominate artery, double aortic arch, or vascular rings have been implicated in TM as well in addition to their extrinsic compression [9, 10].

Preoperative Evaluation

The most common symptom encountered with congenital TM is a barking cough and expiratory stridor. The cough reflex is likely caused by the coaptation of the anterior and posterior tracheal walls. This may also be accompanied by cyanosis, high-pitched breathing, and breath-holding spells. During respiratory exertional activities, these symptoms will worsen as intrathoracic pressure rises, further collapsing the trachea.

Intermittent obstruction can lead to impaired clearance of secretions which may lead to recurrent infections. Additionally, parents may encounter feeding difficulties in infants. They can experience dysphagia, regurgitation, cough, and cyanosis. Respiratory arrest or "death attack" is a reflex thought to be caused by irritation to the trachea from food bolus or bronchoscope which can lead to cardiac arrest [9, 11, 12].

The clinical picture can be divided into mild, moderate or severe TM. Moderate symptoms include stridor, wheezing, infections, and cyanosis. Severe symptoms cause continuous stridor, airway obstruction, and reflex apnea leading to arrest.

Accurate diagnosis of TM is dependent on high index of suspicion based on history, physical exam, and imaging. Due to overlap of many other pulmonary diseases, TM is often misdiagnosed or not diagnosed until later in life. Flow-volume loop can be helpful as it shows decrease in the expiratory phase of the graph and a decreased mid-expiratory/mid-inspiratory ratio [13]. Plain radiographs have only 62 % sensitivity compared to direct bronchoscopy with a child who is spontaneously breathing. Barium esophagography is useful if suspecting tracheoesophageal fistula. CT scans have also been used to diagnose TM with sensitivities reaching 84.6 % [14]. Reconstruction into a three-dimensional model can provide further information for planning surgical correction, especially with the ability to evaluate surrounding vascular structures. However, there are inherent risks associated with exposure of ionizing radiation.

The unique and dynamic compression of the trachea is difficult to capture with CT imaging in young uncooperative patients. Therefore, direct visualization with bronchoscopy remains the gold standard. During the procedure, general inhalation anesthesia is initially used until the trachea is intubated with the bronchoscope. Then the anesthetic is reduced which allows the patient to breath spontaneously and cough to reveal the dynamic compression of the airway. A decrease in the tracheal diameter in the anteroposterior direction by 50 % is considered abnormal [9]. It is essential to decrease any positive pressure from the ventilator as it can stent the floppy trachea open.

Surgical Indications

Technique

The goal of thoracoscopic aortopexy is to elevate the aorta anteriorly toward the posterior surface of the sternum. Since the anterior wall of the trachea is attached to the aorta by the pretracheal fascia, the elevation lifts the trachea thereby increasing the diameter of the tracheal lumen in the anteroposterior direction [3].

Severe symptoms with an accurate diagnosis of TM by bronchoscopy and/or dynamic CT require consideration for surgical repair [15]. Open aortopexy has been well described in various approaches and techniques. Many centers prefer a left lateral muscle-sparing thoracotomy. However, approaches from median full or limited sternotomy have been reported [16].

With the advent of minimally invasive surgery, thoracoscopic approaches from both sides have been reported from many institutions. Advantages include improved patient comfort from small incisions, better postoperative pulmonary efforts, and a superior cosmetic result. A 30-degree laparoscope provides a better operative view since sutures are placed on the “ceiling” [17].

At our institution, we prefer a left-sided thoracoscopic approach. It provides working space for the right-handed laparoscopic needle holder in the left chest. Successful right-sided approach has been published which may reduce possible complications from dissection near the pulmonary trunk [2], though we have not had issues with this. For a left-sided approach, the patient is placed in the supine position with the left side elevated at 15° with a soft roll (Fig. 8.1). CO_2 insufflation of 5 mmHg is achieved with a Veress needle. The pressure is maintained to ensure the increased intrathoracic pressure does not affect ventilation. A total of three 3-mm ports are placed. The 3-mm camera port is placed in the midaxillary line at the fourth intercostal space. The two working ports are placed in the anterior axillary line of the third and sixth intercostal spaces under direct vision.

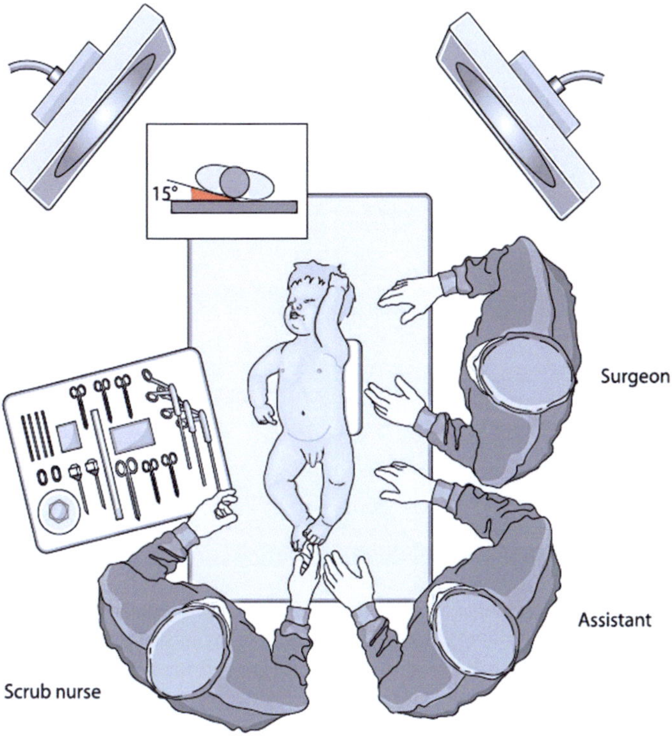

Fig. 8.1. Patient is placed in supine position with the left side elevated 15°. Both surgeon and assistant are positioned on the patient's left side. From Bax K and van der Zee DC [22], reprinted with permission from Springer.

The first view upon entering the thoracic cavity consists of the thymus, heart, and the great vessels. It is important to identify the left phrenic nerve prior to dissection of the pleura (Fig. 8.2a). The nerve can be identified by its posterior course along the pericardium. Next, the left lobe of the thymus overlies the pericardium. The left lobe of the thymus is mobilized and pushed toward the right side of the chest to expose the pericardium (Fig. 8.2b). It is safe to hold the thymus up toward the sternum to allow traction for hook cautery or a 3-mm sealing device to divide the attachments off the pericardium. This will ensure that the dissection will not injure the underlying pericardium or its contents. Once the thymus is mobilized, the pericardium is opened using laparoscopic scissors starting from the aortic root and extending cephalad (Fig. 8.2c). Again, care must be taken to preserve the phrenic nerve.

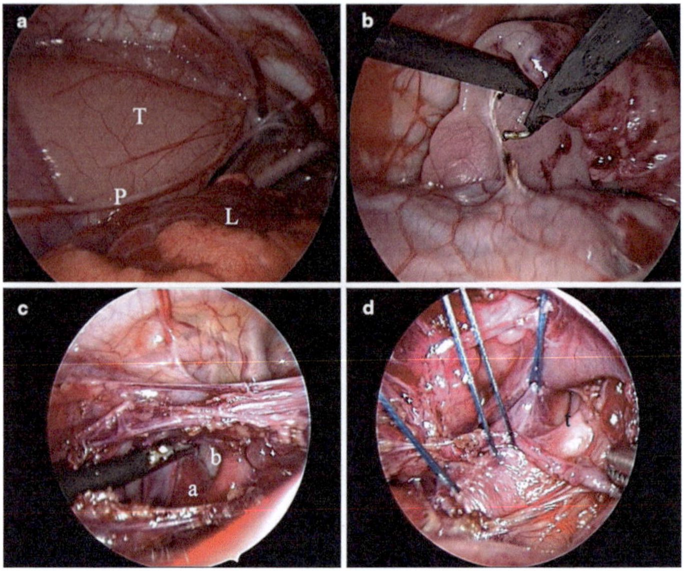

Fig. 8.2. **a** Thoracoscopic view of the left thorax (T, thymus/pericardium; Pn, phrenic nerve; L, left lung). **b** Mobilization of the thymus, T with hook cautery from pericardium, P. **c** Exposure of the aorta (a) and innominate artery (b). **d** Placement of partial thickness traction sutures in aorta, **a**. From van der Zee DC and Straver M [18], reprinted with permission from Springer.

Once the pericardium is adequately opened to reveal the aorta, aortopexy sutures can now be placed. The goal is to approximate the anterior wall of the aorta to the posterior surface of the sternum (Fig. 8.2d). We use a permanent 3-0 polypropylene suture instead of a braided suture to avoid sawing of the aortic wall when elevating the aorta off the trachea; however, vicryl sutures are also used. There are several important points to consider before placement of sutures. The first stitch can inadvertently be placed too close to the aortic valve and coronary arteries. It is also important to ensure that the aorta is not twisted along its long axis [2]. Since the patient is on a 15-degree right tilt, we ensure the sutures on the aorta are at the most anterior portion. Lastly, all sutures are placed through the tunica media of the aorta (partial thickness); sutures through the lumen of the aorta may cause bleeding. A partially straightened needle is passed through a stab incision in the skin. This needle is then grasped with a standard laparoscopic needle holder. The first stitch is placed distal to the

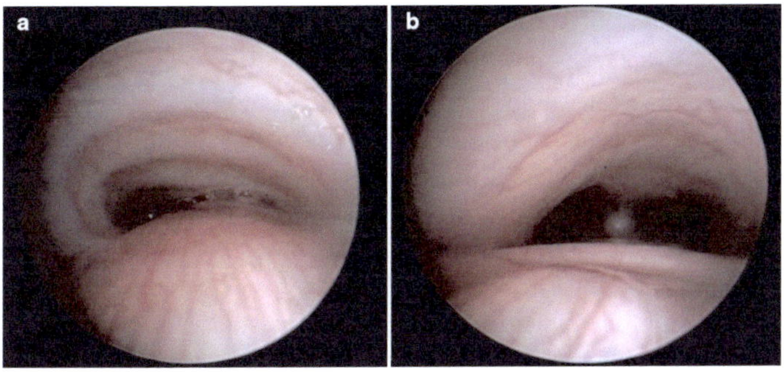

Fig. 8.3. **a** Bronchoscopic view of the trachea before aortopexy. **b** Relief of compression after aortopexy. From van der Zee DC and Straver M [18], reprinted with permission from Springer.

takeoff of the aortic root. The needle is then passed back through the sternum without tying. Securing the aorta to the parasternal tissue has been described but we need to consider the proximity of the left internal mammary vessels as they can be easily injured. A total of 3–8 stitches may be needed to provide adequate traction. We use intraoperative rigid bronchoscopy to guide the number of stitches. The pericardium can also be incorporated into each stitch to act as a pledget [15]. Once the appropriate number of sutures are placed, they are concurrently given traction to approximate the aortic wall to the sternum. A bronchoscope is then inserted to ensure the tracheomalacia is relieved (Fig. 8.3). The sutures are then tied down subcutaneously and ensuring that no aortic twisting has taken place. At the end of the procedure, pneumothorax is evacuated under direct visualization to ensure the left lung inflates adequately. Unless there is an unacceptable amount of bleeding, we do not recommend the routine use of a chest tube. Incisions are closed with 5-0 sutures or simply sealed with surgical glue [17].

Postoperative Care

Patients can be extubated immediately postoperatively. We elect not to place a thoracostomy tube, but if placed, they can be safely removed in 24 h. Ideally, patients are discharged in 3–5 days after resolution of symptoms, pain, and adequate pulmonary hygiene, though other NICU comorbidities often dictate the length of stay.

Outcomes

A single-center study compared the use of stents vs aortopexy. Although stents have been used successfully in vascular and biliary procedures, airway stents have promoted growth of granulation tissue causing obstruction. This typically requires repeat bronchoscopies at regular intervals or permanent removal of stent. At this time, the use of stents is considered an option for palliation of symptoms for inoperable disease [5].

Despite aortopexy being considered the most effective procedure for severe TM resulting in acute life-threatening events (ALTE), there are no randomized controlled trials, and they would be unlikely to be done. Most publications are single center and comprised of small series, but they have shown an immediate and excellent improvement in symptoms of severe TM. A recent review included 581 open and few thoracoscopic cases in literature. Eighty percent of patients had marked improvement in symptoms, 8 % had no improvement, 4 % had worsening of symptoms, and 6 % died. The group with a particularly worse outcome was associated with severe cardiac anomalies or other severe comorbidities [3]. A repeated theme in literature comparing open vs thoracoscopic procedures is the potential to reduce musculoskeletal disorders. Risk of severe deformities like atrophy of the serratus anterior muscle and scoliosis is documented in follow-up pediatric patients after thoracotomy. Muscle-sparing thoracotomy does aid in mitigating the risks of these disorders, but this risk may be further reduced with a thoracoscopic approach [19, 20].

A small, retrospective, single-center series comprising eight patients had recurrence in three of their patients. However, there was a lack of standardization in the cases. One patient who had a recurrence did not have an intraoperative bronchoscopy, and the second patient had a pericardiopexy instead of an aortopexy [21]. At our institution, we do not believe the pericardium has adequate structural integrity to elevate the aorta off the trachea. Nonetheless, as the thoracoscopic approach is further standardized and surgeons become proficient in the technique, we expect to see improved recurrence rates in literature.

Complications

Experts facile in the thoracoscopic approach agree that there is a definite learning curve to performing a successful aortopexy. Similar to open cases, there is a risk of recurrence, pneumothorax, bleeding, pericardial effusion, phrenic nerve palsy, and bleeding. To date, there are no prospective, randomized trials comparing open vs thoracoscopic procedures to see if there is a significant difference. A thoracoscopic view does offer a magnified view of the structures which may reduce complications of bleeding or nerve injury. In addition, we believe the view aids in more accurate placement of sutures on the aorta [3].

Summary

- It is widely accepted that severe tracheomalacia often requires surgical intervention. Aortopexy has proven to provide immediate resolution of the dynamic compression of the trachea when performed well.
- With the availability of small ports, thoracoscopic aortopexy has been shown to provide similar results in patients. As in the open approach, great care must be exercised to identify the surrounding anatomy to prevent inadvertent injury to great vessels or nerves.
- A left-sided thoracoscopic approach will visualize the thymus, heart, and the left phrenic nerve. It is important to identify the nerve before mobilizing the thymus to avoid inadvertent injury.
- The pericardium is opened along the axis of the aorta.
- Partial thickness sutures are placed directly on the anterior wall (tunica media) of the aorta through the sternal body. The aorta is elevated simultaneously, and the sutures are tied down subcutaneously on the anterior aspect of the sternum.
- With simultaneous visualization of the trachea intraoperatively, a surgeon can immediately assess the result of the aortopexy.
- As surgeons overcome the learning curve, the thoracoscopic approach will likely be the preferred approach for most patients with severe TM.

References

1. Dave S, Currie BG. The role of aortopexy in severe tracheomalacia. J Pediatr Surg. 2006;41(3):533–7.
2. Gray F. Thoracoscopic aortopexy for the treatment of pediatric tracheomalacia: a right-sided approach. Oper Tech Thoracic Cardiovasc Surg. 2011;16(4):322–30.
3. Torre M, Carlucci M, Speggiorin S, Elliott MJ. Aortopexy for the treatment of tracheomalacia in children: review of the literature. Ital J Pediatr. 2012;38:62.
4. Weber TR, Keller MS, Fiore A. Aortic suspension (aortopexy) for severe tracheomalacia in infants and children. Am J Surg. 2002;184(6):573–7. discussion 7.

5. Valerie EP, Durrant AC, Forte V, Wales P, Chait P, Kim PC. A decade of using intraluminal tracheal/bronchial stents in the management of tracheomalacia and/or bronchomalacia: is it better than aortopexy? J Pediatr Surg. 2005;40(6):904–7. discussion 7.
6. Boogaard R, Huijsmans SH, Pijnenburg MW, Tiddens HA, de Jongste JC, Merkus PJ. Tracheomalacia and bronchomalacia in children: incidence and patient characteristics. Chest. 2005;128(5):3391–7.
7. Snijders D, Barbato A. An update on diagnosis of tracheomalacia in children. Eur J Pediatr Surg. 2015;25(4):333–5.
8. Wailoo MP, Emery JL. The trachea in children with tracheo-oesophageal fistula. Histopathology. 1979;3(4):329–38.
9. Carden KA, Boiselle PM, Waltz DA, Ernst A. Tracheomalacia and tracheobronchomalacia in children and adults: an in-depth review. Chest. 2005;127(3):984–1005.
10. Johnston RF, Green RA. Tracheobronchiomegaly. Report of five cases and demonstration of familial occurrence. Am Rev Respir Dis. 1965;91:35–50.
11. Filler RM, Rossello PJ, Lebowitz RL. Life-threatening anoxic spells caused by tracheal compression after repair of esophageal atresia: correction by surgery. J Pediatr Surg. 1976;11(5):739–48.
12. Jacobs IN, Wetmore RF, Tom LW, Handler SD, Potsic WP. Tracheobronchomalacia in children. Arch Otolaryngol Head Neck Surg. 1994;120(2):154–8.
13. Abramson AL, Goldstein MN, Stenzler A, Steele A. The use of the tidal breathing flow volume loop in laryngotracheal disease of neonates and infants. Laryngoscope. 1982;92(8 Pt 1):922–6.
14. Boiselle PM, Ernst A. Recent advances in central airway imaging. Chest. 2002;121(5):1651–60.
15. Durkin ET, Krawiec ME, Shaaban AF. Thoracoscopic aortopexy for primary tracheomalacia in a 12-year-old. J Pediatr Surg. 2007;42(7):E15–7.
16. Brawn WJ, Huddart SN. Tracheoaortopexy via midline sternotomy in tracheomalacia. J Pediatr Surg. 1991;26(6):660–2.
17. Perger L, Kim HB, Jaksic T, Jennings RW, Linden BC. Thoracoscopic aortopexy for treatment of tracheomalacia in infants and children. J Laparoendosc Adv Surg Tech A. 2009;19 Suppl 1:S249–54.
18. van der Zee DC, Straver M. Thoracoscopic aortopexy for tracheomalacia. World J Surg. 2015;39(1):158–64.
19. Holcomb 3rd GW, Rothenberg SS, Bax KM, Martinez-Ferro M, Albanese CT, Ostlie DJ, et al. Thoracoscopic repair of esophageal atresia and tracheoesophageal fistula: a multi-institutional analysis. Ann Surg. 2005;242(3):422–8. discussion 8–30.
20. Rothenberg SS. Thoracoscopic repair of esophageal atresia and tracheoesophageal fistula in neonates, first decade's experience. Dis Esophagus. 2013;26(4):359–64.
21. Jennings RW, Hamilton TE, Smithers CJ, Ngerncham M, Feins N, Foker JE. Surgical approaches to aortopexy for severe tracheomalacia. J Pediatr Surg. 2014;49(1):66–70; discussion -1.
22. Bax K, van der Zee D. Aortosternopexy for tracheomalacia. In: Endoscopic surgery in infants and children. Springer; 2008. p. 159.

9. Thoracoscopic Sympathectomy

Wesley Barnes, Zachary Hothem, and Nathan Novotny

Introduction

Historical Background of Thoracic Sympathectomy

Alexander performed the first clinical surgical sympathectomy at the level of the neck in 1889 in an attempt to treat a patient with epilepsy [1, 2]. However, it was not until 1920 that sympathectomy for the management of hyperhidrosis was introduced by Kotzareff [1, 3]. Since that time, a variety of techniques including both open and endoscopic have been described for the performance of a thoracic sympathectomy. During the 1940s, Hughes introduced the concept of thoracoscopic sympathectomy [4]. In 1978, Kux described his large experience with endoscopic thoracic sympathectomy (ETS) for the treatment of hyperhidrosis [5]. With the widespread availability of video-assisted thoracic surgery (VATS) along with piqued physician and patient interest in minimally invasive surgery, thoracoscopic sympathectomy has become the preferred technique for the management of primary palmar and axillary hyperhidrosis.

Epidemiology

Hyperhidrosis (excessive sweating) can be a primary (idiopathic or cryptogenic) disorder, or it can result secondarily from underlying medical conditions or medications. Primary focal hyperhidrosis is defined as excessive, bilateral, and relatively symmetric sweating that may occur in the axillae, palms, soles, or craniofacial region [6]. It is a relatively common disorder. The prevalence of primary focal

D.S. Walsh et al. (eds.), *The SAGES Manual of Pediatric Minimally Invasive Surgery*, DOI 10.1007/978-3-319-43642-5_9

hyperhidrosis has been estimated to range from 0.6 to 3 % of the population, with estimates suggesting that 1.6 % of adolescents and 0.6 % of prepubertal children are affected by this condition [7, 8]. This percentage may be even higher in those of Asian descent [9]. In one study, 65 % of patients undergoing thoracic sympathectomy for hyperhidrosis reported a positive family history, suggesting a hereditary component to the disease [10]. It affects both sexes equally [7]. The age of onset for hyperhidrosis varies by the anatomic site involved. For instance, palmar hyperhidrosis typically presents during childhood or adolescence, whereas those with axillary disease present during adolescence [7, 11, 12]. Axillary disease is the most common and is seen in approximately one-half of patients with hyperhidrosis [6, 7]. Hyperhidrosis of the palms and soles is next most common, affecting approximately one-third of patients [7].

Pathophysiology

The sympathetic and parasympathetic nervous systems are the two main divisions of the autonomic nervous system. The sympathetic nervous system mediates the body's "fight-or-flight" response to environmental stressors. Sympathetic input to blood vessels produces vasoconstriction via smooth muscle fiber contraction. A decrease in this adrenergic activity results in vasodilation. Sweat glands are also primarily innervated by sympathetic nerves, and the release of acetylcholine from postganglionic neurons stimulates these glands to secrete sweat.

Eccrine sweat glands release serous fluid onto the skin to promote cooling via evaporation. These glands are distributed throughout the surface of the skin but are most heavily concentrated in the axillae, palms of the hands, and soles of the feet. Perspiration becomes pathologic when the amount of sweat secreted is greater than that which is needed for physiologic thermoregulation. Although the exact pathophysiology of hyperhidrosis remains unknown, the cause seems to be an abnormal or exaggerated central response to emotional stress [13].

Sympathetic denervation gives increased blood flow to the skin (vasodilation), loss of piloerection, and decreased sweating. The maximal effect of sympathectomy is immediate. Hands become warm, pink, and dry.

Preoperative Evaluation

Clinical Manifestations

Patients are referred to the surgeon because of excessive sweating of the palms, axilla, or face. This referral is often after the patient has failed to respond to topical therapy or other medical treatments. Primary focal hyperhidrosis frequently results in severe social, emotional, and occupational handicaps from an early age. Parents may describe substantial wetness of their child's palms and soles during infancy. Children with palmar hyperhidrosis often saturate everything they touch, thus leading to problems with reading, writing, and other school activities. Antiperspirants are often used on the palms. To avoid the social stigmatization that can be caused by axillary hyperhidrosis, patients will place sanitary pads or rolls of paper towels in their axillae. Excessive perspiration can occur whether the child is calm and resting or emotionally stressed. Adolescence is typically characterized by more intense psychologically and emotionally stressful experiences accompanied by the hormonal changes that result from sexual maturation. Thus, hyperhidrosis often worsens during this stage of life. Because of the embarrassment associated with this disease, some individuals will withdraw from the world by avoiding handshakes, parties, dances, and dating [14]. If not treated, these patients may enter adulthood dreading social interaction and, potentially, avoiding certain professional career choices. Early diagnosis and treatment has the potential to significantly improve quality of life [15].

The diagnostic criterion for primary focal hyperhidrosis includes focal, visible, excessive sweating of at least six months duration without any obvious secondary cause and has at least two of the following features: impairs daily activities, a bilateral and relatively symmetric pattern, frequency of at least one episode per week, an age of onset younger than 25 years, cessation of focal sweating during sleep, or positive family history [6]. It is a diagnosis of exclusion of secondary causes. Generalized sweating suggests a secondary etiology, such as excessive heat, obesity, a neurologic disorder, an endocrinopathy, a malignancy, an infection, or a medication. As it is largely a clinical diagnosis, tests quantifying sweat production are not practical nor are they routinely performed [6].

Indications for Thoracoscopic Sympathectomy

Thoracic sympathectomy has been described for the treatment of a variety of sympathetic disorders. The most common indication in children is for the management of primary focal hyperhidrosis. Other indications, which are much less common in adults and even rarer in children, include complex regional pain syndrome, long QT syndrome, and vasospastic or occlusive disorders (Raynaud's disease, thromboangiitis obliterans). This chapter will primarily focus on the technique of thoracoscopic sympathectomy as it pertains to the management of primary focal hyperhidrosis.

Surgical consultation is generally considered after a child continues to have severe and debilitating symptoms despite other medical therapies (topical antiperspirants, iontophoresis, oral anticholinergics, botulinum toxin injection, etc.) or has not been able to tolerate them. Based upon review of the literature, the Society for Thoracic Surgeons (STS) expert panel proposed that only a small percentage of patients with primary focal hyperhidrosis should be considered for surgical treatment [13]. However, some believe that it should be recommended as first-line therapy for patients with severe palmar hyperhidrosis [16]. Given the ease to which this procedure can be done, the authors here favor the latter approach to this condition. Furthermore, surgery offers the most definitive and long-lasting treatment without the need for repeat injections while also avoiding the systemic side effects associated with oral anticholinergics.

The preoperative evaluation should include confirming the diagnosis of primary focal hyperhidrosis, the anatomic locations involved, and a discussion of the alternatives to surgical therapy along with the potential for surgical complications (compensatory sweating, Horner's syndrome, postoperative pain, possibility of conversion to an open procedure) and for operative failure [13]. According to a STS expert panel, the ideal candidates for thoracoscopic sympathectomy are those who have onset of hyperhidrosis before age 16 years, are younger than 25 years at the time of surgery, have a body mass index (BMI) less than 28, report no sweating during sleep, have no other significant comorbidities, and have a resting pulse greater than 55 beats per minute (as sympathectomy has a partial β-blocker effect on the heart) [13].

Technique

Anatomy

The thoracic paravertebral sympathetic chains descend vertically within each hemithorax covered by the parietal pleura and are positioned anterior to the region bounded by the rib neck and head in most patients [17] (Fig. 9.1). Postganglionic fibers responsible for the innervation of the sweat glands of the palms originate mainly from the second and third thoracic (T2–T3) ganglia, whereas those responsible for innervation of sweat glands in the axillary region originate from the T3–T4 ganglia [18]. In most patients, the sympathetic ganglia are located within their corresponding intercostal space, for example, the T3 ganglion is found between the heads of the third and fourth ribs in the third intercostal space [19, 20].

Multiple aberrant pathways have been described for the thoracic sympathetic chain. The nerve of Kuntz is the most known anatomical variation. It is an alternative sympathetic pathway that directly connects the second

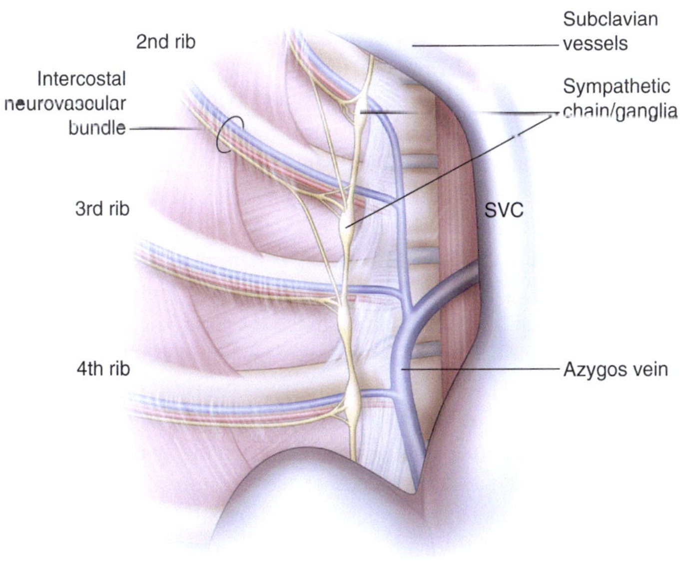

Fig. 9.1. Anatomy of the right thoracic sympathetic chain as seen during thoracoscopic sympathectomy. *SVC*: superior vena cava.

or third thoracic ganglia to the brachial plexus [21]. These anatomical variations are of clinical importance to the surgeon because they provide a route for fibers to bypass the sympathetic chain and may be responsible for the recurrence of symptoms after sympathectomy surgery [22, 23].

Because the terminology used to describe this surgical technique has historically been inconsistent and unclear, an effort has been made to establish an internationally agreed upon nomenclature. The International Society on Sympathetic Surgery (ISSS) and STS committee's consensus was to use a rib-oriented nomenclature. This decision was made because too many patients have mediastinal fat that can obscure clear identification of the specific ganglia and because there are many anatomical variations in the ganglion anatomy [13]. Furthermore, the type of ganglion interruption (clipping, cutting, cauterizing, or removing a segment) should be noted. Thus, if the chain is cauterized on the top of the third rib, the operation should be abbreviated as "cauterized R3, top" [13].

Level of Interruption of the Sympathetic Chain

Historically, palmar hyperhidrosis was treated with transection of the sympathetic chain at R2 and R3, with the addition of R4 if axillary hyperhidrosis was also present. More recent beliefs are that palmar hyperhidrosis can be effectively treated by limiting disruption to a single level, at either R3 or R4, in an effort to minimize side effects and to improve overall quality of life for these patients. Studies have shown that interruption of the sympathetic chain at R4 alone is associated with the lowest incidence of compensatory hyperhidrosis (CH), the fewest regions/sites of CH, and the lowest frequency of excessively dry hands [24, 25]. Multivariate analysis revealed the most important variable influencing patient satisfaction was palmar over-dryness [25]. The satisfaction rate overall was higher in those with slightly moister hands (more common in the R4 group) as opposed to those with excessively dry hands and significantly higher rates of CH (more commonly in R3 group) [24]. Perhaps more importantly, none of the patients undergoing disruption at the R4 level regretted having the operation [25]. Expert consensus reports that two interruptions in the sympathetic chain at R3 and R4 provide the driest hands at the expense of a higher risk of CH. However, the panel's recommendation is for an R3 interruption alone, but goes on to state that R4 interruption is an acceptable alternative in order to limit CH [13]. With this in mind, the options of both an R3 or a R4 disruption can be discussed with parents to allow them to make an educated decision, informing them that an R3 interruption alone tends to provide dry hands, though sometimes overly dry, with an increased risk of CH, whereas an R4 interruption alone has a lower rate of CH but the possibility of continuing to have slightly moister hands than the normal child.

For patients with palmar and plantar hyperhidrosis, expert consensus recommends either R4 interruption alone or R4 and R5 interruptions. To yield the driest feet, this panel endorses two interruptions at R4 and R5. However, disruption at R4 alone may reduce the incidence of CH while still providing satisfactory results [13].

In patients with axillary, palmar-axillary, or palmar-axillary-plantar hyperhidrosis, the optimal operation is an interruption at both R4 and R5 [13]. As with palmar hyperhidrosis, some surgeons favor a single level of interruption, at either R4 [26] or R5 [27], for axillary hyperhidrosis. One study demonstrated a 0 % incidence of CH after R5 interruption with no patient regretting having undergone this procedure [27]. Consent requires a careful discussion of the risks and benefits of the varying levels of interruption and the consequences of aggressive or conservative procedures.

ETS can also be used for patients with severe craniofacial hyperhidrosis and must be distinguished from facial blushing as results for this latter condition are less impressive. Expert consensus recommends R3 interruption alone to reduce the risk of CH and Horner's, which are more common with R2 interruption or R2 and R3 interruptions [13, 27].

Anesthesia

Thoracoscopic sympathectomy is performed under general anesthesia. A single-lumen endotracheal tube (SLT) is sufficient in most cases; however, some surgeons prefer a double-lumen endotracheal tube (DLT). There are pros and cons to both types of tubes. Single-lung isolation is the main advantage offered by a DLT, which decreases motion within the operative field. However, with the use of CO_2 insufflation, positioning, and intermittent breath holding, the lung rarely obscures the surgeon's view to any significant degree. Some authors have employed bronchial blockers successfully. Furthermore, pediatric airway anatomy may only permit the use of the smaller diameter SLT. Larger diameter tubes may increase the likelihood of a sore throat and transient hoarseness in the immediate postoperative period. In general, a DLT is technically more challenging to place, and proper placement should be confirmed both clinically and bronchoscopically. Ultimately, the decision on the type of endotracheal tube depends on individual preference, age of the child, and discussion between the surgeon and anesthesiologist.

Positioning

The patient lies supine in a semi-Fowler position with the head of the bed elevated at 30–45° (Fig. 9.2). This allows gravity to help retract the upper lobes out of the intended operative field and helps to decompress some of the smaller veins coursing near the rib heads. Rotation of the bed toward the contralateral side can also facilitate in this endeavor. Both arms are abducted to 90 degrees and secured to arm boards so as to expose the axillae. The elbows should be padded to avoid postoperative ulnar neuralgia. A roll is placed behind the shoulders to improve access to the upper sympathetic chain. The supine position provides more than adequate exposure and requires no delay for repositioning and re-preparing the opposite chest. Alternatively, some authors prefer a lateral decubitus position with the operating table extended to widen the intercostal spaces. An axillary roll is placed, and the ipsilateral arm is secured to an elevated arm board at a gentle angle. For this positioning, the surgeon stands ventral to the patient with the assistant and video monitor on the opposite side.

Instruments

This procedure requires an operating theater capable of accommodating standard endoscopic equipment. Basic instruments include a 3-mm rigid thoracoscope (either 0- or 30-degree angled lens), a 3-mm hook electrocautery, a 3-mm endoscopic blunt-tipped curved scissors (mini-Metzenbaum-type) with a monopolar cautery attachment, a 3-mm

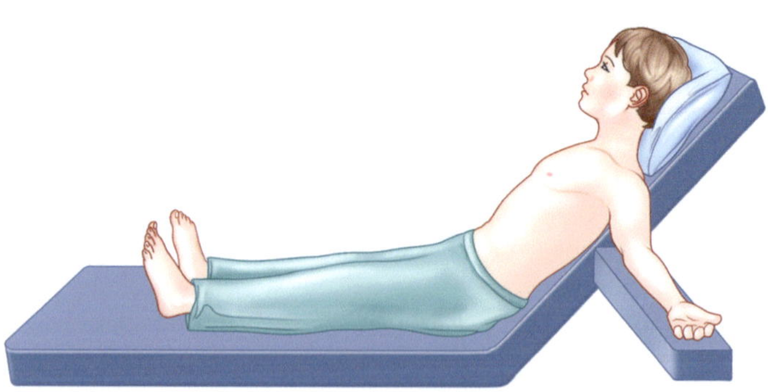

Fig. 9.2. Child in semi-Fowler position with arms abducted.

endoscopic curved dissector, and three 3-mm blunt-tipped trocars. In the unusual event that any significant bleeding is encountered, a suction/irrigation system should be readily available but not opened on the sterile field. Depending on the surgeon's preference for performing interruption of the sympathetic chain, an endoscopic clip applier or the Harmonic scalpel (Ethicon Endo-Surgery, Inc., Cincinnati, OH) can serve as alternatives to hook electrocautery. However, clip appliers and alternate energy devices are not required and may increase the cost of the case.

Steps of the Surgical Procedure

Port Placement

When performing a bilateral procedure, the skin preparation should include the entire anterior thorax with extension to the posterior axillary lines bilaterally as well as both axillary regions. The side on which the operation is commenced varies according to the surgeon's preference. Surgeons have described various techniques employing one-, two-, and three-port sites as well as a multitude of locations for their port placement. The postoperative course of patients with a single 12-mm incision versus multiple 3–5 mm incisions is not significantly different. This chapter will focus on a three-port technique with 3-mm trocar sites, as it offers superior visibility with the ability to retract the lung while cutting and cauterizing.

The first 3-mm blunt tipped trocar is placed in the anterior axillary line within the third, fourth, or fifth intercostal space. Capnothorax is established by insufflating carbon dioxide with a pressure limit of 5 mmHg. This aids in compression and retraction of lung parenchyma while limiting risk of adverse hemodynamic consequences [28]. Next, a 3-mm (or 5-mm to increase illumination and visual quality), 30-degree thoracoscope is introduced. Under direct endoscopic guidance, the second 3-mm blunt-tipped trocar is placed through an incision overlying the fourth, fifth, or sixth intercostal space in the mid-axillary line. The final 3-mm port site is located in the fourth, fifth, or sixth intercostal space near the posterior axillary line.

Exposure of the Thoracic Sympathetic Chain

The sympathetic chain courses cephalad to caudad over the rib heads in the paraspinal region along the posterosuperior aspect of the hemithorax.

In the pediatric patient, it is most often visible through the overlying parietal pleura as a whitish, raised (or multinodular) cord. However, the obese child may have a greater degree of fatty tissue in this area, thus concealing the sympathetic chain. On such occasions, the cord can usually be located by "palpation" with an endoscopic instrument.

Next, the surgeon must identify the correct anatomic rib number in order to define the target levels of the sympathetic chain to be interrupted. The first rib can rarely be seen with the thoracoscope, and so the most cephalad rib visualized will be the second rib. The fatty tissue generally obscures the stellate ganglion and first intercostal space in adults though it is sometimes visible in children. If doubt exists as to the rib enumeration, an intraoperative chest radiograph can help to clarify this anatomy.

Endoscopic shears are used to incise the parietal pleura overlying the rib just lateral to the intended level(s) of sympathetic chain interruption (Fig. 9.3). The chain is then carefully freed from its surrounding tissues with sharp dissection when possible and, if needed, electrocautery.

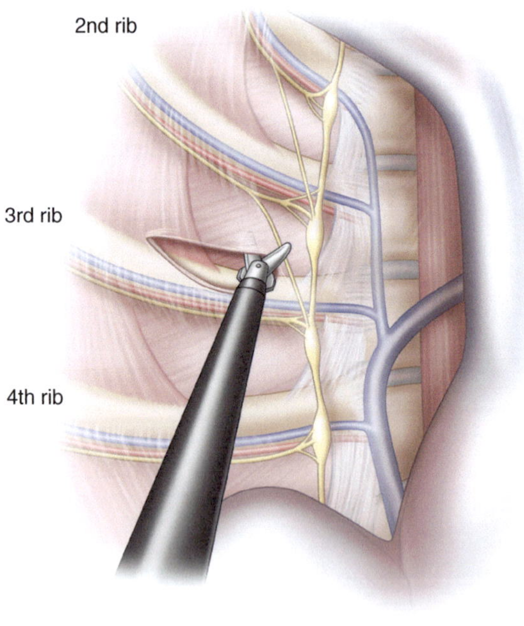

Fig. 9.3. Division of the pleura overlying the top of the third rib so as to expose the underlying sympathetic chain along with any accessory nerves of Kuntz.

To minimize any spread of current toward the stellate ganglion, the surgeon is encouraged to utilize the lowest diathermy setting that can effectively divide the tissue and to employ short "bursts" of cautery current [29]. Fortunately, this is often a fairly avascular plane. However, care must be taken especially in the right chest to avoid avulsing intercostal veins at the T3 and T4 levels, which drain directly into the azygos vein and can bleed significantly when injured [29]. In case of bleeding, hemostasis can often be obtained with direct pressure and/or cautery.

Interruption of the Sympathetic Chain

Upon exposing the target level(s) of the sympathetic chain, the surgeon must decide on the type of interruption to employ (Fig. 9.4). When

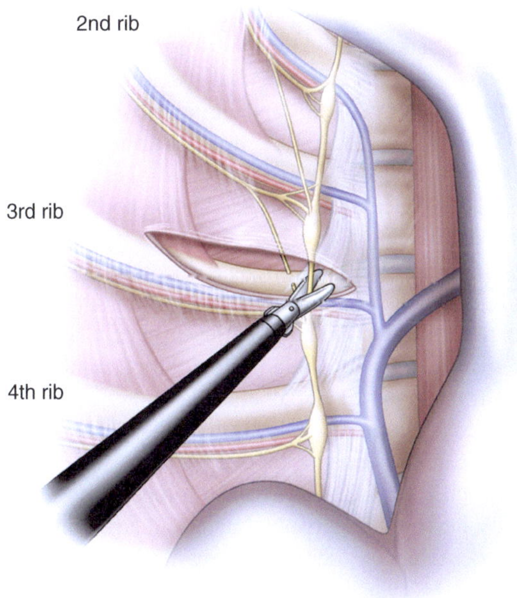

Fig. 9.4. After circumferentially freeing the sympathetic chain from surrounding tissues, the chain is interrupted at the desired level (top of the third rib in this figure). We prefer cutting the sympathetic chain sharply with cold endoscopic shears along the upper border of the rib of the corresponding ganglion. Alternatives for disruption of the sympathetic chain include transection with hook electrocautery, clipping, ablation, and resection.

performing this procedure for hyperhidrosis, the primary objective is to sever the connections between eccrine sweat glands and the sympathetic chain. A variety of methods for chain disruption have been described in the literature, including resection, transection, ablation, and clipping. However, no clear differences have been found among these techniques [13, 30]. Resecting the chain mandates more dissection and increases the potential for trauma to surrounding tissues without any added significant benefit. Some authors report that clipping has the potential for reversal upon clip removal within 10–14 days of the procedure should CH be intolerable [31], but the authors and others are skeptical of this presumption and do not feel clipping should be considered reversible [13]. According to an STS expert consensus panel, the most important factors for achieving a successful operation are that (1) the correct level of division was accomplished and (2) the nerve ends were separated enough to prevent nerve regrowth [13].

Cutting the sympathetic chain sharply with cold endoscopic shears along the upper border of the rib of the corresponding ganglion has proven an effective method. The bleeding is minimal, and, more importantly, this technique avoids any potential spread of current along the chain toward the stellate ganglion and limits the extent of dissection. Furthermore, dividing the chain at the mid- or upper portion of the rib can reduce risk of unintentional injury to the more inferiorly located intercostal vessels. If the chain is transected using hook cautery, then the cutting current should be utilized, or, alternatively, division with the Harmonic scalpel (Ethicon Endo-Surgery, Inc., Cincinnati, OH) may result in less spread to surrounding tissues. Some surgeons routinely monitor sympathetic tone to the hand in the form of a skin temperature probe or a laser Doppler (to determine palmar blood flow) in an effort to objectively confirm adequate sympathetic chain interruption. We do not employ these latter techniques.

Once the sympathetic chain is interrupted, the two ends should be separated from each other to lessen chance of regeneration. This can be accomplished by tucking the nerve end under an adjacent rib or flap of the parietal pleura. Also, consider cauterizing the distal tip of the divided chain with a “hot” Maryland dissector to aid in this endeavor. Avoid cauterizing the proximal end of the divided chain in order to protect the stellate ganglion.

Lung Re-expansion and Wound Closure

Prior to lung re-expansion, hemostasis is ensured and carbon dioxide insufflation is ceased. To help minimize postoperative pain, an intercostal nerve block using a long-acting local anesthetic (i.e., bupivacaine) can easily be performed at this time under thoracoscopic guidance. After the working ports are removed, a small suction catheter (red rubber catheter, feeding tube, or chest tube) is introduced into the thorax through one of these incisions to facilitate evacuation of the capnopneumothorax. The anesthesiologist also assists in lung re-expansion by providing sustained large tidal volumes. When the surgeon is satisfied that the lung is adequately reinflated, the thoracoscope and suction catheter are removed, and the port sites are closed. If 3-mm incisions were employed, skin adhesive is usually all that is needed to seal the incisions. Local anesthetic is injected at the incision sites.

A similar procedure is then repeated on the opposite side for each desired level of chain interruption.

Post-anesthesia Care Unit

In the recovery room, a routine upright chest radiograph is performed to ensure complete lung re-expansion and exclude a significant residual pneumothorax, which is unlikely. However, small apical pneumothoraces that do not require chest tubes are not uncommon. The carbon dioxide within the chest is typically reabsorbed within 3 h. Most patients tolerate this procedure without issue and are discharged home later that same day on an oral pain regimen. We ask patients to limit their activity for 48 h postoperatively and then to gradually increase to regular activity within a week of surgery.

Pearls and Pitfalls

When opening the parietal pleura or dividing the sympathetic chain, the surgeon should avoid the underlying periosteum because damaging it may cause severe sunburn-like pain in the postoperative period [29]. To protect the stellate ganglion from harm, do not carry out any dissection above the superior border of the second rib. Reduce the settings as well as the use of electrocautery during this procedure whenever possible. Also, sharp division or clipping of the sympathetic chain obviates the potential for inadvertent injury to the stellate ganglion due to spread of an electrical current. When dividing the chain sharply, it is important to separate the ends of the nerve adequately using the "tuck" technique described above.

Anatomical variation of the sympathetic chain can increase the likelihood of operative failure or complications. In the child with palmar hyperhidrosis, some authors advocate division of the pleura overlying the bodies of ribs 2 and 3 at least 2 cm lateral to the chain, and any accessory fibers of Kuntz are severed as they are encountered [32–34]. Occasionally, the sympathetic chain may run medial to the rib heads and can increase the probability of an aortic injury in the left chest if caution is not exercised [34]. The surgeon should be aware of the location of the subclavian vessels, azygos vein, hemiazygos vein, thoracic aorta, vagus nerve, and phrenic nerve and take caution to protect them from harm throughout the operation. This procedure usually involves a rather bloodless dissection, but significant bleeding can result from avulsion of intercostal veins draining directly to the azygos vein [20]. Thus, it may be necessary to cauterize or clip some of these vessels while attempting to expose the sympathetic chain. An azygos lobe is an infrequent anatomical variation consisting of an accessory pulmonary lobe at the apex of the lung, which when present may make it difficult or even impossible to accomplish a thoracoscopic sympathectomy [35, 36].

Postoperative Care

Outcomes

Ideally, surgery for primary focal hyperhidrosis should abolish hyperhidrosis but minimize the complications associated with sympathetic denervation of the upper extremity. Overall results from thoracoscopic sympathectomy have mostly been very favorable in this regard. However, the outcomes of this procedure vary according to the anatomic location of sweating and the level of sympathetic chain interruption.

Thoracoscopic sympathectomy has been reported to immediately relieve palmar hyperhidrosis with rates ranging from 94 to 100 % [13, 37]. However, patients undergoing surgery for axillary hyperhidrosis generally have lower immediate success rates (ranging from 77 to 100 %) and higher regret rates when compared to those undergoing surgery for palmar hyperhidrosis [13, 26, 38]. Furthermore, the incidence of long-term recurrent hyperhidrosis has been described between 0 and 65 %—again with higher recurrence rates seen in those being operated for axillary hyperhidrosis [13, 39, 40].

A 2012 study of 453 patients undergoing thoracoscopic sympathectomy for hyperhidrosis found that over 90 % of patients had an immediate and sustained improvement in quality of life until at least the fifth postoperative year [41]. Some researchers feel that thoracoscopic sympathectomy should be done as early as possible because long-term postoperative satisfaction was significantly higher among children less than 14 years (92 %) as compared to patients older than 15 years (81 %) [42]. Another study demonstrated 77 % of children younger than 14 years undergoing thoracoscopic sympathectomy for palmar hyperhidrosis had a great improvement in their quality of life postoperatively [43].

Complications

The main acute complications occurring either intraoperatively or in the immediate postoperative period include hemodynamic instability, pneumothorax requiring chest tube drainage (1 %), pleural effusion (1 %), acute bleeding or delayed hemothorax (1 %), chylothorax, and persistent intercostal neuralgia (<1 %) [13]. Limiting the carbon dioxide insufflation pressure to 5 mmHg should minimize any untoward hemodynamic alterations that might result from mediastinal shift and impaired venous return to the heart. Nevertheless, if the child becomes hypotension, bradycardic, or hypoxic during the conduct of the operation, carbon dioxide insufflation should be discontinued and evacuated while the lung is reinflated by the anesthesiologist. Bleeding and neuralgia can be avoided by careful port placement ensuring avoidance of the intercostal neurovascular bundle running along the inferior aspect of each rib. The majority of pneumothoraces resolve spontaneously, but some may require a chest tube if symptoms are severe. While undertaking bilateral thoracoscopic procedures, remember that the patient may develop a pneumothorax on the first side while the second lung is deflated. Even though this is a rare event, it must be noticed and treated promptly because of potentially fatal consequences. The risk of pneumothorax can be minimized by using blunt-tipped trocars, careful lung manipulation, and appropriate technique during lung reinflation [13].

The most common long-term sequela is compensatory hyperhidrosis (CH) which has been reported with large variation (3–98 %) in the literature [13]. CH is excessive sweating that occurs in areas of the body other than the original problem site, often the trunk or groin. Although the exact mechanism is unknown, it is generally believed to be a thermoregulatory mechanism of compensation for loss of gland secretion from the denervated area. However, newer literature suggests that the changes in sweating patterns can be attributed to a reflex response by the hypothalamus, and thus the term "reflex sweating" may be more appropriate [27].

The rates of CH are quite variable but tend to be lower when ETS is performed for palmar hyperhidrosis versus axillary or facial hyperhidrosis, resulting in decreased satisfaction despite resolution of the initial symptoms [44]. Much of the variability among published rates of CH stems from the heterogeneous patient populations, different level(s) of interruption, and discrepancies in the definition of CH [13]. The severity of CH can be classified as mild (sweating in small amounts without embarrassment), moderate, or severe (sweating in large amounts requiring clothing changes throughout the day) [24]. In one study, a minority of patients who reported moderate-to-severe CH were dissatisfied with the results of their procedure [41]. Interestingly, another study demonstrated a substantial decrease in severe CH following clip removal (median time of 11 months after ETS) with nearly half maintaining resolution of their initial hyperhidrosis [45]. Other authors suggest that children tolerate thoracic sympathectomy better than adults and may have a lower incidence of CH [42, 44]. Literature shows that the most important risk factors associated with bothersome CH include the level of interruption and presence of multiple sweating sites preoperatively (back, buttocks, inguinal folds, and upper thighs) [46]. The data suggest that decreased rates of CH can be accomplished by interrupting the chain at a lower level as well as a single segment and by avoiding the T2 ganglion [13, 24, 47].

Horner's syndrome is another complication which has been reported to occur transiently in 0–23 % of cases often associated with traction injury or inflammation and permanently in 0–6 % of cases [48, 49]. Horner's syndrome consists of miosis, ptosis, hyperemia of the eye, enophthalmos, and anhidrosis of half the patient's face. The greatest risk of injury occurs when dissection is performed above the second rib near the stellate ganglion in cases where the anatomy is incorrectly defined or when managing craniofacial hyperhidrosis. The risk of injury to stellate ganglion can be minimized by maintaining instrumentation below the second rib. However, the surgeon must be especially cautious in the left hemithorax as the stellate ganglion may be more caudal on this side, possibly involving R3 [13]. And as mentioned previously, using the cautery sparingly will help ensure a lower likelihood of inadvertent spread to the stellate ganglion.

Permanent bradycardia has also been reported after surgery for hyperhidrosis as a result of loss of sympathetic fibers traveling through the upper thoracic ganglia to the heart. Fortunately, although there is a decrease in the resting heart rate, patients (excluding competitive athletes) largely remain asymptomatic without a significant change in exercise capacity and the cardiorespiratory response to exercise [50, 51]. However, STS expert consensus recommend the risk of permanent bradycardia be fully discussed with patients who present with a resting heart rate less than 55 beats per minute, as there have been reports of patients requiring a pacemaker [13].

Summary

- Primary focal hyperhidrosis refers to pathologically excessive sweating that may occur in the axillae, palms, soles, or craniofacial region. It can be truly disabling, and so we promote thoracoscopic sympathectomy as early definitive treatment.
- For patients with palmar hyperhidrosis, provide parents the option of an R3 or an R4 disruption after advising them of the overly dry hands and an increased risk of CH seen with a R3 interruption as well as a lower rate of CH but the possibility of slightly moister hands associated with an R4 interruption.
- For patients with an axillary component to their hyperhidrosis, perform an interruption at both R4 and R5 most typically.
- Sharp dissection and interruption of the sympathetic chain is preferred in an effort to reduce risk of inadvertent stellate ganglion injury.
- The "tuck" technique (described above) after burning the distal end is accepted for minimizing nerve regrowth and should be employed whenever possible.
- In general, an interruption at a lower level is associated with decreased rates of CH and Horner's syndrome.

References

1. Hashmonai M, Kopelman D. History of sympathetic surgery. Clin Auton Res. 2003;13 Suppl 1:I6–9.
2. Alexander W. The treatment of epilepsy. Edinburgh: Pentland; 1889.
3. Kotzareff A. Resection partielle du tronc sympathique cervical droit pour hyperhidrose unilaterate (regions faciale, cervicale, thoracique et brachiale droites). Rev Med Suisse Rom. 1920;40:111–3.
4. Hughes J. Endothoracic sympathectomy. Proc R Soc Med. 1942;35(9):585–6.

5. Kux M. Thoracic endoscopic sympathectomy in palmar and axillary hyperhidrosis. Arch Surg. 1978;113(3):264–6.
6. Hornberger J, Grimes K, Naumann M, Glaser DA, Lowe NJ, Naver H, et al. Recognition, diagnosis, and treatment of primary focal hyperhidrosis. J Am Acad Dermatol. 2004;51(2):274–86.
7. Strutton DR, Kowalski JW, Glaser DA, Stang PE. US prevalence of hyperhidrosis and impact on individuals with axillary hyperhidrosis: results from a national survey. J Am Acad Dermatol. 2004;51(2):241–8.
8. Adar R, Kurchin A, Zweig A, Mozes M. Palmar hyperhidrosis and its surgical treatment: a report of 100 cases. Ann Surg. 1977;186(1):34–41.
9. Li X, Chen R, Tu YR, Lin M, Lai FC, Li YP, et al. Epidemiological survey of primary palmar hyperhidrosis in adolescents. Chin Med J. 2007;120(24):2215–7.
10. Ro KM, Cantor RM, Lange KL, Ahn SS. Palmar hyperhidrosis: evidence of genetic transmission. J Vasc Surg. 2002;35(2):382–6.
11. Altman RS, Schwartz RA. Emotionally induced hyperhidrosis. Cutis. 2002;69(5):336–8.
12. Drott C, Gothberg G, Claes G. Endoscopic transthoracic sympathectomy: an efficient and safe method for the treatment of hyperhidrosis. J Am Acad Dermatol. 1995;33(1):78–81.
13. Cerfolio RJ, De Campos JR, Bryant AS, Connery CP, Miller DL, DeCamp MM, et al. The Society of Thoracic Surgeons expert consensus for the surgical treatment of hyperhidrosis. Ann Thorac Surg. 2011;91(5):1642–8.
14. Vazquez LD, Staples NL, Sears SF, Klodell CT. Psychosocial functioning of patients after endoscopic thoracic sympathectomy. Eur J Cardiothorac Surg. 2011;39(6):1018–21.
15. Gelbard CM, Epstein H, Hebert A. Primary pediatric hyperhidrosis: a review of current treatment options. Pediatr Dermatol. 2008;25(6):591–8.
16. Baumgartner FJ, Bertin S, Konecny J. Superiority of thoracoscopic sympathectomy over medical management for the palmoplantar subset of severe hyperhidrosis. Ann Vasc Surg. 2009;23(1):1–7.
17. Wang YC, Sun MH, Lin CW, Chen YJ. Anatomical location of T2-3 sympathetic trunk and Kuntz nerve determined by transthoracic endoscopy. J Neurosurg. 2002;96(1 Suppl):68–72.
18. Schiller Y. The anatomy and physiology of the sympathetic innervation to the upper limbs. Clin Auton Res. 2003;13 Suppl 1:I2–5.
19. Yarzebski JL, Wilkinson HA. T2 and T3 sympathetic ganglia in the adult human: a cadaver and clinical-radiographic study and its clinical application. Neurosurgery. 1987;21(3):339–42.
20. Ramsaroop L, Singh B, Moodley J, Partab P, Satyapal KS. Anatomical basis for a successful upper limb sympathectomy in the thoracoscopic era. Clin Anat. 2004;17(4):294–9.
21. Kuntz A. Distribution of the sympathetic rami to the brachial plexus: its relation to sympathectomy affecting the upper extremity. Arch Surg. 1927;15(6):871–7.
22. Singh B, Moodley J, Ramdial PK, Ramsaroop L, Satyapal KS. Pitfalls in thoracoscopic sympathectomy: mechanisms for failure. Surg Laparosc Endosc Percutan Tech. 2001;11(6):364–7.

23. Ramsaroop L, Partab P, Singh B, Satyapal KS. Thoracic origin of a sympathetic supply to the upper limb: the 'nerve of Kuntz' revisited. J Anat. 2001;199(Pt 6):675–82.
24. Liu Y, Yang J, Liu J, Yang F, Jiang G, Li J, et al. Surgical treatment of primary palmar hyperhidrosis: a prospective randomized study comparing T3 and T4 sympathicotomy. Eur J Cardiothorac Surg. 2009;35(3):398–402.
25. Chang YT, Li HP, Lee JY, Lin PJ, Lin CC, Kao EL, et al. Treatment of palmar hyperhidrosis: T(4) level compared with T(3) and T(2). Ann Surg. 2007;246(2):330–6.
26. Munia MA, Wolosker N, Kauffman P, de Campos JR, Puech-Leao P. A randomized trial of T3-T4 versus T4 sympathectomy for isolated axillary hyperhidrosis. J Vasc Surg. 2007;45(1):130–3.
27. Chou SH, Kao EL, Lin CC, Chang YT, Huang MF. The importance of classification in sympathetic surgery and a proposed mechanism for compensatory hyperhidrosis: experience with 464 cases. Surg Endosc. 2006;20(11):1749–53.
28. Wolfer RS, Krasna MJ, Hasnain JU, McLaughlin JS. Hemodynamic effects of carbon dioxide insufflation during thoracoscopy. Ann Thorac Surg. 1994;58(2):404–7. discussion 7–8.
29. Krasna MJ. Thoracoscopic sympathectomy: a standardized approach to therapy for hyperhidrosis. Ann Thorac Surg. 2008;85(2):S764–7.
30. Yanagihara TK, Ibrahimiye A, Harris C, Hirsch J, Gorenstein LA. Analysis of clamping versus cutting of T3 sympathetic nerve for severe palmar hyperhidrosis. J Thorac Cardiovasc Surg. 2010;140(5):984–9.
31. Hynes CF, Yamaguchi S, Bond CD, Marshall MB. Reversal of sympathetic interruption by removal of clips. Ann Thorac Surg. 2015;99(3):1020–3.
32. Chung IH, Oh CS, Koh KS, Kim HJ, Paik HC, Lee DY. Anatomic variations of the T2 nerve root (including the nerve of Kuntz) and their implications for sympathectomy. J Thorac Cardiovasc Surg. 2002;123(3):498–501.
33. Gossot D, Toledo L, Fritsch S, Celerier M. Thoracoscopic sympathectomy for upper limb hyperhidrosis: looking for the right operation. Ann Thorac Surg. 1997;64(4):975–8.
34. Kim DH, Hong YJ, Hwang JJ, Kim KD, Lee DY. Topographical considerations under video-scope guidance in the T3,4 levels sympathetic surgery. Eur J Cardiothorac Surg. 2008;33(5):786–9.
35. Reisfeld R. Azygos lobe in endoscopic thoracic sympathectomy for hyperhidrosis. Surg Endosc. 2005;19(7):964–6.
36. Kauffman P, Wolosker N, de Campos JR, Yazbek G, Jatene FB. Azygos lobe: a difficulty in video-assisted thoracic sympathectomy. Ann Thorac Surg. 2010;89(6):e57–9.
37. Sinha CK, Kiely E. Thoracoscopic sympathectomy for palmar hyperhidrosis in children: 21 years of experience at a tertiary care center. Eur J Pediatr Surg. 2013;23(6):486–9.
38. Herbst F, Plas EG, Fugger R, Fritsch A. Endoscopic thoracic sympathectomy for primary hyperhidrosis of the upper limbs. A critical analysis and long-term results of 480 operations. Ann Surg. 1994;220(1):86–90.

39. Gossot D, Galetta D, Pascal A, Debrosse D, Caliandro R, Girard P, et al. Long-term results of endoscopic thoracic sympathectomy for upper limb hyperhidrosis. Ann Thorac Surg. 2003;75(4):1075–9.
40. Yazbek G, Wolosker N, de Campos JR, Kauffman P, Ishy A, Puech-Leao P. Palmar hyperhidrosis--which is the best level of denervation using video-assisted thoracoscopic sympathectomy: T2 or T3 ganglion? J Vasc Surg. 2005;42(2):281–5.
41. Wolosker N, de Campos JR, Kauffman P, de Oliveira LA, Munia MA, Jatene FB. Evaluation of quality of life over time among 453 patients with hyperhidrosis submitted to endoscopic thoracic sympathectomy. J Vasc Surg. 2012;55(1):154–6.
42. Steiner Z, Cohen Z, Kleiner O, Matar I, Mogilner J. Do children tolerate thoracoscopic sympathectomy better than adults? Pediatr Surg Int. 2008;24(3):343–7.
43. Neves S, Uchoa PC, Wolosker N, Munia MA, Kauffman P, de Campos JR, et al. Long-term comparison of video-assisted thoracic sympathectomy and clinical observation for the treatment of palmar hyperhidrosis in children younger than 14. Pediatr Dermatol. 2012;29(5):575–9.
44. Bell D, Jedynak J, Bell R. Predictors of outcome following endoscopic thoracic sympathectomy. ANZ J Surg. 2014;84(1–2):68–72.
45. Sugimura H, Spratt EH, Compeau CG, Kattail D, Shargall Y. Thoracoscopic sympathetic clipping for hyperhidrosis: long-term results and reversibility. J Thorac Cardiovasc Surg. 2009;137(6):1370–6. discussion 6–7.
46. Bryant AS, Cerfolio RJ. Satisfaction and compensatory hyperhidrosis rates 5 years and longer after video-assisted thoracoscopic sympathotomy for hyperhidrosis. J Thorac Cardiovasc Surg. 2014;147(4):1160–3. e1.
47. de Campos JR, Kauffman P, Werebe Ede C, Andrade Filho LO, Kusniek S, Wolosker N, et al. Quality of life, before and after thoracic sympathectomy: report on 378 operated patients. Ann Thorac Surg. 2003;76(3):886–91.
48. Ahn SS, Machleder HI, Concepcion B, Moore WS. Thoracoscopic cervicodorsal sympathectomy: preliminary results. J Vasc Surg. 1994;20(4):511–7. discussion 7–9.
49. Kopelman D, Hashmonai M, Ehrenreich M, Bahous H, Assalia A. Upper dorsal thoracoscopic sympathectomy for palmar hyperhidrosis: improved intermediate-term results. J Vasc Surg. 1996;24(2):194–9.
50. Inbar O, Leviel D, Shwartz I, Paran H, Whipp BJ. Thoracic sympathectomy and cardiopulmonary responses to exercise. Eur J Appl Physiol. 2008;104(1):79–86.
51. Noppen M, Dendale P, Hagers Y, Herregodts P, Vincken W, D'Haens J. Changes in cardiocirculatory autonomic function after thoracoscopic upper dorsal sympathicolysis for essential hyperhidrosis. J Auton Nerv Syst. 1996;60(3):115–20.

10. Thoracoscopic Treatment of Pectus Excavatum: The Nuss Procedure

Barrett P. Cromeens and Michael J. Goretsky

Introduction

Epidemiology

Pectus excavatum is the most common chest wall deformity affecting up to 1 % of the population [1–3]. It can be observed at any stage of life from infancy to adulthood but is often noticed during adolescence when accelerated growth exacerbates the defect. The distribution varies by racial demographic in the USA with white infants more commonly affected than black infants [4]. Boys are more commonly affected than girls by as much as 4:1. It is commonly clustered within families with as many as 43 % of patients having some family history of chest wall deformities [5, 6]. Although not proven to be causative, pectus excavatum is observed more often with other musculoskeletal deformities and connective tissue disorders [7, 8].

Pathophysiology

No definitive cause for pectus excavatum has been established. Theories regarding a cause are varied including costochondral dysgenesis, abnormalities of the diaphragm, intrauterine pressure, rickets, genetic predisposition, and abnormalities of the connective tissue [5, 6, 8–12]. The most widely accepted theory was that discordant growth between the ribs and costal cartilages exacerbated by the accelerated growth during adolescence resulted in pushing the sternum inward [10]. This theory has more recently been drawn into question by computed tomography imaging demonstrating

D.S. Walsh et al. (eds.), *The SAGES Manual of Pediatric Minimally Invasive Surgery*, DOI 10.1007/978-3-319-43642-5_10

no difference in costochondral length in laterality of patients with asymmetric defect [13]. There is clustering within families and multiple inheritance patterns have been identified in specific families [5, 6]. However, no specific genetic cause has been identified, and most families with evidence of genetic predisposition demonstrate multifactorial inheritance. Biochemical and genetic analysis of costal cartilages in patients with pectus excavatum have shown differences in makeup and collagen gene regulation compared to the control tissue, but again, no discrete defects have been identified [8, 9, 14]. Further investigation into the genetic and metabolic findings is necessary to elucidate the true cause of this defect.

Preoperative Evaluation

History

Any patient who is referred for pectus excavatum should undergo a full history and physical examination. Presenting symptoms may be varied with the most common being concerns regarding chest wall appearance, shortness of breath and/or chest pain with exercise, and endurance-related issues. Questioning should investigate the progression of the defect, chest pain or shortness of breath at rest or with exertion, fatigue, frequency of upper respiratory infections, palpitations, history of known cardiac or connective tissue disorders, a full family history, and psychosocial factors associated with poor body image. Defects are commonly present during infancy and childhood but often experience rapid progression during adolescence. Some may not manifest until puberty. Patients may experience pain or soreness at the site of the defect as well as subjective exercise fatigue. Cardiac abnormalities and connective tissue disorder are not uncommon with pectus abnormalities, and many patients will have family members that have suffered the same deformities. If surgical correction is anticipated, make sure to investigate metal allergies as patients with metal allergy will require placement of a titanium bar which necessitates preoperative fabrication specific to their anatomy.

Exam

Upon entering the room, first take notice of the patient's general appearance and posture. Patients with this deformity often have an asthenic habitus and slumped posture. In addition to a full physical examination, take a focused examination of the defect. The defect should be examined with the patient lying down and standing upright. Photographs are helpful to track improvements over time if the patient is participating in an exercise and positioning regimen or to compare before and after surgical intervention. Take care to note the extent of the deformity, where it begins superiorly and ends inferiorly, the depth, and look for any asymmetry. These aspects may affect preoperative planning and the necessity for multiple bars. Ensure that the patient does not have Currarino-Silverman deformity where the sternomanubrial joint is prominent with relative depression of the distal sternum. This is often referred to a surgeon as a pectus excavatum but is truly a variant of pectus carinatum. This defect is not amenable to minimally invasive repair. Examine the spine as upward of 15 % will have scoliosis [7]. On cardiac auscultation, listen for systolic clicks or flow murmurs as some patients have associated mitral valve prolapse from anterior compression of the heart from the sternum.

Labs/Imaging/Other Tests

No specific laboratory tests are necessary for pectus excavatum unless patient comorbidities necessitate further workup. All patients who are candidates for the Nuss procedure should have routine metal allergy testing. At present allergEAZE (Smart Practice Dermatology®) dermal patch tests for most of the major and minor components found in the Nuss bar [15]. At a minimum the patient should have an anteroposterior and lateral chest X-ray performed to document the severity of the defect. Numerous measures have been proposed to quantify the severity of a pectus excavatum defect although the most commonly used is the Haller CT index [16]. This method is expressed as a ratio between the transverse and AP diameters of the chest as measured on CT scan or MRI. Although developed with CT scanning, similar measures can be obtained off of conventional radiographs. A ratio of greater than 3.25 is considered severe. Although not required, chest CT or MRI can provide both accurate measures for defect severity and anatomic information specific to the patient, including displacement of mediastinal structures and the extent of cardiac compression. If the patient has a metal allergy, a CT or MRI scan is absolutely necessary as it will be used to design and fabricate their patient-specific titanium implants. Pulmonary function tests should be performed to demonstrate any restrictive or obstructive impairment. Electrocardiogram and echocardiogram should also be performed. Electrocardiogram will demonstrate any conduction abnormalities, while the echocardiogram will evaluate the extent of cardiac compression and any structural abnormalities such as mitral valve prolapse or aortic root dilatation.

Surgical Indications

Criteria for surgical indications in pectus excavatum have been varied in the past, but more objective criteria have been demonstrated and practiced in most centers [2, 17–20]. It is generally agreed that surgery should be avoided in patients with mild-to-moderate defects and should be managed with a rigorous exercise program with postural training. These patients should be followed every 6–12 months to monitor progression. Two or more of the following are considered surgical indications: (1) CT findings showing cardiac or pulmonary compression with a Haller index >3.25; (2) pulmonary function testing consistent with restrictive or obstructive lung disease; (3) cardiac testing revealing cardiac compression, mitral valve prolapse, murmur, aberrant conduction, or displacement; (4) progressive deformity with worsening subjective symptoms; and (5) failure of previous repair [17, 19, 21]. Other considerations include the severity of concerns over body image. Once the decision to operate has been made, appropriate operative timing should be considered. The minimally invasive technique has been applied to patients ranging from 1 year of age to 31 with positive results [22]. The ideal age for minimally invasive repair is early adolescence when the chest is the most flexible (10–14 years) [18]. However, equally good results are obtained in the adult patient, although they may have increased pain and recovery due to their age [22, 23].

Surgical Technique

Special Considerations

As previously mentioned, patients with proven metal allergies should not receive placement of the standard bar. Failure to recognize patients with metal allergy prior to placement results in an inflammatory reaction often confused for infection and may require bar removal [24]. These patients will require a preoperative CT scan or MRI since the titanium bar needs to be custom bent due to the porosity of the metal.

Asymmetric defects and patients with connective tissue disorders are often much more challenging to repair. If there is any doubt that a single bar is not adequate to correct the defect, a second bar should be appropriately placed. Multiple bars are frequently required in patients with a stiff chest (the older patient), asymmetric defects, and saucer/elongated shaped defects.

Instruments

A thoracoscope aids in the dissection and facilitates a safe dissection. Most surgeons will use a 5-mm thoracoscope with a 30-degree lens, but that will be the surgeon preference. As most intrathoracic visualization can be seen through a single right-sided port alone, only one 5-mm trocar should be needed. However, a second trocar should be available in the instance that better left-sided visualization be needed. If bilateral thoracoscopy is performed, care should be taken to avoid bilateral insufflation to minimize a tension physiology. Instruments developed specifically for this procedure include the Biomet® introducer (Biomet Microfixation, Jacksonville, FL) and the bar flipper. The Biomet® introducer is a long narrow blade used for the intrathoracic dissection. The distal end is curved, allowing the introducer to hug the posterior portion of the sternum and make the sharp turn behind the pectus defect. This introducer comes in three sizes and all sizes should be available. The extra-large introducer is very helpful in very deep defects and those with severe torsion. The bar flippers fit on either end of the pectus bar and act as a wrench, allowing the surgeon to flip the bar 180° after its insertion. Other materials that are necessary include appropriately sized pectus bars, bar stabilizers, a Zimmer bar bender, and umbilical tape. The appropriately sized bar should be determined during the preoperative planning phase.

Positioning

The patient is placed in the supine position and secured on the table. General endotracheal anesthesia is induced, and both arms are abducted at the shoulders, allowing access to the lateral chest wall on both sides. Ensure that the arms are adequately abducted so as not to obstruct the thoracoscope once inserted but not so far as to increase the possibility for brachial plexus palsy. With the patient adequately positioned, the chest is sterilely prepped and draped. Draping should be wide from just below clavicles superiorly to below the inferior rib margin inferiorly. Laterally the drapes should be posterior to the mid-axillary line granting adequate access to the lateral chest walls for bar placement. While this is being done, the patient should receive an appropriate dose of a first generation cephalosporin such as cefazolin.

Anatomy

The pectus excavatum deformity involves the sternum and lower costal cartilages; it is rare for the defect to extend above the third costal cartilage. The defects can be midline or asymmetric. The more severe defects will often displace mediastinal structures to the left chest and are the reason for a right-sided surgical approach. With the drapes in place, the external anatomy can be inspected and appropriately marked for bar placement (Fig. 10.1). Meticulous inspection of the anatomy for appropriate placement of the pectus bar is paramount to a successful repair.

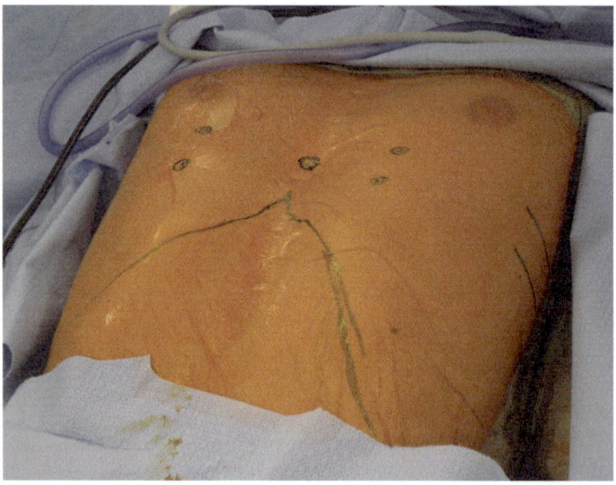

Fig. 10.1. External marking of the pertinent anatomy after the patient is prepped and draped. This patient is marked out for potentially two bars. The deepest point of the defect is noted by the large central point. The inferior costal margin has been marked below for orientation. The intercostal spaces that will be used to pass the pectus bars through the thoracic cavity are also marked. The cephalad intercostal markings correspond with the bar that will pass under the deepest point of the defect. Courtesy of Dr. Brian Kenney at Nationwide Children's Hospital.

First, the deepest portion of the pectus defect should be marked. Next, the horizontal planes that correspond to the intercostal spaces should be marked. It is imperative that if only using one bar that the horizontal plane rests under the sternum, even if the greatest depression is inferior to this. If using two bars it is okay if one does not rest under the sternum. The planned entrance and exit sites should be marked and these MUST be medial to the pectus ridge. If they are lateral to the highest point of the pectus ridge, the muscles will strip and the pectus defect will recur. The incision will be made in the corresponding horizontal plane, usually from the anterior to mid-axillary line.

The size of the bar is selected by measuring from the right to the left mid-axillary line at the greatest depression and subtracting 1–1.5 in. The bar should then be pre-bent for optimal configuration to the patient's chest. A semicircular shape with a short flat central apex and gentle convex curve is most commonly used for all patients. Too angulated or a "tabletop" configuration will make for an unstable bar.

Steps

With the patient positioned, draped, marked, and the pectus bar formed to fit, the surgical procedure can begin. It is beneficial to start with thoracoscopy to confirm the internal anatomy prior to the substernal dissection. A small incision, large enough to accommodate a 5-mm trocar, is placed two intercostal spaces below the right lateral bar incision. The 5-mm trocar is placed and a 5-mm fiber-optic scope with a 30-degree angle of visualization is inserted into the thoracic cavity. Adequate visualization can usually be obtained with controlled ventilation by anesthesiology utilizing lower tidal volumes. CO_2 insufflation of 5–6 mmHg can be utilized to increase visibility. Utilizing external palpation and internal visualization, the intercostal space previously marked for bar insertion is identified. Two lateral transverse incisions are made on either side of the chest wall. The incisions begin at the mid-axillary line and extend anteriorly 2–3 cm. If using two bars, one or two incisions can be made depending on the surgeon preference. The incision is carried down through the subcutaneous tissues to the chest wall. Once down to the chest wall, small subcutaneous flaps are raised circumferentially to accommodate the end of the pectus bar and the bar stabilizers. A subcutaneous tunnel is then created anteriorly along the chest wall extending to the previously marked points medial to the pectus ridge. This will be the site of entry into the thoracic cavity for the pectus bar. If the pectoralis muscle is present in the horizontal plane, it is preferable to make the tunnel beneath the muscle.

With thoracoscopic visualization, a tonsil clamp is used to enter the right side via the previously dissected tunnel. It is imperative to enter the chest medial to the highest point on the pectus ridge. The pectus introducer is then inserted into the pleural cavity through the previous tunnel and advanced beneath the sternum. Once in the thoracic cavity, the introducer is advanced and turned 180° so that the convexity is directed posteriorly and the tip anteriorly (Fig. 10.2). This keeps the tip directed away from the heart and other mediastinal structures, reducing the likelihood for injury. The introducer tip is then used to locate the bloodless dissection plane between the posterior sternum and the pericardium (Fig. 10.3). Using blunt dissection, the introducer is advanced until the left lateral mark on the pectus ridge is identified again through external palpation and internal visualization. The introducer is then advanced through the appropriate intercostal space (medial to the pectus ridge) into the left-sided subcutaneous tunnel and subsequently delivered through the left lateral incision (Fig. 10.4). It is critical to keep the introducer tip in view at all times to minimize cardiac injury. Various techniques of sternal elevation that have been described can facilitate this dissection and are a must if one cannot see the tip [25–27]. Bilateral thoracoscopy can also be utilized if one cannot

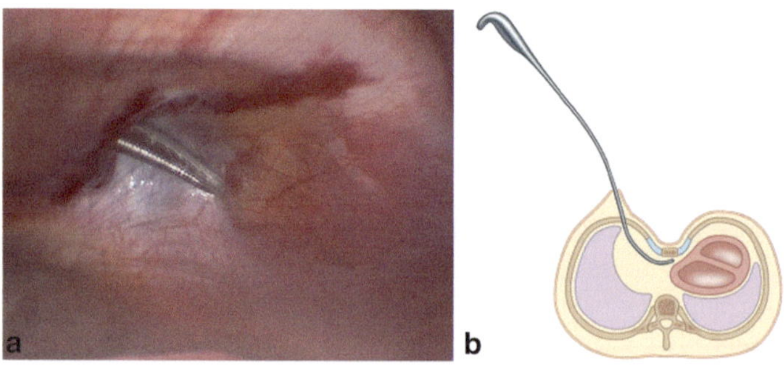

Fig. 10.2. Passing the introducer into the thoracic cavity. (**a**) A tonsil clamp is used to enter the thoracic cavity through the previously determined intercostal space at a point just medial to the pectus ridge. The introducer is passed through the tunnel created by the tonsil clamp with the tip pointed posteriorly and the convexity oriented anteriorly. (**b**) Once the introducer is in the thoracic cavity, it is turned 180° so that the tip is directed anteriorly. This protects the heart and other mediastinal structures during the dissection. This also utilizes the distal curvature of the introducer to make the turn behind the pectus defect. Courtesy of Dr. Brian Kenney at Nationwide Children's Hospital.

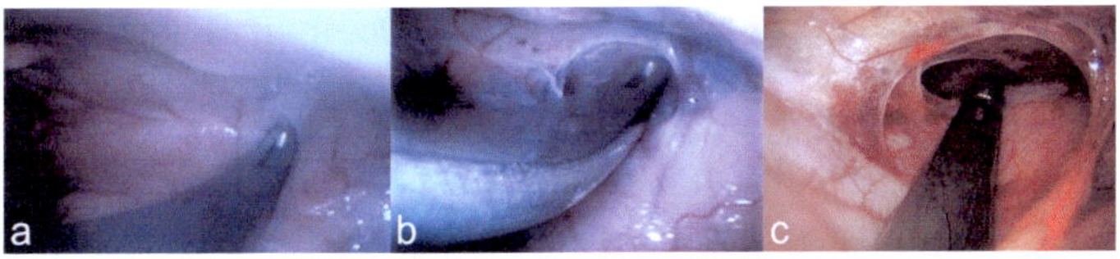

Fig. 10.3. Retrosternal dissection. The tip of the introducer is used to progressively dissect the bloodless plane between the posterior surface of the sternum and the pericardium as shown in panels (**a**) through (**c**). Note that the tip of the introducer is always directed anteriorly and in view at all times so as to avoid cardiac or pericardial injury.

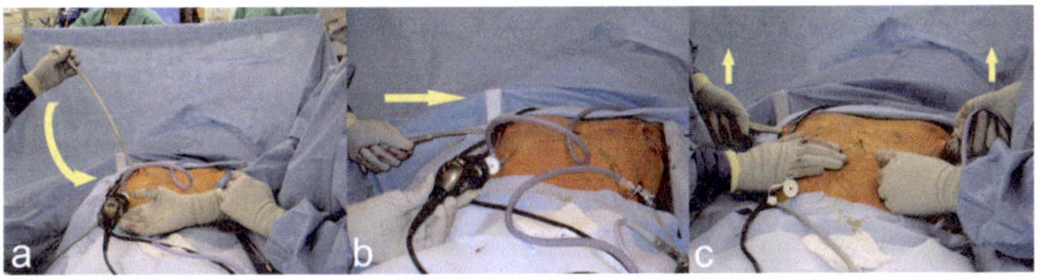

Fig. 10.4. Completion of the intrathoracic dissection. (**a**) With the exit point for the introducer identified, the handle of the introducer is dropped toward the floor, forcing the tip anteriorly through the intercostal space. (**b**) Once through the chest wall, the introducer is advanced through the left-sided subcutaneous tunnel and delivered through the left lateral incision. (**c**) Both ends of the introducer are then grasped and lifted to correct the defect and help remodel the chest wall. Courtesy of Dr. Brian Kenney at Nationwide Children's Hospital.

visualize the space between the heart and sternum in very severe defects with torsion.

With the path of the pectus bar defined by the introducer, the ends of the introducer are grasped by the surgeon and assistant and elevated to correct the depression. This facilitates passing the bar and helps to remodel the chest. In cases with severe torsion and asymmetry, a very stiff chest upon elevating the introducer, or a very long defect that still has a residual depression with the introducer, a second bar should be placed. If a second bar is required, performing the more superior dissection and leaving the introducer in place facilitates the second dissection.

An umbilical tape adequate to traverse the length of the pectus bar path is attached to the islet on the end of the introducer and pulled through the thoracic cavity to the right side of the chest. This will act as a guide for the pectus bar as it is delivered through the tunnel. The umbilical tape is detached from the introducer and tied through the islet of the pectus bar.

Direct visualization with the camera and guidance from the umbilical tape allows the bar to be advanced through the intrathoracic tunnel. Care should be taken to ensure the bar is placed in the correct orientation corresponding to the preoperative molding. The bar should be passed with the convexity directed posteriorly, and once in place, the left and right sides of the bar should match the laterality of the preoperative molding. Once the bar is in place with the ends directed anteriorly, the bar is flipped 180° using even pressure on both ends of the bar using bar flippers (Fig. 10.5). Once the bar is turned, the defect will reverse and the ends should fall within the incisions. The bar should rest laterally on the muscle and not be too tight or too loose. There should be immediate correction of the defect. If there is a residual defect, a second bar is needed and can be placed above or below the initial bar using the same techniques.

Proper securing of the bar is mandatory to minimize flipping. If the first bar appears loose and unstable, then a second bar is required. Only one stabilizer should be placed for each bar to minimize discomfort with growth. In an adult patient who is done growing, bilateral stabilizers are satisfactory but usually not necessary. The stabilizer slides on either end of the bar, perpendicular to its axis, forming a cross. The subcutaneous flaps can be modified in order to accommodate the stabilizers. Once in place, the stabilizer should be affixed to the pectus bar using any permanent suture. If using two bars, the stabilizers should be staggered. Medial fixation further secures the bar [28]. This can be done by visualizing with thoracoscopy and attaching the bar to the underlying ribs using either an absorbable or permanent suture. The use of an absorbable suture will facilitate bar removal. The passage of the sutures is facilitated by using an Endoclose® needle (Covidien, Norwalk, CT) through the lateral thoracic incision under thoracoscopic guidance. Placing numerous absorbable

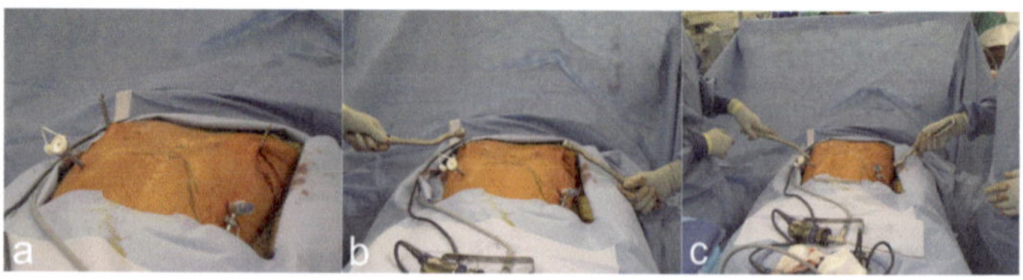

Fig. 10.5. Flipping the bar. (**a**) After the bar has been passed through the intrathoracic tunnel, the ends should be directed anteriorly. (**b**) The bar flippers are placed on either side of the bar. (**c**) Once the bar flippers are in place, even pressure on both ends will be used to flip the bar 180°, resulting in a correction of the defect. Courtesy of Dr. Brian Kenney at Nationwide Children's Hospital.

sutures through all the islets of the bar and stabilizer to the underlying fascia is the final point of fixation (Fig. 10.6).

After adequate hemostasis, the lateral incisions are closed in two layers with subcutaneous absorbable suture, followed by a skin closure of choice. Steristrips and a compressive, sterile dressing are placed. Once the incisions are closed, the CO_2 is evacuated. This can be performed by cutting the tubing to the trocar and placing it in a basin of sterile water that is below the level of the patient to create a water seal. The evacuation of CO_2 is facilitated by placing the patient in Trendelenburg with the left side down and administering multiple positive pressure breaths (Fig. 10.7). The air has been successfully evacuated

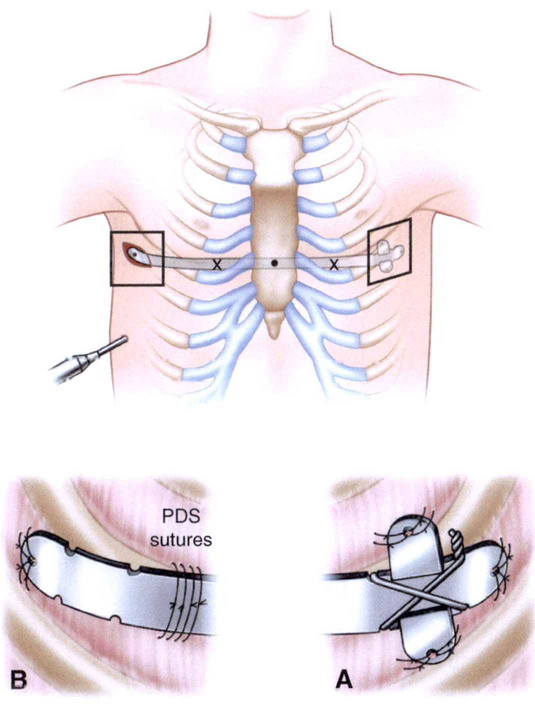

Fig. 10.6. Bar stabilizer and chest wall fixation. (**a**) With the bar in place, a stabilizer should be placed on one end. The stabilizer is affixed to the bar with a nonabsorbable suture. The eyelets in both the stabilizer and bar are used for suture fixation to the chest wall usually with an absorbable suture. (**b**) A third point of fixation is recommended by placing sutures around the bar and rib using thoracoscopic assistance. It is helpful to place these sutures around two separate ribs.

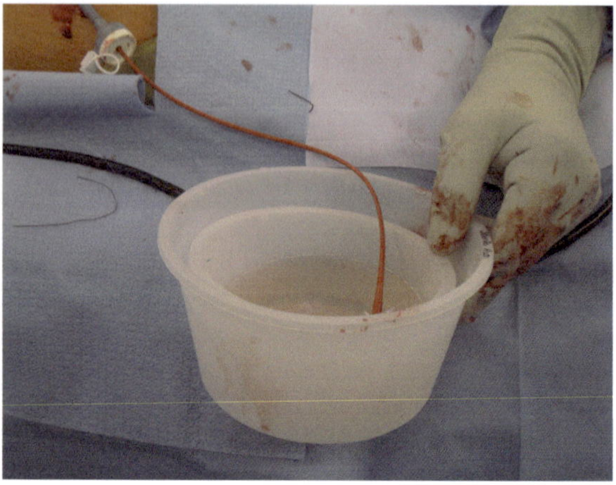

Fig. 10.7. CO_2 evacuation. A red rubber catheter is threaded through the port and placed in a saline or sterile water-filled basin below the level of the patient to create a water seal as shown here. Alternatively, the insufflation tubing for the port can be cut and used in place of the red rubber catheter. Positive pressure breaths are delivered from anesthesia until the CO_2 is evacuated as indicated by cessation of the bubbles. Courtesy of Dr. Brian Kenney at Nationwide Children's Hospital.

from the thoracic cavity when there is cessation of air bubbles. The trocar is removed and the incision closed in the same fashion as the two lateral bar incisions.

Pearls/Pitfalls

Successful repair of the pectus deformity begins with meticulous attention to the individual patient's anatomy and appropriate bar molding. Ensure that the anatomic landmarks stated above are utilized for appropriate placement and that the entrance and exit sites are medial to the greatest apex of the pectus ridge. However, if the defect is not appropriately reversed with the initial attempts, there should be no hesitation to place a second bar if needed. The central portion of the convexity should be relatively flat and should not be in a "tabletop" configuration. Creating a prominent apex increases the risk of bar dislodgment and overcorrection by creation of a pectus carinatum deformity. In asymmetric deformities, complete correction may not be achieved; although the bar placement reverses the sternal depression, it may not reverse the sternal rotation which often occurs in these types of defects. Vigorous elevation of the sternum with the introducer and placing a second bar significantly improves asymmetric defects, and the majority will look significantly better. During the intrathoracic portion of the case, finding the bloodless plane between the posterior surface of the sternum and the pericardium is key to avoiding cardiac injury or the less severe pericardial injury. This is best achieved through adequate visualization which can often be hindered by the more severe defects. Visualization can be improved by either placing a second camera port in the left chest if needed or through sternal elevation. Sternal elevation can be achieved by multiple techniques that have been described elsewhere [25–27]. Some have also suggested the use of a laparoscopic dissector in lieu of the Biomet introducer to dissect in the retrosternal space as it offers more fine and directed dissection [29].

Bar Removal

Bar removal is usually an outpatient procedure. The bars need to be in place for a minimum of 2 years. For complex patients, 3 years is ideal. The patient is brought to the operating room and placed on the table in supine position. The positioning and draping are identical to that for bar placement. Both sides of the chest are entered through the lateral incisions created for initial placement. The bar may have dense scar tissue encapsulating both ends. The incision is carried down through the subcutaneous tissue and surrounding scar tissue until both ends are completely mobilized. It is sometimes required to use a hammer and chisel to mobilize dense calcified scar tissue along with a bone rongeur. The stabilizer is removed first. Once the stabilizer is removed, it is recommended to partially straighten the bar to facilitate removal and minimize cardiac injury and bleeding. The bar should be fairly mobile prior to attempts at removal. This can be facilitated by rocking the bar. With anesthesia giving a positive breath, the bar should slide out easily from the patient's right side. The incisions are closed in two layers with subcutaneous absorbable sutures.

Postoperative Care

Reversal of anesthesia should be smooth so as to avoid bucking or vigorous movement. This increases the risk of dislodgement in the early postoperative period. A postoperative chest X-ray is performed in the post-anesthesia care unit or prior to waking up in the operating room to confirm appropriate bar placement and to ensure adequate evacuation of air. It is rare that a thoracostomy tube be placed for residual pneumothorax. Hospital stay is primarily dictated by control of pain. Any pain control methods within one's armamentarium may be used including patient-controlled analgesia, intravenous and oral narcotics, and nonsteroidal anti-inflammatory drugs. Physical therapy facilitates ambulation on post op day 2. The length of stay should be 4–5 days. The patient can return to school or work in 2–3 weeks with resumption of routine activities in 6 weeks. Resumption of the pectus breathing exercises and aerobic activity are strongly encouraged. After 3 months there are no restrictions except varsity-level contact sports where repetitive direct blows to the chest occur. These should be avoided while the bars are in place. Follow-up should be 2–4 weeks after the initial operation to ensure adequate healing and bar tolerance. They should be followed every year thereafter until the bars are removed.

Outcomes

Initially presented in 1997, the Nuss procedure has since been met with widespread acceptance and use. This has in part been due to the minimally invasive nature of the procedure and promising outcomes. Patient and family satisfaction are high with an expectation of a good or excellent cosmetic result in as much as 96 % of cases [5, 20, 22, 30–32]. Objectively, the minimally invasive approach significantly improves pulmonary function in patients who presented with deficits [33]. Recurrence rates should be low and roughly 1.5 % [22, 32]. A prospective multicenter trial has been performed evaluating the Nuss repair, but could not be compared with the open procedure due to inability to enroll patients in the open arm of the study secondary to patient preference [5].

Complications

Complications can be divided into early and late complications. Postoperative pneumothorax requiring chest tube insertion occurs in approximately 3 % of patients [18, 22]. Other procedure-specific early complications include hemothorax, pleural effusion, pericarditis, and pericardial or cardiac injury. These should occur in less than 1 % of patients. Pericarditis and pleural effusions have been associated with metal allergy and can be reduced through allergy testing [24]. Wound infections should be aggressively treated with adequate drainage and antibiotic therapy until ESR and CRP return to normal so as to avoid seeding of the hardware. Bar removal secondary to infection is rare with aggressive management. By far the most common late complication is bar displacement. Early attempts resulted in bar displacement in as many as 15 % of patients. However, the use of bar stabilizers and other techniques for bar fixation has resulted in reduction of this complication to less than 2 % [18, 19, 22, 28, 32]. Allergy to the bar can present at any time, early or late, and can manifest as a rash, pleural or pericardial effusions, pericarditis, and sterile abscess. These are often managed with oral steroids. It is uncommon that the allergy cannot be controlled requiring removal and replacement with a titanium bar. The routine testing of all patients for metal allergy will minimize this complication [15].

Summary

- Pectus excavatum is the most common anterior chest wall defect.
- This malady can be the source of significant physical and psychosocial morbidity requiring repair.
- The Nuss procedure was proposed as a minimally invasive approach to repair that avoids a large anterior incision and chest wall resection.
- Good or excellent results are achieved in 96 % of patients often with recurrence in only 1.5 %.

References

1. Williams AM, Crabbe DC. Pectus deformities of the anterior chest wall. Paediatr Respir Rev. 2003;4(3):237–42.
2. Adzick NS, Coran AG. Pediatric surgery. Philadelphia: Elsevier Mosby; 2012. Available from: http://VB3LK7EB4T.search.serialssolutions.com/?V=1.0&L=VB3LK7EB4T&S=JCs&C=TC0000629769&T=marc.
3. Westphal FL, Lima LC, Lima Neto JC, Chaves AR, Santos Junior VL, Ferreira BL. Prevalence of pectus carinatum and pectus excavatum in students in the city of Manaus, Brazil. J Bras Pneumol. 2009;35(3):221–6.
4. Chung CS, Myrianthopoulos NC. Factors affecting risks of congenital malformations. I. Analysis of epidemiologic factors in congenital malformations. Report from the Collaborative Perinatal Project. Birth Defects Orig Artic Ser. 1975;11(10):1–22.

5. Kelly Jr RE, Shamberger RC, Mellins RB, Mitchell KK, Lawson ML, Oldham K, et al. Prospective multicenter study of surgical correction of pectus excavatum: design, perioperative complications, pain, and baseline pulmonary function facilitated by internet-based data collection. J Am Coll Surg. 2007;205(2):205–16.
6. Creswick HA, Stacey MW, Kelly Jr RE, Gustin T, Nuss D, Harvey H, et al. Family study of the inheritance of pectus excavatum. J Pediatr Surg. 2006;41(10):1699–703.
7. Shamberger RC, Welch KJ. Surgical repair of pectus excavatum. J Pediatr Surg. 1988;23(7):615–22.
8. Tocchioni F, Ghionzoli M, Messineo A, Romagnoli P. Pectus excavatum and heritable disorders of the connective tissue. Pediatr Rep. 2013;5(3), e15.
9. Fokin AA, Steuerwald NM, Ahrens WA, Allen KE. Anatomical, histologic, and genetic characteristics of congenital chest wall deformities. Semin Thorac Cardiovasc Surg. 2009;21(1):44–57.
10. Sweet RH. Pectus excavatum: report of two cases successfully operated upon. Ann Surg. 1944;119(6):922–34.
11. Brodkin HA. Congenital anterior chest wall deformities of diaphragmatic origin. Dis Chest. 1953;24(3):259–77.
12. Chin EF. Surgery of funnel chest and congenital sternal prominence. Br J Surg. 1957;44(186):360–76.
13. Nakaoka T, Uemura S, Yano T, Nakagawa Y, Tanimoto T, Suehiro S. Does overgrowth of costal cartilage cause pectus excavatum? A study on the lengths of ribs and costal cartilages in asymmetric patients. J Pediatr Surg. 2009;44(7):1333–6.
14. Feng J, Hu T, Liu W, Zhang S, Tang Y, Chen R, et al. The biomechanical, morphologic, and histochemical properties of the costal cartilages in children with pectus excavatum. J Pediatr Surg. 2001;36(12):1770–6.
15. Shah B, Cohee A, Deyerle A, Kelly CS, Frantz F, Kelly RE, et al. High rates of metal allergy amongst Nuss procedure patients dictate broader pre-operative testing. J Pediatr Surg. 2014;49(3):451–4.
16. Haller Jr JA, Kramer SS, Lietman SA. Use of CT scans in selection of patients for pectus excavatum surgery: a preliminary report. J Pediatr Surg. 1987;22(10):904–6.
17. Frantz FW. Indications and guidelines for pectus excavatum repair. Curr Opin Pediatr. 2011;23(4):486–91.
18. Hebra A. Minimally invasive repair of pectus excavatum. Semin Thorac Cardiovasc Surg. 2009;21(1):76–84.
19. Nuss D, Kelly Jr RE. Indications and technique of Nuss procedure for pectus excavatum. Thorac Surg Clin. 2010;20(4):583–97.
20. Nuss D, Kelly Jr RE. Minimally invasive surgical correction of chest wall deformities in children (Nuss procedure). Adv Pediatr. 2008;55:395–410.
21. Kelly Jr RE. Pectus excavatum: historical background, clinical picture, preoperative evaluation and criteria for operation. Semin Pediatr Surg. 2008;17(3):181–93.
22. Kelly RE, Goretsky MJ, Obermeyer R, Kuhn MA, Redlinger R, Haney TS, et al. Twenty-one years of experience with minimally invasive repair of pectus excavatum by the Nuss procedure in 1215 patients. Ann Surg. 2010;252(6):1072–81.

23. Johnson WR, Fedor D, Singhal S. Systematic review of surgical treatment techniques for adult and pediatric patients with pectus excavatum. J Cardiothorac Surg. 2014;9:25.
24. Rushing GD, Goretsky MJ, Gustin T, Morales M, Kelly Jr RE, Nuss D. When it is not an infection: metal allergy after the Nuss procedure for repair of pectus excavatum. J Pediatr Surg. 2007;42(1):93–7.
25. Haecker FM, Sesia SB. Intraoperative use of the vacuum bell for elevating the sternum during the Nuss procedure. J Laparoendosc Adv Surg Tech A. 2012;22(9): 934–6.
26. Jaroszewski DE, Johnson K, McMahon L, Notrica D. Sternal elevation before passing bars: a technique for improving visualization and facilitating minimally invasive pectus excavatum repair in adult patients. J Thorac Cardiovasc Surg. 2014;147(3): 1093–5.
27. Rygl M, Vyhnanek M, Kucera A, Mixa V, Kyncl M, Snajdauf J. Technical innovation in minimally invasive repair of pectus excavatum. Pediatr Surg Int. 2014;30(1): 113–7.
28. Hebra A, Gauderer MW, Tagge EP, Adamson WT, Othersen Jr HB. A simple technique for preventing bar displacement with the Nuss repair of pectus excavatum. J Pediatr Surg. 2001;36(8):1266–8.
29. Noguchi M, Kondoh S, Fujita K. A simple and safe technique for manipulation of retrosternal dissection in the nuss procedure. Eplasty. 2014;14, e8.
30. Nuss D, Kelly Jr RE, Croitoru DP, Katz ME. A 10-year review of a minimally invasive technique for the correction of pectus excavatum. J Pediatr Surg. 1998;33(4): 545–52.
31. Croitoru DP, Kelly Jr RE, Goretsky MJ, Lawson ML, Swoveland B, Nuss D. Experience and modification update for the minimally invasive Nuss technique for pectus excavatum repair in 303 patients. J Pediatr Surg. 2002;37(3):437–45.
32. Sacco Casamassima MG, Goldstein SD, Salazar JH, McIltrot KH, Abdullah F, Colombani PM. Perioperative strategies and technical modifications to the Nuss repair for pectus excavatum in pediatric patients: a large volume, single institution experience. J Pediatr Surg. 2014;49(4):575–82.
33. Lawson ML, Mellins RB, Tabangin M, Kelly Jr RE, Croitoru DP, Goretsky MJ, et al. Impact of pectus excavatum on pulmonary function before and after repair with the Nuss procedure. J Pediatr Surg. 2005;40(1):174–80.

11. Thoracoscopic Approach to Eventration of the Diaphragm

Jingliang Yan and Federico G. Seifarth

Introduction

Diaphragmatic eventration is an abnormal elevation of part or all of the hemidiaphragm. This condition commonly involves the left side but can affect both sides. The congenital form occurs in less than 0.05 % live births and affects males 60–80 % of the time [1–4]. Associations with congenital heart disease [5] and gastric volvulus [6, 7] have been reported.

Despite similar clinical features, the etiologies of the congenital and the acquired forms are two distinct entities. The congenital, "true" diaphragmatic eventration is a structural deficiency of the muscular part of the diaphragm. The muscle fibers of diaphragm are thinned or even absent, and in the most extreme form, it is indistinguishable from congenital diaphragmatic hernia (CDH). Embryological studies suggest this to be a result of failure of muscularization, rather than embryonic component fusion defect [8]. The acquired form, or "diaphragmatic paralysis," is a result of phrenic nerve injury. Common causes are trauma during forceps delivery or injury during cardiac or thoracic surgery [9]. In the acquired form, the muscular portion of the diaphragm is, in fact, intact but dysfunctional.

Diaphragmatic eventration may be discovered as an incidental finding on chest radiographs obtained for other reasons but often presents with various degrees of respiratory distress that may even require mechanical ventilation. The underlying physiology includes ventilation/perfusion mismatch secondary to reduced lung volume on both sides of the thorax. On the diseased side, intra-abdominal contents reduce the space available for lung expansion within the chest cavity. The involved hemidiaphragm

D.S. Walsh et al. (eds.), *The SAGES Manual of Pediatric Minimally Invasive Surgery*, DOI 10.1007/978-3-319-43642-5_11

typically shows paradoxical upward movement during inspiration. The mediastinum shifts toward the contralateral side, compressing the other lung and further decreasing total lung capacity. The lung parenchyma itself is usually not hypoplastic, in contrast to CDH, and there is no pulmonary hypertension. Possible presentations include recurrent pneumonia and symptomatic dysphagia and reflux due to abnormal anatomy of the stomach.

Preoperative Evaluation

Congenital diaphragmatic eventration or hernia may be suspected on prenatal ultrasound after the second trimester. However, the diagnosis is usually suggested by plain X-ray after birth showing an elevated hemidiaphragm. A careful history of prenatal ultrasound showing diaphragmatic abnormalities, traumatic delivery, or prior cardiac or chest surgeries should be sought. On physical exam, paradoxical inward movement of the lower rib cage during inspiration (Hoover's sign) may be seen [10]. A formal PA and lateral chest X-ray should be done. Anatomically, the right hemidiaphragm is normally slightly higher than the left one. Elevation of left hemidiaphragm is suggestive of diaphragmatic eventration; however, this is quite nonspecific as a variety of other conditions may also produce this finding. Fluoroscopy or ultrasound may be utilized to look for paralysis or paradoxical upward movement of the hemidiaphragm during inspiration. While ultrasonography is a very useful tool to evaluate diaphragmatic motility, it can still be difficult to visualize the diaphragmatic dome with that modality. Older children may be asked to fully exhale after a full inhalation to assist with imaging. False negatives may be seen in ventilated patients as positive pressure ventilation tends to flatten the diaphragmatic dome. Once the diagnosis is established, the presence of symptoms guides the need for surgical repair. In the case of possibly reversible phrenic nerve injury, a trial of 2–4 weeks' nonoperative management should be considered. Preoperatively, an echocardiogram (ECHO) should be considered to rule out structural cardiac abnormalities in the congenital form of eventration.

Technique

Special Considerations

The principle of surgical correction centers on creating a taut diaphragm that prevents paradoxical movement during inspiration. Both, thoracic and abdominal approaches have been described, and for each approach, open and minimally invasive techniques are feasible. Traditionally, the surgical repair involves a posterolateral thoracotomy and diaphragmatic plication. In recent years, minimally invasive procedures have gained popularity due to its supposedly lower morbidity, faster recovery, and better wound appearance [11–13]. We favor the thoracoscopic approach, given its superior durability to the laparoscopic repair [14]. Special consideration is given to laparoscopic repair when there is intra-abdominal pathology that needs correction at the same time. In the case of right diaphragmatic eventration, plication should generally be performed thoracoscopically since the liver impedes the laparoscopic view. The video-assisted thoracic surgery (VATS) approach appears also to be safe for patients with congenital heart disease (CHD) who have undergone prior CHD repair [15].

Steps

The thoracoscopic operation is performed under general endotra cheal anesthesia; single-lung ventilation is rarely required. The patient is placed in a near-lateral decubitus position, leaving room for entry into the abdomen if laparotomy is needed (Fig. 11.1). Trocar placements are similar to congenital diaphragmatic repair, with the first 4-mm camera port in the third or fourth intercostal space in the posterior axillary line, and two additional 3-mm working sites (generally no port necessary) at fourth intercostal space anterior axillary line and sixth intercostal space mid-scapular line. Pneumothorax is achieved with 3–5 mmHg of CO_2 insufflation [16]. Intra-abdominal contents are gently reduced with a blunt grasper, taking care not to injure the bowel or any abdominal organ. Diaphragmatic plication is performed similar to an open approach with braided nonabsorbable sutures (Figs. 11.2 and 11.3). Many different ways have also been described to tighten the diaphragm, including “reefing”, “invaginating”, and “pleating”, all with similar results [17, 18].

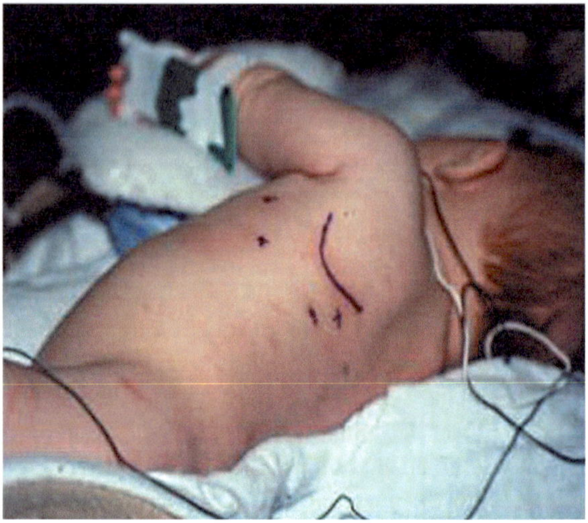

Fig. 11.1. Positioning of the patient in a lateral decubitus position with landmarks (scapular tip and intercostal spaces) cleared marked. From Rothenberg SS. Pediatric Thoracic Surgery. In: Pediatric Thoracic Surgery, Mario Lima, Ed. Springer 2013:63–70. Reprinted with permission.

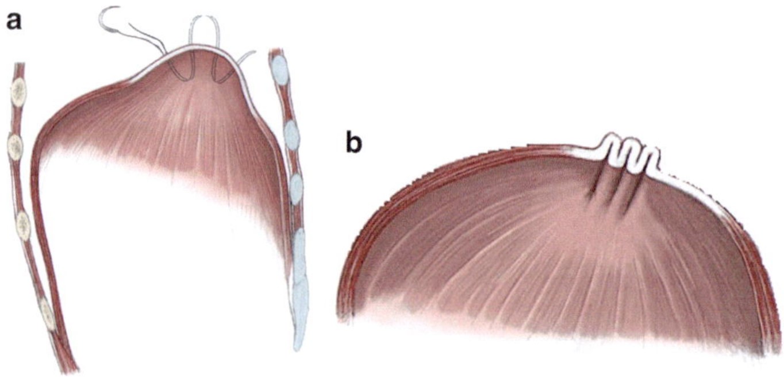

Fig. 11.2. Plication of the diaphragm. Nonabsorbable suture are passed multiple times through the diaphragm and tied (**a**), creating a taut diaphragmatic dome (**b**). From Puri P. Congenital Diaphragmatic Hernia and Eventration. In: Pediatric Surgery, Puri P. and Höllwarth ME, Eds. Springer Surgery Atlas Series 2006: 115–124. Reprinted with permission.

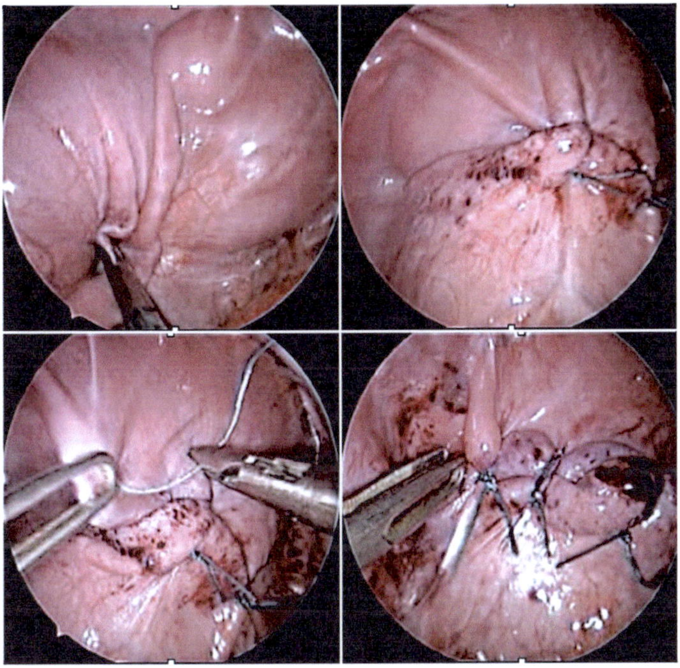

Fig. 11.3. Thoracoscopic view of diaphragmatic plication. From Molinaro F., et al. Diaphragmatic Eventration. In: Pediatric Thoracic Surgery, Mario Lima, Ed. Springer 2013: 233–238. Reprinted with permission.

Suturing technique choices are U stitches, horizontal mattress sutures, continuous running sutures, stapling, or variations of these methods [19]. Care must be taken not to injure or incorporate intra-abdominal organs or to damage branches of the phrenic nerve, which run in a medial to lateral course (Fig. 11.4). For congenital diaphragmatic eventration, the central portion that is severely thinned is usually excised to better visualize the diaphragmatic edge, and subsequent repair is identical to CDH repair with primary closure with nonabsorbable sutures, with the exception that no mesh is used. In the acquired form, no diaphragmatic excision is performed. At the conclusion of the operation, chest tubes are optional and not required routinely.

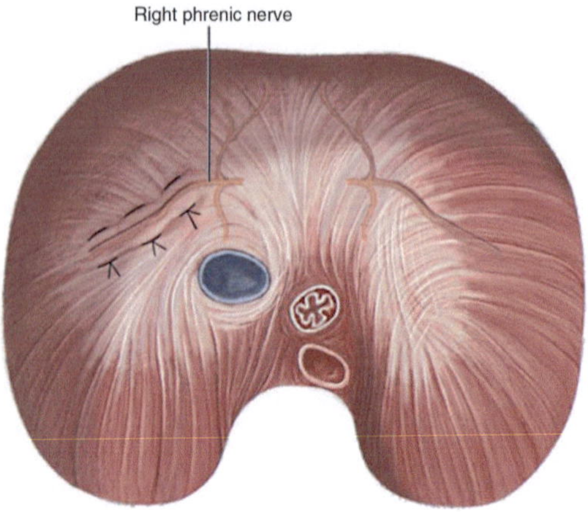

Fig. 11.4. Care is taken not to damage the phrenic nerve, which runs in a medial to lateral course. From Puri P. Congenital Diaphragmatic Hernia and Eventration. In: Pediatric Surgery, Puri P. and Höllwarth ME, Eds. Springer Surgery Atlas Series 2006: 115–124. Reprinted with permission.

Pearls and Pitfalls

- It is important to make sure that there is sufficient diaphragm overlap during repair that it is taut, as muscle fibers stretch invariably and recurrence will ensue.
- Ports must be placed cephalad enough to allow suturing.
- Before suturing it is important to lift the diaphragm off underlying structures like spleen or liver.
- If it is unclear whether bowel or peritoneal organs are involved in the suture line, consider placing a laparoscope.

Postoperative Care and Potential Complications

If patients do not require mechanical ventilation preoperatively, the majority of them (60–100 %) will be successfully extubated either immediately at the conclusion of the surgery or by the end of the day [14, 15, 20]. Infants who require ventilator support prior to surgery can be successfully weaned off ventilator within a week [17]. If a chest tube is inserted during surgery, it should remain until the output becomes less than 20 mL/day. Aggressive pulmonary toilet will aide in re-expansion of the lung. Normal exertion is usually achieved within 1 week of surgery [17, 20]. Feeding can be restarted within 48 h. Surgical treatment is usually very effective with no observed recurrence 1–3 years after the thoracoscopic approach in multiple series [5, 14, 15, 20–22]. The main complications include pneumonia, pleural effusions, and abdominal organ injury. Phrenic nerve injury, although rare, is usually of clinical insignificance.

Summary

- Diaphragmatic eventration can be congenital or acquired, although "true" congenital form is very rare.
- Symptomatic eventration with respiratory distress warrants surgical correction.
- Thoracoscopic diaphragmatic plication to render diaphragm taut is preferred with an excellent result.

References

1. Groth SS, Andrade RS. Diaphragmatic eventration. Thorac Surg Clin. 2009;19(4):511–9.
2. Chin EF, Lynn RB. Surgery of eventration of the diaphragm. J Thorac Surg. 1956;32(1):6–14.
3. Christensen P. Eventration of the diaphragm. Thorax. 1959;14:311–9.
4. McNamara JJ, Paulson DL, Urschel Jr HC, Razzuk MA. Eventration of the diaphragm. Surgery. 1968;64(6):1013–21.
5. Wu S, Zang N, Zhu J, Pan Z, Wu C. Congenital diaphragmatic eventration in children: 12 years' experience with 177 cases in a single institution. J Pediatr Surg. 2015;50(7):1088–92.
6. Oh A, Gulate G, Sherman ML, Golub R, Kutin N. Bilateral eventration of the diaphragm with perforated gastric volvulus in an adolescent. J Pediatr Surg. 2000;35(12):1824–6.
7. Byun J, Kum HY, Noh SY, Kim SH, Jung SE, Lee SC, Park KW. Neonatal gastric perforation: a single center experience. World J Gastrointest Surg. 2014;6(8):151–5.
8. Schumpelick V. Surgical embryology and anatomy of the diaphragm with surgical applications. Surg Clin N Am. 2000;80(1):213–39.
9. Tsugawa C, Kimura K, Nishijima E, Muraji T, Yamaguchi M. Diaphragmatic eventration in infants and children: is conservative treatment justified? J Pediatr Surg. 1997;32(11):1643–4.
10. Hoover CF. The functions of the diaphragm and their diagnostic significance. Arch Intern Med. 1913;12:214–24.

11. Tanaka T, Okazaki T, Fukatsu Y, Okawada M, Koga H, Miyano G, Ogasawara Y, Lane G, Ymataka A. Surgical intervention for congenital diaphragmatic hernia: open versus thoracoscopic surgery. Pediatr Surg Int. 2013;29(11):1183–6.
12. Dingemann C, Ure B, Dingemann J. Thoracoscopic procedure in pediatric surgery: what is the evidence? Eur J Pediatr Surg. 2014;24(1):14–9.
13. Davenport M, Rothenberg S, Crabbe D, Wulkan M. The great debate: open or thoracoscopic repair for oesophageal atresia or diaphragmatic hernia. J Pediatr Surg. 2015;50(2):240–6.
14. Miyano G, Yamoto M, Kaneshiro M, Miyake H, Morita K, Nouso H, Koyama M, Okawada M, Doi T, Koga H, Fukumoto K, Lane G, Ymataka A, Urushihara N. Diaphragmatic eventration in children: laparoscopy versus thoracoscopic plication. J Laparoendosc Adv Surg Tech A. 2014;25(4):331–4.
15. Fujishiro J, Ishimaru T, Sugiyama M, Arai M, Uotani C, Yoshida M, Miyakawa K, Kakihara T, Iwanaka T. Thoracoscopic plication for diaphragmatic eventration after surgery for congenital heart disease in children. J Laparoendosc Adv Surg Tech A. 2015;25(4):348–51.
16. Wulkan M. Atlas of Pediatr Laparosc Thoracosc. 2008;43:261–4.
17. Hu J, Wu Y, Wang J, Zhang C, Pan W, Zhou Y. Thoracoscopic and laparoscopic plication of the hemidiaphragm is effective in the management of diaphragmatic eventration. Pediatr Surg Int. 2014;30:19–24.
18. Snyder CW, Walford NE, Danielson PD, Chandler NM. A simple thoracoscopic plication technique for diaphragmatic eventration in neonates and infants: technical details and initial results. Pediatr Surg Int. 2014;30:1013–6.
19. Calvinho P, Bastos C, Bernardo JE, Eugénio L, Antunes MJ. Diaphragmmatic eventration: long-term follow-up and results of open-chest plicature. Eur J Cardiothorac Surg. 2009;36(5):883–7.
20. Becmeur F, Talon I, Schaarschmidt K, Philippe P, Moog R, Kauffmann I, Schultz A, Grandadam S, Toledano D. Thoracoscopic diaphragmatic eventration repair in children: about 10 cases. J Pediatr Surg. 2005;40:1712–5.
21. Tiryaki T, Livanelioglu Z, Atayurt H. Eventration of the diaphragm. Asian J Surg. 2006;29(1):8–10.
22. Spitz L, Coran A. Operative pediatric surgery. 7th ed. Boca Raton: CRC Press; 2013.

12. Minimally Invasive Approaches to Congenital Diaphragmatic Hernias

Kelly Arps, Priya Rajdev, and Avraham Schlager

Introduction

Epidemiology

Congenital diaphragmatic hernia (CDH) occurs in approximately 1 in 2000–3000 live births [1, 2]. 85 % of cases occur on the left, 13 % occur on the right, and 2 % are bilateral [2]. 70 % of the defects are posterolateral or Bochdalek type, 27 % are anteromedial or the Morgagni type, and the remaining cases are considered complete agenesis [1].

Pathophysiology

CDH is the result of failure of the diaphragmatic musculature to fuse during gestation, allowing herniation of abdominal viscera into the thoracic cavity. Anatomically, this results in pulmonary compression with subsequent hypoplasia and arteriole muscular hypertrophy. Postnatally, decreased surface area and hypertrophied and hyperreactive pulmonary arterioles lead to fixed increased vascular resistance and pulmonary hypertension, the primary source of morbidity and mortality in these patients [1, 3].

D.S. Walsh et al. (eds.), *The SAGES Manual of Pediatric Minimally Invasive Surgery*, DOI 10.1007/978-3-319-43642-5_12

Preoperative Evaluation

History

Approximately 66 % of CDH in the developed world are diagnosed by ultrasound in the prenatal period [1]. 40 % of CDH patients have concurrent congenital anomalies, particularly cardiac defects, which are also detected with prenatal ultrasound [1, 2]. Several prenatal measurements have been proposed for determination of CDH severity: lung to head ratio (LHR), observed to expected LHR, total lung volumes (TLV) by MRI, and observed to expected TLV. Each has significant prognostic association but high interobserver variability [4]. When CDH is diagnosed in utero, delivery at or rapid transfer to a tertiary facility equipped for neonatal intensive care, particularly one with ECMO capabilities, is recommended [3].

Exam

Patients with CDH not diagnosed prenatally generally present with respiratory distress. CDH may be suspected by a paucity of breath sounds on the affected side, shifted heart sounds, or the presence of bowel sounds over the lung fields. The abdominal exam demonstrates a normal to scaphoid abdomen [3]. When the diagnosis of CDH is suspected, respiratory status should be carefully assessed. Tachypnea, cyanosis, delayed capillary refill, and progressive hypoxia are indicators of worsening pulmonary hypertension necessitating prompt resuscitation.

After stabilization of the infant, a full physical exam is used to rule out concurrent anomalies, particularly facial dysmorphism, neurologic defects, genitourinary malformations, digital abnormalities, hypertelorism, or organomegaly, which may prompt diagnostic workup for a systemic genetic syndrome [5, 6].

Imaging

Chest X-ray supports the diagnosis of CDH and demonstrates presence of abdominal viscera in the thoracic cavity. If the diagnosis is uncertain, ultrasound may assist in the diagnosis of right-sided defects in particular by identifying the location of the hepatic vasculature. CT or MRI may be used to evaluate cases in which uncertainty about the diagnosis persists.

Echocardiogram, perhaps the most important part of the evaluation, is performed for assessment of pulmonary hypertension and cardiac function and to rule out concurrent congenital cardiac defects.

Postnatal Management

Clinical respiratory status should be carefully assessed and arterial blood gas should be performed [7]. If respiratory function is compromised, prompt intubation is warranted, as this population is known to recover poorly from hypoxia-induced acidosis [3]. Bag-valve mask should be avoided as inflating the intestines may increase pressure on the compromised lungs [8]. A strategy of permissive hypercapnia provides gentle ventilation to support respiratory function while minimizing the risk of barotrauma [3, 5, 7, 8]. High-frequency oscillatory ventilation (HFOV) is used by many centers as primary therapy or as rescue therapy prior to ECMO cannulation [5, 8]. Vasodilators are used with increasing frequency to treat pulmonary hypertension in affected infants; nitric oxide has failed to demonstrate improved outcomes, but small studies show a mortality benefit with use of sildenafil [9–11]. In severe cases, ECMO is the most effective method of providing cardiorespiratory support. ECMO use has varied widely between centers, from 11 to 58 % historically. Its use contributed significantly to the increase in survival in this population, although improved neonatal ventilator therapy in recent years has decreased the necessity for ECMO [7, 12]. While some choose to perform repair on ECMO, we prefer to wait until after stabilization of the patient following decannulation. These patients generally have larger defects and are more likely to require patch repair. In our experience, thoracoscopic repair after ECMO is feasible, though conversion to laparotomy is more common in this patient subset.

Surgical Indications

CDH was previously treated as a surgical emergency with all patients undergoing repair within the first 24 h of life. Many studies have since demonstrated high rates of respiratory failure and subsequent morbidity and mortality in patients undergoing early repair, prompting most surgeons to delay surgical intervention until respiratory status has been stabilized. Nevertheless, recent data has questioned the actual clinical benefit of the generally accepted delayed repair [13].

Most centers use physiologic criteria to determine readiness of the CDH patient for surgery, whether or not the patient previously required ECMO. Stabilization of respiratory status is determined by minimal clinical evidence of pulmonary hypertension, preductal saturation between 85 and 95 % on <50 % inspired O_2, no preductal or postductal SaO_2 gradient, and/or mean arterial pressure (MAP) that is normal for gestational age [1, 2, 8, 14].

Indications

With rare exception, all CDH patients who are clinically stable to undergo surgical repair are candidates for attempted thoracoscopy. Exceptions include those not able to be weaned off of ECMO and those with unrepaired severe complex cardiac disease or non-resolving pulmonary hypertension [15, 36, 37].

Technique

Special Considerations

Thoracoscopic repairs are more challenging technically and more dangerous for labile infants. CO_2 insufflation increases pressure on hypoplastic lungs. Hypercarbia necessitates increased respiration, increasing the risk of barotrauma, hypoxemia, and acidosis [15].

Patient Positioning and Prep

We will describe the technique for repair of left-sided CDH, as it is the more common type.

1. Place the patient on the operating room table in one of two positions (Fig. 12.1):
   (a) Horizontally at the foot of the bed with the surgeon at the patient's head facing the screen and the assistant at the foot of the bed on the patient's left side
   (b) Longitudinally at the head of the bed with all extraneous pieces of the bed broken down with the surgeon at the patient's head and the assistant on the left

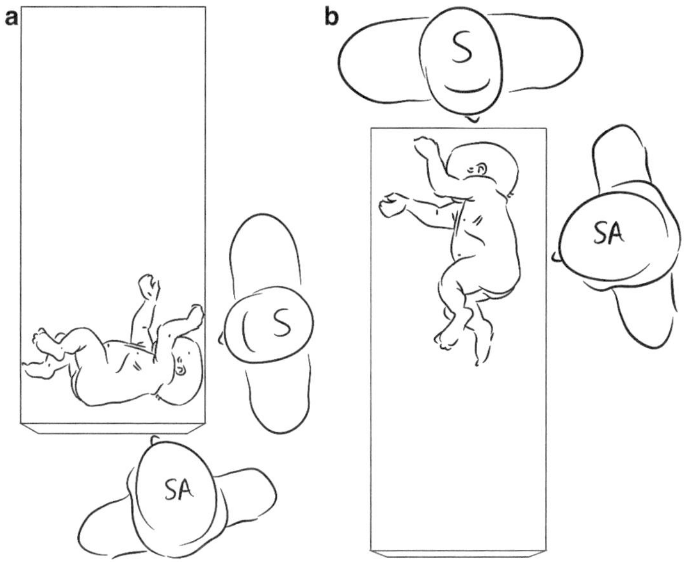

Fig. 12.1. Two variations on standard positioning for thoracoscopic repair of L CDH: option 1 (**a**) and option 2 (**b**).

2. Position the patient in the lateral decubitus position with the affected side up and slightly angled toward supine.
   (a) Coordinate carefully with anesthesia to ensure that the patient's head and the joints of the ET tube connection remain at or slightly below the level of the patient's body so that they will not interfere with or become dislodged during thoracoscopic instrumentation.
   (b) A bronchial blocker is not necessary as the remaining lung on the affected side is hypoplastic and will be further compressed with thoracoscopic insufflation.
3. Place a "jelly roll" to support the posterior aspect of the patient and a cushion between the patient's arms. Use other appropriate cushioning as needed.
   (a) Place the shoulder roll in a readily accessible fashion so that it can be removed and allow sterile repositioning of the patient to a supine position if conversion to subcostal laparotomy is necessary.

(b) Beanbags are often too large for patients of this size and are generally more cumbersome than helpful.

4. Position the arms in a neutral position with respect to abduction/adduction and reaching superiorly at approximately 120° to avoid interference with the ipsilateral port.
5. Tape the hips and ipsilateral shoulder to the bed to further support the patient's position.
6. Prep the left thorax and abdomen from the patient's spine to the anterior midline, superiorly beyond the tip of the scapula and inferiorly to the pelvis. This will allow sterile repositioning without re-prepping if conversion to laparotomy becomes necessary.
7. Drape the patient to expose the left hemithorax in a manner that allows visualization of important landmarks: the ipsilateral nipple, the spine, and the tip of the scapula.

   (a) Place a removable sterile towel over the abdomen during thoracoscopy.

Trocar/Port Placement

1. Access the thorax using the Veress technique. Hold respirations temporarily and place the Veress needle just posteriorly to the tip of the scapula at approximately the fourth intercostal space.
2. Insufflate to a pressure of 3 mmHg at a flow of 1 L/min.

   (a) Warn the anesthesia team to expect a temporary increase in the patient's end-tidal CO_2 that will usually resolve without intervention. Communication with the anesthesia team is essential at this point to ensure that the patient is tolerating the insufflation pressure.

3. If the patient tolerates initial insufflation, raise the pressure to 5 mmHg.
4. Replace the Veress needle with a 4-mm trocar and laparoscope.
5. Place two additional 3.5-mm ports approximately 3 cm on either side of the first port and one to two rib spaces below it (Fig. 12.2).

   (a) Reduce instrument torque with the overlying rib by angling the trocars at a 45° angle or even tunneling a rib space caudad.

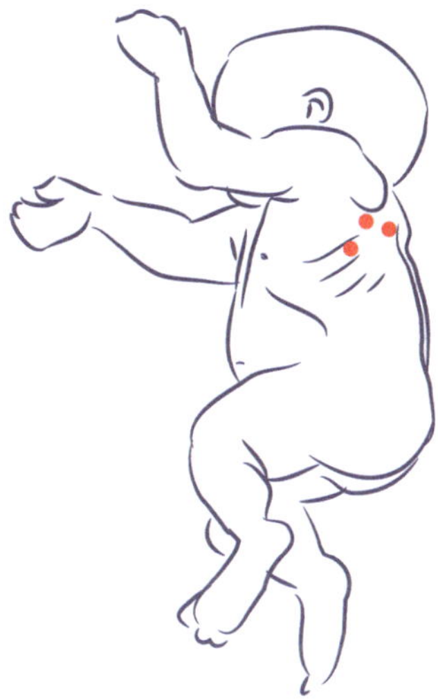

Fig. 12.2. Standard trocar placement for thoracoscopic repair of L CDH.

(b) Place the ports as cephalad as possible to facilitate this angling, enable easier reduction of the abdominal viscera, and allow room for thoracoscopic dissection and repair in an already restricted workspace.
(c) Take care not to place the ports too far medially and laterally as this causes collisions with the patient's arms and increases torque on the instruments when trying to operate in the superior aspect of the surgical field.

Reduction of Abdominal Viscera

1. Use an adjustable grasper and a bowel grasper to gently reduce the abdominal viscera from the chest in the following order: the small bowel, colon, stomach, and spleen (Fig. 12.3a).
   (a) The smaller dimensions of the adjustable grasper facilitate reduction and dissection in the restricted surgical field.
   (b) If necessary, divide diaphragmatic attachments to the colon and other viscera with the hook electrocautery to enable complete reduction of the viscera and unfurling of the diaphragmatic edge.

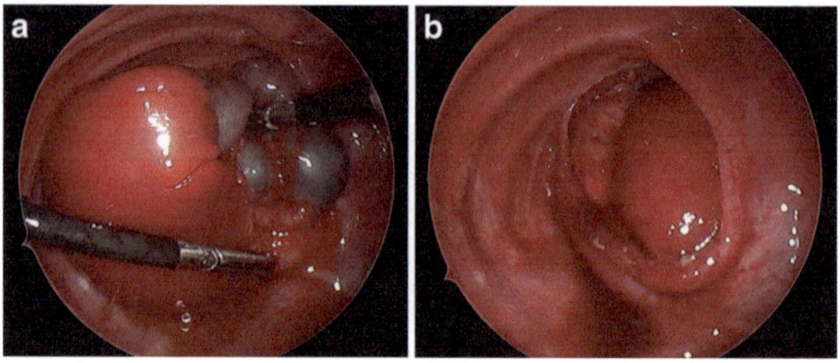

Fig. 12.3. (**a**) Abdominal contents are gently reduced into the abdominal cavity. (**b**) A splenic cap prevents migration of the abdominal contents back into the thoracic cavity during repair.

(c) Use two blunt/atraumatic graspers to reduce the viscera toward the anteromedial or right upper aspect of the field.
(d) Cover the viscera with the splenic cap to prevent the return of the viscera to the chest (Fig. 12.3b).

Diaphragm Repair

1. Place a Surgisis SIS underlay (Cook Medical, Bloomington, IN). It is our practice to do so whether or not a prosthetic patch is required, although at this time evidence is limited regarding its success in reducing recurrence rates. We do not cauterize the edge of the diaphragm peritoneum prior to repair, as there is no well-known evidence that this impacts outcomes.

   (a) Cut the SIS to size, leaving at least 1 cm excess in all directions, and roll it gently.
   (b) Remove one of the two lateral trocars and pass the contralateral grasper transthoracically through the vacant port site.
   (c) Use the grasper to drag the rolled mesh into the thorax (Fig. 12.4).
   (d) Unfurl the SIS on the abdominal side of the diaphragm.
   (e) Fasten the SIS to the diaphragm by including it in every second or third stitch of the diaphragmatic closure.

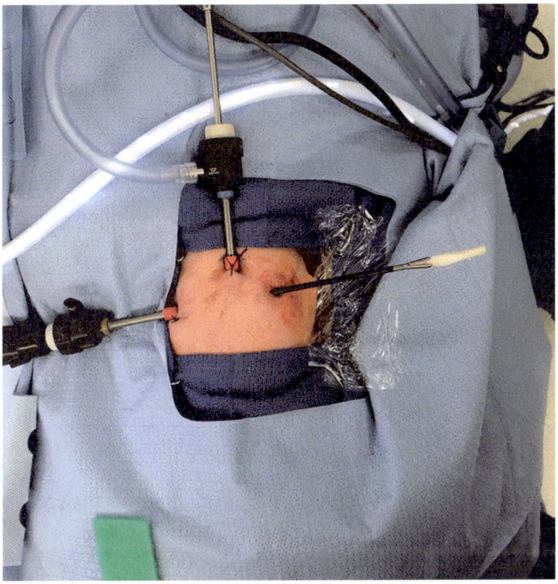

Fig. 12.4. SIS mesh is pulled into the thorax through a vacant port site.

2. Close the diaphragm defect by passing stitches every 8–10 mm. Pass stitches via trocar or transthoracically.

   (a) If placing via trocar, it is our practice to use a 2-0 silk on a ski needle, which can be passed through a 3.5-mm port. The lack of memory in the silk facilitates easier intracorporeal knot tying.
   (b) If placing stitches transthoracically, a standard RB needle may be used rather than a ski needle.

3. Begin primary repair of the diaphragm from the medial to lateral aspect to evaluate whether a patch is required.

   (a) We prefer to begin medially out of concern that although the lateral stitch may successfully approximate the edges of the diaphragm, it may cause undue tension on the repair that only increases upon approximation of the remainder of the diaphragm. By working toward the lateral side, we evaluate whether the lateral edges can be brought together without tension after the rest of the defect is approximated.

(b) Alternatively, the benefit of beginning laterally is that areas of redundancy in the medial diaphragm, if present, can be incorporated into the lateral stitch to re-approximate the lateral defect. This potentially alleviates the need for a prosthetic patch in a subset of patients.
(c) If necessary, ask the assistant to perform external compression of the chest wall when placing lateral stitches, as this is the most challenging part of the repair.
(d) If no patch is necessary, proceed to step 7.

4. If a patch is necessary, begin by placing a pericostal or "rib stitch" to approximate the lateral portion of the defect (Fig. 12.5a). It is easiest to place these first, as they will hang the patch in position while leaving adequate mobility to place the remainder of the stitches. The "rib stitch" may be placed using a variety of techniques:

   (a) *Extracorporeal-assisted rib stitches*. Begin with a 2-mm nick in the skin overlying the anticipated rib (Fig. 12.5b). Place the stitch using one of two devices:

      i. *(Preferred)* Place a Prolene or silk stitch transthoracically using a standard needle driver.

         1. Grasp the needle inside the chest with the intrathoracic needle driver; pass it through the mesh patch and then to the outside of the chest on the other side of the rib (Fig. 12.5c).
         2. When the needle has passed halfway through the chest wall, grasp the tip with the standard needle driver, paying careful attention not to remove it completely from the skin (Fig. 12.5d).
         3. Use a backhand technique to pass the needle driver into the initial 2-mm nick, and tie the stitch (Fig. 12.5e).

      ii. Pass a suture with the needle through the chest wall and the patch using the needle driver. Remove the needle. Place an 18-gauge angiocatheter through the nick on the other side of the rib. At this point, one of two options are possible:

         1. Thread the free end retrograde out of the chest through the angiocatheter (Fig. 12.5f).
         2. Pass a loop of a Prolene or nylon free tie through the angiocatheter and use this to lasso the free end of the stitch (Fig. 12.5g).

iii. Use the Carter-Thomason suture passer (CooperSurgical, Trumbull, CT) to transthoracically place and retrieve a free tie around the rib.

(b) *Completely intracorporeal rib stitches*. Ask the assistant to externally compress the chest wall, and use a sharply angled 18-gauge needle with silk or Prolene suture. This method can be extremely technically challenging with the greatest likelihood of intercostal bleeding.

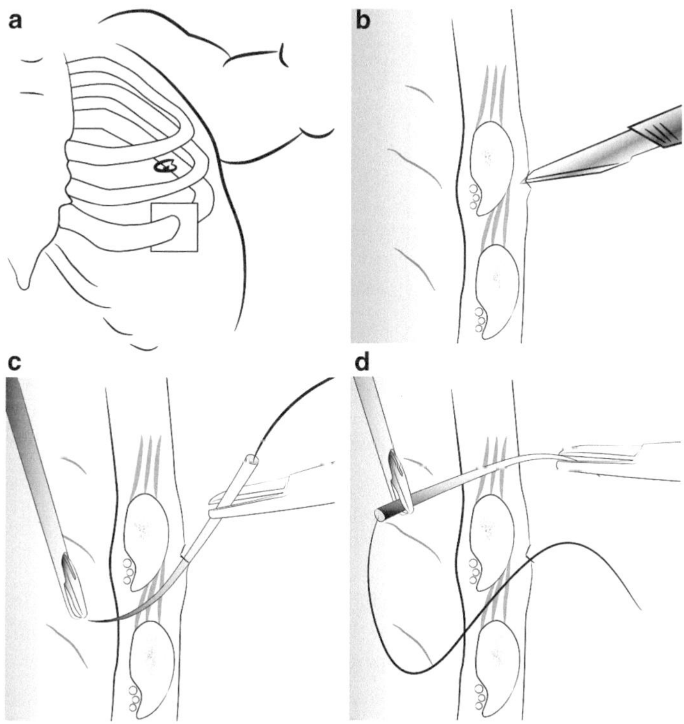

Fig. 12.5. Extracorporeal-assisted rib stitches. (**a**) Location of the rib stitch. (**b**) 2-mm nick overlying the anticipated rib. (**c**) A transthoracic rib stitch is performed by passing the needle from the outside of the body to the thoracic cavity, through the diaphragmatic edge, and (**d**) back outside the thoracic cavity, followed by (**e**) a backhand technique to pass the needle driver into the initial 2-mm nick. (**f**) Alternatively, the free end of the rib stitch is passed back out of the thoracic cavity through an angiocatheter. (**g**) A loop of Prolene or nylon is used to lasso the free end.

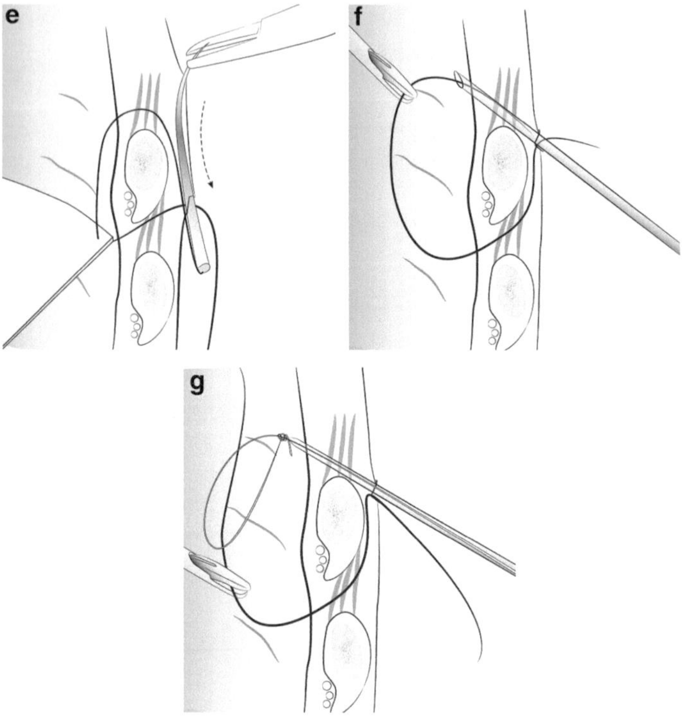

Fig. 12.5. (continued).

5. Prepare a Gore-Tex soft tissue patch (Gore, Newark, DE) and cut it to size.

   (a) Each dimension of the patch should be 5–10 mm longer than the defect in order to recreate the smooth curved contour of a natural diaphragm without undue tension.
   (b) If necessary, enlarge a port site by placing a small nick adjacent to the existing opening in order to accommodate the patch. Pass the patch into the thoracic cavity as described for the SIS mesh above:

      i. Remove one of the two lateral trocars and pass the contralateral grasper transthoracically through the vacant port site.
      ii. Use the grasper to drag the rolled patch into the thorax.

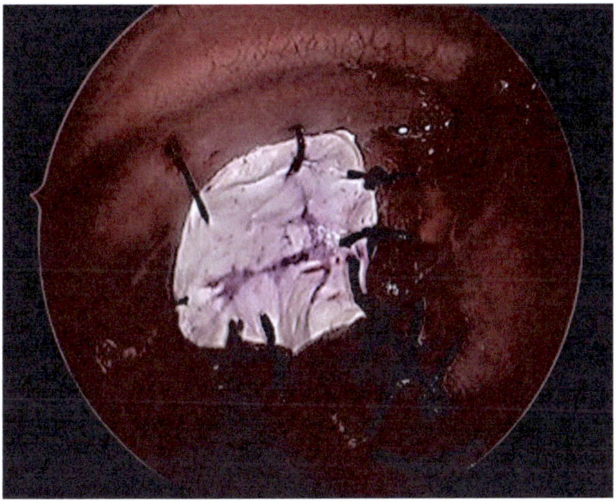

Fig. 12.6. A patch is used to cover the lateral aspect of the diaphragmatic defect.

6. Sew the patch into the remaining diaphragmatic defect (Fig. 12.6).
   (a) It is our practice to sew the patch in an interrupted fashion with approximately 8–10-mm distance in between stitches.
   (b) If a continuous repair is chosen, use multiple continuous segments so that a single break will not unravel the entire repair. Leave a long tail on the individual knots, and sew the tail of one segment to the running stitch on the connecting segment, in order to avoid introducing a loop into the knot.

7. Perform appropriate closure. The necessity of a chest tube for these operations is still a point of debate. If a chest tube is not deemed necessary, remove all trocars, evacuate the CO_2 in the chest, and close the skin.
   (a) If a port site was enlarged to introduce a patch, re-approximate the fascial layer with a single absorbable stitch.
   (b) Seal the trocar sites with Dermabond (Ethicon, Somerville, NJ).

Pearls

- Placement of ports high in the chest and angling inferiorly or tunneling provides the largest operative field while maintaining optimal ergonomics.
- Thoracoscopic insufflation pressures should be in the range of 4–5 mmHg and may often be reduced to 0 after the viscera has been reduced into the abdomen.
- It is often necessary to unfurl the rim of diaphragm and separate it from the abdominal viscera in order to appreciate the actual size of the defect as well as the usage diaphragmatic tissue.
- The patch should be sized to the defect with an additional 5–10 mm in each dimension to create a smooth, curved contour.

Pitfalls

- An initial rise in end-tidal CO_2 is expected after insufflation and may prompt conversion to an open procedure. Give the infant time to acclimate before aborting the thoracoscopic approach.
- Even a small amount of splenic bleeding can greatly obscure the operative field. The spleen should be handled extremely gently.
- The esophagus and aorta are in close vicinity to the repair site and at risk of injury. Pay attention to the insertion of the esophagus and the course of the aorta when suturing the posterior aspect of the defect.

Postoperative Care

Outcomes

Postnatal survival has improved significantly in recent years with the advent of ECMO and advanced neonatal care. Overall survival rates at tertiary centers with these capabilities are reported between 70 and 92 % with better outcomes in infants with isolated CDH [3, 16].

Several factors have been shown to significantly impact CDH survival. The most validated prenatal prognostic measurement is the estimation of the degree of pulmonary hypertension using observed to expected LHR, with estimated 0 % survival if the value is <15 % and >75 % survival for a ratio >45 % [2, 17–20]. Postnatally, average survival is lower in premature infants (53.5 %), and rates decrease with decreasing gestational age [16]. Associated anomalies are a poor prognostic factor; infants with major cardiac defects in particular have a reported 36 % survival rate [3]. In patients with liver herniation, survival was 45 % vs. 93 % in a matching cohort without liver herniation [19]. Survival rates in the ECMO subset range between 50 and 86 % [14, 16, 21, 22].

Complications

Surgical complications include recurrence, tension pneumothorax, intestinal adhesion obstruction, and musculoskeletal deformity.

The primary concern after CDH repair is the risk of hernia recurrence. Recurrence rates have been reported between 10.8 and 41 % overall with a bimodal incidence between 1 and 3 months and between 10 and 36 months after initial repair [23–27]. Large defects requiring synthetic patches and presence of the stomach or liver in the thoracic cavity increase risk of recurrence [23, 24, 28]. Recurrence rates were historically lower after open repair than after thoracoscopy, although improvement in technique has resulted in more similar outcomes in recent years [28, 29]. Recurrences may be repaired laparoscopically or thoracoscopically. It is our practice to repair most of them through the abdomen to achieve better visualization for dissection of the abdominal viscera and safe repair in the setting of thoracic adhesions. When necessary, conversion to an open procedure is performed via a subcostal laparotomy.

Obligate postoperative pneumothorax occurs in nearly all infants after CDH repair. Clinically significant pneumothorax, however, is estimated to occur in up to 30 % of patients, and the percentage of patients requiring intervention is as high as 16.4 % [30–32]. Chylothorax has been reported in 4.6 % of patients postoperatively with higher risk after ECMO use or patch repair [33].

Musculoskeletal deformity is theorized to result from tension of the patch on the growing chest wall, with higher risk in patients with large defects or postoperative empyema [28, 34, 35]. Chest wall deformities, the majority of them pectus excavatum and most of them mild, occur in up to 48 % of patients [28, 35]. Scoliosis is reported in up to 27 % of surviving CDH patients [26, 28, 34].

Intestinal adhesion obstruction after CDH repair is as high as 20 %, a significantly higher rate than in the general pediatric population undergoing laparotomy (2.2 %) [23, 26, 27, 35]. In our experience, the rate of postoperative obstruction is significantly reduced following thoracoscopic repair as compared to open laparotomy.

Summary

- The majority of CDH are the Bochdalek subtype, and left-sided defects are significantly more common than right sided.
- The most common cause of morbidity and mortality in CDH patients is pulmonary hypoplasia and pulmonary hypertension.
- Many cases of CDH are diagnosed prenatally. Postnatally, CDH is suspected by characteristic chest X-ray in the setting of respiratory distress.
- Surgical correction is indicated in all patients with CDH. Surgery is generally delayed, pending stabilization of respiratory status as observed by physiologic criteria.
- The advent of ECMO and improved neonatal care has significantly improved the prognosis of infants with CDH.
- The most common and concerning complication of CDH is recurrence, occurring in the first 3 months of life or between 1 and 3 years in up to 41 % of patients.

References

1. Haroon J, Chamberlain RS. An evidence-based review of the current treatment of congenital diaphragmatic hernia. Clin Pediatr. 2013;52:115–24.
2. Deprest JA, Gratacos E, Nicolaides K, Done E, Van Mieghem T, Gucciardo L, et al. Changing perspectives on the perinatal management of isolated congenital diaphragmatic hernia in Europe. Clin Perinatol. 2009;36:329–47.
3. Hedrick HL. Management of prenatally diagnosed congenital diaphragmatic hernia. Semin Pediatr Surg. 2013;22:37–43.
4. Victoria T, Danzer E, Adzick NS. Use of ultrasound and MRI for evaluation of lung volumes in fetuses with isolated left congenital diaphragmatic hernia. Semin Pediatr Surg. 2013;22:30–6.
5. Wilkinson DJ, Losty PD. Management of congenital diaphragmatic hernia. Paediatr Child Health. 2014;24:23–6.
6. Stoll C, Alembik Y, Dott B, Roth MP. Associated malformations in cases with congenital diaphragmatic hernia. Genet Couns. 2008;19:331–9.
7. Harting MT, Lally KP. Surgical management of neonates with congenital diaphragmatic hernia. Semin Pediatr Surg. 2007;16:109–14.
8. Moya FR, Lally KP. Evidence-based management of infants with congenital diaphragmatic hernia. Semin Perinatol. 2005;29:112–7.
9. The Neonatal Inhaled Nitric Oxide Study Group (NINOS). Inhaled nitric oxide and hypoxic respiratory failure in infants with congenital diaphragmatic hernia. Pediatrics. 1997;99:838–45.

10. Bialkowski A, Moenkemeyer F, Patel N. Intravenous sildenafil in the management of pulmonary hypertension associated with congenital diaphragmatic hernia. Eur J Pediatr Surg. 2015;25:171–6.
11. Hagadorn JI, Brownell EA, Herbst KW, Trzaski AM, Neff S, Campbell BT. Trends in treatment and in-hospital mortality for neonates with congenital diaphragmatic hernia. J Perinatol. 2015;35(9):748–54.
12. Danzer E, Hedrick HL. Controversies in the management of severe congenital diaphragmatic hernia. Semin Fetal Neonatal Med. 2014;19:376384.
13. Moyer V, Moya F, Tibboel R, Losty P, Nagaya M, Lally KP. Late versus early surgical correction for congenital diaphragmatic hernia in newborn infants. Cochrane Datab Syst Rev. 2002;CD001695.
14. Badillo A, Gingalewski C. Congenital diaphragmatic hernia: treatment and outcomes. Semin Perinatol. 2014;38:92–6.
15. Lansdale N, Alam S, Losty PD, Jesudason EC. Neonatal endosurgical congenital diaphragmatic hernia repair: a systematic review and meta-analysis. Ann Surg. 2010; 252:20–6.
16. Logan JW, Rice HE, Goldberg RN, Cotton CM. Congenital diaphragmatic hernia: a systematic review and summary of best-evidence practice strategies. J Perinatol. 2007;27:535–49.
17. Metkus AP, Filly RA, Stringer MD, Harrison MR, Adzick NS. Sonographic predictors of survival in fetal diaphragmatic hernia. J Pediatr Surg. 1996;31:148–51. discussion 151–42.
18. Jani J, Keller RL, Benachi A, Nicolaides KH, Favre R. Gratacos E, et al. Prenatal prediction of survival in isolated left-sided diaphragmatic hernia. Ultrasound Obstet Gynecol. 2006;27:18–22.
19. Hedrick HL, Danzer E, Merchant A, Bebbington MW, Zhao H, Flake AW, et al. Liver position and lung-to-head ratio for prediction of extracorporeal membrane oxygenation and survival in isolated left congenital diaphragmatic hernia. Am J Obstet Gynecol. 2007;197:421–4.
20. Datin-Dorriere V, Rouzies S, Taupin P, Walter-Nicolet E, Benachi A, Sonigo P, et al. Prenatal prognosis in isolated congenital diaphragmatic hernia. Am J Obstet Gynecol. 2008;198:81–5.
21. Antonoff MB, Hustead VA, Groth SS, Schmeling DJ. Protocolized management of infants with congenital diaphragmatic hernia: effect on survival. J Pediatr Surg. 2011; 46:39–46.
22. Rollins MD. Recent advances in the management of congenital diaphragmatic hernia. Curr Opin Pediatr. 2012;24:379–85.
23. Yokota K, Uchida H, Kaneko K, Ono Y, Murase N, Makita S, et al. Surgical complications, especially gastroesophageal reflux disease, intestinal adhesion obstruction, and diaphragmatic hernia recurrence, are major sequelae in survivors of congenital diaphragmatic hernia. Pediatr Surg Int. 2014;30:895–9.
24. Nagata K, Usui N, Terui K, Takayasu H, Goishi K, Hayakawa M, et al. Risk factors for the recurrence of the congenital diaphragmatic hernia-report from the long-term follow-up study of Japanese CDH study group. Eur J Pediatr Surg. 2015;25:9–14.

25. Bagolan P, Morini F. Long-term follow up of infants with congenital diaphragmatic hernia. Semin Pediatr Surg. 2007;16:134–44.
26. Jancelewicz T, Chiang M, Oliveira C, Chiu PP. Late surgical outcomes among congenital diaphragmatic hernia (CDH) patients: why long-term follow-up with surgeons is recommended. J Pediatr Surg. 2013;48:935–41.
27. Moss RL, Chen CM, Harrison MR. Prosthetic patch durability in congenital diaphragmatic hernia: a long-term follow-up study. J Pediatric Surg. 2001;36:152–4.
28. Lally KP, Engle W. Postdischarge follow-up of infants with congenital diaphragmatic hernia. Pediatrics. 2008;121:627–62.
29. McHoney M, Giacomello L, Nah SA, De Coppi P, Kieli EM, Curry JI, et al. Thoracoscopic repair of congenital diaphragmatic hernia: intraoperative ventilation and recurrence. J Pediatr Surg. 2010;45:355–9.
30. Waag KL, Loff S, Zahn K, Ali M, Hien S, Kratz M, et al. Congenital diaphragmatic hernia: a modern day approach. Semin Pediatr Surg. 2008;17:244–54.
31. Migliazza L, Bellan C, Alberti D, Auriemma A, Burgio G, Locatelli G, et al. Retrospective study of 111 cases of congenital diaphragmatic hernia treated with early high-frequency oscillatory ventilation and presurgical stabilization. J Pediatr Surg. 2007;42:1526–32.
32. Boloker J, Bateman DA, Wung J-T, Stolar CJ. Congenital diaphragmatic hernia in 120 infants treated consecutively with permissive hypercapnea/spontaneous respiration/elective repair. J Pediatr Surg. 2002;37:357–66.
33. Levy SM, Lally PA, Lally KP, Tsao K, Congenital Diaphragmatic Hernia Study Group. The impact of chylothorax on neonates with repaired congenital diaphragmatic hernia. J Pediatr Surg. 2013;48:724–9.
34. Vanamo K, Peltonen J, Rintala R, Lindahl H, Jääskeläinen J, Louhimo I. Chest wall and spinal deformities in adults with congenital diaphragmatic defects. J Pediatr Surg. 1996;31:851–4.
35. Peetsold MG, Heij HA, Kneepkens CM, Nagelkerke EF, Huisman J, Gemke RJ. The long-term follow-up of patients with a congenital diaphragmatic hernia: a broad spectrum of morbidity. Pediatr Surg Int. 2009;25:1–17.
36. Gourlay DM, Cassidy LD, Sato TT, Lal DR, Arca MJ. Beyond feasibility: a comparison of newborns undergoing thoracoscopic and open repair of congenital diaphragmatic hernias. J Pediatr Surg. 2009;44:1702–7.
37. Vijfhuize S, Deden AC, Costerus SA, Sloots CE, Wijnen RM. Minimal access surgery for repair of congenital diaphragmatic hernia: is it advantageous?--An open review. Eur J Pediatr Surg. 2012;22:364–73.

13. Thoracoscopic Repair of Esophageal Atresia and Tracheoesophageal Fistula

Ibrahim Abd el-shafy and José M. Prince

Introduction

Esophageal atresia, with or without TEF, occurs in approximately 1/3500 live births. There is a slight male preponderance of 1.26:1. First pregnancy, advanced maternal age, hormonal exposure in pregnancy, and an affected parent and/or siblings are all risk factors. Chromosomal abnormalities, twinning, and associated anomalies are more common than expected. In retrospective studies, only one third of affected infants are identified successfully by prenatal ultrasound. Classically, the diagnosis has been made by the inability to pass a nasogastric tube (NGT) at birth in the setting of excessive drooling, coughing, choking, and regurgitation during feeding. Confirmation of a blind-ending pouch can be made by radiographs showing a coiled NGT at the thoracic inlet. If uncertainty persists in the diagnosis, esophageal atresia can be further characterized by the injection of air or a small amount of dilute contrast into the tube. A child with an esophageal atresia with TEF, type C, will have distal air in the stomach and intestines on X-ray in conjunction with abdominal distention on physical exam. By comparison a patient with a pure esophageal atresia will have a gasless, flat abdomen. Operative intervention for children with pure esophageal atresia typically does not require emergent repair compared to children with esophageal atresia and TEF who do require expeditious operative repair to prevent the development of chemical pneumonitis. Thoracoscopic repair of esophageal atresia and TEF is a safe and effective approach with results equivalent to open repair in some studies. The first reported successful thoracoscopic repair was completed in 2000.

D.S. Walsh et al. (eds.), *The SAGES Manual of Pediatric Minimally Invasive Surgery*, DOI 10.1007/978-3-319-43642-5_13

Preoperative Workup

Children with esophageal atresia and TEF have associated anomalies half of the time, the most common of which are cardiac malformations. It is often seen as part of a nonrandom association of anomalies known as VACTERL (**v**ertebral anomalies, **a**nal atresia, **c**ardiac defects, **t**racheo-esophageal fistula and/or **e**sophageal atresia, **r**enal and **r**adial anomalies, and **l**imb defects). In evaluating a child preoperatively, the echocardiogram is essential to determine the presence of cardiac defects and the location of the aortic arch. The location of the aortic arch might influence the side of the thoracoscopy. The presence of severe cardiac defects could be considered a relative contraindication for a thoracoscopic repair. Some surgeons consider small size between 1500 and 2000 g and severe abdominal distention as relative contraindications. The combination of hemodynamic instability as indicated by significant vasopressor support and severe prematurity with a birth weight less than 1500 g is a contraindication for thoracoscopic repair. Other anomalies such as an imperforate anus or cloacal anomalies are not contraindications to thoracoscopic repair. Preoperative evaluation should also include a chest X-ray and an abdominal radiograph. Absence of air in the abdomen typically represents isolated esophageal atresia without distal TEF.

Operation

There are five main variants of esophageal atresia. This chapter will touch upon operative repair of the most common variant: proximal atresia with a distal TEF type C. Long gap esophageal atresia and pure esophageal atresia will be discussed in a separate chapter reviewing esophageal replacement. Emergent operation for TEF is seldom required, and a period of 1–2 days between initial diagnosis and operation permits for a thorough assessment and preparation of the child. Prior consultation with a pediatric anesthesiologist is critical to establishing a coordinated operative plan.

The patient is initially placed in a supine position for a diagnostic laryngoscopy with rigid/flexible bronchoscopy to evaluate for an H-type fistula. Bronchoscopy also allows for balloon occlusion of the fistula using a small Fogarty catheter or similar. Endotracheal intubation is then performed with the endotracheal tube in the trachea without attempts to perform isolated lung ventilation. Low peak airway pressures and spontaneous ventilation should be utilized until the fistula has been ligated.

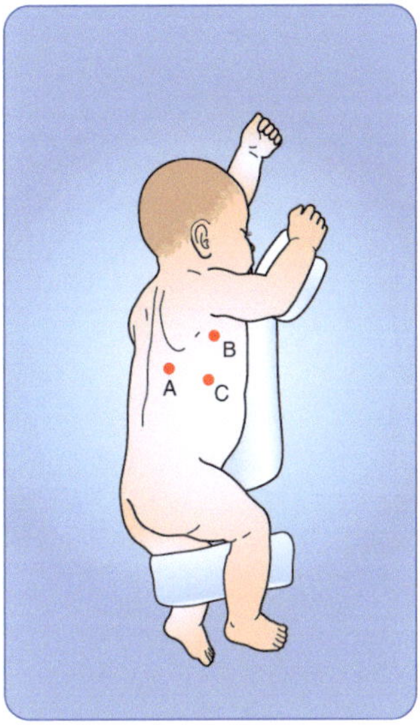

Fig. 13.1. Patient is in the modified prone position with ports as shown. (*A*, *B*) Working ports. (*C*) Camera port.

Consideration should be given for serratus anterior block for regional anesthesia given the potential benefits of decreasing operative pain and narcotic requirement. The patient is then placed in the modified prone position (Fig. 13.1). After positioning, three port sites are selected. Typically, the first port is a 5-mm port near the anterior axillary line approximately by the fifth intercostal space. Often this is the camera port for the 4-mm 30° laparoscope. Two 4-mm ports are placed at the second interspace mid-axillary line and the seventh interspace below or at the posterior axillary line, through which 3-mm instruments will be used. A fourth port is rarely helpful in retracting the lung. Some surgeons prefer to use the most posterior and inferior port for the camera to improve the ergonomic position of the operative surgeon. Initial insufflation should start at 4 mmHg, but if the lung does not collapse to allow adequate visualization, the pressure may be increased to 7–8 mmHg.

The next step is to identify the tracheoesophageal fistula, which can usually be found entering the membranous portion of the trachea superior to the carina (this area is usually delineated by the azygos vein) (Fig. 13.2). Mobilization of the azygos vein with division may be accomplished by the following: hook electrocautery, bipolar sealing device, or 5-mm clips. The vein may be preserved if desired, with a

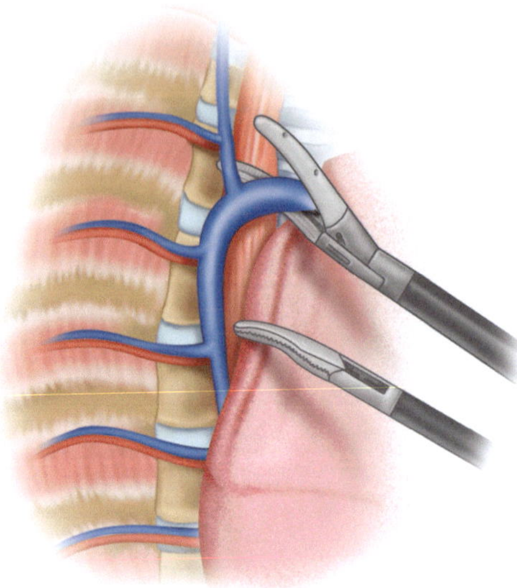

Fig. 13.2. Azygos vein.

suggestion that it might improve the vascularity of the area and decrease the esophageal anastomotic leak rate. The lower esophageal segment is identified and followed to its insertion point on the trachea. The fistula can be either suture ligated or ligated using endoclips. The vagus nerve should be identified to prevent injury. Identification of the upper segment is facilitated by asking the anesthesiologist to place gentle pressure on the naso-esophageal tube. The overlying pleura is then opened. Though not typically required, placement of a stay suture on the lowest aspect of the upper esophageal segment into the NGT may aid in retraction during dissection. Blunt/sharp dissection along the plane between the esophagus and trachea extending into the thoracic inlet completes the mobilization of the upper pouch. An opening and resection of the most distal upper pouch is made to create a wide anastomosis to prevent future stricture formation. The resulting opening may be dilated with the Maryland dissector to improve visualization of the mucosa. The NGT may be advanced to decompress the stomach after the anastomosis is established. The anastomosis is completed using 4-0 or 5-0 absorbable sutures on a small tapered needle in an interrupted manner. (A slipknot approach may be taken with initial approximation. With the second suture, the tension can be increased to gradually bring the ends together

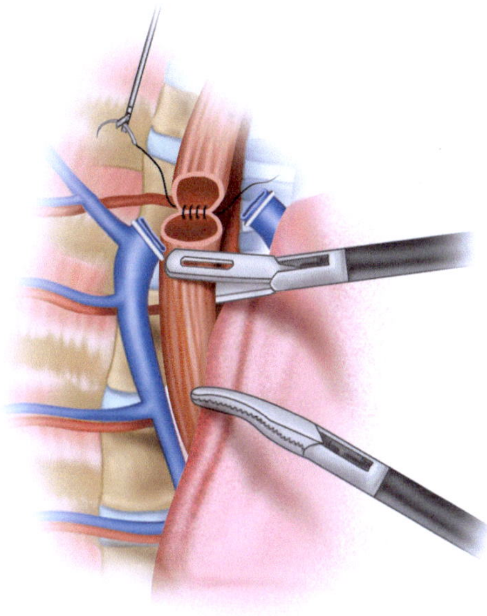

Fig. 13.3. Anastomosis posterior esophageal.

under shared tension.) Alternatively, a traction suture through the chest wall may be used to suspend the two ends of the esophagus to facilitate suturing. The back wall is completed first typically with four interrupted sutures and knots placed intraluminally (Fig. 13.3). Care should be taken to guarantee full-thickness bites that include the mucosa. The nasogastric tube can be used as a guide to suture the anterior wall and prevent inadvertent inclusion of the back wall in the anterior repair. The anterior wall is completed with an additional four interrupted sutures. Under magnification there may appear to be small tears. These tears are usually not clinically relevant but if there is concern, fibrin glue or a pleural patch may be used to bolster the anastomosis. The final step is placement of a chest tube via the lower of the three port sites to facilitate drainage postoperatively.

Postoperative Care

Postoperative care should not differ from open tracheoesophageal fistula repair. It is preferable if the child may be immediately extubated in the operating room. When possible, weaning off ventilator support and removal of the ET tube should be achieved within the first day. Infants with an anastomosis under significant tension, with underlying cardiac disease or with severe prematurity, may require prolonged ventilatory support. Prophylactic antibiotics are given for the first 48 h. On day 5–7 following the operation, we obtain a water-soluble esophagram. In the absence of a leak, oral feeds are initiated and the chest tube is removed the next day. If there is a concern for an anastomotic leak, feeds are held and antibiotic treatment initiated, with a repeat esophagram in 1–2 weeks.

A significant number of neonates have esophageal dysmotility postoperatively, but with time it is less clinically apparent. The latest published series demonstrated a 3.8 % stricture rate requiring endoscopy and dilation. Over half of these neonates develop significant gastroesophageal reflux disease which responds well to H2 blockers.

Pearls

- Consider bronchoscopy for placement of Fogarty catheter to occlude fistula.
- After dividing the fistula, dilating the opening with a Maryland dissector improves visualization of the mucosa and will aid in obtaining full-thickness esophageal tissue when performing the anastomosis.
- If there appears to be significant tension while approximating the two esophageal ends, one may use the slipknot technique and distribute tension to prevent suture tear through.
- Consider transthoracic suture for traction to suspend the two ends of the esophagus to facilitate suturing.

Pitfalls

- Patient selection for thoracoscopic TEF repair should account for low birth weight, or hemodynamic instability, and surgeon experience.
- Failure to communicate and having an inexperienced anesthesiology team reduces the likelihood of success for completing a thoracoscopic TEF repair.
- Do not remove the first suture if you are unable to bring the two esophageal ends together because this may create a tear. Having a gap that can be closed is easier than having a rent.

Summary

- Overall, thoracoscopic repair of TEF offers a safe alternative to open thoracotomy with the potential benefits of reduced risk of scoliosis, less muscle weakness, decreased postoperative pain, and improved cosmetic appearance.
- While requiring more advanced laparoscopic technical skills, this procedure is increasingly used for TEF.

Suggested Reading

1. Keckler SJ, St Peter SD, Valusek PA, Tsao K, Snyder CL, Holcomb 3rd GW, Ostlie DJ. VACTERL anomalies in patients with esophageal atresia: an updated delineation of the spectrum and review of the literature. Pediatr Surg Int. 2007;23(4):309–13.
2. Capizzani T, Hirschl RB, Chillery R. The pediatric chest. Greenfield surgery: scientific principles and practices, 5e.
3. Pretorius DH, Drose JA, Dennis MA, et al. Tracheoesophageal fistula in utero: twenty-two cases. J Ultrasound Med. 1987;6:509–13.
4. Stoll C, Alembik Y, Dott B, et al. Evaluation of prenatal diagnosis of congenital gastro-intestinal atresias. Eur J Epidemiol. 1996;12:611–6.
5. Sparey C, Jawaheer G, Barrett AM, et al. Esophageal atresia in the Northern Region Congenital Anomaly Survey, 1985–1997: prenatal diagnosis and outcome. Am J Obstet Gynecol. 2000;182:427–31.
6. Borruto FA, Impellizzeri P, Montalto AS, Antonuccio P, Santacaterina E, Scalfari G, Arena F, Romeo C. Thoracoscopy versus thoracotomy for esophageal atresia and tracheoesophageal fistula repair: review of the literature and meta-analysis. Eur J Pediatr Surg. 2012;22(6):415–9.
7. Rothenberg SS. Thoracoscopic repair of esophageal atresia and tracheoesophageal fistula in neonates, first decade's experience. Dis Esophagus. 2013;26(4):359–64.
8. McMullen KP, Karnes PS, Moir CR, et al. Familial recurrence of tracheoesophageal fistula and associated malformations. Am J Med Genet. 1996;63(4):525–8.
9. Rothenberg SS. Thoracoscopic repair of esophageal atresia with distal fistula. In: Holcomb, George W, editors. Atlas of pediatric laparoscopy and thoracoscopy. Philadelphia: Saunders/Elsevier; 2008.
10. Rashid KA, Maletha M, et al. Esophageal anastomosis medial to preserved azygos vein in esophageal atresia with tracheoesophageal fistula: restoration of normal mediastinal anatomy. J Neonatal Surg. 2012;1(4):50.

14. Thoracoscopic Approaches to Congenital Lung Lesions

Robert L. Ricca and John H.T. Waldhausen

Introduction

Cystic pulmonary lesions of the newborn are a rare congenital anomaly and in one study were found to have an incidence of 1 per 25,000–35,000 births [1]. These lesions consist of congenital pulmonary airway malformations (CPAMs), bronchopulmonary sequestrations (BPS), and congenital lobar emphysema (CLE). CPAM, previously known as congenital cystic adenomatoid malformation (CCAM), is characterized by a lack of normal alveolarization with an increased number of terminal bronchioles that are cystic in nature. The cysts within these lesions range from less than 1 mm in size to greater than 10 cm. Based upon size of the lesions, CPAMs can be described as macrocystic (lesions greater than 5.0 cm) or microcystic. While the abnormal bronchioles do not participate in normal gas exchange, they maintain their connection with the normal tracheobronchial tree [2, 3]. This communication can lead to overinflation during aggressive attempts at resuscitation in the neonate. Inadequate clearing of normal respiratory bacterial pathogens may lead to recurrent pneumonias [2]. Unlike BPS, CPAMs only receive blood supply from the pulmonary artery. CPAMs may show malignant degeneration if left unresected (pulmonary blastoma and rhabdomyosarcoma in infants and young children, bronchoalveolar carcinoma in older children) [4].

Bronchopulmonary sequestration consists of lung parenchyma that does not communicate with the tracheobronchial tree. These lesions can be extralobar or intralobar. As mentioned previously, the lesion derives its arterial supply from an aberrant systemic vessel [5]. Care must be taken during operative resection to identify and control this vessel as it

D.S. Walsh et al. (eds.), *The SAGES Manual of Pediatric Minimally Invasive Surgery*, DOI 10.1007/978-3-319-43642-5_14

may originate from the abdominal cavity [2]. Similar to CPAM, symptoms of BPS may include respiratory distress and recurrent pneumonia. As in the case of CPAM, elective resection is recommended.

Congenital lobar emphysema is characterized by overdistention of the affected lobe due to emphysematous changes resulting from a variety of causes. This is fundamentally due to normal passage of air into the lung with decreased expulsion of air on expiration. The underlying pathology may be due to abnormal bronchial cartilage, partial obstruction due to inspissated mucous or mucosal proliferation, or external compression of the cartilage. The majority of the cases of CLE affect the left upper lobe [2]. Resection of the emphysematous lobe is dependent upon symptomatology. Unlike CPAM or BPS, children with mild or no symptoms do not require resection.

Prenatal Diagnosis

Pulmonary lesions are routinely diagnosed on prenatal ultrasound. The differential diagnosis includes congenital diaphragmatic hernia, congenital lobar emphysema, bronchopulmonary sequestration, foregut duplication cyst, and mediastinal cystic teratoma. Postnatally they can be confused with congenital diaphragmatic hernia or pneumatocele. Fetal MRI may be used to differentiate between these lesions ultimately allowing for improved prenatal and postnatal care as well as prenatal counseling of the family [6] (Fig. 14.1). The size of the pulmonary lesion is significant prognostically. Compression of the esophagus may lead to polyhydramnios due to abnormal fetal swallowing of amniotic fluid. Compression of the mediastinum by a large lesion may result in compression of the heart and great vessels ultimately leading to hydrops fetalis. CPAM volume ratio (CVR) can be determined using prenatal ultrasound by determining the CPAM volume and dividing by the head circumference to standardize for fetal size. A CVR greater than 1.6 is predictive of increased risk for hydrops [7]. CVR can then be useful for determining which CPAM's require increased level of surveillance prenatally. CPAMs reach maximal growth before 28 weeks of gestation. Following this time period most CPAMs either plateau in size or regress [2].

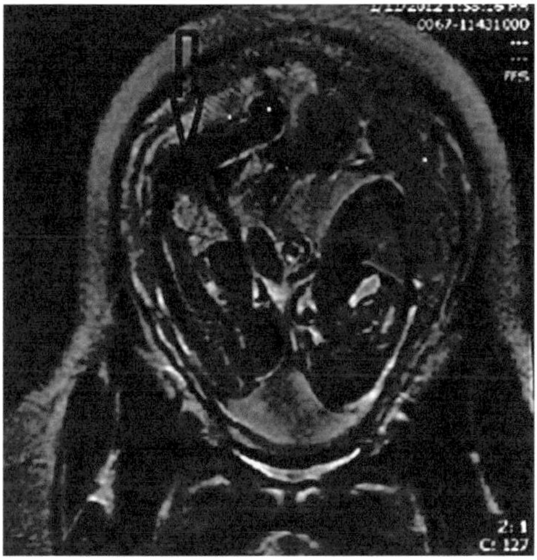

Fig. 14.1. Prenatal MRI of a twin gestation fetus with multilobar CPAM. *Arrow points* to the affected fetus and the lung.

Preoperative Evaluation and Treatment

Management of a fetus with a cystic pulmonary lesion is dependent upon the symptoms present. Prenatal management of CPAM may consist of steroid treatment in fetuses with a CVR greater than 1.4. Betamethasone has been shown to arrest growth of CPAM with subsequent improvement in hydrops symptoms [8]. A fetus that has been diagnosed with a macrocystic CPAM complicated by hydrops may be treated with thoracoamniotic shunting. Microcystic or solid CPAMs that present with hydrops have been approached with fetal surgery [9]. A late gestation fetus with hydrops may benefit from an ex utero intrapartum therapy (EXIT) approach [4, 10]. The fetus with a CPAM without hydrops should be managed with planned delivery and neonatal evaluation and eventual surgery.

All newborns prenatally diagnosed with a congenital pulmonary lesion should have a baseline radiograph at the time of birth. Surgical management should be based upon whether the newborn is symptomatic from the lesion. Infants with hemodynamic or significant respiratory compromise may need immediate resection. Extracorporeal membrane oxygenation (ECMO) has been used in some of these cases [2]. Persistent tachypnea, oxygen requirement, poor weight gain, and inability to feed orally are indications for early resection prior to discharge from the hospital. Asymptomatic children may be discharged and followed up as an outpatient. At our institutions, we typically perform preoperative imaging using computed tomographic scans at 3 months of age. Lesions are typically isolated to a single lobe; however, multilobar CPAM has been documented and will affect surgical decision-making (Fig. 14.2). It may be difficult to differentiate an extralobar sequestration from an intralobar sequestration radiographically. Attention should be paid to look for a systemic blood supply to the lesion to assist in differentiation of CPAM from BPS. Additionally, identification of a subdiaphragmatic feeding vessel will assist with operative planning (Figs. 14.3 and 14.4).

Technique

Resection of pulmonary lesions has been classically performed through a posterolateral thoracotomy. Over the last decade and a half, surgical resection through a minimally invasive approach has become

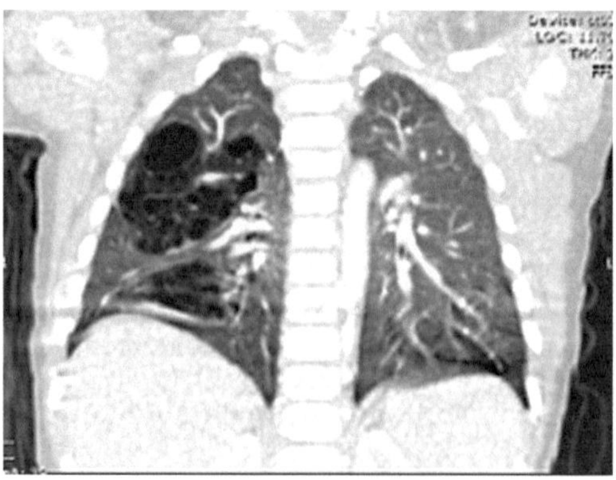

Fig. 14.2. CT scan showing multilobar CPAM involving the entire right lung.

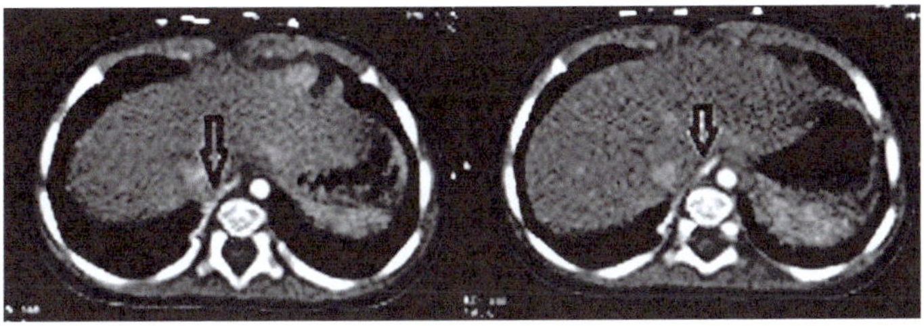

Fig. 14.3. CT scan showing a systemic feeding vessel to a right pulmonary BPS. *Arrow* identifies vessel. This vessel ultimately arose from the celiac plexus.

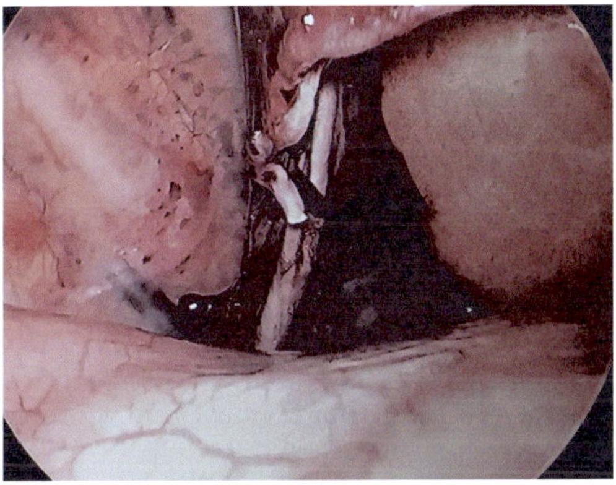

Fig. 14.4. Systemic feeding vessel of intralobar bronchopulmonary sequestration.

more commonplace. We recommend surgical resection, using a minimally invasive approach, when the infant is 3–6 months old. Children who present with infected lesions are recommended to undergo adequate antibiotic therapy for the infection prior to resection of the lesion. Minimally invasive approach is still a viable option in children who have had pneumonia; however, there has been a documented increase in conversion to open thoracotomy in these children [11].

Minimally Invasive Approach

The child should be placed in the lateral decubitus position with the affected side up. Adequate padding of all bony prominences as well as proper positioning of an axillary roll should be ensured. Small gel rolls, placed anteriorly and posteriorly, are adequate to prevent patient movement in younger children. In older children, we use a beanbag underneath the patient as our preferred method of stabilization. Central venous lines, arterial lines, and bladder catheters are not required intraoperatively. Management of the airway requires an anesthesiologist experienced in pediatric airways to ensure adequate single-lung ventilation. A techniques available for isolating the contralateral lung includes double-lumen endotracheal tube in older children and adolescents. In younger children, a Fogarty balloon catheter (Edwards Lifesciences, Irvine, CA) may be used as an endobronchial blocker with placement of a single-lumen endotracheal tube. This technique is more difficult in children less than ~5 kg because the bronchial blocker itself fills much of the lumen of the endotracheal tube making ventilation more difficult. We have passed the blocker extraluminally in order to alleviate this problem. Infants may require main stem intubation of the contralateral bronchus due to the narrow airway [11]. The use of a mild tension pneumothorax may also be useful in helping to collapse the ipsilateral lung and improve visualization. We use a pressure of no more than 4–5 mmHg. Flexible bronchoscopy is necessary to ensure proper placement of the endotracheal tube and bronchial blocker during initial placement and after repositioning of the patient. We do not place epidural catheters for pain management except in rare instances when conversion to an open procedure is needed.

The surgeon and assistant both stand on the same side of the patient depending on the lobe to be resected. We prefer to stand at the front of the patient with the monitor at the patient's back for lower lobes and the reverse for upper lobes. Local anesthetic is infiltrated at each trocar site. A veress needle is used to enter the chest cavity through a Step radially expanding sheath (Medtronic, Minneapolis, MN). Alternatively, a direct cutdown and placement of the initial trocar and reusable trocars may be used. The hemithorax is then insufflated with low-flow, low-pressure carbon dioxide to aid in collapse of the affected lung. This initial entry site is typically through the fifth or sixth intercostal space beneath the tip of the scapula in the anterior axillary line for lower lobes and the posterior axillary line for upper lobes. Entry at this site will allow for visualization of the major fissure and the underlying pulmonary parenchyma [12] (Fig. 14.5). Subsequent ports are then placed such that the camera port overlies the fissure. We typically use three 5-mm ports (two working ports and one camera port). In smaller babies we often use two 3-mm ports and one 5 mm to allow for use of the Ligasure (Covidien Energy Devices, Boulder, CO). For upper lobes all ports are placed in line in the posterior axillary line, while lower lobes have the ports placed in line in the anterior axillary line (Figs. 14.6 and 14.7). A fourth stab incision for insertion of an instrument to assist with parenchymal retraction or suction is placed in the lower chest in the 8–9th interspace. We use the anterior and posterior axillary lines as landmarks because it allows the operating surgeon to place the venous anatomy of the lung lobe between themselves and the monitor while the arterial anatomy is always fixed within the fissure. Alternatively, surgeons may choose to adopt a triangulation method with placement of ports in the anterior, posterior, and midaxillary line using the location of the lesion as the focal point of the triangle.

Resection of pulmonary lesions is typically through formal lobectomy. In the case of multiple lesions affecting multiple lobes, segmental

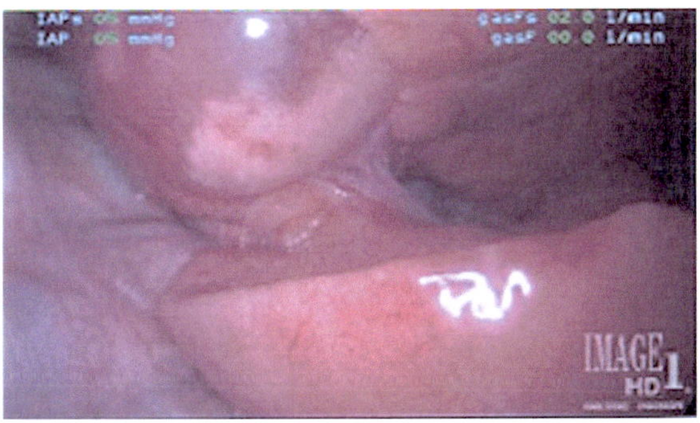

Fig. 14.5. Image on initial entry into thoracic cavity overlying major fissure. Affected lobe is in the superior portion of the image.

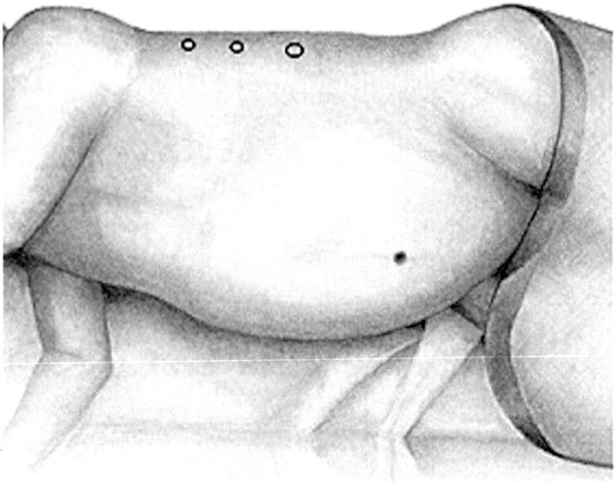

Fig. 14.6. Recommended port placement along posterior axillary line for upper lobe lesions.

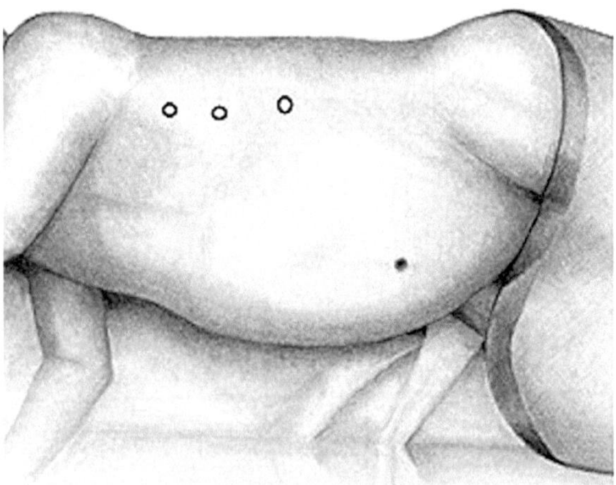

Fig. 14.7. Recommended port placement along anterior axillary line for lower lobe lesions.

resection may be appropriate to preserve pulmonary parenchyma. The steps in dissection vary depending upon the affected lobe and follow the same principles as open thoracotomy [13]. Completion of the major and minor fissure allows for visualization of the pulmonary vasculature and segmental artery branches. Division of the arterial branches is followed by division of the pulmonary veins (Fig. 14.8). Initial division of the pulmonary artery prevents parenchymal congestion and preserves the intrathoracic work space. The Ligasure has proven to be an effective method of dividing pulmonary parenchyma to complete division of the fissure. This device has also been shown to be an effective method of division of pulmonary vessels <7 mm in size. We currently use either the LS 1500 5-mm laparoscopic sealer/divider or the LF 1737 laparoscopic sealer. The LS 1500 has a blunt dolphin-tip while the LF 1737 has a Maryland tip. The Maryland tip we find beneficial for dissection especially around vessels. Multiple vessel sealing devices are available currently (Harmonic, Gyrus, JustRight sealer); however, we have routinely utilized the Ligasure system. For larger vessels, control with an endoscopic hemoclip (Auto Suture ENDO CLIP, Covidien) or with intracorporeal suture ligation followed by division using an energy-based sealing device has been described [11, 14].

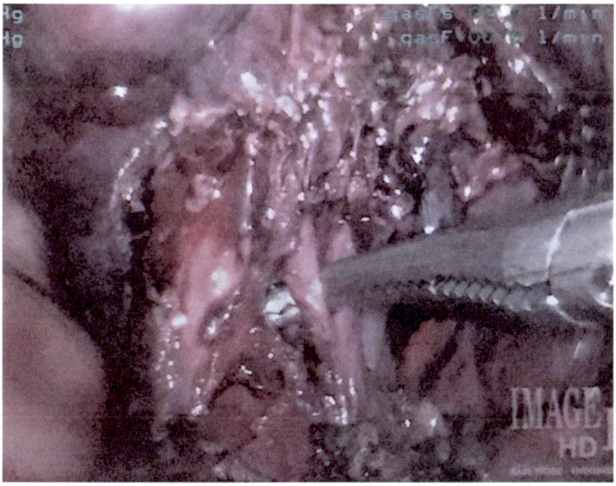

Fig. 14.8. Dissection of segmental vessel using Maryland dissector.

Following division of the pulmonary vasculature, attention is turned to the segmental bronchus. In larger children, an endoscopic stapler can be utilized; however, this may require placement of a 12-mm port. In some instances, the newer 5-mm staplers may be used. In infants we prefer to use a locking hemoclip such as the Hem-o-lok system (Teleflex Medical, Research Triangle Park, NC) [15]. This ensures closure of the bronchus (Fig. 14.9). Alternatively, the bronchus can also be divided and sutured with a monofilament, absorbable suture or closed with an endoloop (Fig. 14.10). After division of the bronchus, the specimen can then be removed by enlarging the most inferior trocar site. We do not routinely utilize an endoscopic pouch for specimen retrieval. An evaluation is then made for any significant bronchial leaks by partially filling the chest with saline and ventilating to a pressure of 20-cm H_2O. If one is discovered, this is suture ligated. An appropriately sized chest tube is placed in the most inferior incision. All wounds are then closed with absorbable sutures. The patient is extubated in the operating room and monitored overnight. We routinely remove the chest tube on the first postoperative day if there is no air leak, with discharge on the same day.

Management of bronchopulmonary sequestration is accomplished in the same manner. Identification of the systemic blood supply is paramount. We typically place a suture ligature or titanium clip (Fig. 14.11) around the artery to ensure adequate control and utilize the Ligasure to divide the vessel. For intralobar sequestration, lobectomy then proceeds

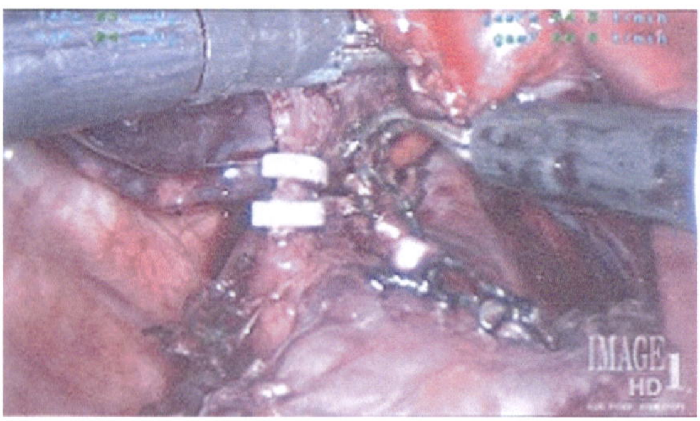

Fig. 14.9. Locking hemoclip in place on bronchus prior to transaction. Vessels have been controlled with silk ties and Ligasure.

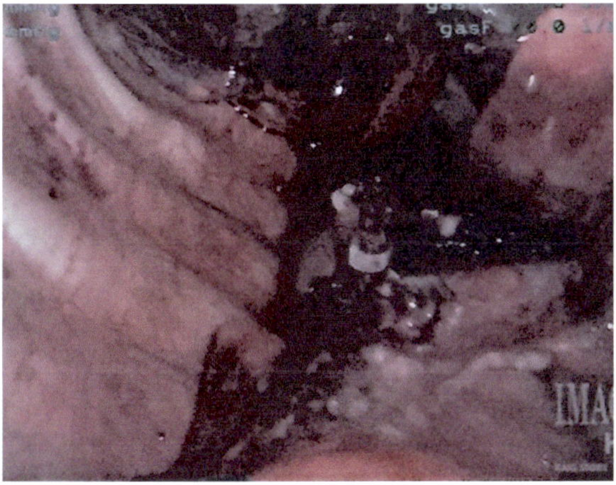

Fig. 14.10. Final operative bed showing bronchus controlled with Hem-o-lok system and control of vessels with suture ligatures in the background.

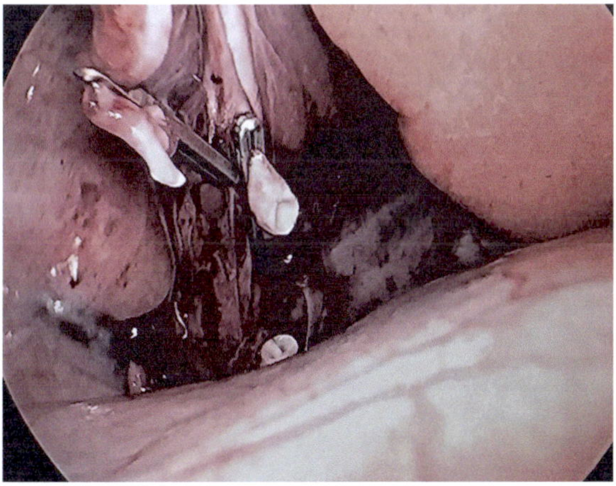

Fig. 14.11. Cut edges of systemic feeding vessel after control with titanium clip and division with scissors.

in the same manner as described previously (Figs. 14.12 and 14.13). For extralobar sequestration, the lesion is invested in the pleura. Resection of the lesion can be accomplished using the Ligasure to divide the pleura without performing a formal pulmonary resection. Chest tubes may not

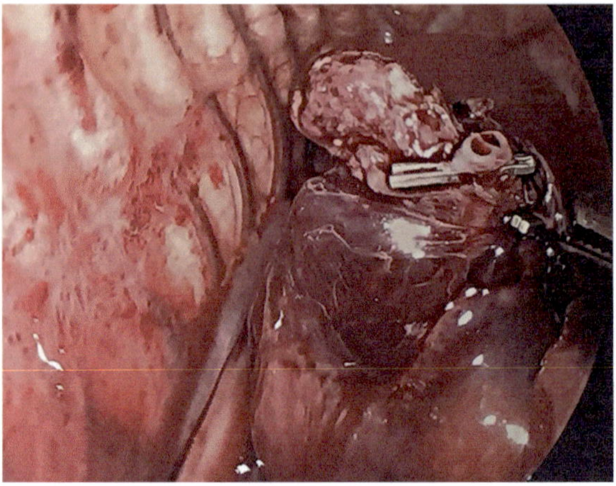

Fig. 14.12. Intralobar bronchopulmonary sequestration showing demarcation after division of systemic feeding vessel allowing for nonanatomic resection.

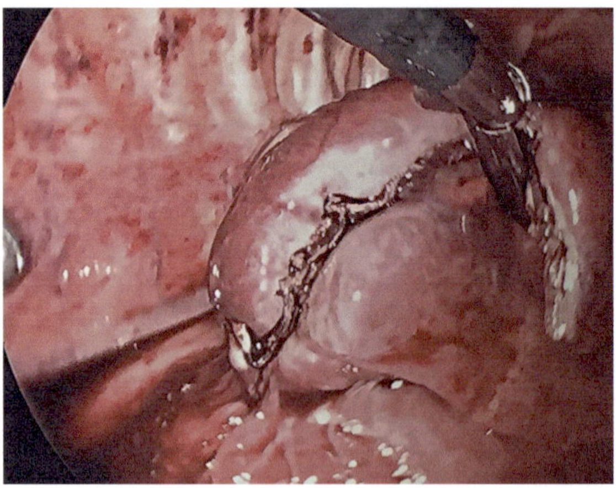

Fig. 14.13. Sealed parenchymal edge after nonanatomic resection using Ligasure LS 1500.

be necessary in these cases and often just evacuate the hemithorax with a rubber catheter prior to final closure.

Recent literature has focused on segmental resection for the treatment of congenital pulmonary lesions. Segmental resection has been an accepted standard in the case of multilobar disease that allows for preservation of pulmonary parenchyma. However, recent literature has suggested that even in the case of focal disease that is peripherally located, segmental resection is a safe alternative. Advocates against nonanatomic resection point to the microscopic disease that may be left behind as it can be difficult to visualize the diseased lung when the lung is deflated [16, 17]. To perform a segmental resection thoracoscopically, port placement proceeds as described previously; however, segmental blood vessels can be divided using a Ligasure. Pulmonary parenchyma can be divided safely with the Ligasure in small patients, obviating the need for an endoscopic stapler (Figs. 14.14, 14.15, and 14.16). We have adopted the use of a fibrin sealant over the cut edge of parenchyma to prevent an air leak. Postoperative management to include chest tube placement remains the same as previously described.

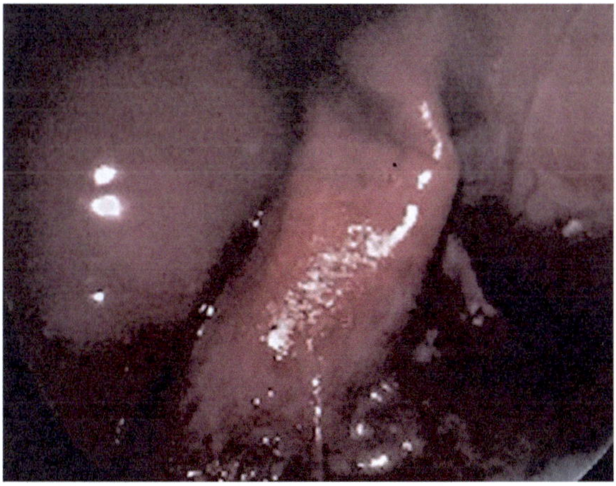

Fig. 14.14. Congenital pulmonary airway malformation (CPAM) amenable to nonanatomic wedge resection with no major bronchial or vascular communications.

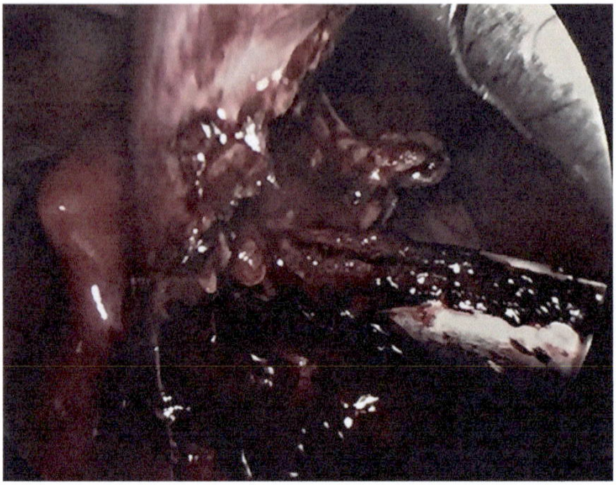

Fig. 14.15. Dissection of pulmonary parenchyma using Ligasure.

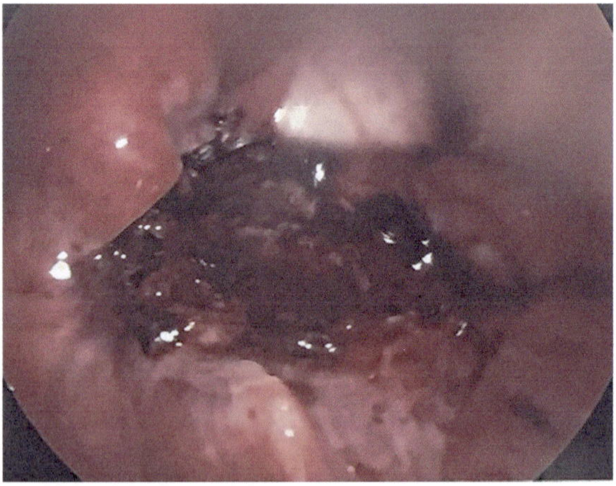

Fig. 14.16. Operative bed after nonanatomic wedge resection of previous CPAM.

Summary

- Thoracoscopic resection of pulmonary lesions is a safe alternative to open resection.
- Despite longer operative times, the minimally invasive approach has been shown in multiple studies to lead to decreased length of hospital stay, a shorter required time for chest tube, and an overall lower post-operative complication rate [18–20].
- Lobectomy remains the current standard of care for resection of pulmonary lesions; however, an increasing body of literature suggests that consideration for segmental resection for peripheral lesions may be a safe alternative with decreased morbidity [16, 17].
- Current limitations for a thoracoscopic approach include patient size and inflammation from recurrent pneumonias making dissection more difficult. However, an attempt at a minimally invasive approach is still recommended in these cases and can be accomplished safely.
- Newborn infants who present with symptomatic lesions may best treated with an open approach depending upon the associated physiologic sequelae.
  - If a child has hemodynamic instability or compromise, an open approach may be the best alternative.
  - For those children with respiratory difficulty or failure to thrive from feeding intolerance, a minimally invasive approach is our preferred operative approach.
- Thoracoscopy in infants and children can be technically demanding but remains a viable option in the management of CCAM in the pediatric population.

The views expressed in this publication are those of the authors and do not necessarily reflect the official policy or position of the Department of the Navy, the Department of Defense, nor the US Government.

References

1. Laberge JM, Flageole H, Pugash D, et al. Outcome of the prenatally diagnosed congenital cystic adenomatoid lung malformation: a Canadian experience. Fetal Diagn Ther. 2001;16:178–86.
2. Adzick NS, Farmer DL. Cysts of the lungs and mediastinum. In: Coran AG, Caldamone A, Adzick NS, et al. editors. Pediatric surgery. 7th ed. Philadelphia: Mosby; 2012. p. 825–35.
3. Stocker JT, Manewell JE, Drake RM. Congenital cystic adenomatoid malformation of the lung: classification and morphologic spectrum. Hum Pathol. 1977;8:155–61.
4. Chiu B, Flake AW. Congenital lung lesions. In: Mattei P, editor. Fundamentals of pediatric surgery. New York: Springer; 2011.
5. Puligandla PS, Laberge JM. Congenital lung lesions. Clin Perinatol. 2012;39:331–47.
6. Pacharn P, Kline-Fath B, Calvo-Garcia M, et al. Congenital lung lesions: prenatal MRI and postnatal findings. Pediatr Radiol. 2013;43(9):1136–43.
7. Crombleholme TM, Coleman BG, Howell LJ, et al. Elevated cystic adenomatoid malformation volume ratio (CVR) predicts outcomes in prenatal diagnosis of cystic adenomatoid malformation of the lung. J Pediatr Surg. 2002;37:331–8.
8. Peranteau WH, Wilson W, Liechty KW, et al. The effect of maternal betamethasone on prenatal congenital cystic adenomatoid malformation growth and fetal survival. Fetal Diagn Ther. 2005;20:74–8.
9. Adzick NS, Harrison MR, Crombleholme TM, et al. Fetal lung lesions: management and outcome. Am J Obstet Gynecol. 1998;179:884–9.
10. Hedrick HL, Flake AW, Crombleholme TM, et al. The EXIT procedure for high risk fetal lung lesions. J Pediatr Surg. 2005;40:1038–43.
11. Seong YW, Kang CH, Kim JT, et al. Video-assisted thoracoscopic lobectomy in children: safety, efficacy, and risk factors for conversion to thoracotomy. Ann Thorac Surg. 2013;95:1236–42.
12. Rothenberg SS. First decade's experience with thoracoscopic lobectomy in infants and children. J Pediatr Surg. 2008;43:40–5.
13. Waldhausen JA, Pierce WS, Campbell DB. Surgery of the chest. St Louis: Mosby Year-Book; 1995.
14. Bignon H, Buela E, Martinez-Ferro M. Which is the best vessel-sealing method for pediatric thoracoscopic lobectomy? J Laparoendosc Adv Surg Tech. 2010;20(4):395–8.
15. Kunisaki SM, Powelson IA, Haydar B, et al. Thoracoscopic vs. open lobectomy in infants and young children with congenital lung malformations. J Am Coll Surg. 2014;218(2):261–70.
16. Bagrodia N, Cassel S, Liao J, et al. Segmental resection for the treatment of congenital pulmonary malformations. J Pediatr Surg. 2014;49:905–9.

17. Rothenberg SS, Shipman K, Kay S, et al. Thoracoscopic segmentectomy for congenital and acquired pulmonary disease: a case for lung-sparing surgery. J Laparoendosc Adv Surg Tech. 2014;24(1):50–4.
18. Vu LT, Farmer DL, Nobuhara KK, et al. Thoracoscopic versus open resection for congenital cystic adenomatoid malformations of the lung. J Pediatr Surg. 2008;43:35–9.
19. Albanese CT, Syorak RM, Tsao KJ, et al. Thoracoscopic lobectomy for prenatally diagnosed lung lesions. J Pediatr Surg. 2003;38:553–5.
20. Koontz CS, Oliva V, Gow KW, et al. Video-assisted thoracoscopic surgical excision of cystic lung disease in children. J Pediatr Surg. 2005;40:835–7.

15. Thoracoscopic Lung Biopsies and Resections in Children

Oliver J. Muensterer

Introduction

Thoracoscopy is less often performed by pediatric surgeons than laparoscopic surgery and has its own set of challenges. The working space in the chest is much smaller than in the abdomen, particularly in newborns and infants. Because dual-lumen endotracheal tubes are not available for small children, the ipsilateral lung often remains ventilated during the procedure, further compromising visibility and working space. Also, lower insufflation pressures are generally used in children to prevent mediastinal shift and hemodynamic instability.

Some lung lesions are easier felt than seen if they lie deep to the pleural surface. For success, preoperative marking may be required. Close interdisciplinary cooperation with interventional radiology is necessary for success.

Nevertheless, a large spectrum of pulmonary lesions lends themselves to thoracoscopic biopsy and resection. Avoiding a thoracotomy in such patients is a major opportunity to decrease postoperative morbidity including pain, scoliosis, scapula alata, and cosmetically conspicuous scars.

Epidemiology

Primary lung tumors are rare in children, the most common ones being carcinoid, inflammatory myofibroblastic tumor, and pleuropulmonary blastoma [1]. Most malignant lung lesions in children are actually metastasis, with secondary lung lesions outnumbering primary tumors almost 12 to 1 [2].

D.S. Walsh et al. (eds.), *The SAGES Manual of Pediatric Minimally Invasive Surgery*, DOI 10.1007/978-3-319-43642-5_15

In one study, blebs and bullae were found incidentally during thoracoscopic sympathectomy for hyperhidrosis in about 6 % of otherwise healthy individuals [3]. Although certain congenital diseases such as Marfan syndrome may increase the risk of spontaneous pneumothorax, the overall incidence of blebs and bullae was similar to the findings in the normal population [4]. Bleb disease is up to ten times more common in boys than in girls, and the annual incidence is about 20/100,000 [5].

Pathophysiology

Tumors of the lung may be neoplastic, granulomatous, or infectious in origin. Although type 1 congenital cystic adenomatoid malformation and pleuropulmonary blastoma share microscopic similarities [6, 7], their genetics make a simple transformation from the former to the latter less likely than previously thought [8]. Pulmonary metastasis of pediatric tumors is most often due to Wilms tumor, osteosarcoma, Ewings, rhabdomyosarcoma, lymphoma, and hepatoblastoma [9]. Benign pulmonary lesions may be infectious or granulomatous in origin and usually measure less than 7 mm in diameter on imaging studies [10].

Blebs occur due to intrinsic structural anomalies of the lung parenchyma and pleura. They are associated with tall stature and lower body mass index [3], although the exact pathomechanism for this association is still unclear.

Preoperative Evaluation

History and Exam

A careful history can hint whether pulmonary nodules are more likely to be neoplastic, granulomatous, or infectious in origin. Previously treated tumors may show their first sign of recurrence in the lung. The travel and family history can give clues toward certain unusual infectious diseases such as tuberculosis or hydatid disease [11]. Other items to query are a history of fever, cough, hemoptysis, or chest pain.

Lung nodules usually cannot be picked up by physical examination. An exception would be decreased breath sounds due to a spontaneous pneumothorax caused by a ruptured bleb or bullae.

Labs and Imaging

Laboratory workup is based on the presumed underlying pathology. It may include urine catecholamines for suspected neurogenic tumors, genetic markers when a syndromic etiology is suspected, or a rheumatologic workup for autoimmune granulomatous disease. Cultures of blood, sputum, or gastric aspirate may be appropriate if the history points toward an infectious entity. Furthermore, antibodies against certain microbes or parasites may be indicated.

Larger pulmonary nodules and blebs may be detected on plain film chest X-ray, but smaller lesions require computed tomography (CT) of the chest. Currently, new rapid magnetic resonance imaging sequences are investigated and show potential for detecting nodules in children over 3 mm in size [12]. While positron emission tomography (PET)/CT was found to detect even small nodules in children with good sensitivity, the specificity regarding histologic diagnosis was low in a well-designed study [13].

Pneumothorax from ruptured blebs is readily visible on plain film radiographs, but the underlying blebs usually require CT imaging (Fig. 15.1).

Surgical Indications

Pulmonary nodules that are increasing in size or associated with other pathologic findings should be biopsied or resected. Generally, thoracoscopy has been used successfully in children for tissue biopsy of lesions such as neuroblastoma, pulmonary metastasis, and lymphoma, with a low conversion rate under 5 % [14]. Patients with Wilms tumor and pulmonary metastasis on CT may be excellent candidates for thoracoscopic resection [15]. However, recurrence rates were high (over 40 %) when osteosarcoma metastasis was approached thoracoscopically [15, 16]. Therefore, thoracoscopy may be a valuable tool for the resection of a variety of nodules but not indicated in cases of metastatic osteosarcoma when complete resection of all lesions is the goal. Another indication for thoracoscopic lung biopsy is interstitial lung disease. Since the underlying disease is diffuse, a wedge resection of an easily accessible lung portion is usually adequate and easier to perform than finding a specific target lesion. If the macroscopic changes are subtle, separate biopsies at different sites can improve the validity of the histologic analysis.

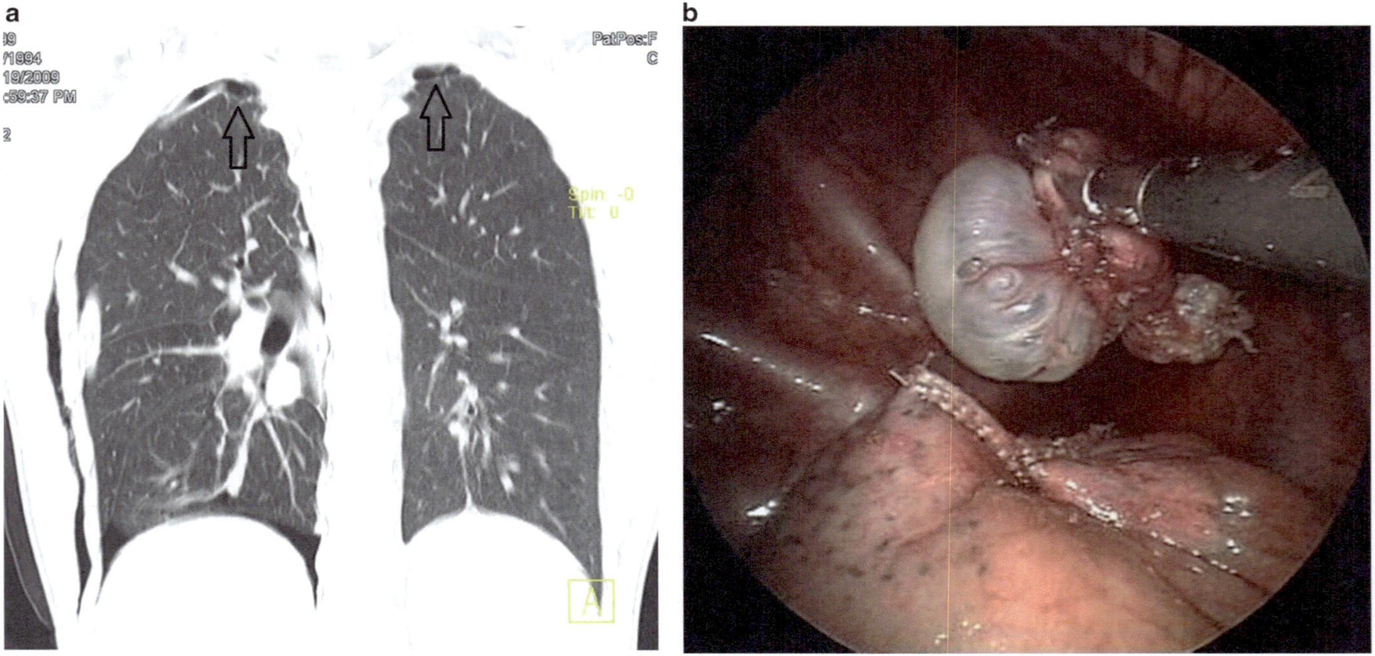

Fig. 15.1. Frontal CT reconstruction of an adolescent boy with right-sided spontaneous pneumothorax and bilateral apical bleb disease (**a**, *arrows*). In this case, bilateral apical bleb resection and pleurectomy were performed (**b**).

In cases of recurrent spontaneous pneumothorax with underlying bleb disease, thoracoscopic resection of the blebs or bullae is indicated. The blebs are usually located in the apical lung portions, but the entire lung should be inspected during the procedure for suspicious lesions. A simultaneous bilateral approach decreases the recurrence rate [17, 18], as does concomitant pleurodesis or pleurectomy of the apical parietal pleura.

Technique

Anatomy

Pulmonary lesions may be present in any of the five lobes. Parietal, peripheral nodules are easier to find thoracoscopically than central ones. Since tactile feedback is limited with thoracoscopy, deep parenchymatous lesions may require preoperative image-guided marking by methylene blue, patient blood, or placement of microcoils [19]. For non-peripheral lesions, it is imperative to recapitulate the vascular and bronchial anatomy beforehand in order to avoid any inadvertent injury or ligation of uninvolved structures or lung segments.

Special Considerations

Single-lung ventilation of the contralateral side is helpful but not mandatory, since the lung in children can be collapsed by insufflating carbon dioxide into the pleural cavity at a pressure slightly above positive end-expiratory pressure (PEEP). Double-lumen endotracheal tubes are not available for small children, so single-lung ventilation is achieved by main stem intubation of the contralateral side under bronchoscopic guidance. Alternatively, a Fogarty catheter can be passed into the ipsilateral main stem bronchus and inflated carefully to block the flow of gas. Care must be taken when repositioning the patient after such interventions, since both the endotracheal tube and the Fogarty catheter may easily dislodge with minimal movement of the head, neck, and torso.

Positioning

Generally, the patient is placed in lateral decubitus position for thoracoscopic lung biopsy. An axillary roll is mandatory, as is careful padding of dependent prominences to avoid pressure sores and nerve injury.

Depending on the location of the lesion, it may be worth angulating the patient more anteriorly than 90° (for posterior lesions) or posterior (for anterior lesions). During the procedure, it is helpful to shift the bed in Trendelenburg or reverse Trendelenburg position, depending on the location of the lesion or lesions. Therefore, the patient should be well secured to the bed. In small children, rolls should be placed on both sides of the torso. A vacuum beanbag may be useful for older children.

Port positioning depends on the location of the lesion. In general, the surgeon, endoscope, target tissue, and main monitor should be in one line, with the grasping port on the surgeon's nondominant hand side slightly beyond the optic port and the working port on the opposite side (triangular configuration). The size of the working port must be chosen to accommodate the selected instruments, depending on the method of resection (stapler, endoscopic loop tie, sealing device).

Instruments

Most thoracoscopic biopsies can be achieved in a three-port, triangulated technique. For children, depending on age, between 2 and 5 mm instruments are mostly adequate and include a Maryland dissector, a blunt grasper, a pair of Metzenbaum scissors, and a hook electrocautery. A 30°- or 45°-angled endoscope is useful to obtain a good view of all aspects of the pleural cavity. The lesion can be isolated from the rest of the lung using either an endoscopic stapler (usually 10–12 mm in diameter but recently also available as a 5 mm device), an endoscopic loop tie (usually 5 mm in diameter), or an advanced bipolar sealer (3–5 mm in diameter). Bronchi cannot be sealed effectively and require loop tie or stapled closure.

Operating Room Setup

As described above, the operating room should be set up so that the surgeon, optic, target lesion, and monitor are all in one line. In case of multiple lesions, this may require adjusting the monitor or changing positions during the procedure. It is helpful to have the surgeon and assistant on one side of the patient if only one monitor is used. For apical lesions, the surgeon and assistant may be better positioned on opposite sides, with the monitor or monitors over the head of the patient.

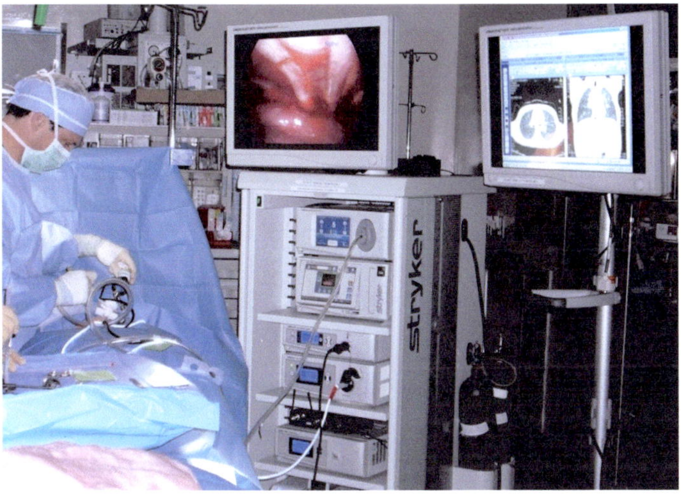

Fig. 15.2. This setup allows the surgeon to view both the thoracoscopic image and the computed tomography scan simultaneously facilitated with exact localization of the target lesion.

Discreet lung lesions may be difficult to localize. Therefore, having the CT and endoscopic image visible to the surgeon at the same time may help with intraoperative orientation (Fig. 15.2).

Operative Steps

- After placement of the trocars and gentle insufflation of the capnothorax, blunt graspers are used to explore the lung and localize the target lesion(s).
- Peripherally located lesions can usually be grasped, retracted and ligated with loop ties (Fig. 15.3), or stapled. It is advisable to use monofilament endoscopic loop ties because braided sutures may rub and twist the lung surface when cinched down.
- When using ties, it is very important that these are placed tightly and securely before transecting the tissue, as loose ties will lead to bleeding and possibly air leak.
- Depending on size, the specimen is removed from the pleural cavity through the largest port site available, either in an endoscopic retrieval bag (mandatory for neoplastic specimens) or directly

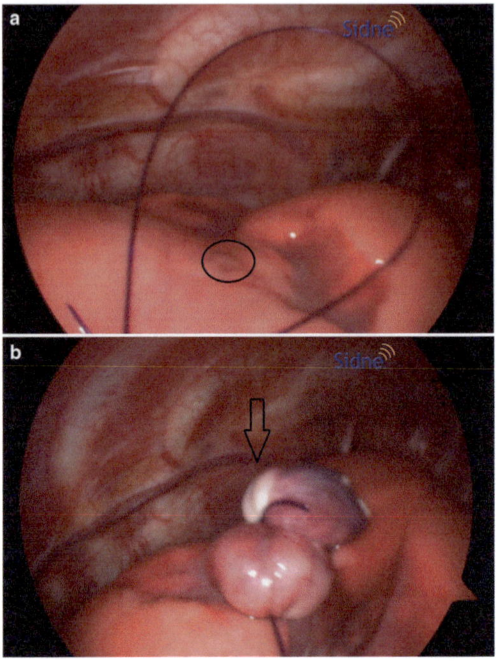

Fig. 15.3. Loop ties are a cost-saving, safe, and efficient alternative to endoscopic staplers for removal of pulmonary nodules (*black oval* in **a**). If the tie appears too close to the lesion for safe resection (*arrow*, **b**), a second tie can easily be placed below.

through the wound. It is helpful to have a camera that will fit a smaller port available so that it can be used during the retrieval process.

- If a pleurodesis or pleurectomy is indicated, it is performed at this time (Fig. 15.4).
- If there is bleeding or a chance of an air leak, an appropriately sized chest tube is placed through one of the port sites under vision and directed either posteriorly (to drain fluid) or anteriorly (to drain gas) under thoracoscopic vision.
- The gas insufflation is stopped, the trocars are opened, and the anesthesiologist is asked to inflate the lung by several Valsalva breaths. Expansion of the entire remaining lung is verified thoracoscopically, then the optic and trocars are removed, and the port sites are closed.

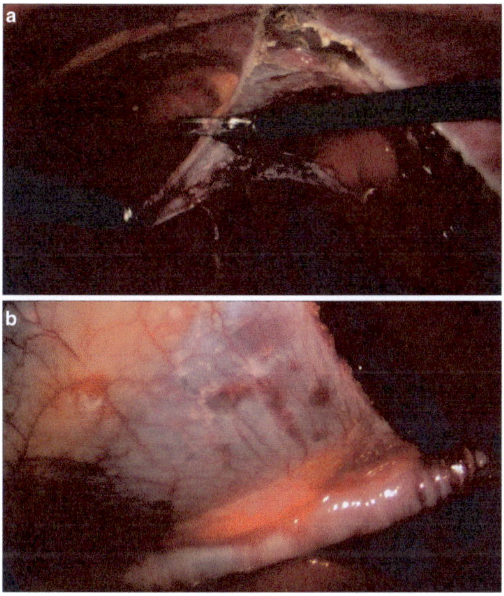

Fig. 15.4. Apical parietal pleurectomy is easily performed by incising the pleura with the electrocautery hook, grasping a loose end (**a**) and then twisting the pleural surface off by turning the instrument in analogy to opening a sardine can (**b**).

Pearls and Pitfalls

- Anticipate that lesions may not be visible thoracoscopically. For any lesion not directly involving the pleural surface of the lung, strongly consider preoperative interventional marking.
- Anticipate and consent for conversion to open thoracotomy if a lesion is not recognizable by thoracoscopy.
- Loop ligation of blebs and bullae is safe, effective, and less costly than using an endoscopic stapler [20]. But make sure that they are securely placed before transecting lung parenchyma.
- Prophylactic treatment of contralateral blebs in patients with primary spontaneous pneumothorax decreases contralateral recurrence [17]. If there are any signs of contralateral blebs on the CT scan, bilateral exploration and apical resection should be performed.
- In case there is a persistent air leak postoperatively, a tautologous blood patch is a useful option [21].

Postoperative Care

Regular diet is given once the patient has recovered from anesthesia. Appropriate analgesics should be administered. In most cases, a combination of oral acetaminophen and ibuprofen is sufficient. Postoperative prophylactic antibiotics are not required unless there is a specific infectious indication.

In most cases, a chest tube is only necessary in select cases when there is any question about potential bleeding or air leak. The chest tube can usually be removed after 24–48 h.

Depending on the condition of the patient, discharge is possible within 1–2 days after the procedure.

Outcomes

Although no formal randomized controlled studies have been published so far comparing open and thoracoscopic resection of intrathoracic lesions in children [22], retrospective studies have found that a thoracoscopic approach was associated with a shorter hospital stay [23] and a lower incidence of scoliosis in children up to 7 years after the procedure [24].

Complications

General complications of thoracoscopic resection of lung lesions in children include bleeding or air leak from the biopsy site. Sometimes, histopathology does not identify the lesion in the biopsied tissue. Therefore, if a lesion cannot be positively identified by thoracoscopy, conversion to the open technique may be necessary to aid with localization through tactile feedback. This should be discussed with the patient and caregivers preoperatively to generate realistic expectations. Also, in equivocal cases, sending the biopsy for frozen section by the pathologist can be helpful to make sure that the correct piece of tissue was resected.

Recurrent pneumothorax after bleb resection is another common complication. The risk of postoperative pneumothorax after wedge resection of bullae has been found to be inversely proportional to patient age, with younger patients experiencing more recurrences [25]. In one study, the most effective intervention to manage spontaneous pneumothorax in minors was thoracoscopic blebectomy using an endoscopic stapling device combined with pleurectomy [26]. This approach yielded a recurrence rate of 11 %, while resection of the bullae with an advanced bipolar sealing device was associated with a 30 % recurrence rate [26]. Simple thoracostomy tube placement and observation led to recurrent pneumothoraces in more than 50 % of cases [25].

Summary

- Thoracoscopic resection of lung lesions in children should become routine for most cases, since morbidity is lower and recovery if faster than after thoracotomy.
- Since tactile feedback is compromised during thoracoscopy, central nodules may not be amenable to thoracoscopy. In such cases, possible conversion should be anticipated.
- Pulmonary osteosarcoma metastasis requiring complete resection is better carried out by an open approach since the lesions are firm and well detectable by palpation.
- Apical bleb resection for spontaneous pneumothorax should be followed by pleurectomy or pleurodesis to decrease the rate of recurrence.

References

1. Yu DC, Grabowski MJ, Kozakewich HP, et al. Primary lung tumors in children and adolescents: a 90-year experience. J Pediatr Surg. 2010;45:1090–5.
2. Dishop MK, Kuruvilla S. Primary and metastatic lung tumors in the pediatric population: a review and 25-year experience at a large children's hospital. Arch Pathol Lab Med. 2008;132:1079–103.
3. Amjadi K, Alvarez GG, Vanderhelst E, et al. The prevalence of blebs or bullae among young healthy adults: a thoracoscopic investigation. Chest. 2007;132:1140–5.
4. Karpman C, Aughenbaugh GL, Ryu JH. Pneumothorax and bullae in Marfan syndrome. Respiration. 2011;82:219–24.
5. MacDuff A, Arnold A, Harvey J. Management of spontaneous pneumothorax: British Thoracic Society Pleural Disease Guideline 2010. Thorax. 2010;65:ii18–31.
6. Nasr A, Himidan S, Pastor AC, et al. Is congenital cystic adenomatoid malformation a premalignant lesion for pleuropulmonary blastoma? J Pediatr Surg. 2010;45:1086–9.
7. Priest JR, Williams GM, Hill DA, et al. Pulmonary cysts in early childhood and the risk of malignancy. Pediatr Pulmonol. 2009;44:14–30.
8. Boucherat O, Jeannotte L, Hadchouel A, et al. Pathomechanisms of congenital cystic lung diseases: focus on congenital cystic adenomatoid malformation and pleuropulmonary blastoma. Paediatr Respir Rev. 2016;19:62–8.

9. Erginel B, Gun Soysal F, Keskin E, et al. Pulmonary metastasectomy in pediatric patients. World J Surg Oncol. 2016;14:27.
10. Breen M, Zurakowski D, Lee EY. Clinical significance of pulmonary nodules detected on abdominal CT in pediatric patients. Pediatr Radiol. 2015;45:1753–60.
11. Cevik M, Boleken ME, Kurkcuoglu IC, et al. Pulmonary hydatid disease is difficult recognized in children. Pediatr Surg Int. 2014;30:737–41.
12. Sodhi KS, Khandelwal N, Saxena AK, et al. Rapid lung MRI in children with pulmonary infections: time to change our diagnostic algorithms. J Magn Reson Imaging. 2016;43:1196.
13. McCarville MB, Billups C, Wu J. The role of PET/CT in assessing pulmonary nodules in children with solid malignancies. AJR Am J Roentgenol. 2013;201:W900–5.
14. Acker SN, Bruny JL, Garrington TP, et al. Minimally invasive surgical techniques are safe in the diagnosis and treatment of pediatric malignancies. Surg Endosc. 2015;29:1203–8.
15. Guye E, Lardy H, Piolat C, et al. Thoracoscopy and solid tumors in children: a multicenter study. J Laparoendosc Adv Surg Tech A. 2007;17:825–9.
16. Yim AP, Lin J, Chan AT, et al. Video-assisted thoracoscopic wedge resections of pulmonary metastatic osteosarcoma: should it be performed? Aust N Z J Surg. 1995;65:737–9.
17. Chou SH, Li HP, Lee JY, Chang SJ, et al. Is prophylactic treatment of contralateral blebs in patients with primary spontaneous pneumothorax indicated? J Thorac Cardiovasc Surg. 2010;139:1241–5.
18. Nathan N, Guilbert J, Larroquet M, et al. Efficacy of blebs detection for preventive surgery in children's idiopathic spontaneous pneumothorax. World J Surg. 2010; 34:185–9.
19. Pursnani SK, Rausen AR, Contractor S, et al. Combined use of preoperative methylene blue dye and microcoil localization facilitates thoracoscopic wedge resection of indeterminate pulmonary nodules in children. J Laparoendosc Adv Surg Tech A. 2006;16:184–7.
20. Liu HP, Chang CH, Lin PJ, et al. Thoracoscopic loop ligation of parenchymal blebs and bullae: is it effective and safe? J Thorac Cardiovasc Surg. 1997;113:50–4.
21. Lillegard JB, Kennedy RD, Ishitani MB, et al. Autologous blood patch for persistent air leak in children. J Pediatr Surg. 2013;48:1862–6.
22. de Lijster MS, Bergevoet RM, van Dalen EC, et al. Minimally invasive surgery versus open surgery for the treatment of solid abdominal and thoracic neoplasms in children. Cochrane Database Syst Rev. 2012;1, CD008403. doi:10.1002/14651858.CD008403.pub2.
23. Petty JK, Bensard DD, Partrick DA, et al. Resection of neurogenic tumors in children: is thoracoscopy superior to thoracotomy? J Am Coll Surg. 2006;203:699–703.
24. Lawal TA, Gosemann JH, Kuebler JF, et al. Thoracoscopy versus thoracotomy improves midterm musculoskeletal status and cosmesis in infants and children. Ann Thorac Surg. 2009;87:224–8.

25. Noh D, Lee S, Haam SJ, et al. Recurrence of primary spontaneous pneumothorax in young adults and children. Interact Cardiovasc Thorac Surg. 2015;21:195–9.
26. Soccorso G, Anbarasan R, Singh M, et al. Management of large primary spontaneous pneumothorax in children: radiological guidance, surgical intervention and proposed guideline. Pediatr Surg Int. 2015;31:1139–44.

16. Thoracoscopic Treatment of Pediatric Chylothorax

J. Eli Robins and Kevin P. Mollen

Overview

Chylothorax is a condition characterized by chyle accumulation in the pleural space. In most instances, this is due to disruption of the thoracic duct or one of its tributaries through congenital anomaly, trauma, or malignancy. Without medical intervention, this uncommon type of pleural effusion can lead to significant morbidity and even mortality due to the loss of essential fats, proteins, electrolytes, and lymphocytes. The vast majority of patients will respond well to nonoperative management, which generally consists of thoracostomy drainage and a period of nothing by mouth (NPO) or a fat-free diet with a goal of decreasing chyle production. Indications for surgical intervention include a failure of medical management or the inability to keep up with nutritional loss [1, 2]. While at one time this required a posterolateral thoracotomy with ligation of the thoracic duct at the level of the diaphragm, advances in thoracoscopy have allowed for a minimally invasive approach.

Congenital chylothorax is a unique presentation of disease, affecting approximately 1 in 7000 births and accounting for the most common cause of pleural effusion in the first few days of life [3]. These cases are caused by congenital defects of the thoracic duct such as absence or atresia, birth trauma, or spontaneous idiopathic formation and are often associated with genetic syndromes including Noonan syndrome, Turner syndrome, and trisomy 21 [3]. Congenital chylothorax is a common manifestation of hydrops fetalis and pulmonary hypoplasia at birth due to impaired venous return and protein loss [4]. In these cases, both antenatal intervention and postnatal care have proven beneficial. The most common cause of chylothorax in older children is surgical disruption of the thoracic

D.S. Walsh et al. (eds.), *The SAGES Manual of Pediatric Minimally Invasive Surgery*, DOI 10.1007/978-3-319-43642-5_16

duct or its tributaries during cardiothoracic surgery [5]. Iatrogenic chylothorax in the pediatric population occurs in 2–4 % of patients undergoing cardiac or esophageal surgery and carries a mortality rate as high as 10 % [6, 7]. Patients with congenital abnormalities such as pulmonary lymphangiomatosis and lymphangiectasia may also present with symptoms later in life [5].

Once the chylothorax is identified, important considerations when deciding upon a treatment plan include prior health conditions, localization of the discharge, and the rate of chyle loss. The clinician must then consider three broad management strategies: (1) nonoperative/medical management, (2) procedural intervention, and (3) treatment of prior health issues such as malignancy or chronic disease [8]. A surgeon will often play a key role in guiding therapy and determining the optimal timing of intervention [1, 2, 8, 9].

Diagnosis and Anatomy

Patients typically present with respiratory distress as with any pleural effusion [10]. The thoracic duct begins at T12, where it ascends from the cisternae chyli in the retroperitoneum. It remains oriented to the right of midline until reaching approximately T6 where it crosses the vertebral body. Superior to T6, the thoracic duct continues its ascent until ultimately connecting with the venous system at the junction of the internal jugular vein and the left subclavian vein. The anatomy of the thoracic duct provides important diagnostic information especially in the case of unilateral perforation. Patients who present with a right-sided pleural effusion generally have a leak inferior to T6 on the right side, while left-sided effusions are usually indicative of a leak above T6. Lesions can also occur bilaterally, which can impact treatment options due to large volume losses.

Pleural fluid must be drained and analyzed for a definitive diagnosis. Typically, there is a milky appearance to the pleural fluid; however, this may also be the case in the setting of empyema. Further, a fasting patient or a patient with reduced intake of dietary fat with chylothorax may exhibit clear pleural fluid. While there are several methods used for analysis, testing the fluid for the presence of chylomicrons is the gold standard. This can be accomplished through lipoprotein analysis or cytological staining using Sudan III [2]. If lipoprotein analysis is not available, triglyceride and cholesterol levels are analyzed. Pleural contents are considered chylous if triglyceride levels are >110 mg/dL and cholesterol levels are <200 mg/dL [11]. If triglyceride levels are <50 mg/dL and cholesterol is

>200 mg/dL and there is an absence of chylomicrons, the effusion is classified as a pseudochylothorax, which is generally associated with chronic diseases such as tuberculosis and rheumatoid arthritis [9]. Low triglyceride levels in the setting of chylothorax may be indicative of fasting or malnutrition, which can accompany iatrogenic or chronic cases, respectively [10, 12].

Imaging

Chylothorax can be evaluated using a variety of imaging modalities, however usually begins with a chest x-ray (CXR) demonstrating a pleural effusion in the affected hemithorax (Fig. 16.1). For older children with nontraumatic etiologies, a CT scan is advised in order to rule out malignancy (Fig. 16.2). If an intrathoracic mass is discovered, treatments such as radiotherapy, chemotherapy, or steroids may be considered to address the chylothorax.

If no identifiable cause of chylothorax is found, investigations into the anatomy of the lymphatic system may be pursued. There are two methods used to visualize the lymphatic system; however, they are rarely performed in the diagnosis of chylothorax. Lymphoscintigraphy confirms the diagnosis of chylothorax by using radiolabeled albumin; however, poor resolution makes visualizing the site of perforation

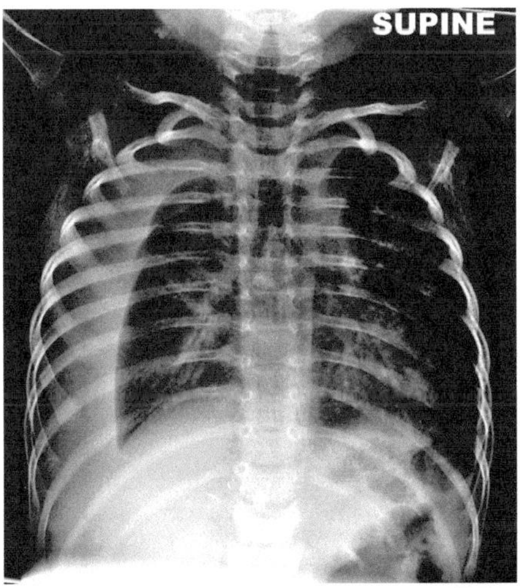

Fig. 16.1. CXR illustrating right-sided chylothorax in an infant.

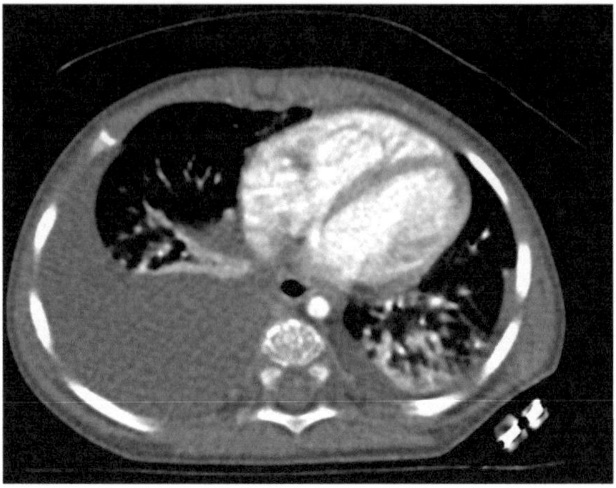

Fig. 16.2. CT illustrating right side dominant bilateral chylothorax in an infant.

difficult [13]. Although more challenging, lymphangiography is still the gold standard due to its accuracy in localizing the site of lymphatic disruption (Figs. 16.3 and 16.4) [13]. Lymphangiography also has the added benefit of causing sclerosant and occlusive effects to the thoracic duct due to the oil-based contrast lipiodol [14, 15]. While doses >20 mL can cause pulmonary arterial embolization, smaller quantities have shown success rates of 50–75 % in resolving chylothorax [16]. Recently, the use of unenhanced MRI with T2-weighted imaging (T2WI) has proven advantageous in the visualization of and preoperative planning for chylothorax [17].

Initial Management

Initial management involves relieving symptoms via drainage and replacing necessary nutrients. Due to the content of chyle, careful monitoring is necessary to avoid hypovolemia, immunosuppression, and significant protein and electrolyte loss [2]. Initial drainage may be performed via thoracentesis, and serial intermittent drainage may be considered. However, early chest tube placement should be considered to allow for complete evacuation of chyle and to facilitate the quantification of the amount and rate of drainage, which may help guide the treatment plan [16]. It is generally accepted that a period of nonoperative management should be pursued in the stable patient with a relatively low-output chylothorax. Some centers would continue with conservative measures if

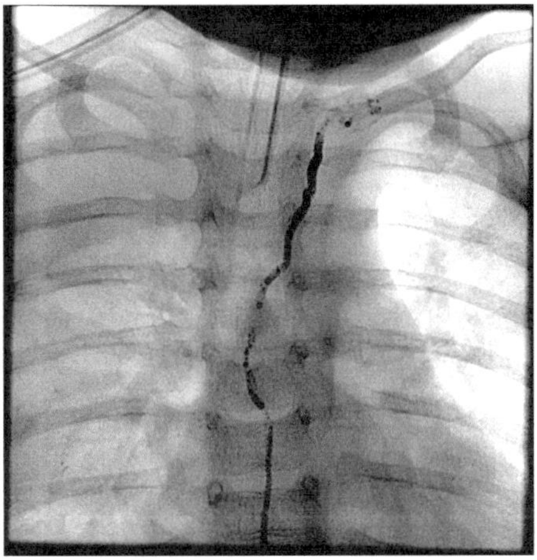

Fig. 16.3. Lymphangiography outlining the thoracic duct.

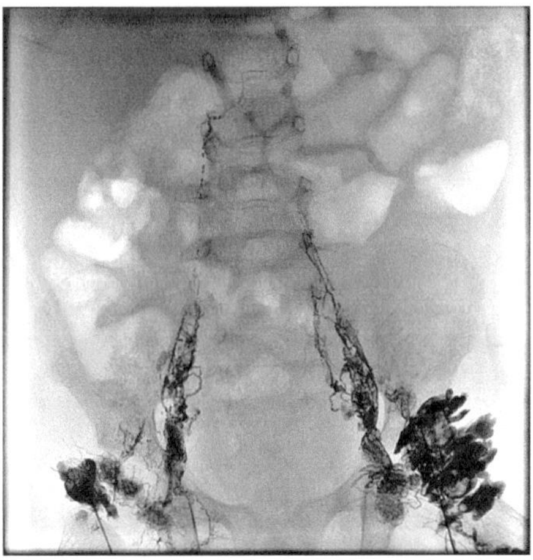

Fig. 16.4. Lymphangiography via injection of inguinal lymph nodes demonstrating no obvious leak.

outputs remained <10 mL/kg/day. Most series describing chylothorax in children suggest a window of 2–4 weeks before operative intervention, due to an 80 % success rate with nonoperative methods [5, 18, 19].

Steps may be taken to reduce chyle production in an effort to reduce pressure in the lymphatic system and allow for natural closure of the leak [1]. Chyle volume can be reduced through the administration of a fat-free diet with or without the addition of medium-chained triglycerides

(MCT). Unlike long-chained triglycerides, MCT are absorbed directly into the portal system, bypassing the lymphatics [8]. This therapy has been shown to resolve up to 50 % of congenital and traumatic chylothorax cases [20]. For infants, initial studies evaluating fat-modified breast milk as an alternative to MCT therapy have demonstrated effectiveness in treating chylothorax. Unfortunately, fat-modified breast milk may slow the growth of the child [21]. In cases of fetal chylous effusion, a low-fat, MCT diet given to the mother has proven effective [22]. If chyle flow does not adequately decrease with MCT, the use of parenteral nutrition with complete bowel rest has proven to further inhibit chyle secretion [23, 24]. If the leak rate exceeds 100 mL/kg body weight per day however, aggressive surgical therapy should be discussed [25]. There is some evidence for the use of somatostatin and its synthetic analogue octreotide in adults, although there is minimal evidence of efficacy in children [18, 26].

Procedural Intervention

There are several treatment options available if a chylothorax ceases to resolve with nonoperative management. These involve the use of targeted therapeutic agents, minimally invasive procedures, and open surgery. Although several treatment plans have been proposed, currently there is no consensus outlining when intervention should be employed. Several studies maintain that the timing of treatment escalation should be case dependent, particularly regarding patients with iatrogenic etiologies and neoplasms [2]. In congenital chylothorax, surgical management is sometimes initiated in as early as 7–10 days after presentation [27]. Successful intervention may decrease the length of hospitalization and reduce the risks of malnutrition and immunosuppression. Surgical success is enhanced when the location of leak is identified preoperatively.

Percutaneous Thoracic Duct Embolization

Percutaneous thoracic duct embolization (TDE) is a rare yet established approach to the treatment of chyle leaks [28]. This procedure uses lymphangiography to guide cisterna chyli or thoracic duct catheterization and embolization [16]. TDE has reported a 70 % success rate, with morbidity less than 2 % and no associated mortality [29, 30]. Rare sequelae include embolization of pulmonary arteries and chylous ascites [31, 32]. Due to the small size of lymphatic vessels, TDE is used much more commonly in adults; however, infants and children have been successfully treated using this method [33]. Embolic materials include dehydrated alcohol, fibrin glue, platinum coils, or a combination, which are delivered via microcatheter to seal the leak site [16].

Surgical Management

Thoracoscopy can be used for both thoracic duct ligation and pleurodesis in chylothorax cases [34–39]. This approach offers several advantages over open thoracotomy including enhanced magnified visualization of anatomy. The origin of the thoracic duct at the diaphragm can be difficult to visualize via an open approach due to its location deep in the surgical field. Further, thoracoscopy increases the likelihood of identifying a discreet leak, thus potentially decreasing the need for extensive dissection. It has proven safer and more cost effective in treating chylothorax in comparison to open thoracotomy [34]. With high efficacy and low morbidity, some have argued that thoracoscopy should be considered earlier on in the treatment of disease [2]. This is highlighted in cases of iatrogenic chylothorax post-esophagectomy, where mortality rates reportedly decrease by up to 40 % when surgical intervention is implemented at diagnosis.

Preoperative Preparation

Medical optimization of volume and nutritional status is key to the success of operative management. Visualization of the thoracic duct during thoracoscopy or an open thoracotomy can be enhanced by the preoperative enteric ingestion of cream, milk, or olive oil. Some have described enhanced visualization of the leak through injection of 1 % Evans blue dye in the thigh [35].

Positioning and Induction of Anesthesia

The procedure is ideally performed under single-lung ventilation. Traditionally, the operation involves three ports with port placement and patient positioning varying depending on the location of the leak [36, 37]. Most commonly, the duct is approached at the level of the diaphragm on the right side. In these cases, the patient is placed in the left lateral decubitus position and rolled forward (modified prone position) in order to enhance exposure of the posterior mediastinum. The right arm is extended in front of or over the head, and an axillary roll is placed. Neither central venous access nor arterial access is generally required for the operation although central venous access is often in place prior to surgery for parenteral nutrition.

Operative Technique

The camera port is placed at the sixth or seventh intercostal space in the posterior axillary line. An instrument port is then inserted under direct vision in the midaxillary line 2–3 interspaces below the camera port, and the final working port is positioned at or above the level of the camera at the mid- to anterior axillary line. Alternatively, the site of chest tube insertion may be used for one of the port sites. Further, if the location of a lymph leak is identified preoperatively or at the time of initial thoracoscopic exploration, port site placement may vary. The surgeon and assistant face the patient and work from anterior to posterior. Low-pressure CO2 insufflation is generally required to collapse the lung with single- or dual-lung ventilation.

The operation begins with a limited exploration of the hemithorax with adhesiolysis as needed and residual fluid evacuation. Then, a thorough evaluation of the vertebra down to the level of the diaphragm is performed. If a distinct source of leakage is identified, then this leak is directly addressed for attempted ligation. A number of means including clipping, suture ligation, or sealing using an energy device can accomplish this. Some surgeons will choose to place fibrin glue at the ligation site [38]. If no distinct area of leakage is identified or the duct cannot be adequately sealed at the source of leakage, then the duct is approached at the level of the diaphragm. The duct should lie posterior and lateral to the esophagus and does require some dissection to visualize. Division of the inferior pulmonary ligament will assist in efforts to identify the duct. If the thoracic duct is not visualized after pleural dissection, mass ligation of the duct and its tributaries has proven useful in management [38]. This involves multiple ligations within the posterior mediastinum once the aorta, azygos vein, and esophagus have been identified and kept out of harm's way. Due to the vast network of tributaries, overall lymphatic flow will not be affected, but the chylothorax should resolve [2, 38]. Ligation at the level of the diaphragm offers the benefit of blocking unrecognized tributaries. Although uncommon in the pediatric population, ligation during esophageal and cardiac surgery surgeries can be used as a prophylactic measure [39].

Pleurodesis is often employed as an adjunct to thoracoscopic duct ligation and has been shown to be both safe and effective in children [5]. During the thoracoscopic approach, mechanical pleurodesis is recommended with particular attention to the inferior thoracic space. This can be accomplished by a number of means including abrasion using a laparoscopic peanut or piece of a scratch pad introduced with a grasper. Partial pleurectomy may also be employed. We do not recommend chemical pleurodesis using talc. Pleurodesis is also a prominent choice when the leak site cannot be identified [2].

In select cases, nonoperative pleurodesis through a chest tube may be considered. This can be accomplished using agents which include tetracycline or bleomycin [27]. Success rates as high as 95 % with limited morbidity have been reported. For neonatal patients, pleurodesis using OK-425 (*Streptococcus pyogenes*) has been implicated in preventing pulmonary hypoplasia and enhancing respiratory function at birth [40]. Case reports have also documented successful intrauterine pleurodesis [41]. Chest tube pleurodesis has been used postoperatively as salvage therapy.

Postoperative Care

Patients should remain NPO postoperatively with a continuation of parenteral nutrition for at least 24–48 h or until evidence of lymphatic leak cessation. A multimodal approach to analgesia using intravenous narcotics, acetaminophen, and NSAIDS is generally employed although a directed nerve block may be considered. Early transition to oral medications is recommended. The chest tube is maintained on suction for a minimum of 48–72 h and should remain in place until the drainage is minimal (<20–50 cc/day of clear fluid/day). The chest tube should be placed on water seal for 24 h prior in removal. If there is no fluid accumulation after 24 h as seen on CXR, the tube may be removed.

Summary

- Chylothorax is a rare condition with a variety of etiologies and treatment options.
- The high success rate accompanying nonoperative management makes it the preferable initial option in the majority of cases.
- Fortunately, if symptoms do not resolve or if lymph losses are great, there are several interventional alternatives available.
- Minimally invasive techniques have dramatically reduced both the morbidity and mortality of disease over the past 60 years.
- While most contend that care must be managed on a case-by-case basis, a large control study focusing on the optimal timing of surgical intervention could further improve outcomes and decrease future morbidity and mortality. In the interim, we propose a new evidence-based algorithm to assist in the management of chylothorax (Fig. 16.5).

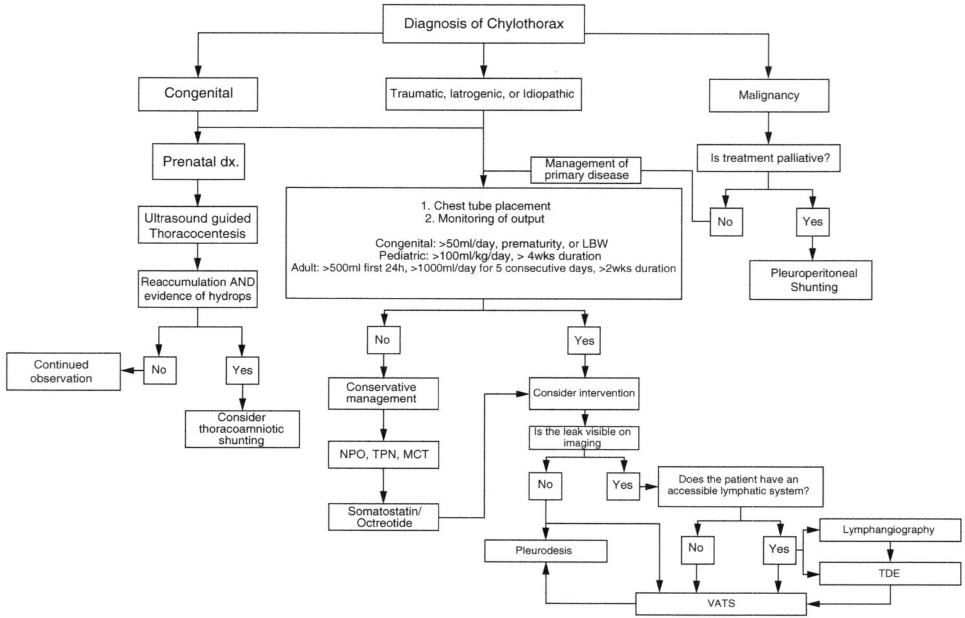

Fig. 16.5. Proposed treatment algorithm for chylothorax. The treatment algorithm depicted outlines management of chylothorax based on etiology, output volume, and duration of effusion. Progression through the diagram occurs following failed treatment, and duration is defined as days under medical management. Decisions concerning operative intervention are often dependent upon practice resources, and therefore the judgment of the surgeon is paramount in management of the condition. *LBW* low birth weight, *NPO* nil per os, *TPN* total parenteral nutrition, *MCT* medium-chained triglycerides, *TDE* thoracic duct embolization, *VATS* video-assisted thoracoscopic surgery.

References

1. Lee H, Gumpeni R, Jain M, Talwar A. Chylothorax: a review of current management strategies. J Resp Dis. 2008;29(8):325–33.
2. Nair SK, Petko M, Hayward MP. Aetiology and management of chylothorax in adults. Eur J Cardiothorac Surg. 2007;32(2):362–9.
3. Downie L, Sasi A, Malhotra A. Congenital chylothorax: associations and neonatal outcomes. J Paediatr Child Health. 2014;50(3):234–8.
4. Dendale J, Comet P, Amram D, Lesbros D. Prenatal diagnosis of chylothorax. Arch Pediatr. 1999;6(8):867–71.
5. Soto-Martinez M, Massie J. Chylothorax: diagnosis and management in children. Paediatr Respir Rev. 2009;10(4):199–207.
6. Mery CM, Moffett BS, Khan MS, Zhang W, Guzmán-Pruneda FA, Fraser Jr CD, et al. Incidence and treatment of chylothorax after cardiac surgery in children: analysis of a large multi-institution database. J Thorac Cardiovasc Surg. 2014;147(2):678–86. e1.
7. Haines C, Walsh B, Fletcher M, Davis PJ. Chylothorax development in infants and children in the UK. Arch Dis Child. 2014;99(8):724–30.
8. McGrath EE, Blades Z, Anderson PB. Chylothorax: aetiology, diagnosis and therapeutic options. Respir Med. 2010;104(1):1–8.
9. Hillerdal G. Chylothorax and pseudochylothorax. Eur Respir J. 1997;10(5):1157–62.
10. Etiology of chylothorax in 203 patients. Mayo Clinic Proc. 2005;80(7):867–70.
11. Staats BA, Ellefson RD, Budahn LL, Dines DE, Prakash UB, Offord K. The lipoprotein profile of chylous and nonchylous pleural effusions. Mayo Clin Proc. 1980; 55(11):700–4.
12. Pleural fluid characteristics of chylothorax. Mayo Clin Proc. 2009;84(2):129–33.
13. Ohtsuka A, Inoue Y, Asano Y, Woodhams R, Shiomi K. Lymphoscintigraphy using dynamic imaging and SPECT/CT in chylothorax. Open J Med Imaging. 2013;3:86.
14. Kos S, Haueisen H, Lachmund U, Roeren T. Lymphangiography: forgotten tool or rising star in the diagnosis and therapy of postoperative lymphatic vessel leakage. Cardiovasc Intervent Radiol. 2007;30(5):968–73.
15. Matsumoto T, Yamagami T, Kato T, Hirota T, Yoshimatsu R, Masunami T, et al. The effectiveness of lymphangiography as a treatment method for various chyle leakages. Br J Radiol. 2009;82(976):286–90.
16. Lyon S, Mott N, Koukounaras J, Shoobridge J, Hudson PV. Role of interventional radiology in the management of chylothorax: a review of the current management of high output chylothorax. Cardiovasc Intervent Radiol. 2013;36(3):599–607.
17. Yu D, Ma X, Wang Q, Zhang Y, Li C. Morphological changes of the thoracic duct and accessory lymphatic channels in patients with chylothorax: detection with unenhanced magnetic resonance imaging. Eur Radiol. 2013;23(3):702–11.
18. Panthongviriyakul C, Bines JE. Post-operative chylothorax in children: an evidence-based management algorithm. J Paediatr Child Health. 2008;44(12):716–21.
19. Milonakis M, Chatzis AC, Giannopoulos NM, Contrafouris C, Bobos D, Kirvassilis GV, et al. Etiology and management of chylothorax following pediatric heart surgery. J Card Surg. 2009;24(4):369–73.

20. Alvarez JF, Kalache KD, Grauel EL. Management of spontaneous congenital chylothorax: oral medium-chain triglycerides versus total parenteral nutrition. Am J Perinatol. 1999; 16(08):0415–20.
21. Kocel SL, Russell J, O'Connor DL. Fat-modified breast milk resolves chylous pleural effusion in infants with postsurgical chylothorax but is associated with slow growth. JPEN J Parenter Enteral Nutr. 2015;5:543.
22. Chylothorax and chylous ascites: Management and pitfalls. Semin Pediatr Surg. 2014; 23(5):298–302.
23. Ramos W, Faintuch J. Nutritional management of thoracic duct fistulas. A comparative study of parenteral versus enteral nutrition. JPEN J Parenter Enteral Nutr. 1986; 10(5):519–21.
24. Robinson C. The management of chylothorax. Ann Thorac Surg. 1985;39(1):90–5.
25. Marts BC, Naunheim KS, Fiore AC, Pennington DG. Conservative versus surgical management of chylothorax. Am J Surg. 1992;164(5):532–5.
26. Cannizzaro V, Frey B, Bernet-Buettiker V. The role of somatostatin in the treatment of persistent chylothorax in children. Eur J Cardiothorac Surg. 2006;30(1):49–53.
27. Favre R, Becmeur F. Surgical management of congenital chylothorax in children. Eur J Pediatr Surg. 2010;20:307–11.
28. Nadolski G, Itkin M. Thoracic duct embolization for the management of chylothoraces. Curr Opin Pulm Med. 2013;19(4):380–6.
29. Marcon F, Irani K, Aquino T, Saunders JK, Gouge TH, Melis M. Percutaneous treatment of thoracic duct injuries. Surg Endosc. 2011;25(9):2844–8.
30. Mauro MA, Murphy KP, Thomson KR, Venbrux AC, Morgan RA. Image-Guided Interventions: Expert Radiology Series. Philadelphia, Pennsylvania: Saunders (2nd Ed.), 2013.
31. Gaba RC, Owens CA, Bui JT, Carrillo TC, Knuttinen MG. Chylous ascites: a rare complication of thoracic duct embolization for chylothorax. Cardiovasc Intervent Radiol. 2011;34(2):245–9.
32. Binkert CA, Yucel EK, Davison BD, Sugarbaker DJ, Baum RA. Percutaneous treatment of high-output chylothorax with embolization or needle disruption technique. J Vasc Interv Radiol. 2005;16(9):1257–62.
33. Itkin M, Krishnamurthy G, Naim MY, Bird GL, Keller MS. Percutaneous thoracic duct embolization as a treatment for intrathoracic chyle leaks in infants. Pediatrics. 2011;128(1):e237–41.
34. Fahimi H, Casselman FP, Mariani MA, van Boven WJ, Knaepen PJ, van Swieten HA. Current management of postoperative chylothorax. Ann Thorac Surg. 2001;71(2): 448–50.
35. Achildi O, Smith BP, Grewal H. Thoracoscopic ligation of the thoracic duct in a child with spontaneous chylothorax. J Laparoendosc Adv Surg Tech A. 2006;16(5):546–9.
36. Graham DD, McGahren ED, Tribble CG, Daniel TM, Rodgers BM. Use of video-assisted thoracic surgery in the treatment of chylothorax. Ann Thorac Surg. 1994; 57(6):1507–12.
37. Kent III RB, Pinson TW. Thoracoscopic ligation of the thoracic duct. Surg Endosc. 1993;7(1):52–3.

38. Slater BJ, Rothenberg SS. Thoracoscopic thoracic duct ligation for congenital and acquired disease. J Laparoendosc Adv Surg Tech A. 2015;25:605–7.
39. Dugue L, Sauvanet A, Farges O, Goharin A, Le Mee J, Belghiti J. Output of chyle as an indicator of treatment for chylothorax complicating oesophagectomy. Br J Surg. 1998;85(8):1147–9.
40. Jorgensen C, Brocks V, Bang J, Jorgensen F, Rønsbro L. Treatment of severe fetal chylothorax associated with pronounced hydrops with intrapleural injection of OK-432. Ultrasound Obstet Gynecol. 2003;21(1):66–9.
41. Leung VK, Suen SS, Ting Y, Law L, Lau T, Leung T. Intrapleural injection of OK-432 as the primary in-utero treatment for fetal chylothorax. Hong Kong Med J. 2012; 18(2):156–9.

17. Treatment of Empyema in Children

Ashwini S. Poola and Shawn D. St. Peter

Introduction

Empyema is defined as the accumulation of pus in a body cavity, derived from the Greek word *empyein* which means to "put pus in." Current medical terminology generally refers to empyema as pus within the pleural space. In childhood, empyema is the most common suppurative complication of community-acquired pneumonia [1]. Other sources include posttraumatic or postoperative hemothorax, sequelae of viral influenza, and esophageal or transdiaphragmatic infectious spread [2]. Although overall rates of bacterial pneumonia have been declining in children, the incidences of complications, such as parapneumonic effusion and empyema, have increased [3]. As a result, there is an evolving discussion over effective treatment protocols for empyema management in the pediatric population.

Pathogenesis

Pleural effusions may develop in the absence of pleural inflammation, identified by worsened physiologic processes such as increased hydrostatic pressure, decreased oncotic pressure, or alterations of lymphatic drainage [4]. However, when the pleura is inflamed or infected as in empyema formation, the interaction of bacteria, lipopolysaccharides, cytokines, and chemokines physically alters pleural permeability and changes pleural fluid components [2]. Specifically, studies have found higher levels of interleukin-8 and TNF-alpha in empyema or complicated effusions [5, 6].

D.S. Walsh et al. (eds.), *The SAGES Manual of Pediatric Minimally Invasive Surgery*, DOI 10.1007/978-3-319-43642-5_17

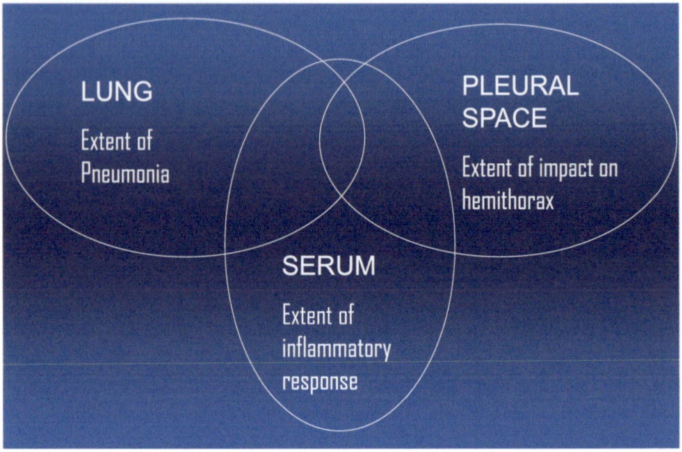

Fig. 17.1. Determinants of overall state of illness in patients with empyema.

The natural progression of parapneumonic pleural disease can be outlined over three to four stages of increasing complexity [7–9]:

1. The *pre-collection* stage is characterized by a localized pleuritis.
2. In the *exudative* stage, a simple effusion forms with clear, free-flowing pleural fluid with a low pleural white blood cell count.
3. The *fibrinopurulent* stage, or complicated parapneumonic effusion, is the classic empyema. Infected pleural space results in a procoagulant environment leading to decreased fibrinolytic activity with a concomitant increase in fibrin deposition. Fibrin acts as the tangible matrix for septations and loculations. This is heralded by an increase in the white blood cell count of the fluid.
4. The *organization* stage, the most advanced phase, results in a thickened rind, which may entrap the lung, manifesting as chronic restrictive lung disease.

Despite being sequentially outlined, there is no certainty that each stage will progress to the next. More importantly, the stage of pleural disease may not relate at all to the degree of physiologic illness. The severity of illness is determined by the extent of underlying parenchymal disease and the extent of intravascular inflammatory response. Patients may be quite systemically ill early in the course of severe pneumonia but clinically stabilized later on in empyema development, which should be considered prior to intervention. The patient should always be viewed considering the layers of processes when treating empyema (Fig. 17.1).

Diagnosis

Clinical Features

The diagnosis is a progressive clinical picture beginning with pneumonia. Patients with an empyema demonstrate some degree of respiratory distress, malaise, persistent fever, and pleuritic chest pain [10–13]. Physical exam reveals diminished breath sounds with dullness to percussion on the affected side indicative of substance within the pleural space.

Laboratory Evidence

Laboratory studies can play a role in the diagnosis of empyema. Serum studies often nonspecifically reflect an infectious process, such as a leukocytosis and elevated inflammatory markers. Pleural fluid findings can be useful. In addition to revealing an exudative process, they have been found to correlate with staging of parapneumonic processes. The Light criteria for complicated parapneumonic effusions include a pH <7.2, lactate dehydrogenase >1000 units, glucose <40 mg/dl or <25 % blood glucose, and Gram stain or culture positive along with loculations or septations proven by imaging [14]. As stages progress from simple to complex, pleural fluid reveals a decrease in glucose and pH while lactate dehydrogenase rises. Multivariate logistic analysis of a retrospective dataset found that pH less than 7.27 in pleural fluid was the only significant factor for the formation of fibrin with/without septations [15]. Similarly, a pleural fluid pH less than 7.1 has been found to result in a sixfold increase in the likelihood of surgical intervention based on retrospective data [16]. Regardless of the findings, in practice once pleural fluid becomes symptomatic, drainage is required.

Radiographic Evidence

Imaging is key in diagnostic evaluation of pleural space disease. Chest X-ray (CXR) is often the initial study and reveals poor penetration on the affected side. It is difficult to distinguish between parenchymal consolidation and pleural fluid using plain radiographs [17]. In a retrospective review of over 300 adult patients, CXR missed all effusions significant enough to warrant drainage by subsequent computed tomography (CT) scans [18]. Decubitus films, however, may be helpful to distinguish between free-flowing and loculated effusion [17]. While CXRs are readily available, adjunct studies are often required.

Ultrasonography (US) is portable, is relatively inexpensive, and involves no radiation. Bedside US assesses both the pleural space, revealing effusions of varying complexity, and the pleura itself (Kearney). Some authors suggest that US is superior to CT in the identification of pleural debris or loculations [19, 20]. It can reliably differentiate between parenchymal and pleural based processes [7]. A post hoc analysis of a prospective trial of pediatric patients studying fibrinolysis against operative debridement revealed 31 children who underwent both CT and US and found that CT offered no diagnostic benefit over US [3]. Two independent series reviewed the implementation of an algorithm using US first in children with complicated pneumonia. Both demonstrated a significant reduction in length of stay as well as a decrease in the use of CT without an increase in the rate of operative management or pleural drainage [21, 22]. In addition to providing accurate, real-time imaging, it can be used to guide percutaneous drainage and catheter placement [23, 24]. The main disadvantages include availability and operator dependence. Regardless, US has been demonstrated as an effective diagnostic tool for empyema management.

Radiation exposure from CT has raised the concern for overall lifetime cancer risk. This is of great concern in the pediatric population, in whom repeat imaging significantly compounds their risk. Nevertheless, CT scans may still be utilized; CT with intravenous contrast effectively differentiates between parenchymal and pleural processes [25]. A small retrospective review comparing US and CT suggested that CT should be used in complex cases only, such as patients undergoing surgery or considered to have parenchymal abscesses or bronchopleural fistulae [20]. Consensus statements are clear; the use of CT should be limited to only when necessary, such as in preoperative planning at surgeon discretion [7, 8].

Management

Empyema management is multifold. The ultimate aim is to return normal thoracic physiology by allowing for full expansion of the lung with the removal of infectious components of the pleural cavity. Treatment options are varied and include antibiotics with or without pleural drainage, intrapleural fibrinolytics via chest drains, or operative debridement via video-assisted thoracoscopic surgery (VATS).

Antibiotics

Historically, the most common causative pathogen in pediatric empyema has been *Streptococcus pneumoniae* [26–29]. While the overall incidence of pediatric community-acquired pneumonia has decreased with the initiation of heptavalent pneumococcal conjugate vaccine (PCV-7), pediatric empyema rates have increased. This has been found to be due to a multitude of organisms, including non-serotype *Streptococcus pneumoniae*, other *Streptococcus* spp., *Staphylococcus aureus*, and unspecified pathogens [29]. Understanding the source will also help reveal the underlying pathogen, e.g., mixed aerobic and anaerobic flora in esophageal rupture cases and subdiaphragmatic sources or *Staphylococcus* spp. in infected posttraumatic or postoperative hemothoraces.

Antibiotic regimens have been classically tailored to what organism is grown on a case-by-case basis, with initial recommendations for broad coverage, particularly for gram-positive organisms. There is little consensus on the duration of agents, particularly once interventions have been done. A retrospective review found that those transitioned to an oral antibiotic regimen after being afebrile, stable from a respiratory perspective and without evidence of loculations, resulted in a decreased hospital stay and financial burden. These patients still underwent approximately 7–14 days of parenteral therapy and, ultimately, were placed on additional 2–4 weeks of enteral therapy [30]. The British Thoracic Society recommended in adult patients a minimum of 3 weeks of oral therapy when the patient showed clinical improvement [31]. The most recent guidelines state a treatment for 10 days after resolution of fever in children treated for empyema complicating community-acquired pneumonia [8, 32]. A prospective, observational study for 7 days of therapy with oral antibiotics after afebrile, off oxygen, and completion of fibrinolysis is underway to help guide future management.

Pleural Drainage

General Principles

After identifying the presence of pleural fluid, the next step in management relies on understanding the nature of the fluid itself—free flowing versus frankly purulent. The need for intervention is dictated by size, symptoms, and presence of septations.

Size classification is difficult to precisely define. In general, small effusions have <1 cm rim of fluid, moderate effusions have 1–2 cm rim, and large effusions have >2 cm rim as seen on decubitus CXR. One pediatric study classified effusions as small, moderate, and large based on the degree of opacification on upright films, <¼ opacification, ¼–½ opacification and >½ opacification, respectively [33]. The authors found small and most moderately sized parapneumonic effusions that could be effectively managed with antibiotics and without drainage procedures without an increase in the length of stay or other complications, suggesting that interventions be based on symptomology versus size criteria alone [33].

Effusion size typically correlates with symptoms. Symptoms precipitating intervention generally include poor feeding intolerance, worsening tachypnea, and increasing oxygen requirement. A retrospective case series in children found respiratory distress on presentation was related to a prolonged stay and higher likelihood for intervention [34]. When symptoms seem to progress, further action is required to manage pleural disease.

Loculated pleural fluid indicates a later pathologic stage of empyema formation. In 2000, the American College of Chest Physicians stated the need for interventional therapy as the stage of parapneumonic effusion increased [35]. This is likely due to disrupted normal fibrinolytic properties in infected pleural fluid. Thus, resolution of septated fibrin matrices or thick pleural peel is unlikely without further intervention past antibiotic treatment [10, 21].

Thoracentesis

The decisional tree for fluid drainage includes the options of single or multiple thoracentesis versus tube thoracostomy. Single thoracentesis can be utilized in the drainage of free-flowing effusions. A prospective, nonrandomized series compared pediatric empyemas treated with repeated US-guided needle aspirations to tube thoracostomy. Thirty-five children underwent repeated needle thoracentesis every other day with an average of 2.4 drainage procedures per patient. This cohort had an overall similar length of stay to those managed with a traditional chest tube [36]. Although less invasive, there is still a requirement for local anesthesia and sedation with each drainage procedure. Practically speaking, while an older child may endure thoracenteses, it is arguable whether this would be tolerable in younger children.

Tube Thoracostomy

The British Thoracic Surgery guidelines recommend chest tube placement when initial thoracentesis fails to adequately drain an effusion to avoid multiple attempts [7]. A retrospective series compared children who underwent chest tube placement on the basis of effusion size and fluid analysis versus those placed only for mediastinal shift or progressively worsening symptoms. The study revealed no difference in hospital stay, suggesting judicious use of chest tubes [37]. Studies evaluating chest tube caliber have revealed catheters as small as 12 French may be used for adequate drainage purposes and for administration of fibrinolytics [38, 39].

Debridement: Surgical Versus Chemical

The definitive management for empyema has traditionally been surgical debridement. While this may be done via open procedures, the current gold standard employs the minimally invasive approach of VATS [40–44]. VATS has resulted in earlier and more complete resolution of empyema than chest tube drainage alone in both retrospective and prospective studies, resulting in shorter hospitalization lengths with primary VATS [45–48]. A retrospective series of 89 children undergoing primary VATS found that only 12 % had a risk of subsequent procedures for ongoing disease or complications [49]. In recent years, the standard of thoracoscopy is being increasingly challenged by chemical debridement as the definitive management for fibrinopurulent pleural space disease.

Chemical fibrinolysis takes advantage of the underlying pathophysiology of empyema formation. Infected pleural fluid allows for increased fibrin deposition, which later forms loculations in complicated effusion. Simply stated, fibrinolytics break down fibrin within the pleural space. Examples include urokinase, streptokinase, and tissue plasminogen activator (tPA). With local instillation, these agents target and liquefy the matrices of pleural debris in empyema and have been shown to be effective in promoting resolution of empyema in multiple series [46–57].

Fibrinolytics have been shown to be superior in chest tube drainage alone in both retrospective and prospective studies by both direct comparison and when used in patients who failed primary chest tube drainage only [50, 51, 54, 56, 57]. Moreover, empyema treatment with fibrinolytics via chest tube has been shown to be more cost effective than solely with chest tube [58].

There is still speculation over the efficacy of one fibrinolytic over another in pleural disease management. In a rabbit model comparing urokinase to streptokinase, there was found to be no overall difference in effect of pus viscosity after treatment [59]. An adult prospective randomized trial comparing these same two agents with empyema demonstrated no difference in disease resolution. Severe allergic reactions were seen in the streptokinase arm, and, thus, the authors concluded favorably for the use of urokinase [60]. As urokinase is no longer available in the United States, tPA has become the most commonly used chemical fibrinolytics. Comparison studies of fibrinolytics have not been done in the pediatric population.

The operative treatment involves placing the patient in lateral position. Lung isolation is not required and the lung will usually be adherent to the chest wall regardless. An initial 5 or 10 mm port is placed below the tip of the scapula and the camera is used to initiate the dissection by sweeping between the lung and chest wall to create enough working space for additional instrument sites. One or two additional ports can be placed with adequate triangulation to get around the entire chest. Through a 10 mm incision, a handheld curved ring tipped grasper can be placed straight into the chest without the port in place to remove large fibrinous chunks. The goal of the operation is to remove or break down the solid components in the pleural space which allows suction of the purulent fluid. It is not advisable to try to remove peel from the lung itself as there can be necrotic and friable areas of lung resulting in a persistent air leak or worse.

There have been three prospective randomized clinical trials comparing fibrinolysis to primary VATS for empyema management in children [61–63]. Two single institution series compared the instillation of three intrapleural doses of fibrinolytic agents to VATS at diagnosis [61, 62]. One utilized urokinase while the other used tPA. Results were highly concordant. Both revealed no difference in hospital length of stay and found VATS to be more expensive. One of these two reported no difference in days of tube drainage, days of fever, and doses of analgesics or oxygen requirements. Failure rates after fibrinolysis requiring salvage VATS was 16.6 % in both studies and is similar to previous studies [61, 62, 64, 65].

More recently, a multicenter randomized clinical trial comparing urokinase to VATS was conducted in 103 children specifically with complicated, septated parapneumonic effusions. Intrapleural urokinase

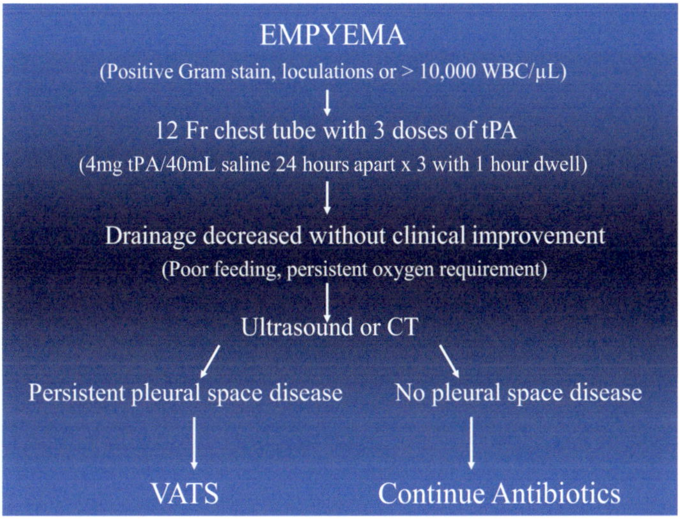

Fig. 17.2. Empyema management algorithm.

was instilled for 3 days every 12 h. The surgical protocol did not include debridement of the pleural peel of the lung. They found no significant difference in overall hospitalization length or postoperative length of stay. Failure rates were similar, 15 % in VATS patients and 10 % in urokinase; only 5 of these 13 total patients requiring salvage thoracoscopy and 8 were treated successfully with repeat fibrinolytics. Three-month radiologic follow-up was considered normal in 66.7 % of VATS and 59.5 % of urokinase patients, again revealing no difference. Overall, urokinase was demonstrated to be as effective as VATS as first-line therapy in treatment of complicated empyema [63].

Based on these studies, there is growing evidence in the efficacy of first-line administration of fibrinolytics in the management of empyema regardless of level of complexity. Current American Pediatric Surgical Association guidelines support this and suggest operative management should be reserved for failure after fibrinolysis [32]. Based on a comprehensive review of the literature, we propose an empyema management algorithm in the pediatric population (Fig. 17.2).

Summary

- The extent of parenchymal and systemic illness determines disease severity more than pleural pathology.
- Ultrasound is an effective, first-line imaging tool for diagnosis and management of empyema. Computed tomography should be reserved for complex pathology.
- There is no consensus on antibiotic duration, but current recommendations range from 7 to 14 days of treatment following resolution of fever.
- Patient's clinical condition, not effusion size, is more important in determining timing of intervention.
- Fibrinolytics are more cost effective and non-inferior to primary video-assisted thoracoscopic surgery; as such, they are an effective first-line management strategy for empyema.

References

1. Durbin WJ, Stille C. Pneumonia. Pediatr Rev. 2008;29(5):147–58.
2. Septimus EJ, et al. Pleural effusion and empyema. In: Mandell, Douglas and Bennett's principles and practice of infectious diseases. 2015, 70. p. 187–210, e2.
3. Jaffe A, Calder AD, Owens CM, et al. Role of routine computed tomography in paediatric pleural empyema. Thorax. 2008;63:897–902.
4. Sahn SA. State of the art: the pleura. Am Rev Respir Dis. 1988;138:184–234.
5. Aleman C, Alegre J, Monasterio J, et al. Association between inflammatory mediators and the fibrinolysis system in infectious pleural effusions. Clin Sci (Lond). 2003;105:601–7.
6. Porcel JM, Vives M, Esquerda A. Tumor necrosis factor-alpha in pleural fluid: a marker of complicated parapneumonic effusions. Chest. 2004;125:160–4.
7. Balfour-Lynn IM, Abrahamson E, Cohen G, et al. BTS guidelines for the management of pleural infection in children. Thorax. 2005;60 Suppl 1:i1–21.
8. Bradley JS, Byington CL, Shah SS, et al. Executive summary: the management of community acquired pneumonia in infants and children older than 3 months of age: clinical practice guidelines by the Pediatric Infectious Disease Society and the Infectious Disease Society of America. Clin Infect Dis. 2011;53:617–30.
9. Hamm H, Light RW. Parapneumonic effusion and empyema. Eur Respir J. 1997; 10:1150–6.
10. Buckingham S, King M, Miller M. Incidence and etiologies of complicated parapneumonic effusions in children. Pediatr Infect Dis. 2003;22:499–504.
11. McLaughlin F, Goldman D, Rosenbaum D, et al. Empyema in children: clinical course and long-term follow-up. Pediatrics. 1984;73:587–93.

12. Goeman A, Kipur N, Toppare M, et al. Conservative treatment of empyema in children. Respiration. 1993;60:182–5.
13. Schultz KD, Fan L, Pinsky J, et al. The changing face of pleural empyemas in children: epidemiology and management. Pediatrics. 2004;113:1735–40.
14. Light RW. Parapneumonic effusions and empyema. Clin Chest Med. 1985;6:55–62.
15. Padman R, King KA, Iqbal S, et al. Parapneumonic effusion and empyema in children: Retrospective review of the duPont experience. ClinPediatr (Phila). 2007;46:518–22.
16. Wong KS, Lin TY, Huang YC, et al. Scoring system for empyema thoracis and help in management. Indian J Pediatr. 2005;72:1025–8.
17. King S, Thomson A. Radiological perspectives in empyema. Br Med Bull. 2002; 61:203–14.
18. Brixey AG, Luo Y, Skouras V, et al. The efficacy of chest radiographs in detecting parapneumonic effusions. Respirology. 2011;16:1000–4.
19. Calder A, Owens CM. Imaging of parapneumonic pleural effusions and empyema in children. Pediatr Radiol. 2009;39:527–37.
20. Kurian J, Levin TL, Han BK, et al. Comparison of ultrasound and CT in the evaluation of pneumonia complicated by parapneumonic effusion in children. AJR Am J Roentgenol. 2009;193:1648–54.
21. Pillai D, Song X, Pastor W, et al. Implementation and impact of a consensus diagnostic and management algorithm for complicated pneumonia in children. J Investig Med. 2011;59:1221–7.
22. Shomaker KL, Weiner T, Esther Jr CR. Impact of an evidence-based algorithm on quality of care in pediatric parapneumonic effusion and empyema. Pediatr Pulmonol. 2011;46:722–8.
23. Balik M, Plasil P, Waldauf P, et al. Ultrasound estimation of volume of pleural fluid in mechanically ventilated patients. Intensive Care Med. 2006;32:318–21.
24. Eibenberger KL, Dock WI, Ammann ME, et al. Quantification of pleural effusions: sonography versus radiography. Radiology. 1994;191:681–4.
25. Brenner DJ, Hall EJ. Computed tomography--an increasing source of radiation exposure. N Engl J Med. 2007;357:2277–84.
26. McIntosh K. Community-acquired pneumonia in children. N Engl J Med. 2002; 346:429–37.
27. Byington CL, Spencer LY, Johnson TA, et al. An epidemiological investigation of a sustained high rate of pediatric parapneumonic empyema: risk factors and microbiological associations. Clin Infect Dis. 2002;34:434–40.
28. Tan TQ, Mason Jr EO, Wald ER, et al. Clinical characteristics of children with complicated pneumonia caused by Streptococcus pneumoniae. Pediatrics. 2002;110:1–6.
29. Grijalva CG, Nuorti JP, Zhu Y, et al. Increasing incidence of empyema complicating childhood community acquired pneumonia in the United States. Clin Infect Dis. 2010;50:805–13.
30. Baranwal AK, Singh M, Marwaha RK, Kumar L. Empyema thoracis: a 10-year comparative review of hospitalised children from south Asia. Arch Dis Child. 2003;88:1009–14.
31. Davies HE, Davies RJO, Davies CWH. Management of pleural infection in adults: British Thoracic Society pleural disease guideline 2010. Thorax. 2010;65(Suppl 2):ii41–53.

32. Islam S, Calkin CM, Goldin AB, et al. The diagnosis and management of empyema in children: a comprehensive review from the APSA Outcomes and Clinical Trials Committee. J Pediatr Surg. 2012;47:2101–10.
33. Carter E, Waldhausen J, Zhang W, et al. Management of children with empyema: pleural drainage is not always necessary. Pediatr Pulmonol. 2010;45:475–80.
34. Soares P, Barreira J, Pissarra S, et al. Pediatric parapneumonic pleural effusions: experience in a university central hospital. Rev Port Pneumol. 2009;15:241–59.
35. Colice GL, Curtic A, Deslauriers J, et al. Medical and surgical treatment of parapneumonic effusions: an evidence based guideline. Chest. 2000;118:1158–71.
36. Shoseyov D, Bibi H, Shatzberg G, et al. Short-term course and outcome of treatments of pleural empyema in pediatric patients: repeated ultrasound-guided needle thoracocentesis vs chest tube drainage. Chest. 2002;121:836–40.
37. Epaud R, Aubertin G, Larroquet M, et al. Conservative use of chest-tube insertion in children with pleural effusion. Pediatr Surg Int. 2006;22:357–62.
38. Rahman NM, Maskell NA, Davies CW, et al. The Relationship between chest tube size and clinical outcome in pleural infection. Chest. 2010;137:536–43.
39. Lin CH, Lin WC, Chang JS. Comparison of pigtail catheter with chest tube for drainage of parapneumonic effusion in children. Pediatr Neonatol. 2011;52:337–41.
40. Wurnig PN, Wittmer V, Pridun NS, et al. Video-assisted thoracic surgery for pleural empyema. Ann Thorac Surg. 2006;81:309–13.
41. Hope WW, Bolton WD, Stephenson JE. The utility and timing of surgical intervention for parapneumonic empyema in the era of video-assisted thoracoscopy. Am Surg. 2005;71:512–4.
42. Olgac G, Fazlioglu M, Kutlu CA. VATS decortication in patients with stage 3 empyema. Thorac Cardiovasc Surg. 2005;53:318–20.
43. Cheng G, Vintch JR. A retrospective analysis of the management of parapneumonic empyemas in a county teaching facility from 1992 to 2004. Chest. 2005;128:3284–90.
44. Tsao K, St Peter SD, Sharp SW, et al. Current application of thoracoscopy in children. J Laparoendosc Adv Surg Tech A. 2008;18:131–5.
45. Kurt BA, Winterhalter KM, Connors RH, et al. Therapy of parapneumonic effusions in children: video assisted thoracoscopic surgery versus conventional thoracostomy drainage. Pediatrics. 2006;118:e547–53.
46. Gates RL, Hogan M, Weinstein S, et al. Drainage, fibrinolytics, or surgery: a comparison of treatment options in pediatric empyema. J Pediatr Surg. 2004;39:1638–42.
47. Aziz A, Healey JM, Qureshi F, et al. Comparative analysis of chest tube thoracostomy and video-assisted thoracoscopic surgery in empyema and parapneumonic effusion associated with pneumonia in children. Surg Infect (Larchmt). 2008;9:317–23.
48. Chiu CY, Wong KS, Huang YC, et al. Echo-guided management of complicated parapneumonic effusion in children. Pediatr Pulmonol. 2006;41:1226–32.
49. Freitas S, Fraga JC, Canani F. Thoracoscopy in children with complicated parapneumonic pleural effusion at the fibrinopurulent stage: a multi-institutional study. J Bras Pneumol. 2009;35:660–8.

50. Yao CT, Wu JM, Liu CC, et al. Treatment of complicated parapneumonic pleural effusion with intrapleural streptokinase. Eur J Cardiothorac Surg. 2005;28: 599–603.
51. Ekingen G, Guvenc BH, Sozubir S, et al. Fibrinolytic treatment of complicated pediatric thoracic empyemas with intrapleural streptokinase. Eur J Cardiothorac Surg. 2004;26:503–7.
52. Kornecki A, Sivan Y. Treatment of loculated pleural effusion with intrapleural urokinase in children. J Pediatr Surg. 1997;32:1472–5.
53. Barbato A, Panizzolo C, Monciotti C, et al. Use of urokinase in childhood pleural empyema. Pediatr Pulmonol. 2003;35:50–5.
54. Cochran JB, Tecklenberg FW, Turner RB. Intrapleural instillation of fibrinolytic agents for treatment of pleural empyema. Pediatr Crit Care Med. 2003;4:39–43.
55. Stringel G, Hartman AR. Intrapleural instillation of urokinase in the treatment of loculated pleural effusions in children. J Pediatr Surg. 1994;29:1539–40.
56. Thomson AH, Hull J, Kumar MR, et al. Randomised trial of intrapleural urokinase in the treatment of childhood empyema. Thorax. 2002;57:343–7.
57. Chen JP, Lue KH, Liu SC, et al. Intrapleural urokinase treatment in children with complicated parapneumonic effusion. Acta Paedtr Taiwan. 2006;47:61–6.
58. Cohen E, Weinstein M, Fisman DN. Cost-effectiveness of competing strategies for the treatment of pediatric empyema. Pediatrics. 2008;121(5):e1250–7.
59. Light RW, Nguyen T, Mulligan ME, Sasse SA. The in-vitro efficacy of varidase versus streptokinase or urokinase for liquefying thick purulent exudative material from loculated empyema. Lung. 2000;178:13–8.
60. Bouros D, Schiza S, Patsourakis G, Chalkiadakis G, et al. Intrapleural streptokinase versus urokinase in the treatment of complicated parapneumonic effusions: a prospective, double-blind study. Am J Respir Crit Care Med. 1997;155(1):291–5.
61. Sonnappa S, Cohen G, Owens CM, et al. Comparison of urokinase and video-assisted thoracoscopic surgery for treatment of childhood empyema. Am J Respir Crit Care Med. 2006;174:221–7.
62. St Peter SD, Tsao K, Spilde TL, et al. Thoracoscopic decortication vs tube thoracostomy with fibrinolysis for empyema in children: a prospective randomized trial. J Pediatr Surg. 2000;35:265–8.
63. Marhuenda C, Barcelo C, Fuentes I, et al. Urokinase versus VATS for treatment of empyema: a randomized multicenter clinical trial. Pediatrics. 2014;134(5):e1301–7.
64. Misthos P, Sepsas E, Konstantinou M, et al. Early use of intrapleural fibrinolytics in the management of postpneumonic empyema. A prospective study. Eur J Cardiothorac Surg. 2005;28:599–603.
65. Doski JJ, Lou D, Hicks BA, et al. Management of parapneumonic collections in infants and children. J Pediatr Surg. 2009;44:106–11.

18. Thoracoscopic Approach to Pediatric Mediastinal Masses

Angela M. Hanna and Brandon VanderWel

Introduction

Mediastinal masses are rare in the pediatric population and may be discovered prenatally, incidentally, or because of symptoms. Advances in ultrasound imaging have led to early diagnosis in the prenatal population. Pediatric patients are often asymptomatic but may have secondary symptoms relating to compression of structures in the mediastinum, such as dysphagia or cough. Masses may be seen on imaging obtained for other reasons and found incidentally. Mediastinal masses are more commonly symptomatic in children than in adults. The pediatric thorax is smaller in size, making the size of a mass needed to produce symptoms significantly smaller than in adults.

There is a wide range of pathology contributing to mediastinal masses. Diagnosis can be made through history, physical exam, laboratory, and radiographic imaging, but final diagnosis may rest with pathologic evaluation. When evaluating a patient with any chest symptoms, mediastinal masses should be on the list of differential diagnoses. Many lesions can be safely resected using minimally invasive techniques. Video-assisted thoracoscopic surgery (VATS), also commonly referred to as thoracoscopic surgery, is an established part of minimally invasive pediatric surgery.

The most common presenting masses categorized by these locations are presented in Table 18.1 [1–3]. Many datasets only include primary tumors of the mediastinum and exclude duplication cysts, which are included in the discussion of this chapter. Thymic masses are mentioned in this chapter but are discussed in more detail in another chapter.

D.S. Walsh et al. (eds.), *The SAGES Manual of Pediatric Minimally Invasive Surgery*, DOI 10.1007/978-3-319-43642-5_18

Table 18.1. Most common mediastinal masses [1–3].

Anterior	Middle	Posterior
Lymphoma	Undifferentiated sarcoma	Neuroblastoma
Germ cell tumor	Lymphoma	Ganglioneuroma
Thymic masses	Foregut duplication cysts	Ganglioneuroblastoma
Undifferentiated sarcoma	Lymphangioma	PNET
Rhabdomyosarcoma	Rhabdomyosarcoma	Lipoma
Lipoma	Hemangioma	Lymphangioma
Hemangioma	Lipoma	Neurofibroma
	Wilms' tumor	Hemangioma
		Rhabdomyosarcoma
		Foregut duplication cysts

Preoperative Evaluation

History and Physical Exam

Young children cannot articulate their sensations, so parents should be asked to give a detailed history. Particular attention should be paid to symptoms of irritability, pain, fevers, fatigue, shortness of breath, stridor, anorexia, exercise intolerance, nausea, vomiting, and bowel movement changes.

Duplication cysts of the mediastinum often become infected and induce fever and cough. Fever and diarrhea can be symptoms of neuroblastoma and often prompt an infectious work-up. Weight loss despite adequate feeding can be an insidious sign of widespread pathology.

Compression of cardiovascular or respiratory structures is a very serious symptom of a mediastinal mass. Compression of the superior vena cava may result in superior vena cava syndrome with significant venous distention of veins superior to the heart. The most common symptoms are dyspnea and fullness of the face. Other symptoms include cough, arm swelling, dysphagia, chest pain, stridor, headache, vision changes, and hoarseness [4].

Patients may also present with heart failure due to compression of one of the great vessels of the heart. Rarely patients will present with paraneoplastic syndromes like opsoclonus-myoclonus syndrome from a neuroblastoma.

Labs

Routine labs including complete blood count, electrolytes, creatinine, liver function tests, and coagulation studies are standard laboratory work-up.

Lactate dehydrogenase may be elevated in lymphoma. Alpha-fetoprotein and beta-human chorionic gonadotropin may be elevated in nonseminomatous germ cell tumors. Neuroblastoma may have elevated catecholamine breakdown products, specifically urinary vanillylmandelic acid (VMA) and homovanillic acid (HVA).

Imaging

A chest x-ray is obtained as a first diagnostic test. An MRI may be helpful to diagnose some lesions, particularly neurogenic tumors. A CT scan is diagnostic for many lesions, and its delineation of structures and anatomic planes is superior for operative planning of lesion resection (Fig. 18.1).

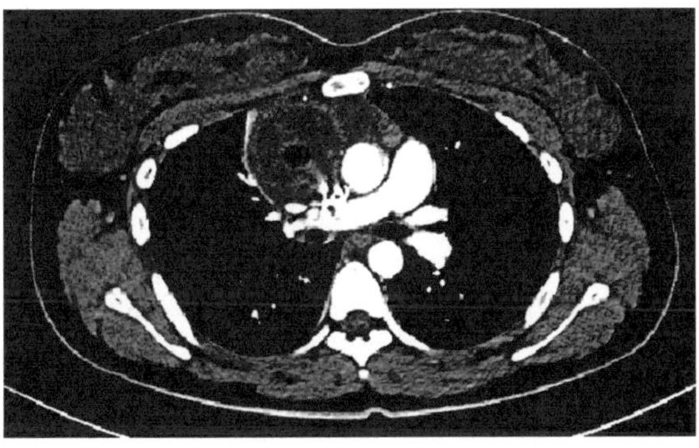

Fig. 18.1. CT scan of a large anterior mediastinal mass [5].

Surgical Indications

When a pediatric mediastinal mass is discovered, a treatment plan should be put into place to diagnose the lesion and treat appropriately. Prenatal diagnosis of a suspicious mediastinal mass should prompt a plan for resection within the first year of life before symptoms develop [6]. Mediastinal masses diagnosed after birth should be treated, especially if symptomatic. Surgery is the primary treatment for all mediastinal masses except for lymphoma, which is treated with chemotherapy, and therefore tissue diagnosis is important to determine appropriate treatment [7]. Some masses may be unresectable at time of diagnosis due to invasion of non-resectable structures and should be biopsied first if possible to make a diagnosis to direct neoadjuvant chemotherapy or radiation.

Large, symptomatic masses should be biopsied under local anesthesia due to the significant risk of cardiovascular collapse under general anesthesia and positive pressure ventilation. Duplication cysts warrant excision as they are often symptomatic from mass effect on surrounding structures, can become infected, and have a potential for malignant transformation [8].

Controversies

Solid Posterior Mediastinal Tumors

The role of minimally invasive surgery for solid posterior mediastinal tumors, including neuroblastoma, ganglioneuroma, and ganglioneuroblastoma, has been an area of considerable debate. Much of the literature about pediatric mediastinal mass survival does not distinguish between thoracotomy and VATS. Temes et al. found a 5-year survival for lymphoma was 74 %, neurogenic tumors 67 %, and germ cell tumor 25 % after treatment with standard of care but did not compare VATS to thoracotomy in patients treated with surgery [9]. Multiple studies demonstrate that thoracic neuroblastoma survival rates are better than abdominal or pelvic neuroblastomas, with survival between 77 and 100 %, but these studies do not compare thoracotomy to VATS [10–13].

Recent retrospective studies comparing VATS resection of neurogenic tumors versus open thoracotomy have reported equivalent rates of recurrence, survival, and disease-free survival with each group having similar tumor characteristics, including size and stage. In addition, thoracoscopic resection compared to thoracotomy has shown decreased perioperative morbidity such as less blood loss, shorter operative times, shorter hospital stay, and shorter duration of chest tube [12, 14–17]. Concerns raised for an increase in port site recurrence have not been supported in the current literature [17].

Pediatric thoracic neurogenic tumors including neuroblastoma, ganglioneuroma, and schwannoma are good candidates for minimally invasive surgery if imaging shows it is resectable. Thoracic neuroblastomas will frequently enter spinal foramina, and aggressive attempts at en bloc resection can result in significant injury and morbidity. Visualization with thoracoscopy is superior and can aid in a safe resection up to the level of the foramina without unnecessary injury [12, 14–16]. It is important to keep this in mind when trying to achieve surgically negative margins as to not cause excessive morbidity, especially for nonmalignant tumors such as ganglioneuromas, as this will not change prognosis or outcomes. Patients with tumors that are not resectable may benefit from biopsy to provide tumor biology and staging to direct neoadjuvant therapy. Biopsy may also be done to direct neoadjuvant therapy in an unresectable tumor that may later become resectable and amenable to minimally invasive resection.

Operative Considerations

Anatomy

Evaluation of the anatomy is critical prior to surgery. Cross-sectional imaging will allow you to assess the extent of disease and determine resectability. Unresectable tumors will invade into the great vessels, pericardium, lung, or spinal cord. Foregut duplication cysts will share a wall with its tissue of origin.

Anesthesia

It is important to have a clear anesthetic plan when preparing for surgery. Having an anesthesiologist experienced with pediatrics and minimally invasive thoracic surgery is recommended. Acceptable perioperative antibiotics include appropriately dosed cefazolin, ampicillin-sulbactam, vancomycin, or clindamycin [18].

General anesthesia is poorly tolerated in children with large mediastinal masses because their airways are more collapsible than those of adults. These factors, combined with decreased muscle tone and the supine position, increase the intrathoracic pressure and can occlude airways or prevent return of blood flow to the heart [19].

It is recommended to have a discussion with the anesthesiologist about the anesthetic plan prior to entering the operating room. Single lung ventilation may be used but is not always necessary. A double lumen tube can be used in children that are 8 years old or large enough for a 6.0 cuffed endotracheal tube, but smaller patients may require either single bronchus intubation or the use of a bronchial blocker. It is recommended that either of these techniques be done under direct visualization and placement confirmed with fiber optic bronchoscope. Insufflation of the thorax with 5–8 mmHg of CO2 is usually well tolerated and is often sufficient to deflate the lung. If insufflation is used, the anesthesiologist should be vigilant about monitoring for tension pneumothorax physiology and be prepared to alert the surgical team to desufflate immediately [20].

Room Setup

The room should be set up to easily transfer the patient to the operating table. Anesthesia is located at the head of the bed. The surgeon stands on the side of the patient opposite the pathology. The assistant stands above or opposite the surgeon. The surgical technologist is positioned near the foot of the bed on the side of the surgeon. It is ideal to have multiple video displays in line with the pathology facing the surgeon and the assistant.

Principles of Patient Positioning

Correct positioning of the patient is critical to the success of the operation. Gravity should be used to optimize exposure. The patient is positioned laterally with the lesion being as perpendicular to gravity as possible. Anterior masses are best approached with the patient in lateral decubitus and rolling the patient to be partially supine. Likewise, exposure to posterior masses benefits from the patient being tilted toward the prone position. Inferior masses benefit from Trendelenburg positioning, while superior masses benefit from reverse Trendelenburg. Towel or gel rolls are helpful in supporting smaller patients, while a beanbag should be considered for larger patients. Ensure that the arms are placed on arm boards and are not under stretch. The break in the surgical bed should be placed at the space between the inferior border of the lateral rib cage and the iliac crest to facilitate opening the rib spaces. A towel roll beneath the small child or neonate may be an adequate alternative to a break in the bed. When the patient is positioned, ensure that there is adequate clearance to manipulate instruments from the desired trocar positions.

Instruments

Standard laparoscopic instruments of appropriate size are sufficient for resection or biopsy of most mediastinal masses. Devices such as monopolar cautery via hook or scissors, a sealing device, or ultrasonic energy device are helpful to work with and can be chosen based on surgeon preference. In smaller kids, 3-mm trocars, instruments, and cameras may be used. There is a 3-mm sealing device that is available and that is helpful in the neonatal population. If a stapling device will be used, it is possible to use a 5-mm stapler, but otherwise consider which 5-mm port may be upsized to a 12-mm port to allow this if necessary. The smaller children have small rib spaces, and posterior rib spaces may be too small to comfortably place a 12-mm trocar. Also consider how you will remove the surgical specimen. Removing the specimen through a 5-mm incision is sometimes possible when the trocar has been removed.

Placing Trocars

Steps for placing trocars will use the same technique for each type of procedure but location of trocars will vary based on location of the mass. Local anesthesia is injected at the site of trocar placement by first feeling the rib inferior to the location with the needle then moving superiorly and injecting the inter-rib space. A small incision is made and the thorax can be entered with an open technique using a curved clamp or with a Veress needle. Insufflation to a pressure of 5 mmHg is tolerated well and assists with lung deflation. If using a Veress needle, dilatable expandable trocars are deployed after insufflation otherwise a regular trocar is placed. Insertion of a 3- or 5-mm 30-degree scope to view the location of the surgical target will help guide subsequent trocar placement. Two additional 3- or 5-mm ports should be placed under direct vision in a position that will allow triangulation. Trocars should be placed at least the distance of a closed fist away from one another, one trocar on the right and left of the camera. When placed under direct visualization, trocars can be placed in the posterior axillary line as high as the scapula allows and as low as the ninth or tenth intercostal space. Additional ports can be placed as needed, or 3-mm instruments can be placed through a stab incision without use of a trocar.

Steps for Thoracoscopic Approach to Mediastinal Mass

Anterior Mediastinal Mass Biopsy or Excision

Anesthesia

From an anesthesia perspective, masses located in the anterior mediastinum are the most problematic, and mediastinal masses overall carry a complication rate from 9.5 to 15% [21, 22]. Retrospective studies of anesthetic complications revealed the strongest predictor of complications to be evidence of tracheal or vascular compression, infection, and three or more respiratory signs or symptoms [22]. Another study found the presence of stridor was the only reliable symptom of prognostic value to predict poor tolerance to general anesthesia [22]. A thorough physical exam should be performed to determine if the patient is a candidate for anesthesia based on symptoms of vascular compression, shortness of breath, stridor, and any ongoing oxygen requirement. If the patient is unsafe for general anesthesia, an open biopsy under local anesthesia should be considered.

Positioning

After induction of general anesthesia, perioperative antibiotics are given, and preparations for single lung ventilation are completed; the patient is placed in the lateral decubitus position, heavily favoring a list to the supine position. The anesthesiologist is instructed to switch to single lung ventilation. A 5-mm trocar placed in the fourth or fifth intercostal space in the posterior axillary line is useful for visualization of lesions in the anterior mediastinum. Triangulating the other two trocars also in a more posterior position will help to work anteriorly. The surgeon will stand on the posterior side of the patient with the assistant standing above or opposite to hold the camera.

Biopsy

See the above anesthesia section for considerations if a patient can safely undergo a biopsy under general anesthesia. After entrance into the chest, attachments can be freed up with sharp and blunt dissection to adequately visualize the lesion. Pleural adhesions are best released with blunt dissection, but it is valuable to have sharp dissection, electrocautery, or an energy device available [23]. When the lesion is encountered, a biopsy location should be chosen that is not in close proximity to any vascular structures. A figure-of-eight silk suture in the biopsy target can facilitate exposure with minimal damage to the specimen [20]. To minimize cautery artifact, sharp dissection should be used to remove the specimen, and then cautery can be used as needed for hemostasis. The specimen will be significantly smaller than what appears on the magnified laparoscope; therefore, it is important to ensure that enough of a specimen is taken to achieve a diagnosis. If there is any question, frozen specimens for pathology are recommended. The specimen can be removed directly through a trocar or through a thoracoscopically deployed specimen bag.

Excision

It is important to consider the biology of the lesion to be excised and the objective achieved by removal of the mass. Compromise on margins in resectable, malignant lesions of the anterior mediastinum, like malignant germ cell tumors, negatively affects prognosis [24]. If a microscopic resection is needed to ensure complete tumor removal, the surgeon should have a low threshold to convert to thoracotomy to ensure a safe, complete resection without excessive morbidity.

The anterior mediastinum contains the thymus, as well as connective and lymph tissue. Dissection of the thymus is safe but should be avoided if unnecessary. Care should be taken to not injure adjacent structures including the internal mammary arteries on the posterior surface of the chest wall and the great vessels and phrenic nerves of the middle mediastinum.

The lesion is visualized and dissected free circumferentially from adjacent structures. Care is taken to protect surrounding structures. Blunt dissection with a grasper or suction catheter can be used for the majority of the dissection. Pleural adhesions can be released with sharp dissection, electrocautery, or an energy device [23]. Most of the dissection can be performed with blunt retraction and judicious use of cautery. Vessels are clipped endoscopically or cauterized. The specimen should be removed en bloc to prevent tumor spillage and spread. The specimen can be placed in an endoscopic bag to prevent potential contamination and tumor spread. Removal of larger specimens will require removal of the trocar and, if needed, extension of the incision.

Middle Mediastinal Mass

Positioning

After induction of general anesthesia, preoperative antibiotics, and preparations for single lung ventilation are completed, the patient is placed in the lateral decubitus position. Most often, access from the right chest will be optimal, but based on anatomy of the lesion, left chest access can be used as well. After the anesthesiologist has confirmed single lung ventilation, a 5-mm trocar in the fourth or fifth intercostal space in the anterior or midaxillary line is useful to start for most lesions in the middle mediastinum, but lesions that abut the anterior mediastinum may be better approached from a more posterior position. Two additional 5-mm ports should be placed under direct vision between the anterior and posterior axillary lines in positions to triangulate the lesion. The surgeon will stand on the posterior side of the patient to maximize visualization with the assistant above or opposite to hold the camera.

Biopsy

Once visualized, the lesion is dissected free from any attachments with sharp and blunt dissection. Pleural adhesions are best released with blunt dissection, as well as electrocautery or energy device [23]. When the lesion is encountered, a biopsy location should be chosen that is not in close proximity to any vascular structures. A figure-of-eight silk suture in the biopsy target can facilitate exposure with minimal damage to the specimen [20]. To minimize cautery artifact, sharp dissection should be used to remove the specimen, and then cautery can be used as needed for hemostasis. The specimen will be significantly smaller than what appears on the magnified laparoscope; therefore, it is important to ensure that enough of a specimen is taken to achieve a diagnosis. If there is any question, frozen specimens for pathology are recommended. The specimen can be removed directly through a trocar or through a thoracoscopically deployed specimen bag.

Excision

Malignant tumors of the middle mediastinum are rarely described as candidates for minimally invasive surgery. Important factors when considering a minimally invasive resection include the biology of the lesion and the objective achieved by removal of the mass.

Another important consideration is the location of the mass in relation to the structures of the middle mediastinum, including the heart, ascending aorta, pulmonary trunk, superior vena cava, phrenic nerves, and left recurrent laryngeal nerve. The thin wall and low pressure of the pediatric pulmonary artery make it a delicate structure, and it should be handled with extreme care.

Blunt dissection with a grasper or suction catheter can be used to dissect the mass from adjacent structures. The pleura can be opened with sharp dissection, electrocautery, or an energy device [23]. An energy device or hook and scissors connected to monopolar cautery is recommended for dissecting the specimen. A sealing device, clips, or stapler can be used to ligate any vessels. The specimen should be dissected and removed en bloc to prevent tumor spillage and spread. The specimen can be placed in an endoscopic bag to prevent potential contamination and tumor spread. The specimen can be removed through a trocar site after removing the trocar. The trocar incision may need to be extended to facilitate specimen extraction.

Posterior Mediastinal Mass

Positioning

After induction of general anesthesia, acceptable perioperative antibiotics, and preparations for single lung ventilation are completed, the patient is placed in the lateral decubitus position with forward lean to expose a significant portion of the back. Before entering the chest, ensure that single lung ventilation has been successfully achieved. A 5-mm trocar placed in the fourth or fifth intercostal space in the anterior to midaxillary line to start will visualize the lesion of the posterior mediastinum. At least two additional 5-mm ports should be placed under direct vision in the anterior axillary line or more anterior location to triangulate the lesion. The surgeon will stand on the anterior side of the patient to be able to maximize working posteriorly with the assistant above or opposite to hold the camera.

Biopsy

The pleura can be opened with sharp dissection to visualize the lesion. Pleural adhesions are best released with blunt dissection, but it is valuable to have sharp dissection, electrocautery, or an energy device available [23]. When the lesion is encountered, a biopsy location should be chosen that is not in close proximity to any vascular structures. To minimize cautery artifact, sharp dissection should be used to remove the specimen, and then cautery can be used as needed for hemostasis. The specimen will be significantly smaller than what appears on the magnified laparoscope; therefore, it is important to ensure that enough of a specimen is taken to achieve a diagnosis. If there is any question, frozen specimens for pathology are recommended. The specimen can be removed directly through a trocar or through a thoracoscopically deployed specimen bag.

Excision

Foregut Duplication Cysts

Upper esophageal lesions are approached from the right chest with the patient in the left lateral decubitus position, while lower esophageal lesions are approached from the left chest. An NG tube is placed in the esophagus and will grossly help with defining the normal esophagus. The lesion is freed up using both blunt dissection and electrocautery. The lesion should be resected in its entirety, including the cyst wall, to prevent recurrence. If there is a common wall shared by the cyst and the esophagus that the cyst cannot be separated from, then every effort should be made to completely resect the mucosal lining and safely obliterate any remaining tissue with cautery. If the common wall is included with the resection, then the esophageal wall should be repaired by using absorbable suture to close the defect transversely, if able, with full thickness, interrupted sutures. If unable to be closed transversely, then the defect can be closed longitudinally but should be performed over a nasogastric tube or bougie to prevent incorporation of the back wall into the suture line and to ensure that the esophagus is not excessively narrowed. Consider performing endoscopy at the end of the surgery to grossly observe patency. A bubble leak test of an esophageal repair can also be performed by insufflating the esophagus with the endoscope and thoracoscopically watching for bubbles from the esophageal repair submerged in saline. Any leaks observed from the esophagus should be repaired primarily (Figs. 18.2 and 18.3).

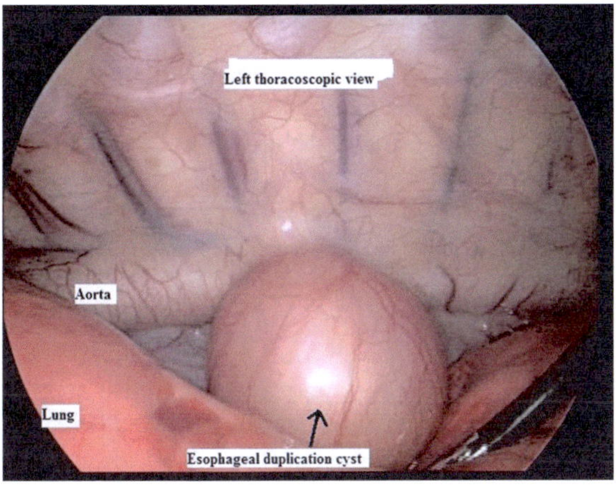

Fig. 18.2. Esophageal duplication cyst denoted by *arrow* [5] (Posterior).

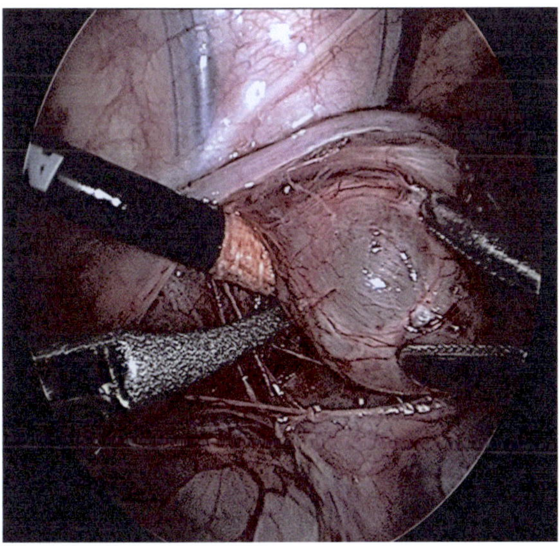

Fig. 18.3. Opening the pleura and dissecting the duplication cyst free [5].

Solid Posterior Mediastinal Tumors

To maximize safety and minimize frustration, ensure that adequate exposure is obtained and the lungs are retracted from the surgical field. A nasogastric tube in the stomach will assist the surgeon by allowing blunt palpation of the esophagus. The pleura is opened sharply, and adhesions can be released with blunt and sharp dissection, using electrocautery [23]. Blunt dissection with a grasper or suction catheter can be used, but sharp dissection will be used for the majority of the dissection. An energy device or scissors connected to monopolar cautery is recommended for dissecting the specimen. Again, it is important to keep in mind that while grossly negative margins are optimal, appropriate margins should be obtained, with care taken to prevent injury leading to significant morbidity, as well as unnecessary injury to surrounding tissue which may contain unseen neurologic structures. When the tumor is completely resected, the lesion should be removed en bloc and placed in an endoscopic bag to minimize the chance of tumor spread. The specimen may be removed through the largest trocar, extending the incision as needed for extraction (Figs. 18.4, 18.5, 18.6 and 18.7).

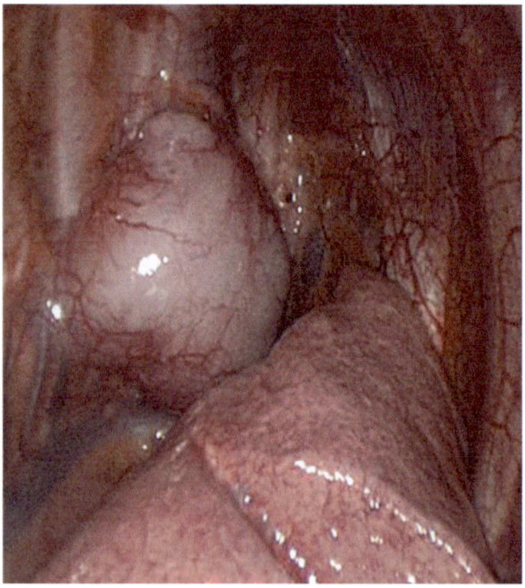

Fig. 18.4. Ganglioneuroma in the posterior mediastinum [5].

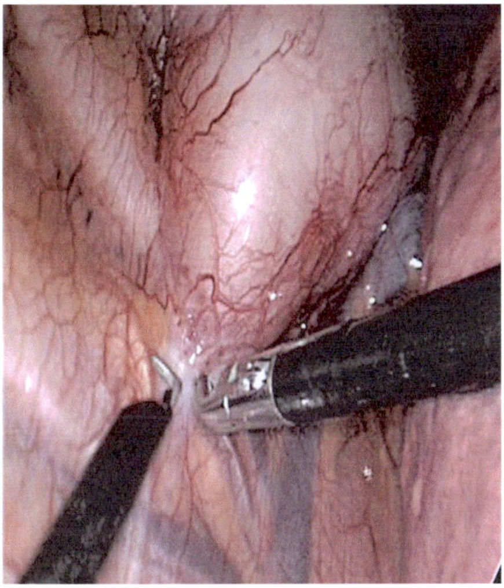

Fig. 18.5. Opening the pleura over a ganglioneuroma using laparoscopic curved dissector and monopolar cautery [5].

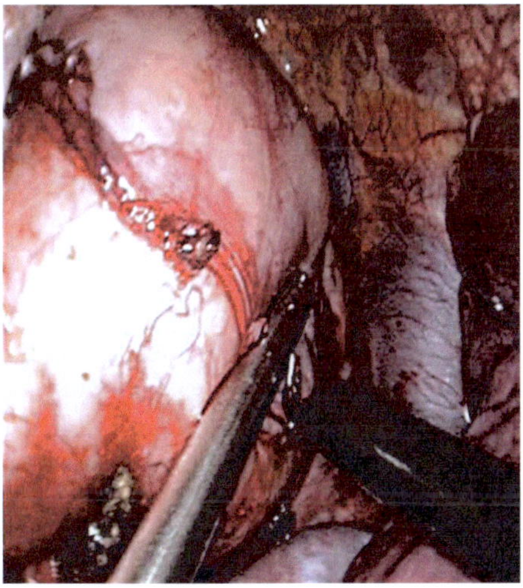

Fig. 18.6. Care is taken to not injure the accessory hemiazygos vein during dissection [5].

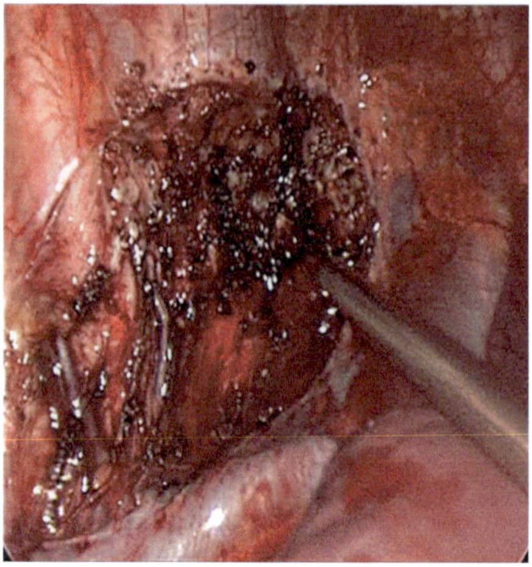

Fig. 18.7. Nonmalignant tumors like this ganglioneuroma should be dissected in a way that minimizes dissection into surrounding structures to ensure minimal morbidity [5].

Conversion to Open

Consider converting to open if there is uncontrollable hemorrhage, inability to ventilate, or poor visualization.

Closure

Placement of a chest drain is largely dictated by the type of tissue dissected. For thoracic surgery that does not injure or resect lung tissue, placement of a chest tube is at the discretion of the surgeon, but it is safe in some cases not to leave a chest tube [25]. Intercostal nerve block with bupivacaine improves pain control. Port sites are closed in layers with absorbable suture.

Pearls/Pitfalls

Pearls

- Correct positioning of the patient and trocars will maximize exposure and retraction.
- Have clear communication with the anesthesiologist regarding single lung ventilation and recognizing tension pneumothorax physiology.
- A 12-mm port may be required for the endoscopic bag device and endoscopic stapler. There are some 5-mm endoscopic bag devices and staplers available.
- Judicious use of monopolar cautery or an energy device will help provide a hemostatic operative field to maximize visualization.
- Consider having endoscopic ultrasound available for identifying the great vessels.
- Aspirate any potential biopsy location with a small needle to prevent biopsy of a vascular structure.
- Confirm with pathology that the specimen is adequate. Utilize frozen sectioning as necessary.
- Patients requiring support with high positive pressure ventilation or significant pulmonary parenchymal disease are more likely to benefit from a chest drain [23].
- Have surgical clips available for hemostasis. Have instruments to convert to open thoracotomy available in the room.
- Place additional 3- or 5-mm ports if dissection is a struggle due to poor triangulation of instruments or insufficient retraction.

Pitfalls

- Bronchial blockers, especially if located in a short right main stem bronchus, may become dislodged and obstruct the entire trachea.
- Excessive intrathoracic pressures may result in tension pneumothorax physiology.
- Identify the phrenic nerve and protect it.
- For biopsy, an adequate amount of tissue for diagnosis is the goal, not complete excision [20].
- If a duplication cyst shares a common wall with the esophagus, be prepared to repair the esophagus [10].

Postoperative Care

Postoperative Course

Patients are admitted to the surgical floor. Pain control with appropriately dosed acetaminophen and ketorolac in infants and young children is usually sufficient. Older children and adolescents may require narcotic medication. No further antibiotics are usually required. Diet may be advanced as tolerated immediately after the operation. Ambulation, as well as incentive spirometry, is encouraged. Chest x-ray is reviewed on postoperative day 1, and if a drain was placed, it is usually removed, sparing excessive output. If a small pneumothorax is identified, it will usually resolve spontaneously. Most patients are discharged by postoperative day 2 [20].

Complications and Outcomes

Postoperative complications include anesthetic respiratory and cardiovascular insufficiency, infection, bleeding, pneumothorax, chylothorax, and injury to surrounding structures. Complication rates of open thoracic surgery for mediastinal masses have been reported as high as 17% with Horner syndrome accounting for approximately and pulmonary complications, chylothorax, scoliosis, and neurologic complications accounting for the remainder [11]. In a series of neurogenic tumor resections with VATS, Fraga et al. reported a complication of Horner syndrome in 12% of patients and no deaths in 16 months of follow-up [12].

Long-term follow-up studies of patients who underwent pediatric thoracotomy report scoliosis developing in over one third of patients [26, 27]. The scoliosis was not severe enough to require treatment but did have a cosmetic morbidity [27]. It may be that the long-term risk of scoliosis development is less using thoracoscopy; however, long-term studies are needed to see if thoracoscopic surgery has a lower correlation to scoliosis.

Meta-analyses and retrospective comparative trials comparing outcomes between the procedures for a variety of pediatric thoracic pathologies concluded that a randomized control trial would be needed to truly compare the two techniques, but VATS was more likely to have less postoperative pain, few days with a chest tube, and shorter hospital stay [28].

Recurrence of foregut duplication cysts is very low and often zero with appropriate resection [23].

Summary

- Minimally invasive approach is reasonable to consider when planning resection of a mediastinal mass.
- Because there is a wide range of pathology, preoperative imaging is key to determine if the mass is resectable and if it involves any major structures.
- Any patient with a mass determined to be resectable should have a thorough evaluation prior to the operating room by an experienced anesthesiologist to develop a safe and effective anesthetic plan.
- General anesthesia should be considered with extreme caution in patients with pulmonary or cardiovascular symptoms.
- Proper patient positioning and trocar placement is critical to setting the stage for a successful VATS.
- Resection of pediatric mediastinal masses can be performed successfully with a minimally invasive approach and is gaining favor due to decreased morbidity, shorter hospital stay, and lower narcotic pain medication requirement.
- As techniques improve, pediatric surgeons' comfort and abilities to treat these lesions in a minimally invasive approach should continue to grow.

References

1. Gun F, Erginel B, Unuvar A, Kebudi R, Salman T, Celik A. Mediastinal masses in children: experience with 120 cases. Pediatr Hematol Oncol. 2012;29(2):141–7.
2. Freud E, Ben-Ari J, Schonfeld T, Blumenfeld A, Steinberg R, Dlugy E, et al. Mediastinal tumors in children: a single institution experience. Clin Pediatr (Phila). 2002;41(4):219–23.
3. Reynolds M. Foregut cysts of the mediastinum in infants and children. In: Shields TW, LoCicero III J, Ponn RB, editors. General thoracic surgery, vol. 2. 5th ed. Philadelphia: Williams & Wilkins; 2000. p. 2393–9.
4. Rice TW, Rodriguez RM, Light RW. The superior vena cava syndrome: clinical characteristics and evolving etiology. Medicine (Baltimore). 2006;85(1):37–42.
5. Photos courtesy of Jose Prince, MD., Long Island, NY.
6. Ballouhey Q, Galinier P, Abbo O, Andrieu G, Baunin C, Sartor A, et al. The surgical management and outcome of congenital mediastinal malformations. Interact Cardiovasc Thorac Surg. 2012;14(6):754–9.
7. Tovar JA. Anterior mediastinal tumors. In: Parikh DH, Crabbe DCG, Auldist AW, Rothenberg SS, editors. Pediatric thoracic surgery. London: Springer-Verlag; 2009. p. 225–31.

8. Sirivella S, Ford WB, Zikria EA, Miller WH, Samadani SR, Sullivan ME. Foregut cysts of the mediastinum. Results in 20 consecutive surgically treated cases. J Thorac Cardiovasc Surg. 1985;90(5):776–82.
9. Temes R, Allen N, Chavez T, Crowell R, Key C, Wernly J. Primary mediastinal malignancies in children: report of 22 patients and comparison to 197 adults. Oncologist. 2000;5(3):179–84.
10. Dutta S, Albanese CT. Thoracoscopic excision of foregut duplications. In: Holcomb III GW, Georgeson K, Rothenberg SS, editors. Atlas of pediatric laparoscopy and thoracoscopy with CD. Elsevier Health Sciences; 2008. p. 279–83.
11. Harble B, Hero B, Berthold F, von Schweinitz D. Characteristics and outcome of thoracic neuroblastoma. Eur J Pediatr Surg. 2002;12(3):145–50.
12. Fraga JC, Rothenberg S, Kiely E, Pierro A. Video-assisted thoracic surgery resection for pediatric mediastinal neurogenic tumors. J Pediatr Surg. 2012;47(7):1349–53.
13. Adams GA, Shochat SJ, Smith EI, Shuster JJ, Joshi VV, Altshuler G, et al. Thoracic neuroblastoma: a Pediatric Oncology Group study. J Pediatr Surg. 1993;28(3):372–7. discussion 7–8.
14. Malek MM, Mollen KP, Kane TD, Shah SR, Irwin C. Thoracic neuroblastoma: a retrospective review of our institutional experience with comparison of the thoracoscopic and open approaches to resection. J Pediatr Surg. 2010;45:1622–6.
15. Lacreuse I, Valla JS, de Lagausie P, Varlet F, H'eloury Y, Temporal G, et al. Thoracoscopic resection of neurogenic tumors in children. J Pediatr Surg. 2007;42: 1725–8.
16. Fraga JC, Aydogdu B, Aufieri R, Silva GV, Schopf L, Takamatu E, et al. Surgical treatment for pediatric mediastinal neurogenic tumors. Ann Thorac Surg. 2010;90:413–8. doi:10.1016/j.athoracsur.2010.04.086.
17. Petty JK, Bensard DD, Partrick DA, Hendrickson RJ, Albano EA, Karrer FM. Resection of neurogenic tumors in children: is thoracoscopy superior to thoracotomy? J Am Coll Surg. 2006;203(5):699–703.
18. Anderson DJ, Sexton DJ. Antimicrobial prophylaxis for prevention of surgical site infection in adults. In: Harris A, editor. UpToDate, Waltham, MA. Accessed 20 Aug 2015.
19. Pearson JK, Tan GM. Pediatric anterior mediastinal mass: a review article. Semin Cardiothorac Vasc Anesth. 2015;19(3):248–54.
20. Little DC, Holcomb III GW. Thoracoscopic biopsy of a mediastinal mass. In: Holcomb III GW, Georgeson K, Rothenberg SS, editors. Atlas of pediatric laparoscopy and thoracoscopy with CD. Elsevier Health Sciences; 2008. p. 275–83.
21. Anghelescu DL, Burgoyne LL, Liu T, Li CS, Pui CH, Hudson MM, et al. Clinical and diagnostic imaging findings predict anesthetic complications in children presenting with malignant mediastinal masses. Paediatr Anaesth. 2007;17(11):1090–8.
22. Ng A, Bennett J, Bromley P, Davies P, Morland B. Anaesthetic outcome and predictive risk factors in children with mediastinal tumours. Pediatr Blood Cancer. 2007; 48(2):160–4.
23. Ponsky TA, Rothenberg SS. Foregut duplication cysts. In: Parikh DH, Crabbe DCG, Auldist AW, Rothenberg SS, editors. Pediatric thoracic surgery. London: Springer; 2009. p. 383–7.

24. Schneider DT, Calaminus G, Reinhard H, Gutjahr P, Kremens B, Harms D, et al. Primary mediastinal germ cell tumors in children and adolescents: results of the German cooperative protocols MAKEI 83/86, 89, and 96. J Clin Oncol. 2000;18:832–9.
25. Ponsky TA, Rothenberg SS, Tsao K, Ostlie DJ, St Peter SD, Holcomb GW. Thoracoscopy in children: is a chest tube necessary? J Laparoendosc Adv Surg Tech A. 2009;19 Suppl 1:S23–5.
26. Westfelt JN, Nordwall A. Thoracotomy and scoliosis. Spine (Phila Pa 1976). 1991;16(9):1124–5.
27. Durning RP, Scoles PV, Fox OD. Scoliosis after thoracotomy in tracheoesophageal fistula patients. A follow-up study. J Bone Joint Surg Am. 1980;62(7):1156–9.
28. Dingemann C, Ure B, Dingemann J. Thoracoscopic procedures in pediatric surgery: what is the evidence? Eur J Pediatr Surg. 2014;24(1):14–9.

19. Minimally Invasive Approaches to Esophageal Disorders: Strictures, Webs, and Duplications

Timothy D. Kane and Nicholas E. Bruns

Introduction

Disorders of the esophagus in infants and children are comprised of acquired and congenital conditions. The most common acquired problems of the esophagus are strictures secondary to caustic ingestion or postoperative esophageal anastomotic complications. Esophageal webs or distal congenital stenosis on the esophagus are very rare but often require intervention secondary to feeding difficulties in these children. Duplications of the esophagus are often asymptomatic and found incidentally when radiographic imaging of the chest or barium esophagram is performed for unrelated indications. The diagnosis of each of these will be outlined together since the workup is similar with a few exceptions. The general operative management of each condition will be discussed individually.

Esophageal Strictures and Webs

Strictures are most commonly secondary to caustic ingestion or esophageal anastomotic complications following esophageal atresia repair or esophageal resection. Esophageal webs or congenital esophageal stenosis are rare with an estimated incidence of 1 in 25,000–50,000 individuals [1]. Webs typically occur in the upper third of the esophagus and present with dysphagia and infant refusal of solid foods [2]. Congenital esophageal stenosis may usually be managed by esophageal dilation [1–3] using techniques as described above, but some may require resection depending upon the etiology of the stenosis [4].

D.S. Walsh et al. (eds.), *The SAGES Manual of Pediatric Minimally Invasive Surgery*, DOI 10.1007/978-3-319-43642-5_19

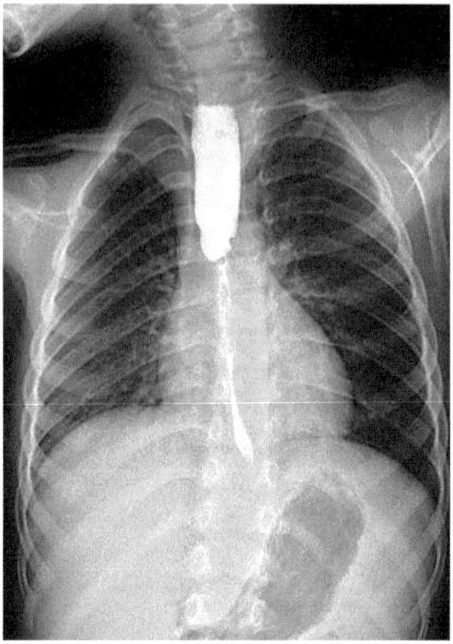

Fig. 19.1. Short esophageal stricture secondary to caustic ingestion in a 5-year old that was recalcitrant to esophageal dilatation.

Preoperative Evaluation

A child with known caustic ingestion should be evaluated for esophageal stricture at a month following ingestion regardless of symptoms. If there has been inability to feed the child during the time prior to this interval, a nasogastric or surgical gastrostomy should have been placed. The majority of children will present with progressive dysphagia (with or without weight loss) and vomiting. Similarly, an infant or child who has undergone esophageal anastomosis for esophageal atresia or segmental esophageal resection will present with dysphagia or emesis if a significant anastomotic stricture develops.

Common signs and symptoms of esophageal stricture include drooling, feeding intolerance, emesis, and dysphagia. In general, laboratory studies are not helpful. If there has been long-standing feed intolerance, it may be prudent to evaluate for electrolyte disturbances.

Barium esophagram is the primary study needed to assess strictures whether they are from caustic injury or postsurgical (Figs. 19.1, 19.2 and 19.3). Double endoscopy (under fluoroscopy) via oropharynx and gastrostomy is also useful to assess stricture length (Figs. 19.4 and 19.5).

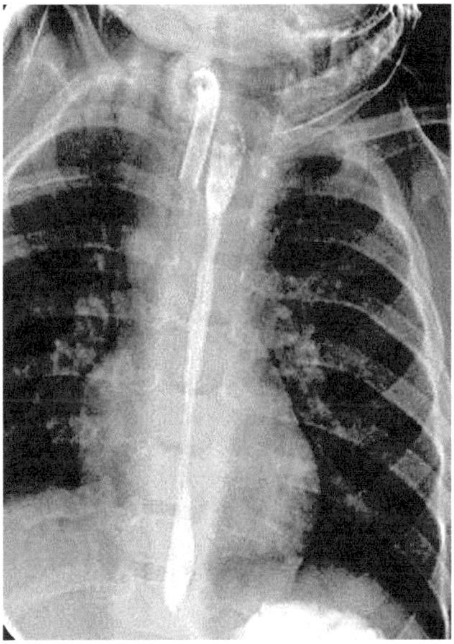

Fig. 19.2. Long esophageal stricture secondary to accidental caustic ingestion in an 18-month-old infant.

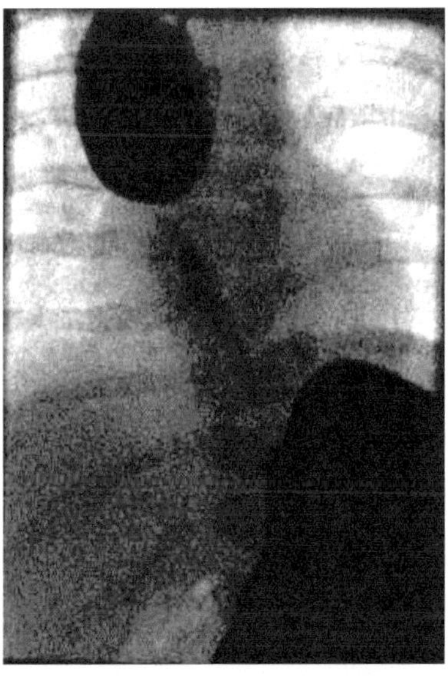

Fig. 19.3. Postoperative anastomotic stricture in a patient with pure esophageal atresia.

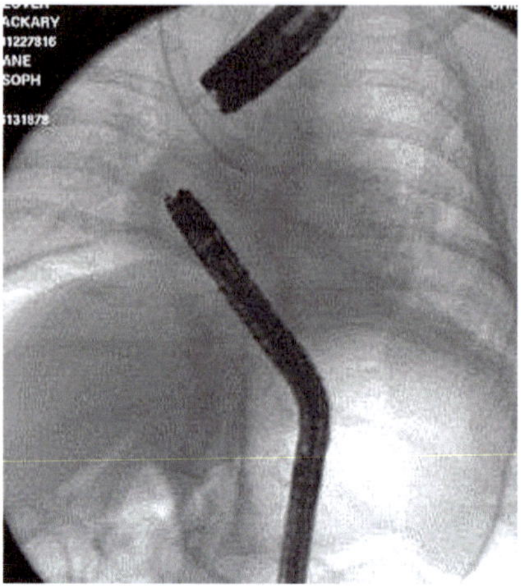

Fig. 19.4. Double endoscopy with endoscopes introduced via oropharynx and gastrostomy tube.

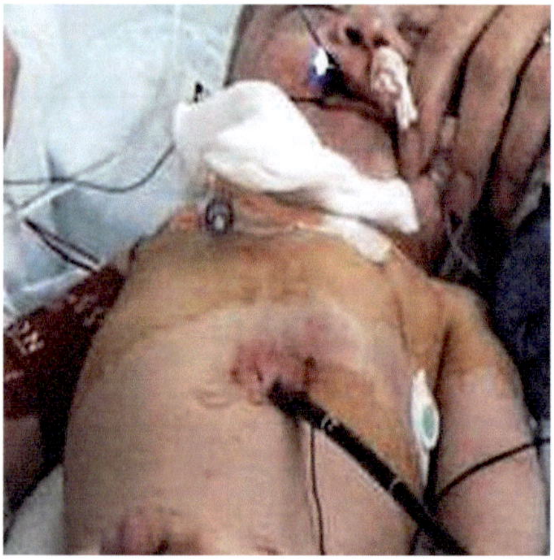

Fig. 19.5. Endoscope passed via gastrostomy up into mouth to access esophagus with a string, guidewire, or dilators.

Surgical Indications

Surgical indications for caustic esophageal strictures include symptomatic stricture requiring dilation, strictures refractory to endoscopic dilation, and inability to reinitiate oral feeding. Long strictures of the esophagus with inability to achieve oral feeding and long-term risk of esophageal cancer (2–30 %) [5, 6].

Surgical indications for managing anastomotic strictures include the same indications as for caustic strictures. The surgical approaches to esophageal strictures include multiple dilation techniques, segmental resection, or, in severe cases, esophageal replacement. The authors' preferred esophageal substitute is the stomach, which is performed by minimally invasive esophagectomy with gastric pull-up when indicated and possible [7–9]. Multiple esophageal replacement techniques are discussed in depth in Chap. 20. Esophageal resection and anastomosis may be achieved using a thoracoscopic approach for short segment strictures [10].

Esophageal Dilation

Special Considerations

Antegrade dilation can generally be performed and is preferred. In the presence of a gastrostomy, retrograde dilation may also be performed, if necessary, such as when access to the mouth is impaired.

Bougienage dilation utilizes Maloney or Hurst dilators and requires the need to negotiate across a stricture. This technique often "shears" the mucosa during dilation, as evidenced by blood is seen on dilator. These dilators are blunt tipped (and less rigid) and thus may not enable passage across tight strictures with a proximally dilated esophagus.

Balloon dilation is performed with controlled-radial-esophageal (CRE) dilators, which are very effective in dilation of esophageal strictures (Figs. 19.6 and 19.7). Fluoroscopy may be a useful adjunct when using radiopaque contrast to distend the balloon dilator.

Tucker dilators, while no longer manufactured, are useful for retrograde esophageal dilation. Now filiform dilators with followers may be used for narrow strictures requiring retrograde or antegrade dilation [11].

Technique

The patient is placed in supine position on a fluoroscopy compatible table. Care is taken to protect the face and mouth from trauma. The Olympus GIF 180 (9.3 mm OD) and GIF XP 160 (4.9 mm OD) (Olympus America, Center Valley, PA) are used depending on the size of the patient. As described above, fluoroscopy, Maloney, Hurst and Tucker dilators, and filiform dilators and followers should be available depending on the technique elected.

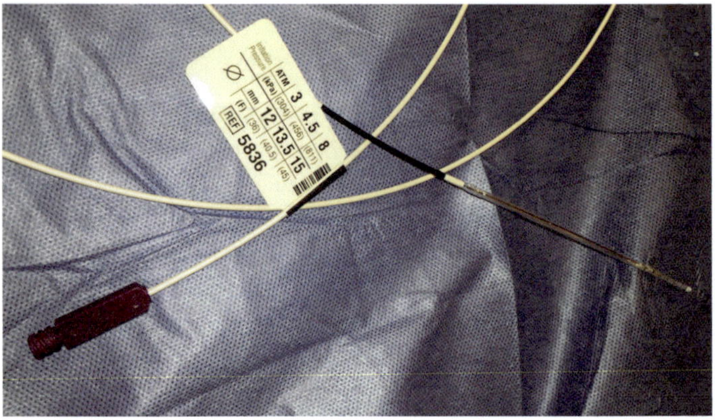

Fig. 19.6. Controlled radial esophageal (CRE) dilator. Balloon pressure/diameter (atmospheres (ATM)/diameter and French guide).

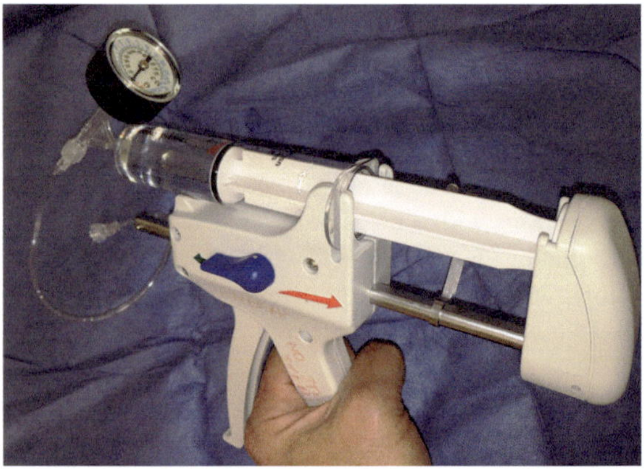

Fig. 19.7. Handgun for CRE dilator.

- Flexible endoscope is introduced orally to assess the stricture. The markings on the scope can assist in identifying the depth of the stricture from the teeth and estimating the appropriate depth of passage of the dilators to maximize stricture dilation but minimize accidental gastric perforation.
- The CRE dilator may be passed through the working channel of the scope (9.3 mm OD) or alongside endoscope (4.9 mm OD). Both fixed balloons on the end of the wire and balloons that can be passed over a guidewire can be utilized, depending on surgeon preference. Both are

available in a variety of diameters and should be affixed to a handheld manometer for safe usage. The packaging of the CRE selected should be consulted for correlating the balloon diameter to the appropriate inflation pressure.
- Contrast may be injected into the esophageal lumen or injected into the dilating balloon and observed under fluoroscopy. Fluoroscopy images may show a waist on the balloon at the initiation of balloon dilation and loss of the waist at the completion of the dilation, demonstrating efficacy.
- Inflate balloon to indicated diameter and manometer pressure and hold for 1 min before releasing the pressure. The dilation is generally repeated at least twice or increased to a larger diameter and pressure for sequential enlargement. If necessary, the balloon may be exchanged for a larger diameter balloon to achieve an appropriate diameter at the site of the stricture.
- Caution should be used on dilating an esophagus further once blood has been seen on a withdrawn dilator.
- Consider repeating your endoscopy or performing an on-table contrast esophagoscopy after dilation to reassess the stricture, evaluate the esophagus distal to the stricture for secondary concerns, and ensure no perforation of the esophagus or stomach is identified.

Pearls/Pitfalls

- Tight, short strictures with proximal esophageal dilation may be difficult to access from the oropharynx.
- If the patient has a gastrostomy tube, retrograde access with passage of a guidewire will enable the passage of serial dilators retrograde and subsequently in an antegrade manner.
- A chest radiograph in the recovery room with mediastinal air should prompt evaluation for an esophageal leak with a contrast study.

Postoperative Care

Most dilations may be performed as an outpatient procedure. Depending upon the severity and length of the stricture, repeated dilations may be necessary. Dilations are generally started at 4–6 weeks following injury or anastomosis creation. There is no standard for length of interval or rate of diameter increase, and, although technical success is high, there is also a high recurrence rate [12]. Dilations may be done every 2 weeks for severe strictures or as needed for less severe ones.

There is no role for esophageal stents although adjuvant application of topical agents (e.g., Mitomycin C, steroids) following dilation may be of benefit [13].

Esophageal perforation risk is 15–25 % but likely much less with advent of balloon dilation techniques [5]. Other possible complications include creation of false esophageal lumen, pneumothorax, and mediastinitis.

Esophageal Resection with Primary Anastomosis

Special Considerations

Short strictures of the esophagus, which do not respond to dilation, may be considered for resection with primary anastomosis. Distal and very proximal strictures are technically more challenging to resect and anastomose using MIS techniques. Segmental strictures are typically approached by right thoracoscopy with the exception being for very distal esophageal strictures, where left thoracoscopy affords better exposure.

Technique

The patient is placed in lateral decubitus with side of approach upright for thoracoscopic approaches (or supine for abdominal and cervical approaches).

Standard 3.5-mm or 5-mm laparoscopic/thoracoscopic instruments (depend on size of child) should be available, including Maryland® dissectors, DeBakey graspers, Ligasure™ device (Medtronic, Minneapolis, MN), and hook cautery. A flexible endoscope should be available in the case of segmental resection.

- Flexible endoscopy is first used to identify the stricture. The scope is left in place to serve as a marker.
- Right thoracoscopy is performed with 3–4 ports in anterior and midaxillary line.
- The stricture is identified thoracoscopically, and the esophagus is circumferentially dissected with cautery or bluntly, taking care to exclude the vagus nerves.
- The esophagus is encircled with Penrose® drain for retraction. Once fully exposed, the stricture is resected sharply.

- An interrupted, end-to-end anastomosis is performed with absorbable braided suture under limited tension. The endoscope is used to visualize the anastomosis, and a test for a leak can be performed before it is removed.
- A nasogastric tube may be placed across the anastomosis under direct vision, and a chest tube can be placed adjacent to the anastomosis to control any leakage in the immediate postoperative period.

Pearls/Pitfalls

- The light on thoracoscope can be turned off, and endoscope light turned on "transilluminate" to identify the stricture.
- Braided suture is easier to tie intracorporeally.
- Stay sutures can be placed to assist anastomosis and relieve tension.

Postoperative Care

An esophagram is performed 5–7 days postoperatively dependent upon the clinical course. Tension-free anastomoses should not require subsequent dilation. Complications include anastomotic leak, stricture, and gastroesophageal reflux.

Gastric Pull-Up

Special Considerations

Long or multiple esophageal strictures are best managed with esophageal replacement. Esophageal replacement for long gap esophageal atresia may be performed using MIS (laparoscopy, +/– thoracoscopy, and cervical esophagogastric anastomosis).

Technique

The patient is placed in lateral decubitus for thoracoscopic approaches (or supine for abdominal and cervical approaches). Patient repositioning is necessary during gastric pull-up (lateral then supine), unless a transhiatal approach is used where the patient remains supine (abdominal and cervical incisions only). Instrumentation is the same as for esophageal resection, except that an Endostapler® (Medtronic, Minneapolis, MN) is also necessary to create a gastric conduit.

- Thoracoscopy is performed, typically beginning in the right chest utilizing 3–4 ports. If visualization is impaired by the inflating lung, CO2 at a low pressure (4–6 mmHg) can push the lung away without hemodynamic compromise.
- Dissect out the esophagus from the diaphragm to the thoracic inlet. Stay directly on the esophagus to avoid injury to the thoracic duct, membranous trachea, and lung, especially if adhesions are present.
- Encircle esophagus with Penrose® drain and place it high in the thoracic inlet for future use. The instruments and trocars can now be removed, and the chest port sites can be closed, leaving a thoracostomy tube in place.
- Reposition the patient supine and initiate laparoscopy using 3–4 ports, similar to those used in a fundoplication.
- If a gastrostomy tube is in place, it should first be taken down, and the gastrostomy closed. First, divide the short gastric vessels, well away from the gastroepiploic vessels, as the conduit is based on this blood supply. Next, divide the gastrohepatic ligament and open the lesser sac to dissect the stomach distally to pylorus. A Kocher maneuver further frees the duodenum to create the necessary length for the pull-up.
- Divide the left gastric artery and vein with either a stapler, a clip, or a Ligasure®, depending on the size of the structures. Multiple firings of an Endostapler® from lesser curve toward the Angle of His and fundus are used to tubularize the gastric conduit. Continuing distally on the stomach, a pyloroplasty is performed to improve gastric emptying.
- The esophageal hiatus is now opened anteriorly to accommodate conduit. After pulling the conduit through the hiatus, attach the fundus area to the esophageal remnant with sutures for subsequent pull-up into a neck incision.
- Leave the trocars in abdomen and perform a cervical incision, most commonly on the right side. Dissect out esophagus from neck and retrieve Penrose® drain from thoracic inlet. Dissect and widen the thoracic inlet to allow space for conduit in the neck. Hegar dilators can be useful for this maneuver.
- Next, divide the proximal esophagus at area of the intended anastomosis. The distal esophagus with the attached conduit can now be pulled up into the neck. Care should be taken to ensure there is not a twist in the conduit during this maneuver. An end-to-end cervical esophagogastric

anastomosis is now performed. A passive drain should be left in the neck adjacent to the anastomosis.

- Attention is returned to the abdomen, and laparoscopy is now repeated. The conduit is sutured to the hiatus with 2–3 sutures to prevent herniation through this space.
- A surgical jejunostomy tube should now be placed for nutrition. The gastric remnant resulting from the tubularization can be removed just prior to closure of the port sites.

Pearls/Pitfalls

- Pure esophageal atresia patients may be approached using laparoscopy with cervical incision (transhiatal pull-up).
- If a prior fundoplication has been done, this must be taken down to create the gastric conduit.
- Either abdominal or thoracic approaches may be performed using open techniques if conversion proves necessary.

Postoperative Care

Long-term conduit function is generally good with no need for revision. Dilations are required in cases of reflux-related strictures of cervical esophagogastric anastomoses. Complications include anastomotic leak, gastroesophageal reflux, esophagogastric anastomotic stricture, and airway injury.

Esophageal Duplications

Preoperative Evaluation

Duplications of the esophagus may be intramural or extramural and occasionally extend below the diaphragm if large. As it is rare to have a communication between the duplication and the native esophagus, most patients are asymptomatic. Those who do have symptoms present with infection, chest pressure, pain, or cough. A barium esophagram will identify an intramural duplication (Fig. 19.8) but possibly miss an extramural cyst where 3D imaging such as computed tomography or magnetic resonance imaging is required. Additional background information on

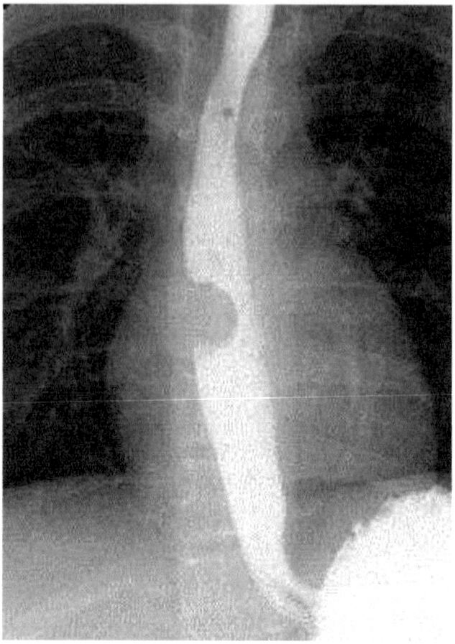

Fig. 19.8. Appearance of an intramural esophageal duplication cyst on esophagram.

duplications can be found in Chaps. 18 and 27 of this text; as such, this section will focus on the technical aspects of resection of esophageal duplications.

Surgical Indications

The presence of a lesion alone is an indication for surgery. Lesions may become infected, and there is a small but real risk of malignancy developing within the duplication.

Special Considerations

Cysts may be intramural or extramural and will rarely communicate with the esophageal lumen. Duplication cysts may be located at any level of the esophagus.

Technique

The patient is positioned in right or left lateral decubitus depending upon location of the lesion. Instrumentation is the same as for MIS gastric pull-up.

- After positioning, a large bougie or endoscope is placed through the esophagus into the stomach. Thoracoscopy is performed, and dissection begins along the cyst or esophagus to visualize the lesion.
- Extramural cysts may be removed for the surrounding attachment with hook cautery or energy devices assuring that esophageal lumen is not entered (Fig. 19.9). If esophageal lumen is entered, this should be closed with absorbable suture.
- If cyst is intact, it may be drained in order to reduce its size for extraction.
- Intramural cysts require opening the longitudinal muscle of the esophagus (Fig. 19.10). This layer may be left open following resection, and the endoscope will confirm submucosal integrity (Fig. 19.11).
- Pediatric esophageal duplication cysts that communicate to the esophagus can be treated by endoscopically dividing the common wall with a needle knife, allowing the duplication to drain internally [14].

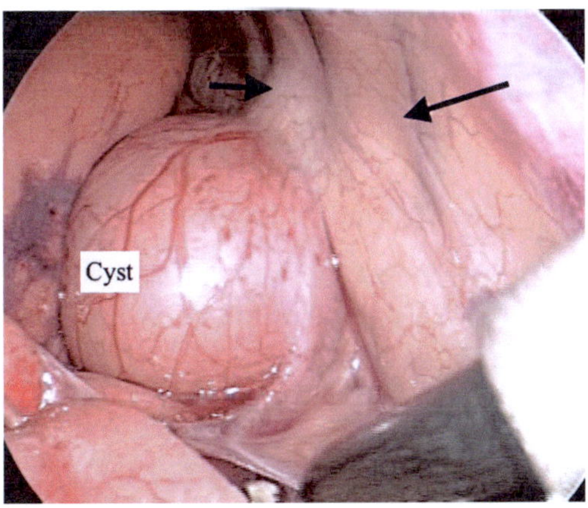

Fig. 19.9. Thoracoscopic view of a left extramural esophageal duplication cyst coming off esophagus (*short arrow*) with adjacent aorta (*long arrow*).

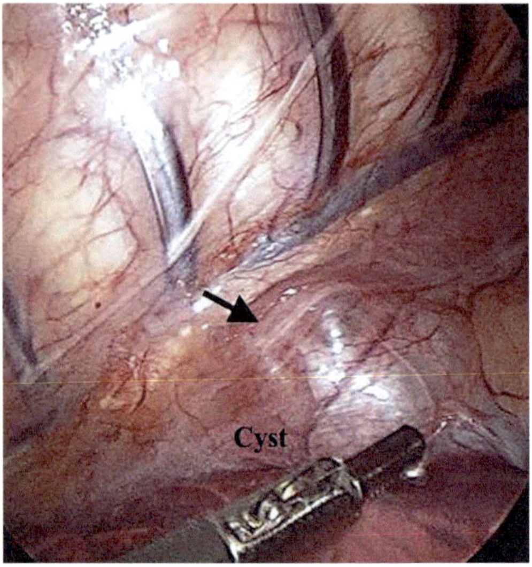

Fig. 19.10. Right thoracoscopic initial view of an intramural esophageal duplication cyst.

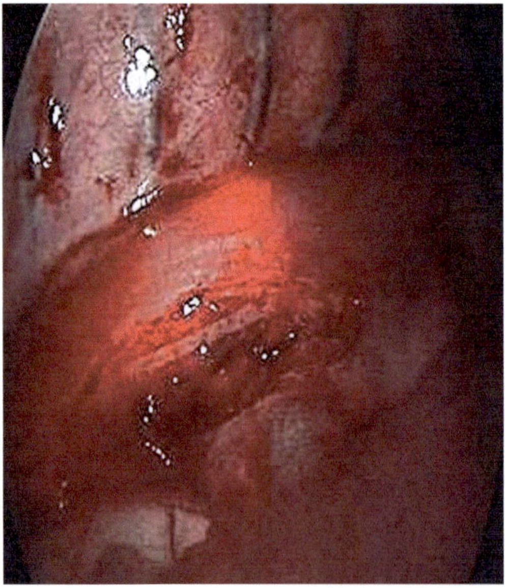

Fig. 19.11. View of intramural esophageal duplication cyst post resection with endoscope in esophagus.

Pearls/Pitfalls

- A postoperative esophagram to evaluate for a leak is required only if endoscope is not used during resection.
- Endoscopy assists with identifying cyst using transillumination [15].

Postoperative Care

The outcomes are generally very good. There have been no recurrences reported. Complications of the procedure include esophageal perforation, leak, and cyst rupture.

Summary

- Pediatric esophageal strictures frequently may be treated with endoscopic dilation. Thoracoscopic resection with anastomosis or esophageal replacement should be reserved for complicated cases.
- Pediatric esophageal duplication cysts may be treated thoracoscopically and should typically not require segmental resection of the esophagus so long as careful attention is given to assure submucosal integrity.
- Endoscopic treatment of duplication cysts that communicate with the esophagus has been described via needle knife drainage.

References

1. Savino F, Tarasco V, Viola S, Locatelli E, Sorrenti M, Barabino A. Congenital esophageal stenosis diagnosed in an infant 9 month of age. Ital J Pediatr. 2015; 41:72. doi:10.1186/s13052-015-0182-y.
2. Patel PC, Yates JA, Gibson WS, Wood WE. Congenital esophageal webs. Int J Pediatr Otorhinolaryngol. 1997;42(2):141–7.
3. Jones DW, Kunisaki SM, Teitelbaum DH, Spigland NA, Coran AG. Congenital esophageal stenosis: the differential diagnosis and management. Pediatr Surg Int. 2010;26(5):547–51.
4. Takamizawa S, Tsugawa C, Mouri N, Satoh S, Kanegawa K, Nishijima E, Muraji T. Congenital esophageal stenosis: therapeutic strategy based on etiology. J Pediatr Surg. 2002;37:197–201.
5. Eliçevik M, Alim A, Tekant GT, Sarimurat N, Adaletli I, Kurugoglu S, Bakan M, Kaya G, Erdogan E. Management of esophageal perforation secondary to caustic esophageal injury in children. Surg Today. 2008;38(4):311–5.

6. Zhang X, Wang M, Han H, Xu Y, Shi Z, Ma G. Corrosive induced carcinoma of esophagus after 58 years. Ann Thorac Surg. 2012;94(6):2103–5.
7. Nwomeh BC, Luketich JD, Kane TD. Minimally invasive esophagectomy for caustic esophageal stricture in children. J Pediatr Surg. 2004;39(7):e1–6.
8. Kane TD, Nwomeh BC, Nadler EP. Thoracoscopic-assisted esophagectomy and laparoscopic gastric pull-up for lye injury. JSLS. 2007;11(4):474–80.
9. Ng J, Loukogeorgakis SP, Pierro A, Kiely EM, De Coppi P, Cross K, Curry J. Comparison of minimally invasive and open gastric transposition in children. J Laparoendosc Adv Surg Tech A. 2014;24(10):742–9.
10. Malek MM, Shah SR, Katz AL, Kane TD. Multimedia article: endoscopically guided thoracoscopic esophagectomy for stricture in a child. Surg Endosc. 2010;24(1):219. doi:10.1007/s00464-009-0545-9.
11. Baird R, Laberge JM, Levesque D. Anastomotic stricture after esophageal atresia repair: a critical review of recent literature. Eur J Pediatr Surg. 2013;23(3):204–13.
12. Doo EY, Shin JY, Kim JH, Song HY. Oesophageal strictures caused by the ingestion of corrosive agents: effectiveness of balloon dilatation in children. Clin Radiol. 2009;64(3):265–71.
13. Rosseneu S, Afzal N, Yerushalmi B, Ibarguen-Secchia E, Lewindon P, Cameron D, Mahler T, Schwagten K, Kohler H, Lindley KJ, Thomson M. Topical application of mitomycin-C in oesophageal strictures. J Pediatr Gastroenterol Nutr. 2007;44(3): 336–41.
14. Walsh DS, Harris AS, Dokler ML, George DE. Endolumenal management of tubular esophageal duplications. Society of American Gastrointestinal and Endoscopic Surgeons; 2012. Epublished at: http://thesagesmeeting.org/endolumenal-management-of-tubular-esophageal-duplications/.
15. Davenport K, Mollen KP, Rothenberg SS, Kane TD. Experience with endoscopic and endoscopic-assisted management of pediatric surgical problems: results and lessons. Dis Esophagus. 2013;26(1):37–43.

20. Esophageal Replacement Surgery in Children

Ian C. Glenn, Mark O. McCollum, and David C. van der Zee

Introduction

Long-gap esophageal atresia (EA) is the most common indication for esophageal replacement in the pediatric population. The term "long gap" is not rigorously defined. Qualitatively, it refers to any EA in which the two ends may not initially be easily approximated [1]. However, not all patients with long-gap EA will require esophageal replacement, due to the success of so-called delayed primary repair [2–5] or traction technique [6, 7].

Before the subject of esophageal substitution is more deeply explored, it must be emphasized that the majority of surgeons will agree that all reasonable attempts should be made to use the patient's native esophagus prior to progressing to esophageal replacement [2, 3, 8–12].

Epidemiology

Esophageal atresia, with or without tracheoesophageal fistula (TEF), is a congenital disease with incidence of approximately 1 in 2500–4000 live births [13]. Pure esophageal atresia is much rarer, occurring in 1 in 40,000 live births or 8% of all EA cases [14] although a higher incidence of proximal fistula has been described [15]. EA may be seen with the VACTERL (vertebral, anorectal, cardiac, tracheoesophageal, renal, and limb deformities) association or less commonly the CHARGE association (coloboma, heart defects, atresia choanae, retarded growth and

D.S. Walsh et al. (eds.), *The SAGES Manual of Pediatric Minimally Invasive Surgery*, DOI 10.1007/978-3-319-43642-5_20

Table 20.1 Incidence of esophageal atresia by Gross classification [16]

Gross type	Incidence (%)
C	86
A	7
E	4
B	2
D	<1

development, genital hypoplasia, and ear deformities) and Potter's syndrome (Table 20.1).

In terms of genetic disorders, EA is also associated with trisomies 18 and 21, as well as the chromosomal deletions 22q11 and 17q22q23.3.

Pathophysiology

The pathophysiologies of both EA and TEF are intimately related and are due to malformation of the foregut. The etiology is incompletely understood and is most certainly multifactorial. In experimental models the Sonic hedgehog gene, and other genes involved in related signaling pathways, has been implicated [16].

Embryologically, the primitive foregut is derived from the endoderm and forms around 4–6 weeks gestational age. The respiratory diverticulum forms from the cranial foregut and will later give rise to two lung buds. The ventral tubular structure will give rise to the trachea and the dorsal structure the esophagus. It is postulated that either the respiratory system grows away from the foregut, forming a separate structure, or that the structures grow in parallel with a caudocranial separation forming and ultimately dividing the two. As the cranial foregut is developing, the stomach develops from the caudal foregut. While the esophagus elongates in the caudal direction, its lumen decreases in size until it is almost obliterated [17]. Normally, the lumen will reform following fusion of the esophagus and stomach. When the esophagus does not appropriately elongate (and/or the respiratory bud does not properly elongate), EA and/or TEF develop [18].

Preoperative Evaluation

History

When diagnosed prenatally, EA is typically discovered via ultrasound. Magnetic resonance imaging may also be used, particularly when there is a high suspicion for abnormality [19]. Suggestive sonographic findings include microgastria or absent gastric bubble, upper pouch sign (dilated proximal esophageal pouch), and polyhydramnios [20]. Pure EA is associated with polyhydramnios in approximately 87 % of cases, but EA with distal TEF only has polyhydramnios in 50 % of cases [13]. Despite the increasing use and accuracy of antenatal ultrasound, EA is diagnosed prenatally in 20–34 % of cases [13]. Postnatal signs and symptoms of esophageal atresia include inability to swallow, feeding intolerance, and respiratory distress.

Exam

A thorough physical exam should be performed, particularly given the fact that EA is associated with other congenital anomalies in 48–55 % of cases [13], the most common of which is the VACTERL association [21]. Common symptoms of esophageal atresia are coughing and choking, particularly when feeding. Signs of EA include inability to pass orogastric or nasogastric tubes as well as difficulty swallowing.

Labs

Laboratory examination is not required in the diagnosis of esophageal atresia. However, blood work including complete blood count, comprehensive metabolic panel, coagulation profile, and blood type with crossmatching should be obtained preoperatively, as well as to potentially screen for other congenital abnormalities. Metabolic derangements may need to be corrected prior to surgery.

Imaging

Plain film radiography is often diagnostic of esophageal atresia as well as tracheoesophageal fistula. Common radiographic findings of pure EA include air in the proximal esophageal pouch without distal

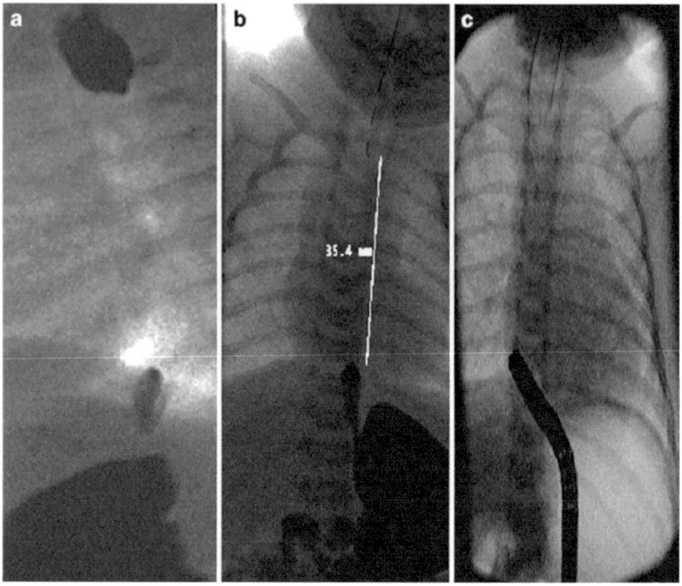

Fig. 20.1. The gap-o-gram provides an accurate representation of the distance between the proximal and distal esophageal portions. Radiopaque objects, and/or contrast, are placed in both ends of the esophagus. Ideally, tension is applied to lessen the distance between the ends (as will ultimately be done in surgery when approximating the ends of the esophagus). From Pediatric Thoracic Surgery, Esophageal Replacement, 2009, pp. 321–333, Pattillo JC. With permission of Springer.

bowel gas and coiling of the nasal or orogastric tube in the proximal esophageal pouch. If a coincident TEF is present, there may be gas present in the stomach and distal bowel, although this may not be apparent on the initial X-ray. Patients who are unable to undergo immediate primary anastomosis will require gastrostomy tube placement for feeding purposes. In these patients, a "gap-o-gram" or gap study can be performed for operative planning and further characterization of the atresia, including measurement of the length between the esophageal ends (Fig. 20.1). A passive gap study is performed by injecting contrast into the proximal esophageal pouch (typically via nasoesophageal tube) and into the stomach and/or distal esophageal pouch via the gastrostomy tube [22]. Alternatively, an active, or dynamic, gap study is performed using fluoroscopy while applying controlled tension with radiopaque instruments placed in both esophageal ends, in order to stretch the two esophageal ends closer together [10]. This study is more predictive of the true gap that will be encountered intraoperatively after esophageal mobilization but carries the risk of pushing up the fundus instead of the distal esophagus, giving a false-positive impression of the length of the distal esophagus or hollow viscus perforation.

At a later stage contrast imaging through the gastrostomy is indicated in patients who may undergo jejunal interposition in order to rule out malrotation or congenital short bowel [23–25].

Other Tests

Due to the strong association between EA and cardiac defects, a transthoracic echocardiogram should be routinely performed on patients who are diagnosed with EA. Approximately 1.8–5 % of patients with EA/TEF have a right-sided aortic arch, which may impact surgical approach to repair of the EA [16, 26, 27].

Tracheoscopy and bronchoscopy are obligatory preoperatively in determining the presence of fistulae and their related characteristics, such as tracheomalacia [16, 28].

Surgical Indications

All patients with esophageal atresia require repair. However, as discussed earlier, correction with native esophagus should be attempted first. In patients with a history of esophageal atresia and primary repair, indications for esophageal substitution relate to complications with the native esophagus, such as leaks, strictures, refractory gastroesophageal reflux, and recurrent tracheoesophageal fistula that precludes the use of the native esophagus [9].

Additional indications for pediatric esophageal replacement include caustic ingestion and peptic stricture. Although the overall incidence of caustic ingestion has continued to decline, there remain regional demographics where there are a substantial number of caustic ingestions, usually related to lye (sodium hydroxide) ingestion. This declining trend has been largely attributed to the usage of child-resistant lids on caustic products.

Technique

Special Considerations

Tracheoesophageal fistula is often coincident with EA and must be definitively diagnosed or ruled out prior to planned repair of EA. In those patients with multiple defects, there must be strong coordination of consulting services, including anesthesiology, cardiology, neonatology, and other relevant services, to determine the proper order of surgical interventions.

In patients with suspected or confirmed EA, a Replogle suction catheter should be placed in the proximal esophageal pouch to prevent aspiration of oral secretions. Additionally, patients with EA who are not able to undergo immediate repair will require gastrostomy tube placement.

There is debate as to whether patients awaiting delayed primary anastomosis should have a cervical esophagostomy (commonly known as a cervicostomy or "spit fistula") placed as opposed to long-term esophageal pouch suction. It is our opinion that suction alone should be implemented to keep all options open. Placement of cervical esophagostomy risks damaging the recurrent laryngeal nerve. Furthermore, the cervicostomy effectively increases the length of the gap between the esophagus and stomach [29]. Thus, if a patient receives a cervical esophagostomy and later requires esophageal replacement, jejunal interposition can be made technically much more challenging, potentially requiring microvascular anastomosis [30], or impossible. While it has been advocated that cervical esophagostomy allows for patient discharge from the hospital, it has been demonstrated that patients may safely stay at home with proximal pouch suction [31].

Anatomy

The posterior mediastinum is the location of the native esophagus and is the shortest distance between the neck and abdomen for an esophageal replacement. Furthermore, this location minimizes lung compression by the conduit. This is the preferred location for the conduit.

In the past the retrosternal position has been described for various conduits [32, 33]. It may be technically less challenging than posterior mediastinal placement and was said to avoid tedious dissection in patients who have had caustic ingestions, peptic esophageal strictures, or prior cardiothoracic surgeries. Thoracotomies at that time were still high-risk procedures.

The retrohilar, or transpleural, approach is also considered technically less challenging than posterior mediastinal placement. This method is primarily of historical significance. It requires a thoracotomy to be performed and will inevitably lead to some lung compression.

Important considerations when deciding the ideal conduit route include maintenance of some anatomic normalcy, patient anatomic variations (e.g. dextrocardia, right-sided aortic arch), prior thoracic surgeries or other inflammatory processes in the chest (e.g. caustic ingestion), technical difficulty, lung compression, and prevention/reduction of gastroesophageal reflux.

Consideration should be given to remaining extrapleural during the thoracic portions of the surgery. This may be exceedingly difficult in the youngest of patients, however.

Positioning

Due to surgery being performed in both the abdomen and thorax or neck, multiple positions may be required during the operation. Generally, the supine position is used for both open abdominal and laparoscopic surgery. For thoracoscopy, the patient is placed in the left lateral decubitus semi-prone position. For thoracotomy, the left lateral decubitus position is used (Figs. 20.2 and 20.3).

Instruments

In neonatal thoracoscopy, 3-mm instruments are used. In older children, 5-mm instruments are longer and may allow for better access to structures in the relatively larger thoracic cavity. The existence of a 3-mm laparoscopic vessel sealer and 5-mm laparoscopic stapler has proven invaluable.

Steps

This chapter is intended for those rare circumstances in which the native esophagus alone is insufficient to correct the problem, and delayed primary anastomosis after 3 months or the traction technique is not possible. Please refer to other chapters in this text that discuss surgical cor-

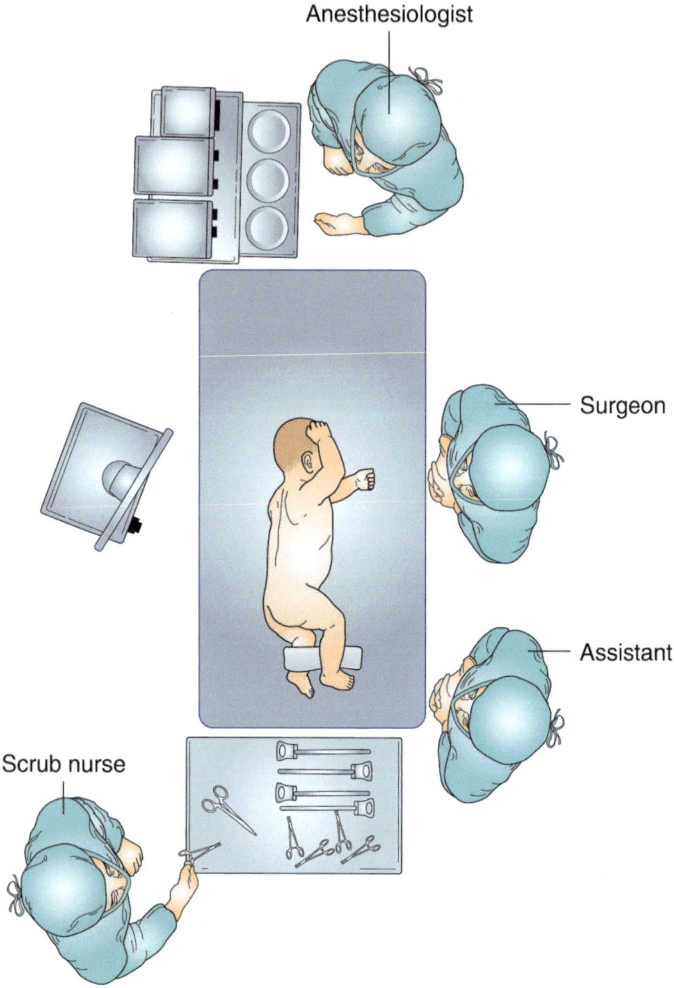

Fig. 20.2. Demonstration of patient positioning and surgeon location for thoracoscopic repair of long-gap esophageal atresia. Note that the patient is placed in a 45° left lateral decubitus position (semi-prone).

rection of esophageal atresia using the native esophagus. It is the opinion of the authors that jejunal interposition should be the esophageal substitution operation of choice, followed by gastric transposition or gastric tube interposition. The last resort would be colonic interposition.

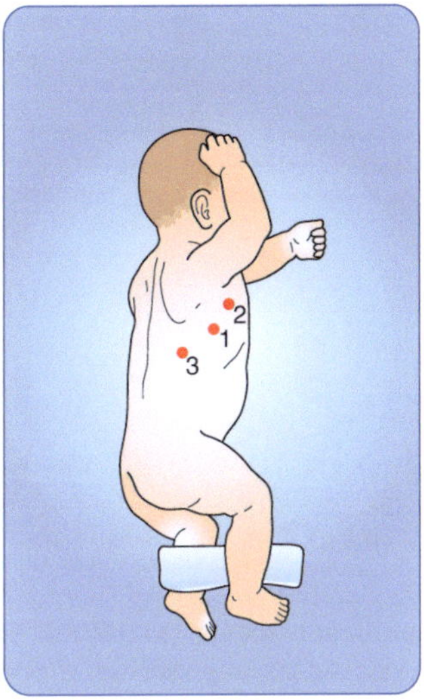

Fig. 20.3. Trocar placement for thoracoscopic repair of long-gap esophageal atresia. The thoracoscope (#1) is inserted approximately 1-centimeter inferior and anterior to the tip of the scapula, and working instruments are placed in positions #2 and #3.

Small Bowel Interposition (Fig. 20.4)

Jejunum, and rarely ileum, has many distinct advantages and nowadays is the esophageal replacement conduit of choice for most. The jejunum is similar in size to the native esophagus and occupies less space in the chest than the much larger stomach. This helps to minimize restrictions on the pulmonary system. Unlike other substitution choices, the small bowel retains peristaltic activity, thus avoiding many of the late complications seen with the stomach and colon, such as stasis and reflux [34]. Jejunal interposition is considered the most technically difficult operation of the esophageal replacement choices, and the blood supply tends to be more tenuous. It also involves three anastomoses. The ability to perform the surgery may be limited by prior surgeries, such as cervical esophagostomy, or congenital anomalies, such as intestinal malrotation.

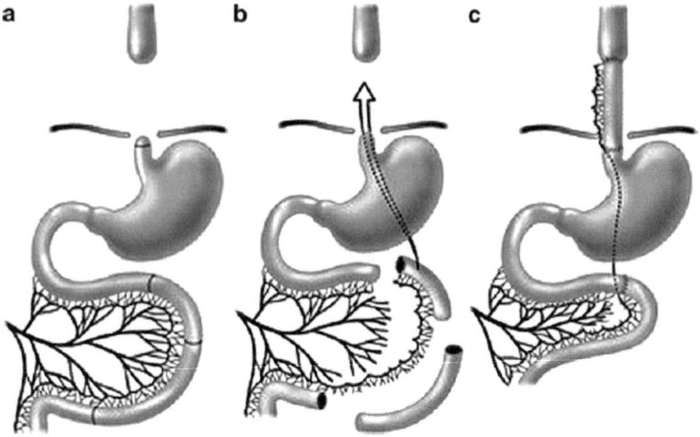

Fig. 20.4. Jejunal transposition is shown. (**a**) Suitable portion of small bowel is chosen. (**b**) While the vasculature is preserved, a portion of small bowel is removed to provide additional length. (**c**) The segment of small bowel is passed into the chest in an anteperistaltic fashion. Small bowel continuity is restored. From Pediatric Thoracic Surgery, Esophageal Replacement, 2009, pp. 321–333, Pattillo JC. With permission of Springer.

Jejunal interposition may be used to replace the length of the esophagus or to bridge a smaller, subtotal portion of the esophagus. The use of "free" segments of small bowel, requiring a microvascular anastomosis, has been described in the pediatric literature [34, 35] but is much more commonly seen in adult populations, due to the difficulty of performing such an anastomosis in a pediatric patient. A pedicled graft is much more commonly used [25].

Jejunal interposition is performed as a single-stage operation and can be performed as early as 1 month of age [29, 36].

Following induction of anesthesia, prepping, and draping, if applicable, the cervical esophagostomy is taken down. Next, right thoracoscopy is performed, with the patient in the left lateral prone position, to determine if small bowel interposition will be feasible and the length of small bowel which will be required is sufficient. If small bowel interposition is to be performed, a right posterolateral thoracotomy is performed, and the distal esophagus is dissected to allow easy passage of the jejunum into the thorax. The proximal esophagus is maximally prepared to facilitate the proximal anastomosis. The skin is reapproximated, and the patient is placed into the supine position.

The second step is to perform a midline laparotomy. It is the opinion of the authors that mobilizing the jejunal segment laparoscopically would carry an excessively high risk of compromising the vascular supply to the bowel. The gastrostomy tube is removed and the gastrostomy is closed.

The superior portion of the neoesophagus will be a point just distal to the first feeding artery from the ligament of Treitz. The jejunum is transected distal to the ligament of Treitz and at the level of the third major mesenteric branch to the bowel. The "excess" jejunum is discarded and small bowel continuity restored. The first two mesenteric branches are ligated, with care taken to leave the peripheral arcades intact.

The phrenoesophageal ligament is divided, and the gastroesophageal junction and proximal stomach are mobilized. The jejunal segment is introduced into the retrohilar portion of the chest, in a retrocolic, retrogastric fashion via the esophageal hiatus with stay sutures.

The patient is placed in the right lateral decubitus position, and the thoracotomy incision is reopened. The jejunum is anastomosed with the proximal and distal esophagus in an interrupted fashion using braided, absorbable suture. Nasogastric tube is placed, as well as a chest tube, prior to closure of the chest and abdomen. A gastrostomy or jejunojejunostomy can be performed for feeding.

Gastric Transposition (Also Referred to as Gastric Pull-Through or Pull-Up) (Fig. 20.5)

Not all patients will be suitable candidates for small bowel interposition. Intestinal malrotation has an increased incidence in patients with EA, and these patients may have vascular anatomy that is prohibitive to performing small bowel interposition. These patients are better served with a gastric conduit for esophageal replacement [23–25]. Advantages of gastric transposition include robust blood supply, the relative ease of bringing the stomach into the chest, and the presence of only one anastomosis. Of note, gastric transposition is the only esophageal replacement surgery that is able to be performed in its entirety in a minimally invasive fashion. Disadvantages involve the large size of the stomach, lack of peristalsis, and gastric reflux [37]. Patients who have had cervical esophagostomy will require takedown of the stoma and a subsequent cervical anastomosis, which will require an open approach. Discussion of this technique has been described by multiple authors [38–40] and will not be discussed herein.

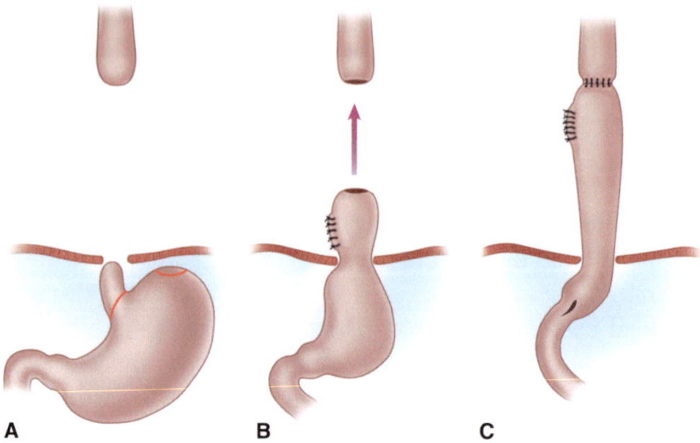

Fig. 20.5. Gastric transposition for esophageal replacement. (**a**) Stomach is mobilized laparoscopically. (**b**) The stomach is pulled into the right hemithorax and the distal esophageal stump removed. (**c**) The cervical esophagus is anastomosed to the gastric fundus, and laparoscopic pyloroplasty is performed.

Following induction of anesthesia, placement of the patient in the supine position, prepping, and draping of the patient, laparoscopic entry into the abdomen is obtained in a fashion similar to that used for a Nissen fundoplication.

The G-tube is removed and the gastrostomy is closed. The abdominal wall defect previously containing the G-tube is used as an additional laparoscopic port site. The stomach is completely mobilized, including division of the gastrocolic and gastrohepatic ligaments. Traction sutures are placed in the distal esophageal stump after it too has been mobilized. The left gastric and gastroepiploic arteries are ligated along with the short gastric vessels. Care is taken to preserve the right gastric and gastroepiploic arteries. The esophageal hiatus is dilated, and the stomach, with attached distal esophagus, is passed into the right hemithorax.

The patient is placed in the 45-degree left lateral decubitus position, and the right hemithorax is entered thoracoscopically, in the fashion traditionally used for EA repair. With the use of traction sutures, the stomach is brought into the posterior mediastinum. The distal esophagus is resected from the stomach, and esophagogastrostomy is performed with a single layer of absorbable suture (typically 4–0 or 5–0). A 360-degree gastric fundoplication around the anastomosis may be performed [41].

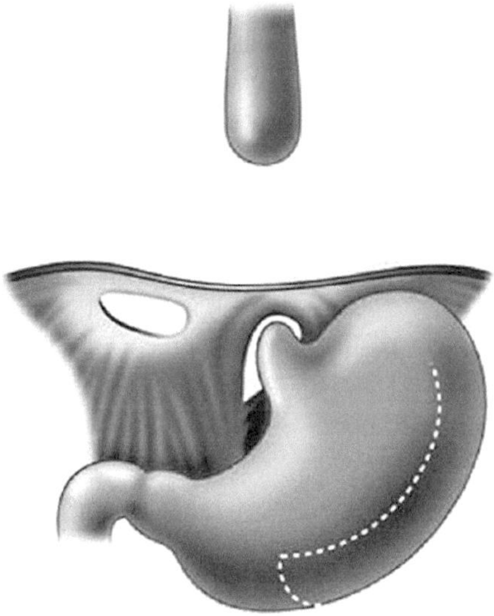

Fig. 20.6. Reversed gastric tube. The greater curvature of the stomach is used to form the reversed gastric tube for esophageal replacement. From Pediatric Thoracic Surgery, Esophageal Replacement, 2009, pp. 321–333, Pattillo JC. With permission of Springer.

The patient is returned to the supine position, and attention is returned to the abdomen. The gastric antrum is fixed to the crura with nonabsorbable suture, and a Heineke-Mikulicz pyloroplasty may be performed, although there is no consensus as to the advantage of a pyloroplasty. Feeding tube jejunostomy may be performed prior to closure of the abdomen.

Gastric Tube Interposition (or Gastric Tube Esophagoplasty) (Fig. 20.6)

There are have been numerous reports on various types of gastric tube conduits for the use in esophageal atresia [42–45], but none have been performed in children in a minimally invasive fashion, as many date from a time prior to the era of minimally invasive surgery. An open technique favored by the authors, reversed gastric tube (RGT), is presented.

Advantages of the gastric tube interposition include avoidance of exposure of a small bowel or colonic conduit to refluxed gastric secretions, a single anastomosis (which is typically intrathoracic), and a smaller volume conduit when compared with gastric transposition. It should be noted that in a patient in whom the G-tube is very close to the greater gastric curvature, RGT may not be possible. The RGT has the disadvantage of being antiperistaltic, but isoperistaltic gastric tubes have been described [42, 44–46].

Following induction of anesthesia, placing the patient in the supine position, prepping, and draping of the patient, a midline laparotomy incision is performed. The gastrostomy tube is removed, and the gastrostomy is closed. The gastrocolic ligament is divided, with care taken to not excessively ligate the gastroepiploic arcade. Additionally, the phrenoesophageal ligament is divided, and the gastroesophageal junction and proximal stomach are mobilized. The distal esophageal stump is removed from the stomach.

A cervical incision is mandatory for taking down cervical esophagostomy and in cases where there is an extremely short proximal esophageal pouch.

The gastric conduit will start a minimum of 2 cm from the pylorus. At this location, the right gastroepiploic artery is divided, and a longitudinal incision through the anterior and posterior gastric walls is performed. A luminal obturator (frequently a 20–24 French chest tube) is placed in the stomach along the greater curvature to ensure adequate internal diameter. A GIA stapler is fired parallel to the greater curvature (approximately 2 cm from the "edge") to create the gastric conduit. The short gastric vessels are divided with care taken to protect the spleen and the staple lines are oversewn. The hiatus is enlarged, and the neoesophagus is passed through the esophageal hiatus into the posterior mediastinum (Fig. 20.7).

The patient is placed in the left lateral decubitus position, and a right posterolateral thoracotomy is performed. The upper pouch is mobilized, and esophagogastric anastomosis is performed with a single layer of 5–0 monofilament absorbable sutures.

A pyloroplasty is performed, and the tube gastrostomy or jejunostomy is performed prior to closure of the abdomen.

Colonic Interposition (Fig. 20.8)

The colon should be considered the last choice for esophageal replacement conduit. Disadvantages include lack of peristaltic activity, requirement for three anastomoses, and long-term complications related to excessive redundancy of the conduit, stricture, and gastric reflux.

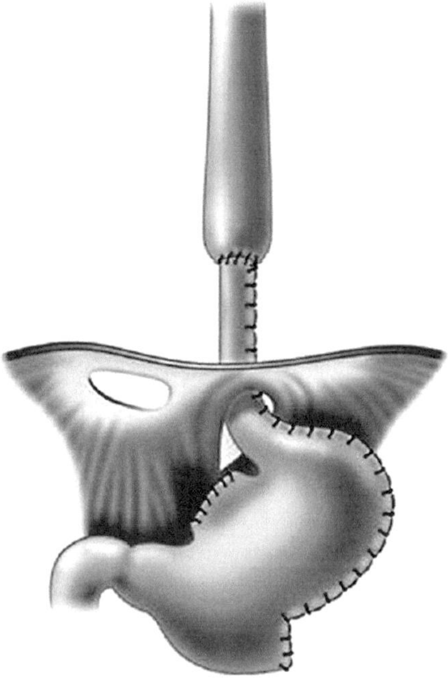

Fig. 20.7. The reversed gastric tube traverses the esophageal hiatus. The cervical esophagus and neoesophagus are anastomosed in the chest. From Pediatric Thoracic Surgery, Esophageal Replacement, 2009, pp. 321–333, Pattillo JC. With permission of Springer.

Laparoscopic-assisted colonic transposition has been described, and the use of the transverse colon as a conduit will be discussed below [47]. The left, transverse, or right colon (as well as left or right colon in conjunction with transverse colon) may be used for esophageal replacement performed in an open fashion. The transverse colon has the advantage of being narrower than other portions of colon and better at propelling solids [33].

Following induction of anesthesia, placement in the supine position, prepping, and draping of the patient, the abdomen is entered laparoscopically in a fashion similar to that used for a Nissen fundoplication. The gastrostomy tube is removed and the gastrostomy is closed. The associated abdominal wall defect is used as an additional trocar site. If a cervical esophagostomy is present, it may be taken down at this time as well.

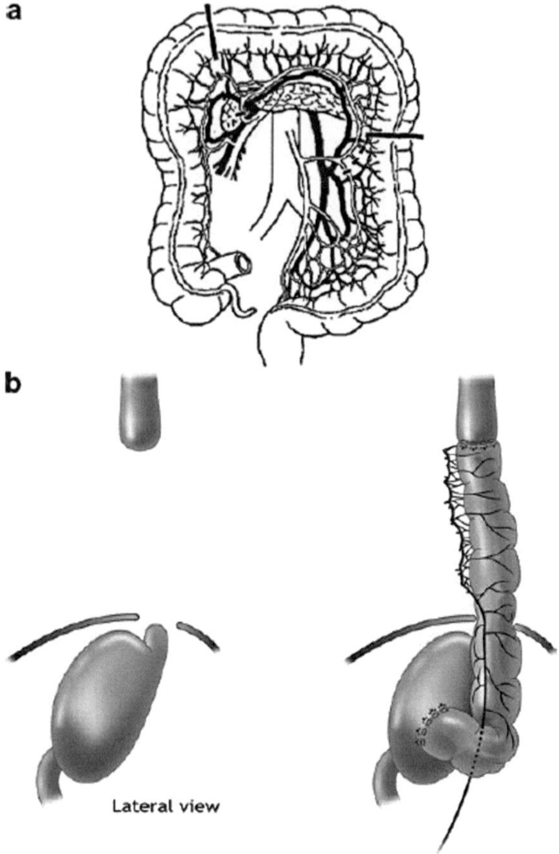

Fig. 20.8. Colonic interposition. (**a**) A suitable portion of colon is chosen, preferably anteperistaltic. Ascending or descending colon may be used instead of the transverse colon. (**b**) The colon is passed into the chest. Here, retrogastric placement is shown. From Pediatric Thoracic Surgery, Esophageal Replacement, 2009, pp. 321–333, Pattillo JC. With permission of Springer.

The diaphragmatic hiatus is enlarged, and the distal esophageal stump is fully mobilized. Transhiatal dissection is carried superiorly into the mediastinum anterior to the aorta while attempting to remain extrapleural. The short gastric vessels are divided as the colonic conduit will ultimately be in a retrogastric position.

A right cervical, supraclavicular incision is performed (if the patient had a left cervical esophagostomy, that incision alternately will be used) and the proximal esophagus mobilized. The mediastinal tunnel is developed to connect with the tunnel started from the abdomen.

Returning to the abdomen, the splenic and hepatic flexures are mobilized. The goal is for the transverse colon segment to have dual blood supply from the left colic artery and marginal paracolic arcade (via the sigmoid artery) [33]. With that in mind, the middle colic vessels are ligated, along with the marginal artery of the colon. The umbilical incision is enlarged, and the entirety of the transverse colon is exteriorized. The transverse mesocolon and greater omentum are divided as needed, and the proximal and distal ends of the transverse colon are divided to provide an appropriate length of conduit. An umbilical tape, or similar, is tied to the proximal colon to function as a traction suture. Colonic continuity is restored and the colon returned to the abdomen, with the conduit placed in the retrogastric position. The proximal stomach is next exteriorized and the distal esophageal stump resected. The distal end of the colonic conduit is anastomosed to the stomach in a running fashion with braided, absorbable suture, preferably at the prior G-tube site, in an isoperistaltic fashion. A 180-degree fundoplication is performed and the stomach returned to the abdomen. Laparoscopy is resumed and a pyloroplasty performed.

The proximal colon is passed superiorly, via the posterior mediastinum, until it is able to be grasped via the cervical incision. From the abdomen, the crura are reapproximated and fixed to the colonic conduit with permanent sutures. The esophagocolostomy is performed with braided, absorbable sutures. The colon may be fixed to the thoracic inlet with permanent sutures. A drain is left in the neck.

Pearls/Pitfalls

As emphasized previously, every effort should be taken to preserve the maximum amount of native esophagus. This often requires patience. Natural esophageal growth can be significant over the first 3 months of life. Natural elongation of distances of three to five vertebral bodies in length is not uncommon and can obviate the need for esophageal replacement.

Patients who have failed (delayed) primary anastomosis and/or esophageal lengthening procedures should be referred to tertiary centers with significant experience in esophageal replacement [48, 49].

A contrast study to determine the length of bowel and mechanical bowel preparation should be performed prior to esophageal replacement surgery regardless of the conduit which has been selected. In the event of unexpected problems, multiple options should be available.

Extreme care should be taken to prevent injury to the recurrent laryngeal nerve and thoracic duct when operating in the chest and neck.

Postoperative Care

All patients undergoing esophageal replacement surgery should be monitored in an intensive care setting in the immediate postoperative period.

Outcomes

The majority of published data regarding outcomes in esophageal replacement consists of small case series which tend to have significant variation in their results, likely due to the small number of patients involved in each study. Furthermore, the methodologies across studies are heterogeneous, which prevents strong conclusions from being drawn, and almost all studied open surgery as there is very limited data on minimally invasive surgery. Due to these limitations, the data presented here is confined to comparative studies [49–52]. Unfortunately, none of these studies compares all four techniques.

Tannuri and colleagues [50] retrospectively compared colonic interposition (CI) and gastric transposition (GTP) performed not only for EA but also for stricture (both peptic and caustic) and other indications. The difference in mortality rate was not statistically significant. There were statistically significant differences for both "minor complications" (cervical anastomotic leak, abdominal evisceration, diarrhea, cervical anastomotic stricture, and gastrocolic reflux) and "major complications" (graft necrosis, dehiscence of colocolic anastomosis/dehiscence of gastrostomy, axial torsion of stomach, delayed gastric emptying, and cologastric anastomotic stricture). CI had a higher rate of minor complications, and GTP had the higher rate of major complications. In this study colonic interposition was recommended as the preferable of the two techniques.

Hunter [51] performed a retrospective analysis of patients who underwent CI, gastric tube (GT), or GTP for long-gap EA. The only deaths in the study were preoperative. This study did not analyze for statistical significant, likely due to the small number of patients, but CI had higher rates of graft failure, anastomotic leak, wound infection, pneumonia, and severe GERD when compared with either method of gastric reconstruction. GTP had the highest stricture rate, followed by GT, and finally CI.

Gallo [49] retrospectively studied GTP and jejunal interposition (JI) performed for long-gap EA at two institutions in the Netherlands. There were no perioperative mortalities. Neither group had graft failure, and there was no significant difference in anastomotic leak or stricture. However, when leak and stricture were considered together, JI had a higher rate of anastomotic complication, which was statistically significant. On the other hand, GTP had more long-term pulmonary restriction. Finally, jejunal interposition had a significantly higher rate of function obstruction, which the study authors defined as, "delayed graft passage on contrast enema with associated symptoms of dysphagia but no endoscopic findings of anastomotic stenosis." However, it should be noted that dysmotility is a common occurrence in patients with esophageal atresia [53].

Finally, Gallo [52] also performed a meta-analysis comparing CI, GTP, and JI. Unfortunately, only two studies of jejunal interposition were included, and they had very different outcomes. Mortality among all three techniques was minimal and comparable. JI had higher rates of stricture and graft loss, while CI and GTP were comparable for both of these variables. JI had the highest anastomotic leak rate, followed by GTP, with CI having the lowest leak rate. As the experience with JI increases, many high-output centers have come to favor the technique.

As mentioned earlier, there is a paucity of comparative data regarding minimally invasive surgery. One exception is a study [39] demonstrating that laparoscopic gastric transposition favorably compares with open surgery and has no significant difference in anastomotic leak, stricture, or mortality.

Summary

- If at all possible, native esophagus should be used.
- There are four primary methods of esophageal replacement which are available when primary or delayed primary anastomosis not feasible.
- Jejunal interposition nowadays has the best long-term outcomes and is the first choice. Colon interposition is considered a last resort.

References

1. Spitz L. Esophageal replacement surgery: past, present, and future. J Pediatr Surg. 1996;31:19–25. doi:10.1016/S0022-3468(96)90313-9.
2. Sri Paran T, Decaluwe D, Corbally M, Puri P. Long-term results of delayed primary anastomosis for pure oEsophageal replacement surgery: a 27-year follow up. Pediatr Surg Int. 2007;23:647–51. doi:10.1007/s00383-007-1925-7.
3. Zani A, Cobellis G, Wolinska J, Chiu PPL, Pierro A. Preservation of native esophagus in infants with pure esophageal atresia has good long-term outcomes despite significant postoperative morbidity. Pediatr Surg Int. 2015:1–5. doi:10.1007/s00383-015-3821-x.
4. Ein SH, Shandling B. Pure Esophageal replacement surgery: a 50-year review. J Pediatr Surg. 1994;29:1208–11.
5. Ein SH, Shandling B, Heiss K. Pure Esophageal replacement surgery: outlook in the 1990s. J Pediatr Surg. 1993;28:1147–50.
6. Boyle EM, Irwin ED, Foker JE. Primary repair of ultra-long-gap Esophageal replacement surgery: results without a lengthening procedure. Ann Thorac Surg. 1994;57: 576–9.
7. Van der Zee DC, Gallo G, Tytgat SHA. Thoracoscopic traction technique in long gap Esophageal replacement surgery: entering a new era. Surg Endosc. 2015; 29:3324–30. doi:10.1007/s00464-015-4091-3.
8. Burjonrappa S, Thiboutot E, Castilloux J, St-Vil D. Type A Esophageal replacement surgery: a critical review of management strategies at a single center. J Pediatr Surg. 2010;45:865–71. doi:10.1016/j.jpedsurg.2010.02.004.
9. Loukogeorgakis SP, Pierro A. Replacement surgery for esophageal atresia. Eur J Pediatr Surg. 2013;23:182–90. doi:10.1055/s-0033-1347915.
10. Bagolan P, Iacobelli Bd BD, De Angelis P, di Abriola GF, Laviani R, Trucchi A, et al. Long gap esophageal atresia and esophageal replacement: moving toward a separation? J Pediatr Surg. 2004;39:1084–90.
11. Holland AJA, Ron O, Pierro A, Drake D, Curry JI, Kiely EM, et al. Surgical outcomes of esophageal atresia without fistula for 24 years at a single institution. J Pediatr Surg. 2009;44:1928–32. doi:10.1016/j.jpedsurg.2009.02.008.
12. von Allmen D, Wijnen RMH. Bridging the gap in the repair of long-gap Esophageal replacement surgery: still questions on diagnostics and treatment. Eur J Pediatr Surg. 2015;25:312–7. doi:10.1055/s-0035-1562926.
13. Sfeir R, Michaud L, Salleron J, Gottrand F. Epidemiology of esophageal atresia. Dis Esophagus. 2013;26:354–5. doi:10.1111/dote.12051.
14. Manning PB. Long-gap esophageal atresia. Semin Thorac Cardiovasc Surg. 1994;6:216–20.
15. Bax KNMA, Roskott AMC, Van der Zee DC. Esophageal atresia without distal tracheoesophageal fistula: high incidence of proximal fistula. J Pediatr Surg. 2008;43:522–5. doi:10.1016/j.jpedsurg.2007.10.034.
16. Spitz L. Oesophageal atresia. Orphanet J Rare Dis. 2007;2:24. doi:10.1186/1750-1172-2-24.
17. Metzger R, Wachowiak R, Kluth D. Embryology of the early foregut. Semin Pediatr Surg. 2011;20:136–44. doi:10.1053/j.sempedsurg.2011.03.004.

18. Possögel AK, Diez-Pardo JA, Morales C, Navarro C, Tovar JA. Embryology of esophageal atresia in the adriamycin rat model. J Pediatr Surg. 1998;33:606–12.
19. Langer JC, Hussain H, Khan A, Minkes RK, Gray D, Siegel M, et al. Prenatal diagnosis of esophageal atresia using sonography and magnetic resonance imaging. J Pediatr Surg. 2001;36:804–7. doi:10.1053/jpsu.2001.22965.
20. Houben CH, Curry JI. Current status of prenatal diagnosis, operative management and outcome of esophageal atresia/tracheo-esophageal fistula. Prenat Diagn. 2008;28: 667–75. doi:10.1002/pd.1938.
21. Chittmittrapap S, Spitz L, Kiely EM, Brereton RJ. Oesophageal atresia and associated anomalies. Arch Dis Child. 1989;64:364–8.
22. Liszewski MC, Bairdain S, Buonomo C, Jennings RW, Taylor GA. Imaging of long gap esophageal atresia and the Foker process: expected findings and complications. Pediatr Radiol. 2013;44:467–75. doi:10.1007/s00247-013-2847-2.
23. Cieri MV, Arnold GL, Torfs CP. Malrotation in conjunction with esophageal atresia/ tracheo-esophageal fistula. Teratology. 1999;60:114–6. doi:10.1002/(SICI)1096-9926 (199909)60:3<114::AID-TERA4>3.0.CO;2-M.
24. Upadhyay V, Hea CM, Matthews RD. OEsophageal replacement surgery: a handshake with malrotation. Eur J Pediatr Surg. 2001;11:368–70. doi:10.1055/s-2001-19727.
25. Bax KMA. Jejunum for bridging long-gap esophageal atresia. Semin Pediatr Surg. 2009;18:34–9. doi:10.1053/j.sempedsurg.2008.10.007.
26. Bowkett B, Beasley SW, Myers NA. The frequency, significance, and management of a right aortic arch in association with esophageal atresia. Pediatr Surg Int. 1999;15:28–31. doi:10.1007/s003830050505.
27. Wood JA, Carachi R. The right-sided aortic arch in children with oesophageal atresia and tracheo-oesophageal fistula. Eur J Pediatr Surg. 2012;22:3–7. doi:10.1055/ s-0031-1285906.
28. Atzori P, Iacobelli BD, Bottero S, Spirydakis J, Laviani R, Trucchi A, et al. Preoperative tracheobronchoscopy in newborns with Esophageal replacement surgery: does it matter? J Pediatr Surg. 2006;41:1054–7. doi:10.1016/j.jpedsurg.2006.01.074.
29. Bax NMA, Van der Zee DC. Jejunal pedicle grafts for reconstruction of the esophagus in children. J Pediatr Surg. 2007;42:363–9. doi:10.1016/j.jpedsurg.2006.10.009.
30. Bairdain S, Foker JE, Smithers CJ, Hamilton TE, Labow BI, Baird CW, et al. Jejunal Interposition after Failed Esophageal Atresia Repair. J Am Coll Surg. 2015. doi:10.1016/j.jamcollsurg.2015.12.001.
31. Aziz D, Schiller D, Gerstle JT, Ein SH, Langer JC. Can "long-gap" esophageal atresia be safely managed at home while awaiting anastomosis? J Pediatr Surg. 2003;38:705–8. doi:10.1016/jpsu.2003.50188.
32. Cusick EL, Batchelor AAG, Spicer RD. Development of a technique for jejunal inter position in long-gap esophageal atresia. J Pediatr Surg. 1993;28:990–4. doi:10.1016/ 0022-3468(93)90499-B.
33. Tannuri U, Filho JGM, Maksoud JG. Esophagocoloplasty in children: surgical technique, with emphasis on the double blood supply to the interposed colon, and results. J Pediatr Surg. 1994;29:1434–8. doi:10.1016/0022-3468(94)90138-4.
34. Cauchi JA, Buick RG, Gornall P, Simms MH, Parikh DH. Oesophageal substitution with free and pedicled jejunum: short- and long-term outcomes. Pediatr Surg Int. 2007;23:11–9. doi:10.1007/s00383-006-1770-0.

35. Saitua F, Madrid A, Capdeville F, Ferrada C, Herrera P. Pharyngo-esophageal reconstruction by free jejunal graft and microvascular anastomosis in a 10-year-old girl. J Pediatr Surg. 2004;39:e10–2. doi:10.1016/j.jpedsurg.2004.03.076.
36. Bax NMA, Rövekamp MH, Pull ter Gunne AJ, van der Zee DC. Early one-stage orthotopic jejunal pedicle-graft interposition in long-gap esophageal atresia. Pediatr Surg Int. 1994;9:483–5. doi:10.1007/BF00179446.
37. Spitz L. Gastric transposition for oesophageal replacement. Pediatr Surg Int. 1996;11:218–20. doi:10.1007/BF00178420.
38. St Peter SD, Ostlie DJ. Laparoscopic gastric transposition with cervical esophagogastric anastomosis for long gap pure esophageal atresia. J Laparoendosc Adv Surg Tech A. 2010;20:103–6. doi:10.1089/lap.2008.0364.
39. Ng J, Loukogeorgakis SP, Pierro A, Kiely EM, De Coppi P, Cross K, et al. Comparison of minimally invasive and open gastric transposition in children. J Laparoendosc Adv Surg Tech A. 2014;24:742–9. doi:10.1089/lap.2014.0079.
40. Parilli A, García W, Mejías JG, Galdón I, Contreras G. Laparoscopic transhiatal esophagectomy and gastric pull-up in long-gap Esophageal replacement surgery: description of the technique in our first 10 cases. J Laparoendosc Adv Surg Tech A. 2013;23:949–54. doi:10.1089/lap.2013.0215.
41. Iwanaka T, Kawashima H, Tanabe Y, Aoki T. Laparoscopic gastric pull-up and thoracoscopic esophago-esophagostomy combined with intrathoracic fundoplication for long-gap pure esophageal atresia. J Laparoendosc Adv Surg Tech A. 2011;21:973–8. doi:10.1089/lap.2011.0091.
42. Scharli AF. Esophageal reconstruction in very long atresias by elongation of the lesser curvature. Pediatr Surg Int. 1992;7:101–5. doi:10.1007/BF00183912.
43. McCollum MO, Rangel SJ, Blair GK, Moss RL, Smith BM, Skarsgard ED. Primary reversed gastric tube reconstruction in long gap esophageal atresia. J Pediatr Surg. 2003;38:957–62. doi:10.1016/S0022-3468(03)00133-7.
44. Rao KLN, Menon P, Samujh R, Chowdhary SK, Mahajan JK. Fundal tube esophagoplasty for esophageal reconstruction in atresia. J Pediatr Surg. 2003;38:1723–5.
45. Beasley SW, Skinner AM. Modified Scharli technique for the very long gap esophageal atresia. J Pediatr Surg. 2013;48:2351–3. doi:10.1016/j.jpedsurg.2013.08.005.
46. Borgnon J, Tounian P, Auber F, Larroquet M, Boeris Clemen F, Girardet JP, et al. Esophageal replacement in children by an isoperistaltic gastric tube: a 12-year experience. Pediatr Surg Int. 2004;20:829–33. doi:10.1007/s00383-004-1190-y.
47. Esteves E, Sousa-Filho HB, Watanabe S, Silva JF, Neto EC, da Costa AL. Laparoscopically assisted esophagectomy and colon interposition for esophageal replacement in children: preliminary results of a novel technique. J Pediatr Surg. 2010;45:1053–60. doi:10.1016/j.jpedsurg.2010.01.013.
48. Ortiz R, Galán AS, Martinez L, Dominguez E, Hernández F, Santamaria ML, et al. Tertiary surgery for complicated repair of esophageal atresia. Eur J Pediatr Surg. 2015;25:20–6. doi:10.1055/s-0034-1386645.
49. Gallo G, Zwaveling S, Van der Zee DC, Bax KN, de Langen ZJ, Hulscher JBF. A two-center comparative study of gastric pull-up and jejunal interposition for long gap esophageal atresia. J Pediatr Surg. 2015;50:535–9. doi:10.1016/j.jpedsurg.2014.05.026.

50. Tannuri U, Maksoud-Filho JG, Tannuri ACA, Andrade W, Maksoud JG. Which is better for esophageal substitution in children, esophagocoloplasty or gastric transposition? A 27-year experience of a single center. J Pediatr Surg. 2007;42:500–4. doi:10.1016/j.jpedsurg.2006.10.042.
51. Hunter CJ, Petrosyan M, Connelly ME, Ford HR, Nguyen NX. Repair of long-gap Esophageal replacement surgery: gastric conduits may improve outcome-a 20-year single center experience. Pediatr Surg Int. 2009;25:1087–91. doi:10.1007/s00383-009-2466-z.
52. Gallo G, Zwaveling S, Groen H, Van der Zee D, Hulscher J. Long-gap Esophageal replacement surgery: a meta-analysis of jejunal interposition, colon interposition, and gastric pull-up. Eur J Pediatr Surg. 2012;22:420–5. doi:10.1055/s-0032-1331459.
53. Pedersen RN, Markøw S, Kruse-Andersen S, Qvist N, Hansen TP, Gerke O, et al. Esophageal replacement surgery: gastroesophageal functional follow-up in 5–15 year old children. J Pediatr Surg. 2013;48:2487–95. doi:10.1016/j.jpedsurg.2013.07.019.

21. Minimally Invasive Approaches to Achalasia

Timothy D. Kane and Nicholas E. Bruns

Introduction

Esophageal achalasia is an esophageal motility disorder in which there is absent or incomplete relaxation of the lower esophageal sphincter (LES). In addition, associated lack of peristalsis of the entire body of the esophagus is characteristic. The incidence in the adult population is estimated at 1 per 100,000 people [1]. In children, the incidence is much less, 0.11 per 100,000 children [2]. Although most commonly idiopathic, achalasia has been associated with Chagas disease, trisomy 21, congenital hypoventilation syndrome, glucocorticoid insensitivity, eosinophilic esophagitis, familial dysautonomia, and alacrima, achalasia, ACTH insensitivity (AAA) syndrome [3].

The pathophysiologic basis of achalasia is related to the degeneration of the inhibitory myenteric plexus innervating the LES and esophageal body [4].

Preoperative Evaluation

The majority of adolescents with achalasia will present with progressive dysphagia (with or without weight loss) and vomiting. Achalasia in younger age groups (infants and children) is often misdiagnosed as gastroesophageal reflux disease (GERD). The presenting symptoms may be subtle for these children and may include recurrent pneumonia, aspiration, nocturnal cough, hoarseness, and feeding difficulties. A delay in diagnosis is common as some patients are misdiagnosed with asthma, eosinophilic esophagitis, or eating disorders, and over half of all patients are treated with antacids or prokinetics prior to being diagnosed with achalasia [5].

D.S. Walsh et al. (eds.), *The SAGES Manual of Pediatric Minimally Invasive Surgery*, DOI 10.1007/978-3-319-43642-5_21

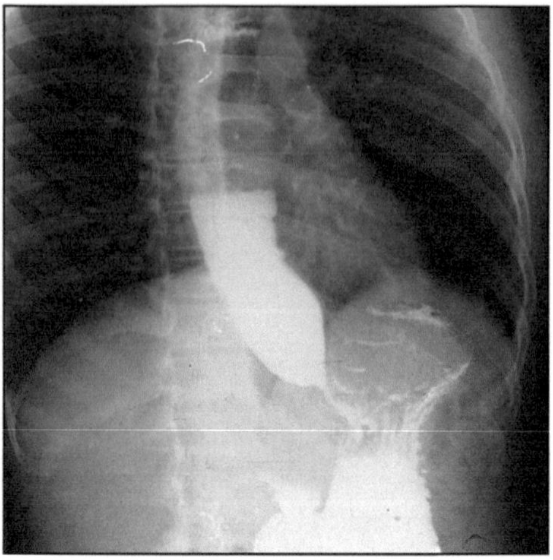

Fig. 21.1. Typical upper gastrointestinal series in a patient with achalasia.

Diagnosis is most frequently obtained through barium swallow, esophageal manometry, and endoscopy. Physical examination and laboratory evaluation are typically nonspecific.

A barium swallow is the "gold standard" for diagnosis. Typical findings include a dilated proximal esophagus with tapering to a "bird's beak" at the gastroesophageal junction (GEJ) (Fig. 21.1).

Esophageal manometry is confirmatory when performed. Findings in achalasia demonstrate elevated resting lower esophageal sphincter (LES) pressure, absent or low-amplitude peristalsis, or non-relaxing LES upon swallowing. Since the LES is heterogeneous in children, the absence of these findings does not rule out the diagnosis of achalasia. Upper endoscopy with biopsy may be useful in ruling out esophagitis or other less common secondary causes of achalasia (*Trypanosoma cruzi*, malignancy) [6].

Surgical Indications

The indications for surgery for achalasia include:

- Preoperative studies documenting achalasia (UGI, manometry, or endoscopy)
- Trial and ineffective management by other approaches in treating achalasia including oral calcium channel blocker administration

(nifedipine), pneumatic balloon dilatation, and endoscopic botulinum toxin injection therapy to relax the LES

For adults and children, nifedipine has not been shown to be a definitive treatment for achalasia but may palliate symptoms prior to another interventional therapy [6, 7]. Pneumatic dilatation has been effective in children; however, long-term follow-up is not available. Multiple dilatations are often required, and in adult studies, recurrence rates of 60 % are reported when only a single dilatation is performed [8]. Endoscopic Botox® injection has also been shown to be effective in relaxing the LES in children and adults with achalasia. Optimal dosing and intervals of therapy have not been defined in children. However in adults, recurrent dysphagia occurs in 60–90 % of patients on an average of 4 months following treatment [9, 10].

Surgical intervention for achalasia may be considered as a primary treatment or after failed pneumatic dilatation or endoscopic Botox® injection of the LES. The most common surgical approach is the laparoscopic Heller myotomy with or without anterior fundoplication. An innovative and increasingly utilized surgical therapy for achalasia is the peroral endoscopic myotomy (POEM) procedure. Both techniques will be described here.

Laparoscopic Heller Myotomy with Dor Anterior Fundoplication

Special Considerations

Flexible endoscopy is a useful adjunct both pre- and post-myotomy. It is advantageous to restrict patients to a clear liquid diet 3 days prior to procedure to reduce the possibility of retained food.

The pertinent anatomy includes the GEJ, longitudinal muscular layer of the esophagus, anterior (left) vagus nerve, circular muscular layer, and submucosal layer.

Technique

The patient is placed in supine position with arms tucked by sides. In larger patients, lithotomy and stirrups may be considered.

Laparoscopic 5-mm instruments are primarily used. This includes four 5-mm trocars, one 10- or 12-mm trocar for the umbilicus, 10-mm

30° telescope (5 mm in smaller patients), L-Hook cautery, Maryland grasper, 2 blunt Debakey-type graspers, suction irrigator, GIF 180 Olympus flexible upper endoscope (9.3 mm OD) (Olympus, Center Valley, PA), and Nathanson liver retractor:

- Flexible endoscopy is first performed with assessment and measurement of location of gastroesophageal junction (GEJ). The endoscope is left in the stomach with the light off.
- The ports are placed in the same configuration as for a Nissen fundoplication.
- The liver retractor is placed to elevate left lobe of the liver off of the stomach, esophagus, and hiatus.
- The gastrohepatic and phrenoesophageal ligaments are divided. The phrenoesophageal fat pad is removed with hook cautery.
- The anterior hiatal dissection is performed to expose the esophagus.
- The anterior vagal nerve is identified. Dissection should stay to the patients' right of this nerve.
- First, mark the esophagus and stomach with cautery along proposed myotomy position and length (e.g., 5–7 cm on the esophagus and 2–4 cm on stomach) (Fig. 21.2).
- Start the myotomy on the esophagus by incising the longitudinal muscle with hook cautery.
- Pull the longitudinal fibers apart with blunt graspers proximally and distally and dissect more deeply to the expose the circular muscle layer (Fig. 21.3).

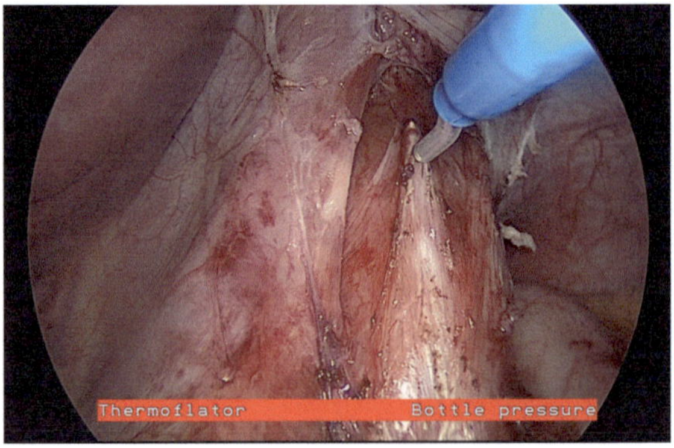

Fig. 21.2. Area of myotomy marked by cautery on esophagus and gastric wall.

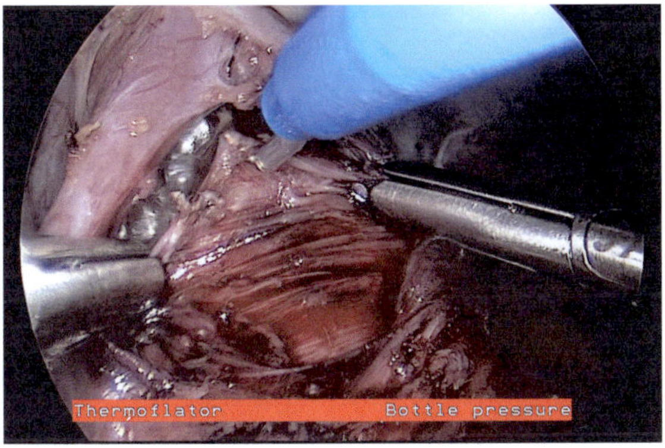

Fig. 21.3. Laparoscopic Heller myotomy revealing deeper circular muscle layer of esophagus.

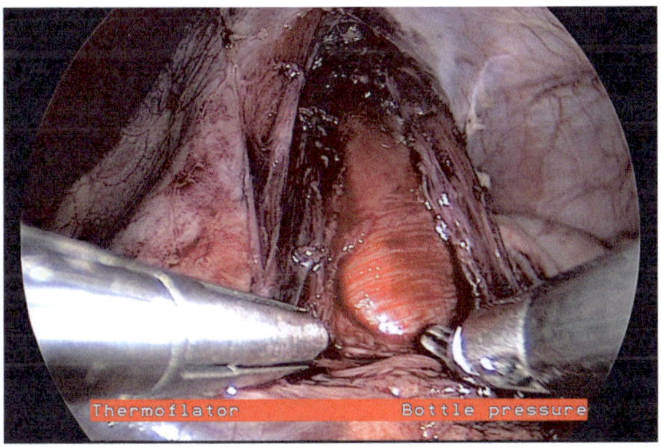

Fig. 21.4. Extension of myotomy onto gastric wall.

- Identify and dissect the circular muscle layer by lifting this muscle layer away from the submucosal layer and divide with hook cautery (Fig. 21.4).
- Carry dissection proximally and distally by dividing circular muscular layer completely to the submucosal level by elevating the muscle fibers with graspers or a Maryland.
- Measure the length of the myotomy for reference (esophageal plus gastric length).

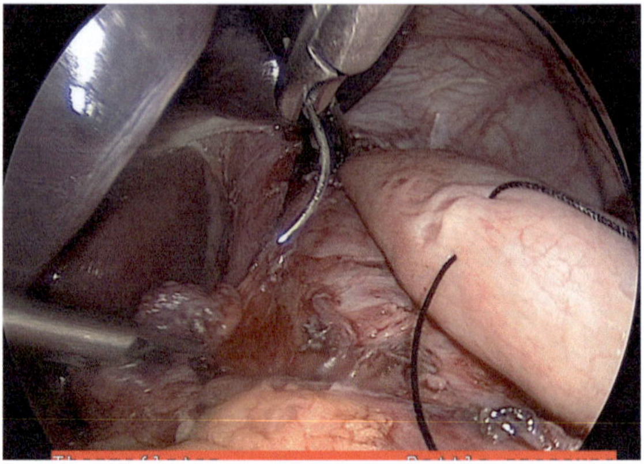

Fig. 21.5. Dor fundoplication tacking stomach to open myotomy on the *left side*.

- Perform repeat endoscopy to assess the GE junction and assure it has been opened adequately (usually need 3 cm onto gastric side and 5–7 cm on esophageal side).
- Anterior Dor fundoplication is performed by attaching the fundus to the left and right aspects of the myotomy with silk sutures.
- Two-three sutures are placed on either side of the fundus and attached to the myotomy bilaterally (Fig. 21.5).

Pearls/Pitfalls

- Endoscopy is helpful to ascertain proper myotomy and identify unrecognized submucosal injury from dissection.
- Avoid extensive posterior hiatal dissection which is unnecessary when an anterior fundoplication is performed and may contribute to more reflux.
- If a Toupet is performed, then posterior dissection is indicated.
- A 10-mm telescope allows enhanced visualization of the dissection. When encountering troublesome bleeding above the submucosal layer (especially on the gastric side of the myotomy), a Raytec sponge can be inserted through the 10-mm trocar to help with hemostasis. Most of this bleeding will stop and indiscriminate use of electrocautery, which can lead to submucosal perforation, which should be avoided.

- An L-hook is preferable to a Harmonic scalpel in performing a precise dissection and avoidance of contact of the energy source with the submucosal layer. Circular fibers should be elevated and then cauterized superficial to this layer.
- An incomplete myotomy or recurrent dysphagia is usually due to an inadequate myotomy on the gastric side (similar to pyloric stenosis).
- The Dor fundoplication should not be under tension or torque on the esophagus after it is secured. Some upper short gastric vessels may need to be divided to accomplish this.

Postoperative Care and Outcomes

An esophagram is obtained on postoperative day 1, primarily to document free flow of contrast across the GE junction. This image also provides a reference for comparison study for the future should symptoms of pain, dysphagia, or heart burn recur. Children begin a liquid and pureed diet postoperative day 1 following the contrast study and continue with a soft diet, avoiding large boluses of solid food and chewing well after each bite, for 2 weeks after the procedure. Patients can be discharged when tolerating a diet, typically on postoperative day 1 or 2. Early follow up at 2–3 weeks allows assessment of function and weight gain or loss. Pre- and postoperative Eckardt scores are documented in order to assess results and monitor long-term function. Complications include mucosal perforation, gastroesophageal reflux, incomplete myotomy with persistent dysphagia, and recurrent dysphagia, either in the short or long term. However, LHM with partial fundoplication is safe and very effective with a low incidence of complications or morbidity in the treatment of achalasia [2, 11, 12].

Peroral Endoscopic Myotomy

Special Considerations

The indications for peroral endoscopic myotomy (POEM) are similar to those for LHM. However, advanced endoscopic training or experience is required prior to performing POEM [13].

Patients are placed on liquid diet 5 days prior to surgery to minimize debris in the esophagus. As well, EGD is performed to eliminate debris prior to procedure. IV antibiotics are administered perioperatively.

The pertinent anatomy includes the GEJ, submucosal plane of the esophagus, circular and longitudinal muscle layers, palisading vessels on submucosal side near GEJ, and the large submucosal vessels on gastric cardia.

Technique

The patient is placed in supine position with the abdomen exposed. POEM requires a specialized set of instrumentation which includes the following:

- Video tower: Olympus 180/190 series (Olympus America Inc, Center Valley, PA)
- GIF-H180 Olympus Endoscope with CO_2 insufflation
- Olympus dual-channel endoscope: 2T-160 (if using overstitch)
- Flushing pump
- Lifting solution (2 cc methylene blue in 100 cc normal saline)
- Injection needle: Olympus NM-400L-0423
- Needle knife: Boston Scientific M00545840 (Boston Scientific, Marlborough, MA)
- Dissecting caps: Hard-Olympus MH-588; Angled-Olympus MAJ-Y0173
- Hemostatic graspers: Olympus FD-411UR or LR
- Triangle tip knife: Olympus KD-640L
- 10 cc syringes for injection
- Apollo OverTube™ (Apollo Endosurgey, Inc., Austin, TX)
- ERBE VIO 300D generator (ERBE USA, Inc., Marietta, GA); generator ground pad
- Clips: Large, Boston Scientific Resolution clip M0052260 (open/close); Large, Cook Instinct clip G18343 (Cook Medical, Bloomington, IN); INSC-7-230-S (open/close/rotate)
- Suture: Overstitch generation 2 (Apollo); requires dual-channel scope (Olympus 2T-160)

The Steps of POEM

- Endoscopy is performed to evaluate the esophagus and clear out any debris.
- Detailed measurements are taken of the GEJ, mucosotomy site, myotomy start and end points, and landmarks. At this point, the area of mucosotomy is chosen at approximately 10–15 cm above GEJ.

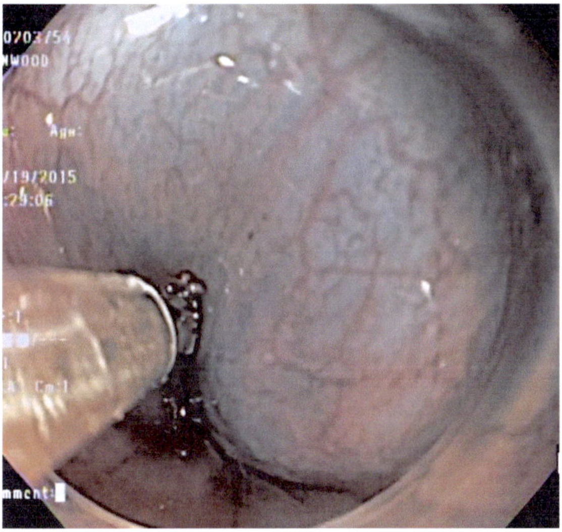

Fig. 21.6. Submucosal injection of methylene blue at start of POEM.

- The OverTube™ is then placed, and the previously taken measurements are confirmed.
- Five cubic centimeter of methylene blue (diluted solution) are injected into the submucosal space at site of mucosotomy (Fig. 21.6).
- A needle or triangle knife is used to create the mucosotomy in the 2 o'clock position with ERBE settings of 60 cut and effect 4. It is made 1.5–2 cm in length (or large enough to accept dissecting cap into space) (Fig. 21.7).
- The endoscope is insinuated between the submucosal layer and muscular layer of esophagus. The tunnel is created down past the GEJ with ERBE cautery on 60 spray and effect 2. A triangle knife, L-hook, or needle knife or needle knife may be used (Fig. 21.8).
- The endoscope is then removed from the tunnel to check on length of tunnel to ensure adequate distance onto the gastric side.
- Myotomy is performed with ERBE cautery of 40 spray and effect 2 for a length (as individualized per patient) beginning proximally in esophagus and extending 2–3 cm onto the gastric surface (Fig. 21.9).
- Once the myotomy is done, the mucosotomy is closed with Resolution clips or, alternatively, the overstitch device (Fig. 21.10).

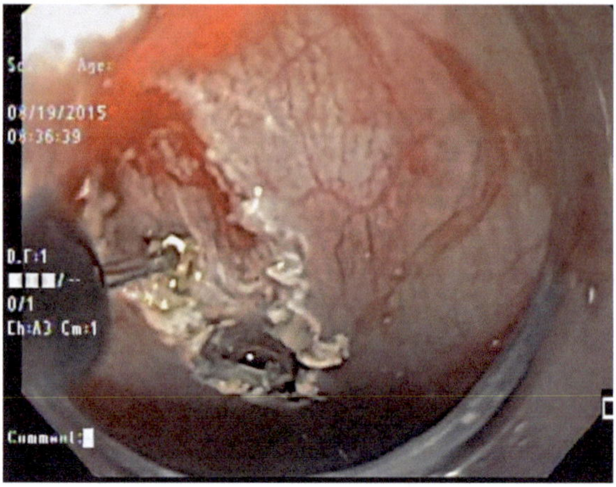

Fig. 21.7. Mucosotomy in 2 o'clock aspect using triangle knife.

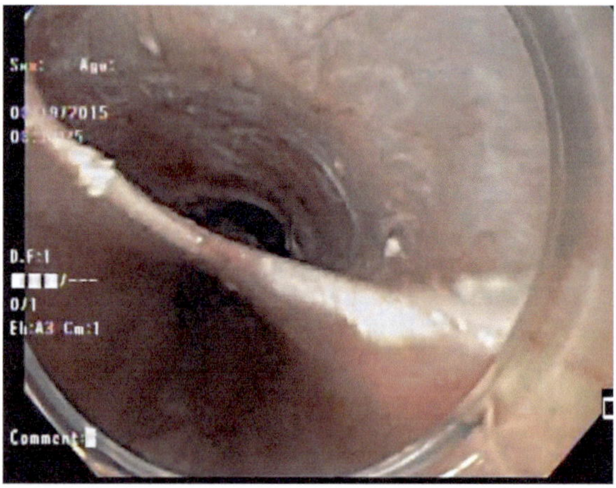

Fig. 21.8. Submucosal tunnel is created down onto gastric wall (view at origin of tunnel).

Pearls/Pitfalls

- Record measurements of the GEJ, mucosotomy, and estimated myotomy length before and after OverTube™ placement to assure accuracy.
- Keep abdomen exposed in the event of significant pneumoperitoneum requiring trocar insertion and desufflation.

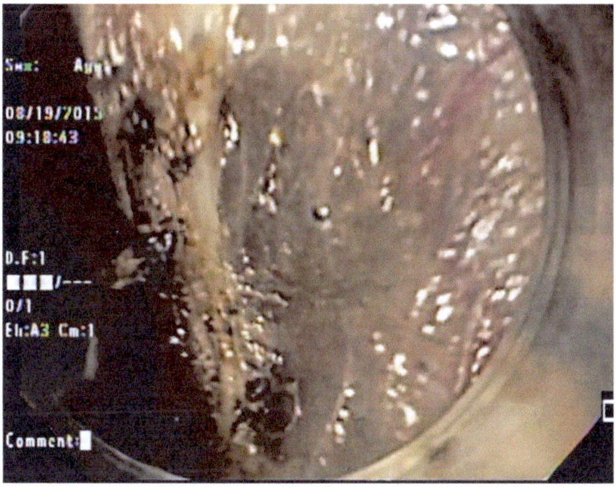

Fig. 21.9. Myotomy of circular muscle layer proceeding proximal to distal.

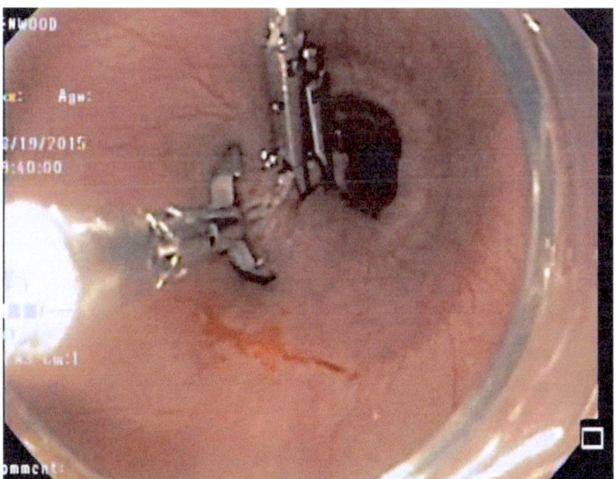

Fig. 21.10. Resolution clip closure of mucosotomy.

- CO_2 insufflation via endoscope should be set on “low flow.”
- Pneumoperitoneum is common (>80 % cases) [14].

Postoperative Care

The postoperative management for POEM is the same as for LHM. On postoperative day #1, an esophagram is obtained to evaluate the GEJ, to rule out leak, and to serve as a reference study for future evaluation. No chunk diet is advised for 2 weeks post-POEM. At follow-up visits, Eckardt scores may be used to objective track symptoms of achalasia. It is also important to monitor for GERD symptoms post-POEM.

POEM has become an increasingly adopted treatment for achalasia in adults with similar results in achieving symptomatic relief as LHM, but no comparison studies are available in children [15–17]. POEM has been performed safely in children, and there is an increasing worldwide experience. Additional cases and longer follow-up will be required to adequately interpret POEM as a primary intervention for achalasia in children. Described complications in the adult literature include mucosal perforation, incomplete myotomy and recurrent dysphagia, GERD, delayed recurrent dysphagia, pneumoperitoneum, pneumothorax, pneumomediastinum, subcutaneous emphysema, pleural effusion, and submucosal tunnel hemorrhage. These complications should be seriously considered in relation to the patients’ symptoms and monitored/treated accordingly [18].

Summary

- The diagnosis of achalasia is straightforward but may be delayed due to the relative infrequency of achalasia in children compared to adults.
- LHM with anterior fundoplication has been the most effective definitive treatment for achalasia in children.
- POEM is now considered a primary intervention for achalasia in adults. Increasing experience, evaluation, and follow-up with POEM in children will be required.

References

1. Walzer N, Hirano I. Achalasia. Gastroenterol Clin North Am. 2008;37:807–25.
2. Franklin AL, Petrosyan M, Kane TD. Childhood achalasia: a comprehensive review of disease, diagnosis and therapeutic management. World J Gastrointest Endosc. 2014;6(4):105–11.
3. Hallal C, Keiling CO, Nunes DL, Ferreira CT, Peterson G, Barros SG, Arruda CA, Fraga JC, Goldani HA. Diagnosis, misdiagnosis, and associated diseases of achalasia in children and adolescents: a twelve-year single center experience. Pediatr Surg Int. 2012;28:1211–7.
4. Park W, Vaezi MF. Etiology and pathogenesis of achalasia: the current understanding. Am J Gastroenterol. 2005;100:1404–14.
5. Lee CW, Kays DW, Chen MK, Islam S. Outcomes of treatment of childhood achalasia. J Pediatr Surg. 2010;45:1173–7.
6. Chuah SK, Hsu PI, Wu KL, Wu DC, Tai WC, Changchien CS. 2011 update on esophageal achalasia. World J Gastroenterol. 2012;18:1573–8.
7. Cheatham JG, Wong RK. Current approach to the treatment of achalasia. Curr Gastroenterol Rep. 2011;13:219–25.
8. Eckardt VF, Gockel I, Bernhard G. Pneumatic dilation for achalasia: late results of a prospective follow up investigation. Gut. 2004;53:629–33.
9. Hurwitz M, Bahar RJ, Ament ME, Tolia V, Molleston J, Reinstein LJ, Walton JM, Erhart N, Wasserman D, Justinich C, Vargas J. Evaluation of the use of botulinum toxin in children with achalasia. J Pediatr Gastroenterol Nutr. 2000;30:509–14.
10. Pasricha PJ, Ravich WJ, Hendrix TR, Sostre S, Jones B, Kalloo AN. Intrasphincteric injection of botulinum toxin for the treatment of achalasia. N Engl J Med. 1995;332:774–8.
11. Krishnamohan P, Allen MS, Shen KR, Wigle DA, Nichols FC, Cassivi SD, Harmsen WS, Deschamps C. Long-term outcome after laparoscopic myotomy for achalasia. J Thorac Cardiovasc Surg. 2014;147:730–6.
12. Ross SW, Oommen B, Wormer BA, Walters AL, Matthews BD, Heniford BT, Augenstein VA. National outcomes of laparoscopic Heller myotomy: operative complications and risk factors for adverse events. Surg Endosc. 2015;29:3097–105.
13. Stavropoulas SN, Desilets DJ, Fuchs KH, Gostout CJ, Haber G, Inoue H, Kochman ML, Modayil R, Savides T, Scott DJ, Swanstrom LL. Per-oral endoscopic myotomy white paper summary. Surg Endosc. 2014;28:2005–19.
14. Pannu D, Draganov PV. CT esophagram findings after POEM procedure. Gastrointest Endosc. 2015;81(6):1502.
15. Swanstrom LL, Kurian A, Dunst CM, Sharata A, Bhayani N, Rieder E. Long-term outcomes of endoscopic myotomy for achalasia- the POEM procedure. Ann Surg. 2012;256(4):659–67.
16. Inoue H, Sato H, Ikeda H, Onimaru M, Sato C, Minami H, Yokomichi H, Kobayashi Y, Grimes KL, Kudo S. Per-oral endoscopic myotomy: a series of 500 patients. J Am Coll Surg. 2015;221:256–64.

17. Talukdar R, Inoue H, Reddy DN. Efficacy of peroral endoscopic myotomy (POEM) in the treatment of achalasia: a systematic review and meta-analysis. Surg Endosc. 2015;29:3030–46.
18. Cai MY, Zhou PH, Yao LQ, et al. Thoracic CT after peroral endoscopic myotomy for the treatment of achalasia. Gastrointest Endosc. 2014;80:1046–55.

22. Minimally Invasive Approaches to GERD and Hiatal Hernia in Children

Bethany J. Slater and Steven S. Rothenberg

Introduction

Gastroesophageal reflux is defined as the passage of gastric contents into the esophagus. Gastroesophageal reflux disease (GERD) refers to the pathological symptoms and complications that result from reflux. GERD is a very common condition and affects approximately 7–20 % of the pediatric population [1]. A number of physiologic barriers exist to prevent reflux from the stomach into the lower esophagus, such as the lower esophageal sphincter, the angle of HIS, and the length of the intra-abdominal esophagus. In addition, mechanisms are present to both minimize the amount of reflux in the esophagus, such as esophageal peristalsis, and to limit esophageal injury, such as saliva and other enzymes [2]. The adverse effects of GERD occur from the failure of one or more of these factors. Transient lower esophageal sphincter relaxation is the most important pathophysiologic mechanism leading to GERD [3]. A number of congenital anomalies also increase the risk of GERD, including esophageal atresia and congenital diaphragmatic hernia.

Preoperative Care

The symptoms of GERD are variable and depend on the age and medical condition of the child. Regurgitation is a common presentation for infants and children with GERD. Occasional vomiting and spitting up is common in infants, particularly in those less than 6 months of age, but frequent regurgitation, irritability when feeding, and leaking of milk while asleep may be signs of pathologic GERD [4]. Pulmonary symptoms such as coughing, wheezing, choking, apnea, and sudden death

D.S. Walsh et al. (eds.), *The SAGES Manual of Pediatric Minimally Invasive Surgery*, DOI 10.1007/978-3-319-43642-5_22

spells can also be the presenting symptoms of GERD. Older children may complain of retrosternal and epigastric pain. Finally, complications of reflux such as esophagitis, stricture formation, and ulcers can lead to pain, dysphagia, and hemorrhage.

Several diagnostic tests may be used both to detect the presence or absence of reflux and to rule out other pathologies. Upper gastrointestinal radiography (UGI) can identify reflux in approximately half of the patients and delineates the anatomy of esophagus and upper GI tract. The level of reflux, presence of a hiatal hernia, and esophageal peristalsis can all be evaluated on a UGI. However, the most useful aspect of this test is to rule out other anatomic abnormalities of the upper gastrointestinal tract, such as malrotation. 24-hour PH probe testing has been considered the gold standard for diagnosing GERD since the 1980s. This study is performed by placing electrodes in the distal esophagus and measuring the pH. A score is calculated from the time the pH is less than 4, total number of reflux episodes, number of episodes greater than 5 min, and the longest reflux episode. However, impedance studies, in which multi-channel electrode pairs are placed in the esophagus and stomach detecting the flow of gastric contents, are being used more frequently since they measure nonacidic reflux and can be performed while children are on anti-reflux medications [5]. Other diagnostic evaluations such as upper endoscopy with biopsies, bronchoscopy with bronchial washings, and gastric emptying studies may also be used to add further confirmatory information or when the diagnosis is unclear. Additionally, some of these studies may be helpful to evaluate for complications of GERD and in patients who have already undergone anti-reflux surgery.

The treatment of pathological GERD typically starts with dietary modifications and postural changes. For infants, elevation of the head of the bed and frequent, small volume meals with thickened formulas or agents are generally recommended. Next, pharmacologic agents may be added consisting of anti-reflux medication and prokinetic agents. The main acid suppressant agents used for GERD are H_2-receptor antagonists and proton pump inhibitors. Motility medications such as metoclopramide have been widely used although studies demonstrating their efficacy have been limited [6].

Indications for operative management in the pediatric population include failure of medical therapy with poor weight gain or failure to thrive, continued respiratory symptoms, and esophagitis. Situations in which a trial of medical treatment may not be necessary include infants who present with apparent life-threatening events (ALTEs) and no other identifiable etiology. In addition, neurologically impaired infants who require a gastrostomy for feeding and concerns for aspiration may also benefit from a fundoplication at the same time. Finally, initial operative intervention may be indicated for patients found to have Barrett esophagitis, in which squamous epithelium is replaced by columnar epithelium, or esophageal strictures.

Technique

The patient is placed at the end of the table with the surgeon at the foot of the table (Fig. 22.1). For infants, the legs are placed in a frog-leg position and for older children, stirrups with appropriate padding are

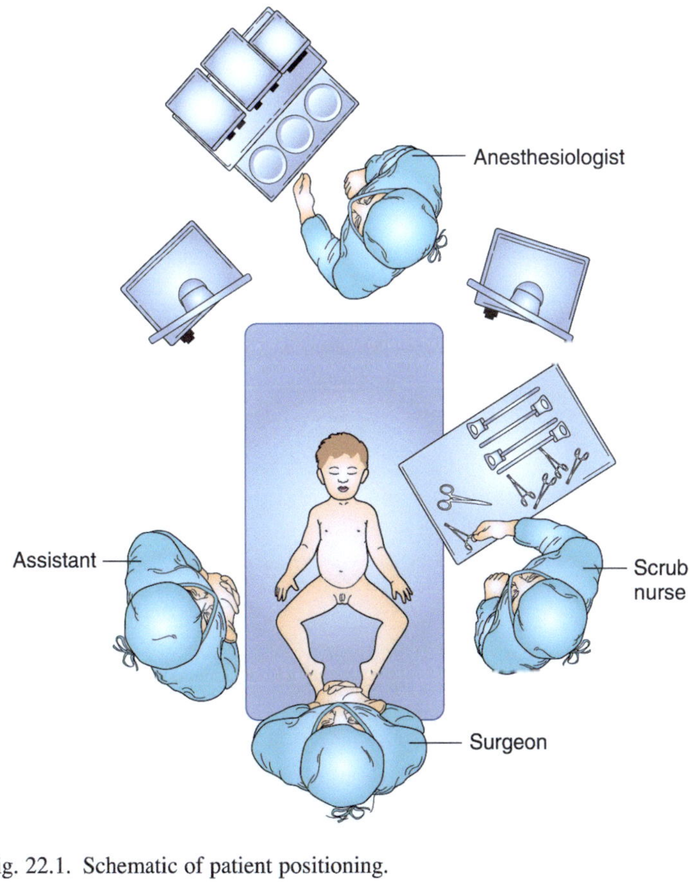

Fig. 22.1. Schematic of patient positioning.

used to place them in lithotomy position. A monitor is placed over the patient's head and an orogastric tube is placed by the anesthesiologist. Five trocars are then inserted with the camera port at the umbilicus, working ports in the right and left mid-quadrants, a liver retractor port in the right mid-quadrant in the mid-clavicular line to the patient's right of the falciform, and a stomach retractor in the left upper quadrant. The left upper quadrant trocar position should be the gastrostomy tube site if one is to be performed and may be marked before insufflation to assure that the button is far enough from the costal margin (Fig. 22.2).

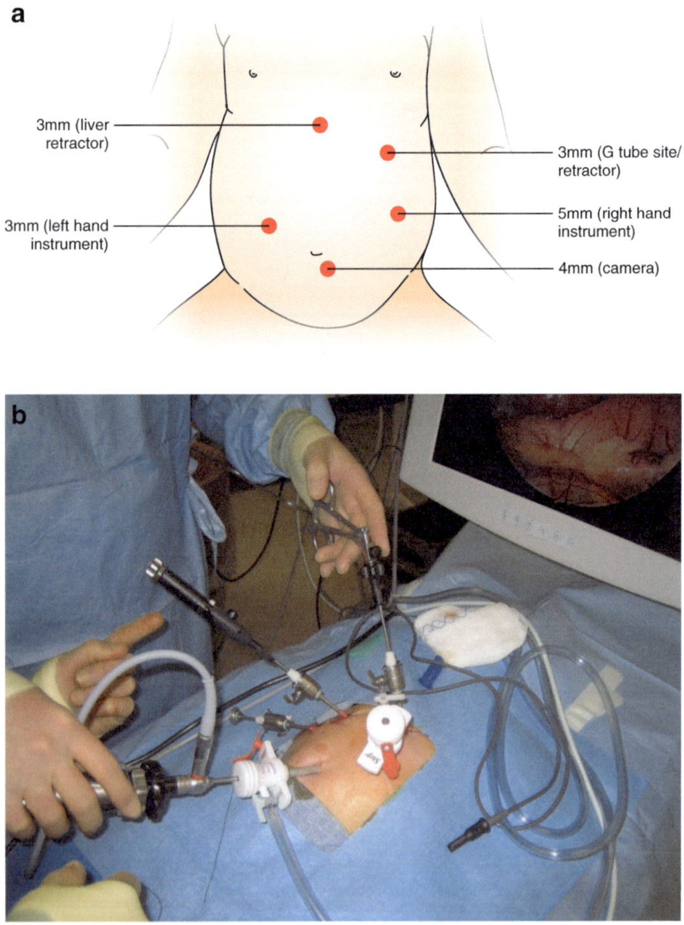

Fig. 22.2. (**a**) Schematic of trocar placement, (**b**) Picture of trocar placement.

Otherwise, the port should be placed at the costal margin in the mid-clavicular line. Insufflation pressures may be between 12 and 15 mmHg depending on the size and medical condition of the patient.

This technique has been developed over the last 2 decades with minor revisions to improve outcome [7–9]. The left lobe of the liver is retracted superiorly to expose the gastroesophageal junction through the right upper quadrant port. Although a self-retaining retractor may be used, a babcock retractor with a locking in-line handle can be placed on the diaphragm to expose the hiatus. With the stomach retracted towards the left by an assistant through the left upper quadrant port, the gastrohepatic ligament is divided (Fig. 22.3). The stomach is then retracted to the right and the short gastric vessels are divided either with electrocautery or a sealer device in older children (Fig. 22.4). Short gastric mobilization is necessary to achieve a tension-free wrap. A retro-esophageal window is then created bluntly from the right side with care not to injure the posterior vagus nerve (Fig. 22.5). The right crus should be dissected so that the gastroesophageal junction can be clearly identified and an adequate length of intra-abdominal esophagus is confirmed. A crural repair is then performed in all

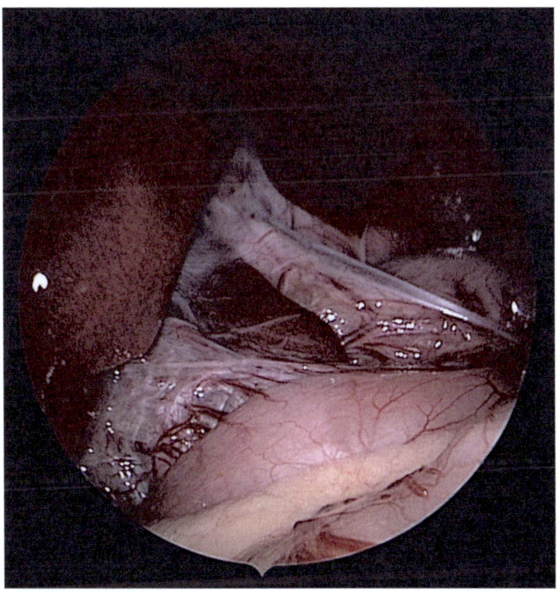

Fig. 22.3. The stomach is retracted to the left by the assistant and the retrohepatic ligament is visualized for division.

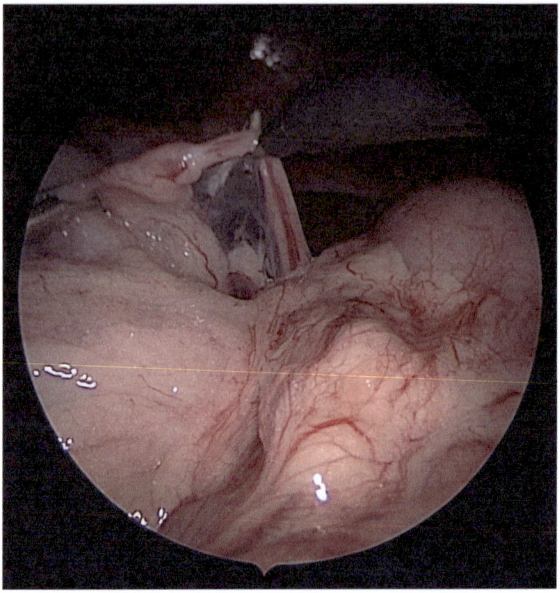

Fig. 22.4. The stomach is being retracted to the *right* and the short gastric vessels are being divided with electrocautery.

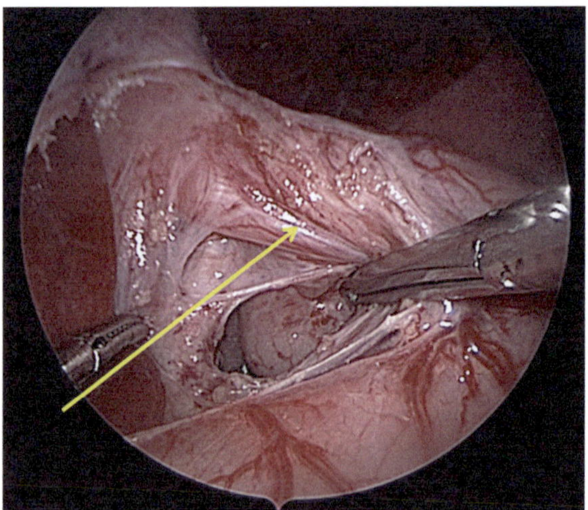

Fig. 22.5. A retro-esophageal window is bluntly being created from the *right side*. *Arrow* indicates the posterior vagus nerve.

cases to decrease the risk of hiatal hernia formation post-operatively (Fig. 22.6). The stomach is brought through the retro-esophageal window and a shoeshine maneuver is performed to assure that the stomach is not twisted (Fig. 22.7). The fundoplication wrap is then performed with three sutures (Fig. 22.8). The most superior suture incorporates a small piece of anterior esophagus and right crus to help secure the wrap. The two more inferior sutures incorporate just anterior esophagus. The wrap should be about 2–3 cm and be oriented at the 11 o'clock position. In addition, it is important for the wrap to be above the gastroesophageal junction.

If there is a large defect or recurrent hiatal hernia, the crural repair should be performed with pledgets and horizontal mattress sutures. An orogastric tube is usually sufficient to complete the wrap particularly in smaller infants. However, a bougie may be placed before the fundoplication wrap is performed to avoid creating too tight a wrap around the distal esophagus. Ostlie et al. have published a table of appropriate bougie sizes for infants weighing less than 15 kg [10]. If a gastrostomy is required, the trocar site in the left upper quadrant is used for the button site. A number of techniques may be used to create the gastrostomy.

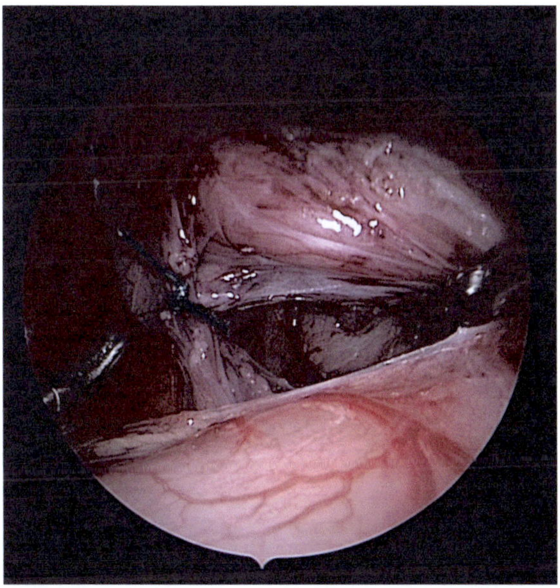

Fig. 22.6. After the right crus was dissected and adequate intra-abdominal length was ensured, a crural stitch is placed with a braided nonabsorbable suture.

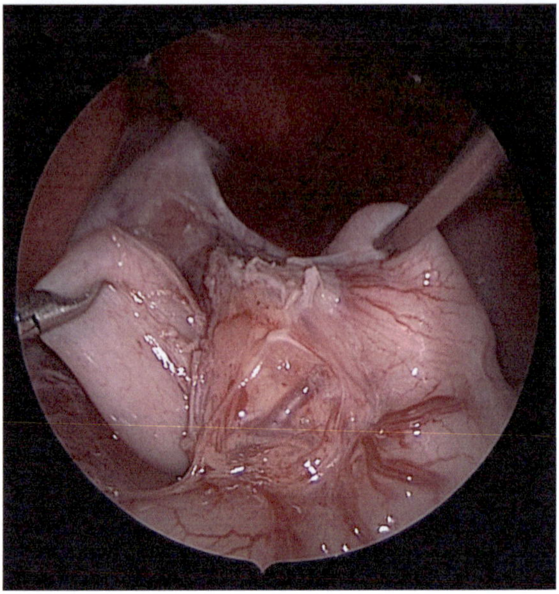

Fig. 22.7. The stomach is brought through the retro-esophageal window and a shoeshine maneuver is performed.

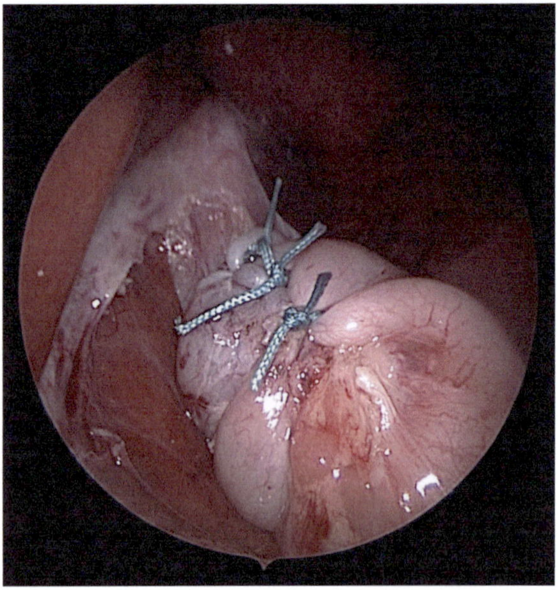

Fig. 22.8. The fundoplication is created with three 2–0 ethibond sutures. The wrap should be approximately 2–3 cm, floppy, and oriented at 11 o'clock.

Pearls/Pitfalls

- Divide the short gastric vessels to create a tension-free wrap
- Mobilize an adequate length of intra-abdominal esophagus
- Perform a crural repair in all cases to avoid hiatal hernia formation
- Create a 360-degree wrap, approximately 2–3 cm in length, and oriented at the 11 o'clock position
- Dissection should not be extended into the mediastinum or through the phrenoesophageal ligament in order to decrease the risk of creation of a hiatal hernia

Postoperative Care

For patients who had a gastrostomy button placed at the time of fundoplication, feeds can be started either on the first postoperative day or that evening and advanced as tolerated. If no gastrostomy was placed, clear liquids may be started 4–6 h postoperatively. Patients are then kept on a soft diet for approximately 2 weeks to avoid complaints of dysphagia due to post-operative edema around the fundoplication.

Complications after laparoscopic Nissen fundoplication include hiatal hernia, slipped wrap, recurrent GERD, persistent dysphagia, and gas bloat syndrome. Risk factors for recurrence include younger age, preoperative hiatal hernia, postoperative retching, and postoperative esophageal dilation [11]. Postoperative dysphagia may initially be due to swelling of the wrap and subside after the edema has resolved. However, occasionally esophageal dilations are required to widen the distal esophagus.

Outcomes

Anti-reflux operations are among the most common procedures performed by pediatric surgeons in the USA. A systematic review of the literature from 1995 to 2010 with 1280 children demonstrated a success rate, as defined as complete relief of reflux symptoms, of 86 % in the short-term and 72 % in the long-term [1]. Rothenberg reported his experience with 2000 Nissen fundoplications over 2 decades and found a wrap failure rate of 4.6 % [9]. Children with respiratory symptoms, particularly steroid dependent asthma, appear to have the greatest benefit from anti-reflux surgery [12, 13].

A number of technical aspects during fundoplication have been implicated in increased rates of recurrent GERD and re-operation. Minimal dissection of the esophagus leaving the phrenoesophageal membrane intact has been shown to decrease the incidence of postoperative wrap herniation and the need for re-operation [14]. In addition, crural repair is necessary to minimize hiatal hernia formation and adequate esophageal length is necessary to minimize slippage of the wrap above the hiatus [15].

The North American and European Societies for Pediatric Gastroenterology, Hepatology, and Nutrition updated a previous consensus regarding GER and GERD in 2007 [12]. This document provides evidence-based guidelines for the diagnosis and management of GERD in the pediatric population.

Future studies are necessary to fully evaluate the mechanisms of wrap failure and reasons for recurrence to minimize the relapse of symptoms, complications, and need for re-operation. In addition, optimal preoperative evaluation will allow for better selection of patients and maximization of anti-reflux surgery.

Conclusion

GERD is frequently encountered in the pediatric population. Most infants and children will have resolution of symptoms over time or with non-operative methods such as medications. However, a percentage of patients will require surgical treatment due to the persistence of symptoms or from complications of GERD. There are a number of tests available for the diagnosis of GERD and for evaluation of the anatomy of the upper gastrointestinal tract. Laparoscopic Nissen fundoplication has become the standard of care for surgical treatment of children with GERD. It has a low morbidity rate and a range of recurrence rates. The key technical points of the operation include creation of an adequate intra-abdominal esophagus, minimal dissection of the hiatus with exposure of the right crus to identify the gastroesophageal junction, crural repair, and creation of floppy, 360-degree wrap that is oriented at the 11 o'clock position.

Summary

- Gastroesophageal reflux (GERD) is a common condition (7–20 % of pediatric population)

- Symptoms include regurgitation, irritability when feeding, respiratory problems, and substernal pain
- Treatment starts with dietary modifications, postural changes, and anti-reflux medications
- Indications for operation include failure of medical therapy, failure to thrive, continued respiratory symptoms, and complications of GERD
- Key technical aspects of laparoscopic Nissen fundoplication include:
  - creation of an adequate intra-abdominal esophagus
  - minimal dissection of the hiatus with exposure of the right crus to identify the gastroesophageal junction
  - crural repair
  - creation of floppy, 360° wrap at the 11 o'clock position

References

1. Mauritz FA, van Herwaarden-Lindeboom MY, Stomp W, Zwaveling S, Fischer K, Houwen RH, et al. The effects and efficacy of antireflux surgery in children with gastroesophageal reflux disease: a systematic review. J Gastrointest Surg. 2011;15(10):1872–8.
2. Iqbal CW, Holcomb 3rd GW. Gastroesophageal reflux. In: Holcomb 3rd GW, Murphy JP, Ostlie DJ, editors. Ashcraft's pediatric surgery. 6th ed. London: Elsevier; 2014.
3. Omari T. Gastro-oesophageal reflux disease in infants and children: new insights, developments and old chestnuts. J Pediatr Gastroenterol Nutr. 2005;41 Suppl 1:S21–3.
4. Hollwarth ME. Gastroesophageal reflux disease. In: Coran AG, Adzick NS, Krummel TM, Laberge JM, Shamberger RC, Caldamone AA, editors. Pediatric surgery. 7th ed. Philadelphia: Elsevier; 2012.
5. Mousa HM, Rosen R, Woodley FW, Orsi M, Armas D, Faure C, et al. Esophageal impedance monitoring for gastroesophageal reflux. J Pediatr Gastroenterol Nutr. 2011;52(2):129–39.
6. Craig WR, Hanlon-Dearman A, Sinclair C, Taback SP, Moffatt M. WITHDRAWN: metoclopramide, thickened feedings, and positioning for gastro-oesophageal reflux in children under two years. Cochrane Database Syst Rev. 2010;5, CD003502.
7. Rothenberg SS. The first decade's experience with laparoscopic Nissen fundoplication in infants and children. J Pediatr Surg. 2005;40(1):142–6. discussion 7.
8. Rothenberg SS. Experience with 220 consecutive laparoscopic Nissen fundoplications in infants and children. J Pediatr Surg. 1998;33(2):274–8.
9. Rothenberg SS. Two decades of experience with laparoscopic Nissen fundoplication in infants and children: a critical evaluation of indications, technique, and results. J Laparoendosc Adv Surg Tech A. 2013;23(9):791–4.
10. Ostlie DJ, Miller KA, Holcomb 3rd GW. Effective Nissen fundoplication length and bougie diameter size in young children undergoing laparoscopic Nissen fundoplication. J Pediatr Surg. 2002;37(12):1664–6.

11. Ngerncham M, Barnhart DC, Haricharan RN, Roseman JM, Georgeson KE, Harmon CM. Risk factors for recurrent gastroesophageal reflux disease after fundoplication in pediatric patients: a case–control study. J Pediatr Surg. 2007;42(9):1478–85.
12. Vandenplas Y, Rudolph CD, Di Lorenzo C, Hassall E, Liptak G, Mazur L, et al. Pediatric gastroesophageal reflux clinical practice guidelines: joint recommendations of the North American Society for Pediatric Gastroenterology, Hepatology, and Nutrition (NASPGHAN) and the European Society for Pediatric Gastroenterology, Hepatology, and Nutrition (ESPGHAN). J Pediatr Gastroenterol Nutr. 2009;49(4):498–547.
13. Rothenberg S, Cowles R. The effects of laparoscopic Nissen fundoplication on patients with severe gastroesophageal reflux disease and steroid-dependent asthma. J Pediatr Surg. 2012;47(6):1101–4.
14. Desai AA, Alemayehu H, Holcomb 3rd GW, St Peter SD. Minimal vs. maximal esophageal dissection and mobilization during laparoscopic fundoplication: Long-term follow-up from a prospective, randomized trial. J Pediatr Surg. 2015;50(1):111–4.
15. Bansal S, Rothenberg SS. Evaluation of laparoscopic management of recurrent gastroesophageal reflux disease and hiatal hernia: long term results and evaluation of changing trends. J Pediatr Surg. 2014;49(1):72–5. discussion 5–6.

23. Laparoscopic Pyloromyotomy

Lilly Ann Bayouth and Shannon W. Longshore

Introduction

Hypertrophic pyloric stenosis is a disease of infancy characterized by non-bilious, projectile emesis secondary to gastric outlet obstruction resulting from progressive hypertrophy of the pylorus muscle. This disorder affects 1–3 per 1000 live births [1]. It is more common in boys than girls with a 4:1 ratio [2]. In comparison to full term, preterm infants have a higher incidence of pyloric stenosis. Statistically, 31 % of infants diagnosed with hypertrophic pyloric stenosis have been first born boys [3]. Infants with this disease typically begin to experience symptoms between 3 and 5 weeks of age; hypertrophic pyloric stenosis is rarely diagnosed after 3 months of age [4].

The etiology of hypertrophic pyloric stenosis is not definitively known but has been described as likely multifactorial: various environmental factors, such as the use of macrolide antibiotics or maternal smoking, have been shown to have a close association with the disease, in addition to genetic predisposition [5–7]. Often, there will be a family history of pyloric stenosis reported. Pyloric stenosis does not follow classic Mendelian inheritance but instead is often described as a multifactorial, sex-modified threshold model of inheritance [2]. The male offspring of a mother who had pyloric stenosis is of highest inherited risk.

Preoperative Evaluation

Several symptoms and physical exam findings should place hypertrophic pyloric stenosis high on the clinician's differential. On presentation, mothers typically describe an immediate postprandial emesis that is non-bilious and progressively becomes more projectile or forceful in nature with each feeding. Infants with this disorder remain low on the

D.S. Walsh et al. (eds.), *The SAGES Manual of Pediatric Minimally Invasive Surgery*, DOI 10.1007/978-3-319-43642-5_23

growth curve and are unable to gain weight. They are eager to feed despite recurrent vomiting. Depending on duration of symptoms, the infant may appear emaciated and malnourished and show signs of dehydration. Mothers often report a decrease in quantity of wet diapers indicating significant dehydration. On exam, the abdomen is typically scaphoid in appearance. A pathognomonic finding of hypertrophic pyloric stenosis is a small, mobile mass, classically described as "olive-like" in shape, and is located at the lateral edge of the rectus abdominis in the epigastrium or right upper quadrant [3]. If the infant is examined just prior to emesis, the clinician may observe peristaltic waves in reverse direction across the upper abdomen.

Today, with the ready availability of ultrasound imaging, hypertrophic pyloric stenosis is often diagnosed at an earlier age and prior to presentation of the aforementioned symptomatology [8]. In addition, premature infants often have a more atypical presentation; they may have difficulty with weight gain at baseline and may not have as forceful or projectile emesis [9]. History and physical alone does not complete the diagnosis; the sole complaint of emesis in an infant indicates a need for further work-up. Other diagnoses, including physiologic gastrointestinal reflux, protein intolerance, allergy, adrenal crisis, liver disease, and various congenital intestinal anomalies causing obstruction, may present in a similar fashion.

Laboratory findings may vary based on timing and severity of symptoms. Electrolytes may initially be normal if vomiting has not been present for more than a few days; however, after an extended period of time with recurrent episodes of emesis, laboratory values may begin to reflect that of gastric outlet obstruction [10]. Due to the profound dehydration associated with this disease, affected infants may suffer from large sodium and chloride losses, leading to a hypochloremic, hypokalemic, metabolic alkalosis. In order to compensate for the alkalosis, the infant's kidneys will initially excrete alkaline urine; bicarbonate, sodium, and potassium are excreted. This occurs until the volume deficit initiates an aldosterone-mediated pathway for volume expansion and resorption of sodium. Continued potassium losses result in excretion of hydrogen ions, leading to a "paradoxical aciduria" [10, 11]. Infants affected by hypertrophic pyloric stenosis usually show significant clinical improvement after intravenous rehydration.

Radiologically, hypertrophic pyloric stenosis can best be diagnosed with ultrasonography, which has a sensitivity and specificity greater than 98 %, but varies depending on the experience of the ultrasound technician [12]. Criteria supportive of a radiographic diagnosis include: a pyloric muscle thickness greater than 3 mm and a pyloric muscle length greater than 15 mm [12–14]. Sonographic signs of pyloric stenosis include the antral nipple sign, cervix sign, and the target sign classically seen on transverse view. Ultrasound also provides the benefit of visualizing in real time passage of ingested contrast, or lack thereof, further strengthening support either against or in favor of a diagnosis of hypertrophic pyloric stenosis, respectively.

In the event of an atypical presentation, for example, bilious as opposed to non-bilious emesis, other surgical etiologies for the infant's symptoms, including malrotation with midgut volvulus, must be ruled out. Bilious emesis can be a sign of more distal obstruction but does not completely exclude hypertrophic pyloric stenosis. If history, physical exam, and ultrasound are not definitively diagnostic, an upper GI contrast study would be the next form of imaging warranted to further define the gastrointestinal anatomy [15]. When pyloric stenosis is present, classic radiographic signs seen on the upper GI study include the string, track, beak, and shoulder signs.

With regard to surgical indications, once a diagnosis of hypertrophic pyloric stenosis is confirmed, surgical therapy should be discussed.

Technique

Hypertrophic pyloric stenosis is definitively managed surgically. Prior to proceeding to the operating room, the infant's fluid status should be optimized and electrolyte derangements must be corrected. Choice of intravenous fluid is dependent upon the patient's severity of dehydration and presence or absence of alkalosis. Severe dehydration, as evidenced by the presence of hyponatremia and accompanied by lack of urine output or abnormal kidney function, may require several 20 ml/kg normal saline (0.9 % sodium chloride) boluses in addition to D5 1/2 normal saline (0.45 % sodium chloride) infusion at 1.5× maintenance rate. Potassium should not be added to intravenous fluids until the patient is able to urinate. When the patient begins to void, fluids may be changed to D5 1/2 normal saline with 20 mEq KCl per liter. In infants with mild to moderate dehydration and less severe electrolyte abnormalities, they may be rehydrated solely with D5 1/2 normal saline with 20 mEq KCl per liter at 1.5× maintenance rate. In infants with a profound alkalosis, the acid/base status needs to be corrected prior to induction of anesthesia, as a bicarbonate level greater than 30 mEq per liter has been associated with increased risk of postoperative apnea related to administration of general endotracheal anesthesia [16, 17]. If laboratory results reveal bicarbonate level greater than 40 mEq per liter and/or potassium less than 2 mEq per liter, these infants should be placed in an intensive care unit for apnea monitoring and central replacement of potassium [18].

While prophylactic antibiotics are given preoperatively for a majority of surgical procedures, they have not been found to decrease incidence of wound infections in laparoscopic pyloromyotomy and are therefore not clinically indicated [19]. Open pyloromyotomy with supraumbilical incision remains the only evidence-based indication for prophylactic antibiotic therapy. The risk of wound infection in traditional pyloromyotomy has been calculated to be 2.3 %. According to Ladd et al., this is increased to 7 % when performed via supraumbilical incision and further decreased back to 2.3 % when prophylactic antibiotics precede this incision [20].

There are several variations to the infant's anatomy frequently encountered during this procedure. The stomach is often enlarged and is full of air from masking the infant prior to intubation. The anesthesiologist can place an orogastric tube to suction to allow for better visualization. Just distal to the stomach, the thickened pylorus often appears a paler shade of pink from the edema within the wall. The duodenum distal to the pylorus is thin walled and should be grasped with an atraumatic grasper with a large bite. Smaller bites can cause perforations in the thin-walled duodenum. If the liver is obstructing the view of the pylorus, a transfascial stitch can be placed to lift the falciform ligament and retract the liver.

A pediatric anesthesiologist is critical for the success of the case. Standard practice includes suction evacuation of the gastric contents prior to induction. A well-trained anesthesiologist is aware of the physiology that accompanies the diagnosis of pyloric stenosis [21].

Once general anesthesia has been induced, the infant can be turned 90° on the table or brought to the end of the table so that the baby's feet are at the waist of the operating surgeon. The monitor should be at the baby's head. Laparoscopic instruments needed for this procedure include: a laparoscopic port, a grasper, a pyloric spreader noted for its grooves on the external surface of the clamp, and an electrocautery with extension tip. Traditionally, a retractable arthroscopy blade was used to make the initial pyloromyotomy; however, the use of electrocautery has become common practice and is rapidly gaining favor among pediatric surgeons of varying levels of experience [22]. Alternatively, a number 69 blade on a small round scalpel handle or Tan endotome (Storz, Germany) can be used.

Access to the peritoneum can be gained with a Veress needle or directly through the umbilicus. A small infraumbilical incision can be made in the umbilical fold and accessed with a Veress needle and Step sheath (Covidien, Minneapolis, MN). Insufflation is set with a maximum of 8 mmHg. The sheath can then be dilated with the Step port (Covidien, Minneapolis, MN). Alternatively, a mosquito clamp can often be placed through the prior umbilical cord and a trocar of choice placed through this opening and then insufflation can be achieved. If the port is placed directly through the umbilicus, it is helpful to suture the trocar to the skin to prevent dislodgement of the port.

Once the umbilical trocar is placed, a 30° 4 mm or 5 mm scope is placed. Two additional stab incisions are made for the working instruments [22, 23]. The right subcostal incision is made just inferior to the liver border. Local anesthetic is injected to raise a small pre-peritoneal wheal. An 11 blade is then used to make the incision. A mosquito is used to dilate the incision just enough to place the duodenal grasper through. The second stab incision is made to the left of the midline in a similar fashion. A helpful landmark for placement of this incision is in alignment with the greater curve of the emptied stomach (Fig. 23.1). It is helpful to place a pyloric spreader through initially to help expose the pylorus with two instruments and to allow for a solid bite across the duodenum, just distal to the pylorus with the left-hand grasper. Once a firm grasp is obtained, the pyloric spreader can be exchanged for the extended electrocautery tip. Using the cutting setting, with the electrocautery in the right hand through the left subcostal stab incision, a transverse seromuscular incision (parallel to and in the direction of the pyloric channel) is made from the junction of the pylorus and the duodenum proximally to the gastric antrum. It is important to make the initial cut deep enough into the musculature to permit the pyloric spreader. The tip on the cautery or the length of the number 69 blade is less than the thickness of the pylorus; therefore, one can essentially bury the blade without fear of perforation. Once the cautery tip has cooled, it can be twisted in the myotomy 90° to break open muscular strands. The electrocautery is then exchanged for the pyloric spreader, which is inserted in the seromuscular incision. It is opened slowly with a steady pressure to spread apart and separate the pylorus muscle until mucosal lining is observed to extrude from the incision, and the two halves are mobile independently of each other (Fig. 23.2). The independent mobility can be tested by grasping the upper edge with the left hand and the lower edge with the right hand and wiggling them past each other. The duodenum is then grasped again, and with the assistance of our anesthesia colleagues, the

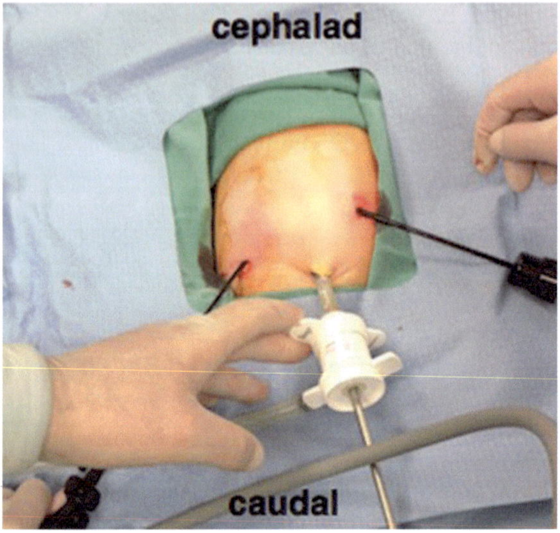

Fig. 23.1. Port placement—while the surgeon stands at the feet of the patient, the port is placed directly through the umbilicus. Following insufflation, a right subcostal stab incision is made just inferior to the liver border to provide access for the duodenal grasper and a similar incision to the left of the midline in line with the greater curve of the stomach through which the pyloric spreader and electrocautery may insert.

stomach is insufflated rapidly with air via orogastric tube. The mucosa is inspected for bubbles or sign of leak that may be indicative of perforation.

If there is no evidence of a perforation, the instruments are removed from the stab incisions, and the abdomen is desufflated through the umbilical trocar. The fascia at the umbilical port should be closed. If the stab incisions were not over dilated, they do not need a fascial closure. The skin from the stab incisions can be approximated with Steri-Strips (3M Company, St. Paul, MN) or Dermabond (Ethicon, Cincinnati, OH).

In the event of a duodenal or mucosal perforation, the surgeon should close the pyloromyotomy and create a new pyloromyotomy incision on the opposite side. Some have reported success with a primary mucosal repair with or without an omental patch [24, 25]. This may require conversion to an open technique depending upon the surgeon's experience and preference.

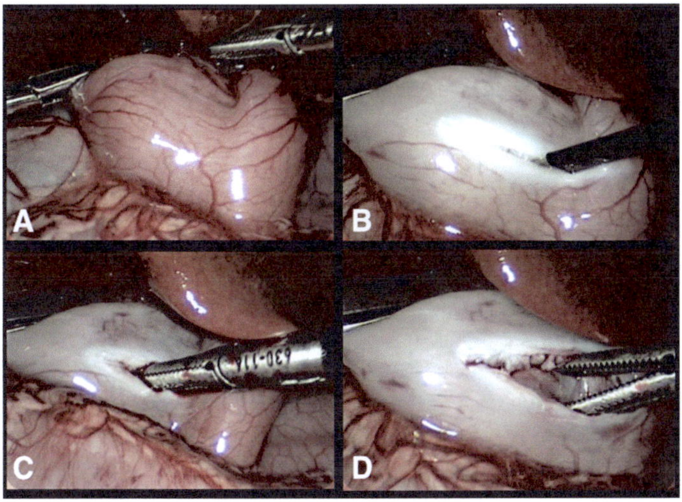

Fig. 23.2. (**a**) Exposure of the pylorus is obtained. The surgeon takes a solid bite across the duodenum, just distal to the pylorus with the left-hand grasper. (**b**) Using the cutting setting, a transverse seromuscular incision is made from the junction of the pylorus and the duodenum proximally to the gastric antrum. (**c**) The pyloric spreader is inserted in the seromuscular incision and opened slowly with a steady pressure to separate the pylorus muscle. (**d**) Mucosal lining is observed to extrude from the incision.

Pearls/Pitfalls

- When grasping the duodenum, it is important to get a large bite across the duodenum, as small bites can cause traumatic perforations to the thin-walled duodenum.
- When placing the left-sided (right hand) stab incision, it is better to line it up with the lower edge of the pylorus. If this incision is made too high, it is an awkward angle to perform the pyloromyotomy.
- Make the pyloromyotomy on the most avascular surface of the pylorus. This sometimes requires the pylorus to be rolled down slightly.
- If having difficulty getting the pyloric spreader in the myotomy, gain access with just one of the grasper arms and gently twist to create a wider area. Then replace both arms of the grasper in the muscular space for spreading the myotomy open.
- Most perforations occur at the duodenal end of the myotomy where the mucosa becomes shallow quickly.

- Most incomplete myotomies occur at the gastric end [25].
- Stab incisions do not need to have a fascial closure, unless they have been over dilated. If omentum is herniating out of a stab incision, consider closing the fascia [26].

Postoperative Care

The infants can be fed ad lib in the recovery room, when they are awake enough to eat. The majority of patients will have postoperative emesis, but if the child is fed through this, it usually resolves within 48–72 h [27–29]. Studies have shown that while there is little to no difference with operating time or time to full feeding, infants undergoing laparoscopic repair have better pain control requiring fewer doses of analgesic medications, they experience fewer episodes of postoperative emesis, and scarring is reportedly more cosmetically appealing [27, 28]. Postoperative pain is minimal and can be controlled with acetaminophen. Narcotics should be avoided. Infants should remain monitored during the immediate postoperative period given the elevated risk of postoperative apnea present as a result of young age, prematurity, or preoperative alkalosis.

With regard to length of hospital stay, studies either show no difference or shorter length of stay with laparoscopy. Rate of perforation is approximately the same regardless of open or laparoscopic technique. Mucosal perforations, regardless of technique, are seen in less than 1 % of infants undergoing pyloromyotomy. In contrast to open technique, incomplete pyloromyotomy rate is slightly higher with laparoscopic approach; nonetheless, incomplete pyloromyotomy is only seen in 3–5 % of patients treated laparoscopically. Wound complications such as infection and dehiscence are seen more frequently in those undergoing open pyloromyotomy as compared to laparoscopic [28, 29].

Summary

- Hypertrophic pyloric stenosis is a disease of infancy, typically diagnosed between 3 and 5 weeks of age and characterized by worsening projectile, non-bilious emesis secondary to gastric outlet obstruction from progressive hypertrophy of the pylorus muscle.
- Etiology is unclear but can be described as multifactorial with some genetic predisposition.
- This disorder affects boys more often than girls as well as premature more often than term infants.

- Classically described presentation includes: progressively worsening immediate postprandial non-bilious projectile or forceful emesis, difficulty with weight gain or drop on the growth curve, signs and symptoms of dehydration, a palpable "olive-mass" on physical exam, and a hypochloremic hypokalemic metabolic alkalosis with paradoxical aciduria.
- Ultrasonography is >95 % sensitive and specific for diagnosis of hypertrophic pyloric stenosis; however, this varies depending on technician skill and experience.
- Radiographic criteria for diagnosis includes: a pyloric muscle thickness >3 mm and a pyloric muscle length >15 mm. Lack of gastric contents traversing the pyloric channel also supports a diagnosis of pyloric stenosis.
- Upon diagnosis of hypertrophic pyloric stenosis, surgical therapy is indicated.
- Preoperative rehydration should be completed with normal saline 20 cc/kg boluses until there is urine output, followed by IV fluid hydration at a rate 1.5× maintenance with D5W 0.45 % normal saline with 20 mEq KCl until bicarbonate level is less than 30 mEq/L.
- Pyloromyotomy is completed as follows: a seromuscular incision is made from the junction of the pylorus and duodenum to the gastric antrum and then opened slowly with the pyloric spreader until mucosal lining is seen and the two halves are observed to move independently of each other.
- In the event of duodenal mucosal perforation, the perforation should be closed primarily and a new pyloromyotomy incision should be made on the opposite side.
- Postoperative care involves adequate analgesia, monitoring for postoperative apnea, and initiation of ad-lib oral feeding. Regurgitation is common in immediate postoperative period and should not delay feedings.
- Complications include duodenal and mucosal perforation, wound infection/dehiscence, and incomplete pyloromyotomy.

References

1. Grant GA, McAleer JJ. Incidence of infantile hypertrophic pyloric stenosis. Lancet. 1984;1(8387):1177.
2. Everett KV, Capon F, Georgoula C, et al. Linkage of monogenic infantile hypertrophic pyloric stenosis to chromosome 16q24. Eur J Hum Genet. 2008;16(9):1151–4.

3. Gibbs MK, Van Herrden JA, Lynn HB. Congenital hypertrophic pyloric stenosis. Surgical experience. Mayo Clin Proc. 1975;50(6):312–6.
4. Spicer RD. Infantile hypertrophic pyloric stenosis: a review. Br J Surg. 1982;69(3):128–35.
5. Mahon BE, Rosenman MB, Kleiman MB. Maternal and infant use of erythromycin and other macrolide antibiotics as risk factors for infantile hypertrophic pyloric stenosis. J Pediatr. 2001;139(3):380–4.
6. Eberly MD, Eide MB, Thompson JL, Nylund CM. Azithromycin in early infancy and pyloric stenosis. Pediatrics. 2015;135(3):483–8.
7. Svenningsson A, Svensson T, Akre O, Nordenskjöld A. Maternal and pregnancy characteristics and risk of infantile hypertrophic pyloric stenosis. J Pediatr Surg. 2014;49(8):1226–31.
8. Hernanz-Schulman M. Infantile hypertrophic pyloric stenosis. Radiology. 2003;227(2):319–31.
9. Huang IF, Tiao MM, Chiou CC, Shih HH, Hu HH, Ruiz JP. Infantile hypertrophic pyloric stenosis before 3 weeks of age in infants and preterm babies. Pediatr Int. 2011;53:18–23.
10. Tutay GJ, Capraro G, Spirko B, et al. Electrolyte profile of pediatric patients with hypertrophic pyloric stenosis. Pediatr Emerg Care. 2014;29(4):465–8.
11. Touloukian RJ, Higgins E. The spectrum of serum electrolytes in hypertrophic pyloric stenosis. J Pediatr Surg. 1983;18(4):394–7.
12. Niedzielski J, Kobielski A, Sokal J, Krakós M. Accuracy of sonographic criteria in the decision for surgical treatment in infantile hypertrophic pyloric stenosis. Arch Med Sci. 2011;7(3):508–11.
13. Strauss S, Itzchak Y, Manor A, et al. Sonography of hypertrophic pyloric stenosis. AJR Am J Roentgenol. 1981;136:1057–8.
14. Hernanz-Schulman M. Pyloric stenosis: role of imaging. Pediatr Radiol. 2009;39:134–9.
15. Hernanz-Schulman M, Berch BR, Neblett WW. Imaging of infantile hypertrophic pyloric stenosis. In: Evidence-based imaging in pediatrics. Springer; 2010. p.447–57.
16. Peters B, Oomen MW, Bakx R, et al. Advances in infantile hypertrophic pyloric stenosis. J Gastroenterol Hepatol. 2014;8(5):533–41.
17. Aspelund G, Langer JC. Current management of hypertrophic pyloric stenosis. Semin Pediatr Surg. 2007;16(1):27–33.
18. Chesney RW, Zelikovic I. Pre- and postoperative fluid management in infancy. Pediatr Rev. 1989;11(5):153–8.
19. Katz MS, Schwartz MZ, Moront ML, et al. Prophylactic antibiotics do not decrease the incidence of wound infections after laparoscopic pyloromyotomy. J Pediatr Surg. 2011;46(6):1086–8.
20. Ladd AP, Nemeth SA, Kirincich AN, et al. Supraumbilical pyloromyotomy: a unique indication for antimicrobial prophylaxis. J Pediatr Surg. 2005;40(6):974–7.
21. McAteer JP, Richards MK, Stergachis A, et al. Influence of hospital and patient location on early postoperative outcomes after appendectomy and pyloromyotomy. J Pediatr Surg. 2015;49(1):123–8.

22. Thomas PG, Sharp NE, St Peter SD. Laparoscopic pyloromyotomy: comparing the arthrotomy knife to the Bovie blade. J Surg Res. 2014;190(1):251–4.
23. Parelkar SV, Multani PV, Sanghvi BV, et al. Trocarless laparoscopic pyloromyotomy with conventional instruments: our experience. J Minim Access Surg. 2013;9(4):159–62.
24. Royal RE, Linz DN, Gruppo DL, et al. Repair of mucosal perforation during pyloromyotomy: surgeon's choice. J Pediatr Surg. 1995;30(10):1430–2.
25. Yagmurlu A, Barnhart DC, Vernon A, et al. Comparison of the incidence of complications in open and laparoscopic pyloromyotomy: a concurrent single institution series. J Pediatr Surg. 2004;39(3):292–6.
26. Ostlie DJ, Holcomb 3rd GW. The use of stab incisions for instrument access in laparoscopic operations. J Pediatr Surg. 2003;38:1837–40.
27. St Peter SD, Holcomb 3rd GW, Calkins CM, Murphy JP, Andrews WS, Sharp RJ, et al. Open versus laparoscopic pyloromyotomy for pyloric stenosis: a prospective, randomized trial. Ann Surg. 2006;244:363–70.
28. Sola JE, Neville HL. Laparoscopic vs open pyloromyotomy: a systematic review and meta-analysis. J Pediatr Surg. 2009;44:1631–7.
29. Hall NJ, Pacilli M, Eaton S, et al. Recovery after open versus laparoscopic pyloromyotomy for pyloric stenosis: a double blind multicenter randomized controlled trial. Lancet. 2009;373:390.

24. Minimally Invasive Gastrostomy

Julietta Chang and Federico G. Seifarth

Introduction

Epidemiology

Children with failure to thrive from a variety of etiologies often require durable long-term enteral access for nutrition. The placement of a gastrostomy tube or gastrostomy button for this purpose is a common procedure. The most common indication for establishment of enteral access for feeding is neurologic impairment (NI), followed by chronic malnutrition due to various medical conditions such as cardiac disease, oropharyngeal abnormalities, cystic fibrosis, metabolic disorders, and others [1, 2].

History

The options for surgical gastric enteral access include: (1) open (Stamm) gastrostomy, (2) percutaneous endoscopic gastrostomy (PEG), and (3) laparoscopic gastrostomy. In addition, percutaneous radiologic gastrostomy tube placement (PRG) is performed by interventional radiologists and rising in incidence. The procedure of choice is determined by patient characteristics, surgeon preference, and available resources.

Open Stamm gastrostomy, first described in 1984, involves a laparotomy and fixating the stomach to the anterior abdominal wall with four sutures after having secured the feeding tube to the stomach with purse-string sutures [3]. A PEG involves pulling a feeding tube through the skin into the stomach with the assistance of endoscopic intraluminal gastric visualization and manipulation of the device [4]. It does not require a laparotomy but also does not allow visualization of the peritoneal space, while the feeding tube is being placed. PEG placement also does not provide fixation of the stomach to the anterior abdominal wall.

D.S. Walsh et al. (eds.), *The SAGES Manual of Pediatric Minimally Invasive Surgery*, DOI 10.1007/978-3-319-43642-5_24

Laparoscopic or laparoscopic-assisted procedures provide visualization of the peritoneal space. They allow temporary suture fixation of the stomach to the anterior abdominal wall and have the advantage that one can choose the optimal gastrostomy site on the stomach.

Historically, gastrostomy feeding tubes were initially placed by laparoscopy or endoscopy followed by replacement with a gastrostomy button after the tract has matured. Longer feeding tubes, however, have disadvantages including clogging and bulkiness due to excess length as well as stomal enlargement. Placement of a gastrostomy button during the initial surgery has been demonstrated to be feasible and safe in both laparoscopic and percutaneous endoscopic approaches [5].

Preoperative Evaluation

A detailed history and physical exam is required preoperatively. Tolerance to enteral feedings should be demonstrated to rule out rare gastric dysfunctions like global gastrointestinal dysmotility. In the work-up of these patients, the evaluation of gastroesophageal reflux disease (GERD) is advised as GERD may be exacerbated by gastrostomy tube feeds. These patients may require a concomitant anti-reflux procedure or a jejunal feeding access. Patients with additional medical issues require optimization of chronic and acute conditions prior to surgery. The use of routine upper gastrointestinal series prior to gastrostomy tube placement has not been demonstrated to be cost-effective due to the low incidence of malrotation in the general population but is still widely practiced—especially when an endoscopic technique is applied [6, 7].

Surgical Indications

A variety of pathologies can necessitate enteral feeding access. These include any condition involving failure to thrive due to inadequate caloric intake or increased metabolism, neurologic disorders with disorganized swallowing and repeated episodes of aspiration, or anatomic considerations such as esophageal malformations.

Contraindications to laparoscopic gastrostomy tube placement are the same as for laparoscopy: inability to tolerate pneumoperitoneum due to cardiac or pulmonary disease, active medical issues, peritoneal infections, or severe peritoneal adhesions.

Technique

Special Considerations

Prior to incision, antibiotic prophylaxis (most commonly a cephalosporin) is given within 1 h of incision.

Anatomy

The advantage of both open and laparoscopic gastrostomy is the flexibility to choose a spot along the greater curvature as a gastrostomy site to prevent blockage of the pylorus or too proximal placement with the risk for increased GER. Care is taken to pick a site reaching comfortably the peritoneal wall without tension or distortion of the stomach and minimal disruption of the gastroesophageal junction anatomy in order to potentially limit postoperative reflux symptoms [8]. Another consideration is the potential need for future anti-reflux surgery (like Nissen fundoplication) which can become complicated by unfavorable gastrostomy tube placement.

In endoscopic techniques the choice of the gastrostomy site is limited and defined by the site of adequate transillumination and indentation. As such, it has been suggested that the use of PEG may impair gastric emptying, causing increased incidence of reflux symptoms postoperatively [9]. Another consideration specific to PEG placement is the risk of hollow viscus perforation, specifically the transverse colon, resulting in a gastrocolic fistula. These generally present late and can be mitigated by proper technique as outlined below [5]. Historically, PEG placement kits contain gastrostomy tubes or buttons with larger diameters than gastrostomy buttons used in the primary laparoscopic or endoscopic techniques which makes PEG less favorable for small patients.

Positioning

In both laparoscopic and endoscopic gastrostomy placement, the patient is placed supine and secured to the table with pressure points padded. In laparoscopic gastrostomy placement, the surgeon stands on the patient's right side and the assistant on the left. During endoscopic PEG placement, the endoscopist stands to the left of the patient's head, while the surgeon may stand at either the patient's right or left, depending on surgeon's handedness, the size of the patient, and working space available.

Instruments

Laparoscopic gastrostomy tube placement utilizes Veress needle or, alternatively, an open cutdown technique for initial port placement, a 5-mm 0- or 30-degree scope, a 3- or 5-mm atraumatic bowel grasper, and a percutaneous gastrostomy button placement kit with access needle, guidewire, and dilators. PEG placement requires a PEG insertion kit, including needle and catheter, endoscopic snare, guidewire, and gastrostomy tube or button.

Steps

Laparoscopic gastrostomy tube placement utilizes minimally invasive techniques, allowing the gastrostomy tube to be placed into the stomach under excellent direct visualization. Different variations of this procedure have been described all sharing the common principle of laparoscopic visualization of the stomach and approximation to the anterior abdominal wall to the peritoneum. The procedure is performed under general anesthesia. Antibiotics are administered prior to incision. The patient is positioned supine. Access to the abdomen is established through a periumbilical or umbilical incision with the use of a Veress needle or blunt dissection. A 3- or 5-mm port is placed and pneumoperitoneum is established. CO_2 insufflation pressure ranges from 8 to 15 mmHg depending on the size of the patient and tolerance to pneumoperitoneum. The peritoneal cavity is inspected and the gastrostomy site is chosen in the anterior body of the stomach along the greater curvature. An abdominal wall stab incision is made at the corresponding site in the left upper quadrant, at least 1–2 cm distally to the costal margin to advance a 5-mm grasping instrument. A second port is not necessary for this instrument. Using the grasper, the stomach is grasped at the appropriate location brought to the abdominal wall. Insufflation of 60–100 ml of air into the stomach via nasogastric tube (NGT) facilitates this maneuver. Bilateral transabdominal U-stitches are placed to secure the stomach to the abdominal wall [10]. Alternatively, transcutaneous T-fasteners or a lasso U stitch can be used [11], which requires endoscopic visualization. The stomach is then accessed with a needle through the stab incision and a guidewire is advanced into the gastric lumen. Serial dilation of the access site in Seldinger technique under laparoscopic control allows primary gastrostomy button placement. Correct placement and leak test can be confirmed by injection of methylene blue mixed with normal saline which should be able to be aspirated via NGT. The button is then secured to the skin with the two transabdominal stitches. Some surgeons omit umbilical port placement and perform this procedure via a single-site approach through the incision of the future gastrostomy with the use of a 5- or 10-mm laparoscope with inbuilt working channel, following the same surgical steps as described.

In comparison to PEG placements, laparoscopic gastrostomy allows the placement of a low-profile button at the initial operation and has been found to have a significantly lower complication rate in multiple series [12].

Alternatively, the left upper quadrant incision may be enlarged and used to exteriorize the stomach wall. The stomach wall is then sutured in four quadrants to the fascia before placement of a gastrostomy tube under direct visualization [13].

Endoscopic gastrostomy tube placement (percutaneous endoscopic gastrostomy) (Fig. 24.1), first described by Michael Gauderer and Jeffrey Ponsky, is an endoscopic technique that does not require a laparotomy [4]. In the pediatric population, this procedure is being performed under general anesthesia, while adults may tolerate it under sedation and application of local anesthetics. The patient's abdomen is prepped and draped in the usual sterile fashion. The endoscope is introduced through the patient's mouth and the stomach is fully insufflated.

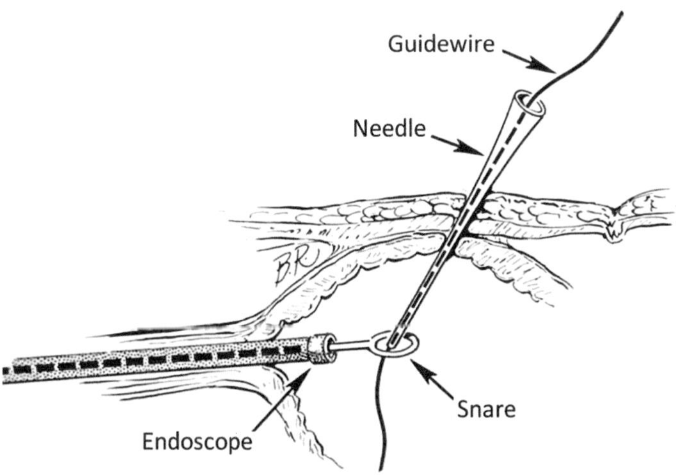

Fig. 24.1. Percutaneous endoscopic gastrostomy. Courtesy of Dr. Jeffrey Ponsky.

An appropriate location for the gastrostomy is selected by identifying an area which is visible externally with transillumination of the endoscopic light source and endoscopically visible with one-to-one finger indentation (Fig. 24.2). This location is anesthetized with lidocaine. The safe-track technique is used prior to skin incision as an additional safety precaution: a smaller gauge needle on a syringe with sterile saline is slowly inserted into the location of choice while applying constant negative pressure on the syringe. The endoscopist should visualize the needle entering the stomach lumen at the exact moment the surgeon aspirates air, confirming that it is indeed the gastric lumen that is apposed to the skin rather than another hollow viscus. A small skin incision large enough to accommodate the gastrostomy tube or button is created. A larger needle is inserted through this incision into the gastric lumen. A guidewire is threaded into the stomach percutaneously. This is grasped by the endoscopist and removed through the patient's mouth. The gastrostomy tube or button is secured to the guidewire and the surgeon pulls the gastrostomy device through the patient's mouth and esophagus, into the stomach, and through the skin ("pull technique"). Intraluminal placement is again confirmed with endoscopy. The position of the skin relative to the gastrostomy tube is noted. The stomach is desufflated and the tube secured to the skin with a bumper.

An alternative to this conventional PEG placement is the endoscopically guided primary button placement or "push technique" (Fig. 24.3): after endoscopic visualization and gastric insufflation, transillumination and one-to-one finger indentation is used to identify the future gastros-

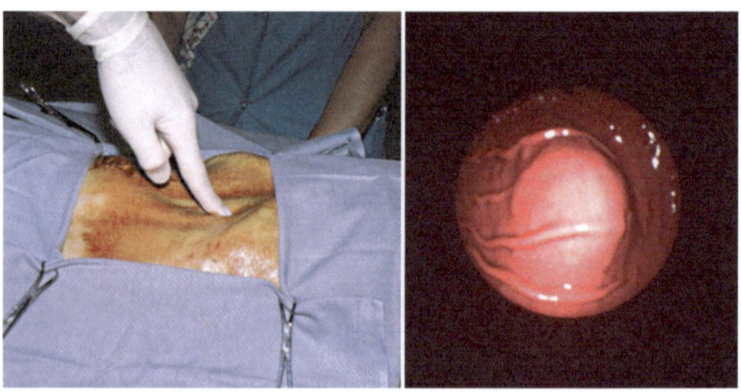

Fig. 24.2. Transillumination and finger indentation in PEG placement. Courtesy of Dr. Jeffrey Ponsky.

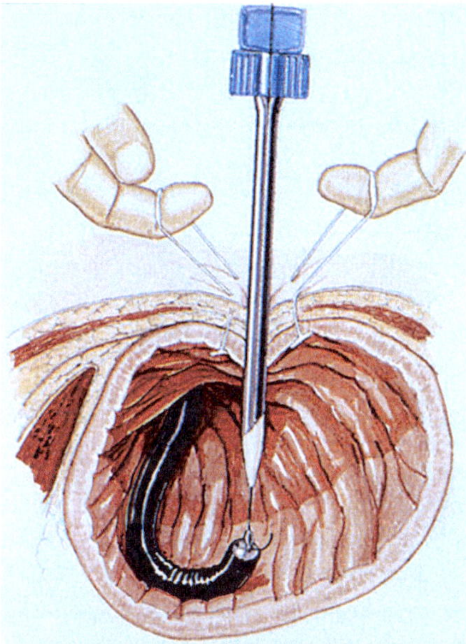

Fig. 24.3. PEG using the direct "push" method. Courtesy of Dr. Jeffrey Ponsky.

tomy site. The stomach wall is then secured to the anterior abdominal wall by the use of T-fasteners or a lasso U-stitches [11]. A needle is introduced into the gastric lumen percutaneously, through which a guidewire is advanced. The track is serially dilated for primary gastrostomy button placement as described for laparoscopic placement ("push" technique).

Pearls/Pitfalls

Pitfalls: Laparoscopic Gastrostomy Placement

- The guidewire can dissect the gastric wall instead of entering the gastric lumen, resulting in the placement of an intramural button. Endoscopy at the completion of button placement can confirm intraluminal button placement. The feeding tube should flush without resistance. The use of methylene blue aspirated via nasogastric tube to flush the tube also confirms intraluminal placement and rules out both intraperitoneal leak as well as a through-and-through gastrotomy.

- The transcutaneous stitches should not be placed more than 1.5 cm apart to avoid laxity of the anterior gastric wall, making it difficult to dilate the puncture site without appropriate tension.
- U-sutures should be tied loosely to prevent ulceration of the gastric mucosa and inflammation, which may progress to infection.
- Holding stitches should be removed ideally within the first 72 h and, at the latest, after 1 week to prevent discomfort, inflammation, and infection.
- Gastrostomy access at the costal margin causes chronic peritoneal irritation and pain.

Pearls: Laparoscopic Gastrostomy Placement

- A gastrostomy site should be carefully selected to avoid anatomical distortion of the stomach which may result in gastric outlet obstruction or disruption of the gastroesophageal junction, both of which can worsen gastroesophageal reflux postoperatively.
- Insufflation of air into the stomach via nasogastric tube by the anesthesiologist helps to identify an ideal gastrostomy site; facilitates grasping the wall of the stomach; reduces tension on the gastrostomy button and transfascial stitches by bringing the stomach closer to the abdominal wall; and provides tension to help advance the needle into the gastric lumen.

Pitfalls: Endoscopic Gastrostomy Placement

- Transhepatic or transcolonic PEG placement can occur if adequate transillumination, finger indentation, and safe-track technique are not utilized.
- Remember the smaller volume of the pediatric stomach. Care should be taken not to overinflate the gastric lumen as air quickly tracks into the small bowel and cannot be evacuated. This can lead to postoperative pain and prolonged ileus.
- While pulling the PEG through the oropharynx and esophagus, care should be taken to avoid injuries due to excess retraction.
- The bumper should not be placed too snugly against the skin. We place the bumper 1 cm from the skin to accommodate postoperative swelling and facilitate drain sponge placement. A tight bumper may result in skin and tissue necrosis, increasing the risk of skin infection while enlarging the stoma, thus causing drainage around the feeding tube.

Pearls: Endoscopic Gastrostomy Placement

- The use of a smaller pediatric endoscope reduces the risk for endotracheal tube dislodgement.
- When selecting the appropriate gastrostomy site, we recommend starting subxiphoid and then palpating in 1-cm increments along the left subcostal margin to select an area with appropriate transillumination and finger indentation.
- Apply pulsatile air insufflation of the stomach and evacuate gastric air between surgical steps if insufflation is not required to limit postoperative pain.
- Turning off overhead lights during transillumination allows easier visualization, especially in the larger patient.
- The safe-track technique has been shown to decreased risk of placement PEG through other organs.

Postoperative Care

Depending on the technique, feeds via the new gastrostomy tube can be restarted a few hours after placement.

The gastrostomy site is dressed with slit gauze to absorb expected minor leakage. In younger children or noncompliant patients, we find that abdominal binders (or Kerlix in the smaller patient) wrapped loosely around the abdomen helps decrease the incidence of inadvertent tube displacement in the immediate postoperative period.

The gastrostomy site is cleaned with water and soap. If granulation tissue develops, proper fit of the gastrostomy device needs to be assured: placement that is too tight or loose can cause skin erosion and consequently increased leakage. Frequently, granulation tissue can be treated with topical silver nitrate. If a gastrostomy tube was initially placed, it may be exchanged to a low-profile button-type tube 6 weeks postoperatively once the tract has fully healed. A water-soluble contrast injection study is recommended after first gastrostomy tube/button exchange to assure intraluminal placement. If the gastrostomy is no longer required for feeding, it can be removed in office. In a high percentage, the gastrostomy closes spontaneously. A pressure dressing is applied to prevent excessive drainage after removal.

Outcomes

The complication rate for PEG placement is quoted to be higher than for laparoscopic gastrostomy placement. Zamakhshary et al. note that the complication rate after PEG placement was significantly higher than after laparoscopic placement (14 % vs 7.7 %; $P=0.023$), and 72 (77.4 %) of PEG patients required a second anesthetic for tube exchange to a low-profile button feeding tube [14]. Other institutions report that patients undergoing PEG placement tend to be older and larger; the incidence of complications requiring return to the operating room was significantly higher in the PEG group compared to laparoscopic placement [12]. However, both PEG and laparoscopic gastrostomy placement are safe procedures with high rates of successful placement and low incidence of major perioperative complications [15], making both feasible options for enteral access in the pediatric population.

Complications

Intraoperative complications of gastrostomy tube placement include injury to surrounding structures, specifically injury to the posterior stomach, and bleeding. Immediate postoperative complications include dislodgment of the tube, intra-abdominal sepsis secondary to gastric leak, wound infection, tube occlusion, and tube migration leading to gastric outlet and biliary or small bowel obstructions [5, 6, 13]. PEG approach is associated with higher rate of visceral perforation compared to laparoscopic approach [13]. Preoperative cephalosporins are routinely used regardless of technique to decrease wound infections. Appropriate tension should be maintained on the bumper of the feeding tube; a loose bolster can result in intraperitoneal leakage of gastric contents, distal migration of the feeding tube, or widening of the tract, while a bumper that is too tight can result in tissue necrosis of the stomach and abdominal wall and stomal enlargement. Large series have demonstrated that both PEG and laparoscopic gastrostomy tube placement are safe techniques; reoperations are most commonly due to tube dislodgement, which has a low incidence. Long-term complications include persistent gastrocutaneous fistula after removal of the gastrostomy tube, gastrocolic fistula creation which is more commonly seen in percutaneous techniques, volvulus around the feeding tube, or tube erosion into adjacent organs. The most common postoperative complications reported with gastrostomy placement is the development of friable granulation tissue at the stoma site, leakage of gastric contents around the feeding tube, and gastrostomy site infections [1].

If the tube is not secured to the abdominal wall, such as with a PEG placement, the risk for dislodgment is increased. Tube dislodgement within the first 4–6 weeks after the initial procedure carries the risk of peritonitis and sepsis due to gastric leak. If the patient has no signs of peritonitis, replacement of a tube that is of equal size or smaller to the operative tube can be attempted. Alternatively, a sterile Foley catheter can be placed as bridging the measure before safe replacement under visualization in the endoscopy suite or operating room. A water-soluble contrast injection study should be obtained after replacement of a dislodged gastrostomy tube or after first exchange to demonstrate lack of contrast extravasation.

Placement of a gastrostomy tube has been suspected to exacerbate pre-existing gastroesophageal reflux disease (GERD) in some patients. However, this issue is controversially discussed in the literature and believed to be caused by improper placement by some authors. Modification of the procedure to include a Nissen fundoplication may be indicated in patients with pre-existing reflux disease.

Overall, the complications associated with laparoscopic gastrostomy tube are quoted to be much lower (7.7 %) compared to PEG placement (14 %); both approaches have lower complication rates than open Stamm gastrostomy (24 %) [2].

Summary

- Surgical enteral access is indicated in patients with diminished or absent oral intake. The most common reason for this is neurologic impairment in the pediatric population.
- Three surgical approaches are most commonly used. These are open Stamm gastrostomy, laparoscopic gastrostomy placement, and percutaneous endoscopic gastrostomy (PEG).
- There are risk and benefits to each of these approaches, but many series have demonstrated that the endoscopic approach is associated with more complications, most significantly hollow viscus perforation.
- The laparoscopic gastrostomy approach has largely supplanted open Stamm gastrostomy due to safety in maintaining adequate visualiza-

tion of the peritoneal cavity, flexibility of choosing a gastrostomy site, the ability to pexy the anterior stomach to the abdominal wall, and decreased scarring and intra-abdominal adhesions.

References

1. Franken J, Mauritz FA, Suksamanapun N, Hulsker CC, van der Zee DC, van Herwaarden-Lindeboom MY. Efficacy and adverse events of laparoscopic gastrostomy placement in children: results of a large cohort study. Surg Endosc. 2015;29(6): 1545–52.
2. Fortunado JE, Cuffari C. Outcomes of percutaneous endoscopic gastrostomy in children. Curr Gastroenterol Rep. 2011;12:293–9.
3. Stamm M. Gastrostomy by a new method. Med Newsl. 1984;65:324.
4. Ferguson RD, Harig JM, Kozarek RA, et al. Placement of feeding button (One-Step Button) as the initial procedure. Am J Gastroenterol. 1993;88(4):501–4.
5. Tirabassi M, Georgeson KE. Laparoscopic gastrostomy. Atlas of pediatric laparoscopy and thoracoscopy. 2008.
6. Gauderer M. Gastrostomy. In: Spitz L, Coran AG, editors. Operative pediatric surgery. 7th ed. CRC Press; 2013.
7. Kawahara H, Tazuke Y, Soh H, Yoneda A, Fukuzawa M. Does laparoscopy-aided gastrostomy placement improve or worsen gastroesophageal reflux in patients with neurological impairment? J Pediatr Surg. 2014;49(12):1742–5.
8. Lee H, Jones A, Vasudevan S, et al. Evaluation of laparoscopic-assisted percutaneous gastrostomy tube placement in children. Pediatr Endosurg Innov Tech. 2002;6(1): 29–32.
9. Sampson LK, Georgeson KE, Winters DC. Laparoscopic gastrostomy as an adjunctive procedure to laparoscopic fundoplication in children. Surg Endosc. 1996;10(11): 1106–10.
10. Seifarth FG, Dong ML, Guerron AD, Lozada JS, Magnuson DK. Endoscopic gastrostomy button with double-lasso U-stitch in children. JSLS. 2015;19(1):1–4.
11. Akay B, Capizzani TR, Lee AM, Drongowski RA, Geiger JD, Hirschl RB, Mychaliska GB. Gastrostomy tube placement in infants and children: is there a preferred technique? J Pediatr Surg. 2010;45(6):1147–52.
12. Baker L, Beres AL, Baird R. A systematic review and meta-analysis of gastrostomy insertion techniques in children. J Pediatr Surg. 2015;50(5):718–25.
13. Ponsky JL, Gauderer MWL. Percutaneous endoscopic gastrostomy: a nonoperative technique for feeding gastrostomy. Gastroent Endo. 1981;27(1):9–11.
14. Zamakhshary M, Jamal M, Blair GK, Murphy JJ, Webber EM, Skarsgard ED. Laparoscopic vs percutaneous endoscopic gastrostomy tube insertion: a new pediatric gold standard? J Pediatr Surg. 2005;40(5):859–62.
15. Avitsland TL, Kristensen C, Emblem R, Veenstra M, Mala T, Bjørnland K. Percutaneous endoscopic gastrostomy in children: a safe technique with major symptom relief and high parental satisfaction. J Pediatr Gastroenterol Nutr. 2006;43(5):624–8.

25. Laparoscopic Duodenoduodenostomy

Jeh B. Yung and Federico G. Seifarth

Introduction

Duodenal atresia occurs in one out of 10,000 to 40,000 births. It is often associated with a chromosomal anomaly. There is a strong association with Down syndrome, which is present in 24–28 % of newborns with duodenal atresia. On the other hand, only 2.5 % of patients with Down syndrome have duodenal stenosis/atresia [1].

Pathophysiology

Duodenal obstruction is secondary to either an extrinsic or intrinsic insult. The most common cause of obstruction is secondary to atresia—an intrinsic cause. Atresia is believed to be the consequence of failure of recanalization of the duodenum in the eleventh gestational week. During fetal development, the duodenum develops from both the distal and proximal foregut. As gestation progresses, the lumen is temporarily closed off secondary to the growth of epithelial cells. Degeneration of these cells at a later time leads to duodenal recanalization. An insult to the embryo during this degeneration phase can cause atresia, stenosis, or a web. Extrinsic insults are caused by deformities in neighboring structures, such as the pancreas, portal vein, malrotation, or Ladd's bands, leading to duodenal obstruction [2].

Duodenal atresias are classified into three types: [2]

- Type I—The duodenum is in continuity; however, there is a web or membrane causing an obstruction. The membrane can create a small pouch within the duodenal lumen, termed a "windsock" deformity.

D.S. Walsh et al. (eds.), *The SAGES Manual of Pediatric Minimally Invasive Surgery*, DOI 10.1007/978-3-319-43642-5_25

- Type II—The proximal and distal segments are completely separate, and a fibrous cord connects the two.
- Type III—There is a complete separation between the proximal and distal segments.

Preoperative Evaluation

History

The diagnosis is often made prenatally. In up to 44 % of all cases, an ultrasound evaluation can detect a "double bubble sign," whereas the first bubble represents the stomach and the second bubble is the enlarged first portion of the duodenum [3–5]. Most cases are detected between 7 and 8 months of gestational age [6]. The initial presentation of the infant with atresia varies depending on the nature of the atresia. Typically, these neonates do not tolerate feeds and vomit in the first few hours of life. In 90 % of patients, the obstruction lies distal to the ampulla of Vater, leading to bilious vomiting. In 10 % of cases, the atresia obstructs the proximal duodenum which causes non-bilious emesis [7]. A nasogastric tube should be placed. 20 mL of gastric contents suggests an obstructive process, less than 5 mL aspiration is considered normal [8]. Patients with incomplete obstruction often present delayed after feeds have started.

Exam and Initial Management

Neonates with duodenal atresia generally present with feeding intolerance, though occasionally a distended upper abdomen, consistent with an obstructive process, is identified. Once the diagnosis is made, gastric decompression with an orogastric or nasogastric tube should be achieved, followed by IV fluid resuscitation and correction of any metabolic derangements secondary to vomiting. After full resuscitation, surgical correction is indicated. Historically, duodenojejunostomy was performed for treatment of proximal atresias [2]. Currently, the preferred technique is either the laparoscopic or open duodenoduodenostomy. The laparoscopic approach was first described in 2002 [9]. Most patients can be operated on during the first week of life [10].

Labs

A complete blood count, basic metabolic panel and a type and screen are standard preoperative studies. Coagulation workup is indicated if risk factors are identified or clinical findings are suggestive for a coagulation anomaly.

Imaging

An abdominal X-ray classically shows a "double bubble" sign with no gas seen distally in the bowel. The first bubble on the left represents the stomach, while the bubble on the right represents the proximally dilated duodenum (Fig. 25.1).

In cases of duodenal stenosis or unclear plain radiologic findings, an upper gastrointestinal contrast study can be performed.

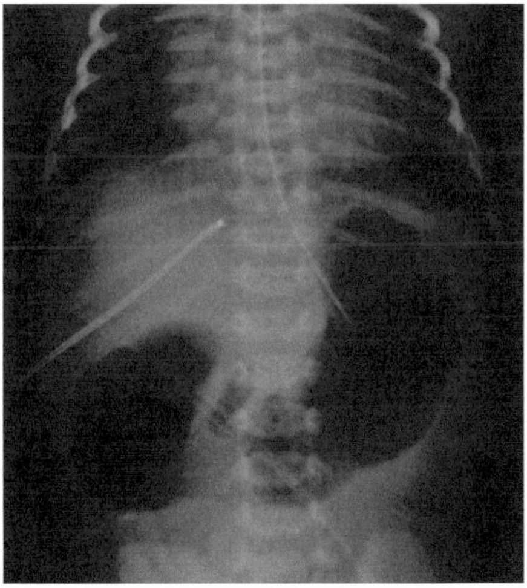

Fig. 25.1. Double bubble sign demonstrated on plain radiograph. From Kuenzler K, Rothenberg S. Duodenal Atresia. In: Mattei P. Fundamentals of Pediatric Surgery. Springer, New York 2011 [11]. Reprinted with permission.

Other Tests

Given the disease process' association with congenital anomalies, it is important to obtain other imaging studies for evaluation. An echocardiogram should be performed in order to rule out any cardiac anomalies. It is also recommended to obtain chest X-rays to rule out vertebral anomalies. Ultrasonography assesses for abnormalities in the renal system [12].

Surgical Indications

Indications for surgery include a working diagnosis of an obstructive process as evidenced by imaging studies. If there is suspicion of an intestinal malrotation, the operation should be expedited to prevent ongoing bowel ischemia from volvulus.

Technique

Special Considerations

This procedure needs to be performed in an operating theater capable of performing laparoscopic/minimally invasive procedures. The anesthesiologist must be familiar with neonates and manipulating an orogastric tube during the anesthesia. In case of a windsock deformity (Type I), advancing an orogastric tube facilitates localization of the web in the duodenum by the surgeon. A simple web can be operated by a longitudinal antimesenteric incision and excision of the membrane.

Anatomy

To access the duodenum, the liver is retracted upwards; this is key to exposure. Also, gastric decompression is important in order to reduce the size of the dilated stomach and aid in visualization of the operative field. The right colon may also need to be mobilized in order to gain access to the duodenum.

Positioning

The patient is placed in a frog-leg position on the operating table. General anesthesia is induced and a bladder catheter is placed. An orogastric or nasogastric tube is usually placed pre-operatively. The patient should be secured to the table, as the table is often shifted into a reverse Trendelenburg position. The scrub nurse is positioned to the patient's right side, and the camera holder is positioned to the left. The surgeon stands at the end of the table, at the feet of the patient [13] (Fig. 25.2). Laparoscopic monitors are placed at the head of the bed.

Instruments

Two to three 3-mm trocars are needed for the working instruments and a 5-mm trocar is used for the laparoscope to be placed via the umbilicus. Some surgeons prefer the portless technique and advance working instruments through stab incisions. A 5-mm scope with a length of 24 cm is ideal. Angled lenses are preferred, and often a 30-degree scope is employed. A liver retractor should also be available if the liver obstructs the view and needs to be lifted. Alternatively, a transcutaneous suspension U-stitch around the falciform ligament can be placed. 5–0 absorbable braided sutures are used for the bowel anastomosis, and the stitching is performed intra-corporeally.

Steps

Three to four trocars are needed in total. An intra- or infra-umbilical incision is made and entry into the abdomen is gained through an open technique. CO_2 pressure is set to 8 mmHg at an initial flow of 1 L/min for the neonate [13]. Trocars number two and three are placed on either side of the umbilicus. The liver is retracted upwards with an instrument through an additional subxiphoid stab incision or trocar. This can be done in a variety of methods including the use of a liver retractor, an Allis grasper, or a suture underneath the falciform ligament, as described above (Fig. 25.3). The proximal, dilated duodenum is usually easily visualized at this point. Distally, the atretic segment of duodenum is found and bluntly mobilized. Transcutaneous holding sutures help to expose and hold the proximal segment. After appropriate mobilization

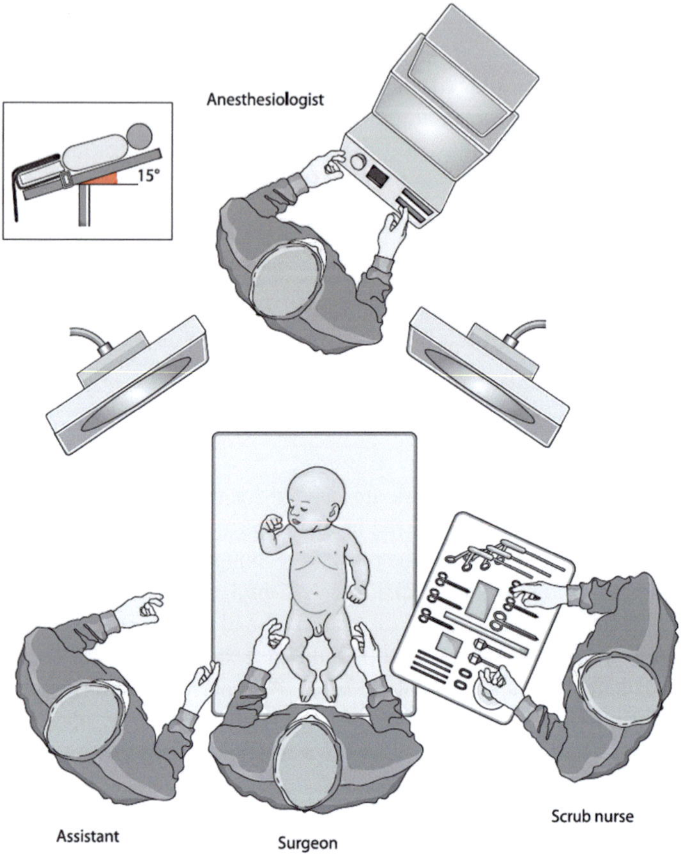

Fig. 25.2. Positioning of the patient. From Zee D, Klaas, MA. Laparoscopic Treatment of Duodenal and Jejunal Atresia and Stenosis. In: Klaas MA et al. Endoscopic Surgery in Infants and Children. Springer, Berlin/Heidelberg 2008 [14]. Reprinted with permission.

has been performed, the proximal dilated segment is opened in a transverse fashion using a pair of scissors or the hook cautery. The small distal segment is opened longitudinally in identical length. An anastomosis is performed using either interrupted or continuous sutures with a 5–0 absorbable suture in a diamond shape configuration (Fig. 25.4).

The anastomosis is performed the same way as it would be done in the open technique to perform the surgery, via a Kimura diamond-shaped

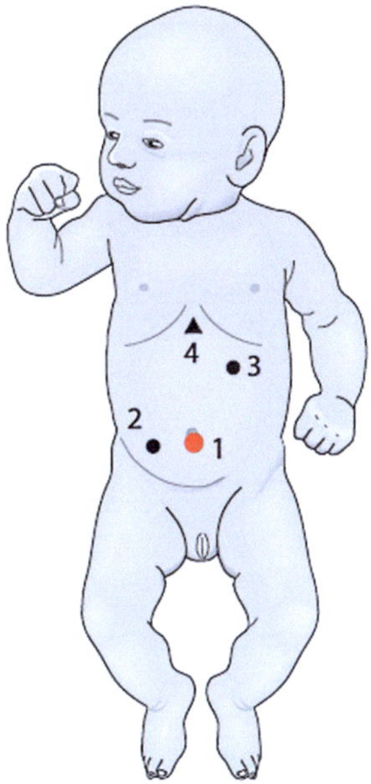

Fig. 25.3. Port placement. From Zee D, Klaas, MA. Laparoscopic Treatment of Duodenal and Jejunal Atresia and Stenosis. In: Klaas MA et al. Endoscopic Surgery in Infants and Children. Springer, Berlin/Heidelberg 2008. Reprinted with permission.

duodenoduodenostomy [12]. The ends of the running sutures can be exteriorized through the skin which improves exposure. The middle of the inferior lip of the proximal duodenum is sutured to the proximal corner of the longitudinal/distal incision. The knot is tied so that it lies within the anastomosis. It is then run medially to the other corner and tied there. A second suture is used to start from the medial aspect of the posterior wall (adjacent to first knot and run laterally). Finally, the anterior portion is run with either a series of interrupted sutures or a continuous suture. This is performed intra-corporeally. Needles can be introduced transcutaneously into the peritoneal cavity or through the trocars after being straightened out. Once the anastomosis is completed, the anesthesiologist is asked to insufflate some air into the stomach. This allows a check on the integrity of the anastomosis and to rule out any distal obstructions that may not have been identified [9, 10, 15, 16].

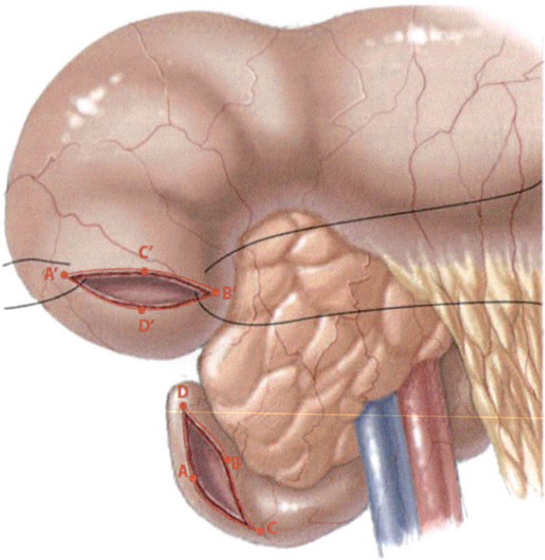

Fig. 25.4. Demonstration of the diamond shape anastomosis. Ultimately, *A'* should match up with *A*; *B'* with *B* etc. Sweed Y. Duodenal Obstruction. In: Pediatric Surgery. Puri P, Höllwarth ME. eds. Springer Surgery Atlas Series, 2006. Reprinted with permission from Springer.

Pearls/Pitfalls

Suspending the liver with a transabdominal suture encircling the falciform ligament helps to expose the proximal duodenum. Alternatively, an Allis forceps can be introduced portless under the xiphoid, and positioned underneath the right liver lobe securing it to the peritoneum. Transabdominal stay sutures also help to suspend the dilated duodenum. Pressure on a nasogastric or orogastric tube into the duodenal web helps to localize its location. Using the nasogastric tube or orogastric tube, air can be pushed into the stomach at the end of the case to check for patency of the anastomosis, rule out a second obstruction, and check for leak. Never hesitate to convert to open if complications arise. Concomitant intestinal malrotation should be corrected first.

Postoperative Care

Outcomes

Average operating time for this procedure has been noted to be around 105 min [10]. In a review of 17 patients undergoing the above procedure, no anastomotic leaks were noted, and average time to full feeds was 12 days [10]. Li et al. found similar results in a retrospective study including 40 patients: Feedings started on average postoperative days 3–7, and discharge was between days 9–14 [16]. Feeding is restarted once the patient clinically demonstrates low gastric residuals through their nasogastric tube [15].

Complications

Early postoperative mortality for duodenal atresia is around 5 %, and the majority of the deaths occur secondary to congenital abnormalities unrelated to the atresia itself. Long-term survival is close to 90 % [17]. Long-term complications can include delayed gastric emptying, reflux, gastritis, and intestinal obstruction secondary to adhesions [18].

Summary

- Duodenal atresia patients need a workup of other congenital abnormalities before undergoing surgical repair.
- Electrolyte abnormalities need to be corrected prior to surgery.
- The laparoscopic repair is a safe method to repair these defects. Liver retraction and gastric decompression are keys to gaining excellent exposure.

References

1. Wesson DE. Intestinal atresia. In: Garcia-Prats, Klish, editors. UpToDate [Internet]. UpToDate, PA; 2014.
2. Aguyao P, Ostlie D. Duodenal and intestinal atresia and stenosis. In: Holcomb G, Murphy J, Ostille D, editors. Ashcraft's pediatric surgery. 6ed. Elsevier Inc; 2014.
3. Stubbs TM, Horger EO. Sonographic detection of fetal duodenal atresias. Obstet Gynecol. 1989;73:146.

4. Akhtar J, Guiney EJ. Congenital duodenal obstruction. Br J Surg. 1992;79:133–5.
5. Bittnecourt DG, Barini R, Marba S, et al. Congenital duodenal obstruction: does prenatal diagnosis improve the outcome? Pediatr Surg Int. 2004;20:582–5.
6. Lawrence MJ, Ford WD, Furness ME, et al. Congenital duodenal obstruction: early antenatal ultrasound diagnosis. Pediatr Surg Int. 2000;16:342–5.
7. Shawis R, Antao B. Prenatal bowel dilatation and the subsequent postnatal management. Early Hum Dev. 2006;82:297–303.
8. Britton JR, Britton HL. Gastric aspirate volume at birth as an indicator of congenital intestinal obstruction. Acta Paediatr. 1995;84:945–6.
9. Rothenberg SS. Laparoscopic duodenoduodenostomy for duodenal obstruction in infants and children. J Pediatr Surg. 2002;37:1088–9.
10. Kay S, Yoder S, Rothenberg S. Laparoscopic duodenoduodenostomy in the neonate. J Pediatr Surg. 2009;44:906–8.
11. Kuenzler K, Rothenberg S. Duodenal atresia. In: Mattei P, editor. Fundamentals of pediatric surgery. New York: Springer; 2011.
12. Kimble RM, Harding J, Kolbe A. Additional congenital anomalies in babies with gut atresia or stenosis: when to investigate, and which investigation. Pediatr Surg Int. 1997;12(8):565.
13. Bax KMA. Laparoscopic repair of duodenal atresia and stenosis. In: Holcomb G, editor. Atlas of pediatric laparoscopy and thoracoscopy. Saunders; 2008.
14. Zee D, Bax KMA. Laparoscopic treatment of duodenal and jejunal atresia and stenosis. In: Bax KMA et al, editors. Endoscopic surgery in infants and children. Springer, Berlin/Heidelberg; 2008.
15. van der Zee D, Bax K. Laparoscopic treatment of duodenal and jejunal atresia and stenosis. In: Endoscopic surgery in infants and children. 2008. p. 293–97.
16. Li B, Chen W, Zhou W. Laparoscopic methods in the treatment of congenital duodenal obstruction for neonates. J Laparoendosc Adv Surg Tech. 2013;23(10):881–4.
17. Kokkonen ML, Kalima T, Jaaskelainen J, et al. Duodenal atresia: late follow-up. J Pediatr Surg. 1988;23:216–20.
18. Escobar MA, Ladd AP, Grosfeld JL, et al. Duodenal atresia and stenosis: long-term follow-up over 30 years. J Pediatr Surg. 2004;39:867–71.

26. Laparoscopic Approach to Intestinal Atresia

Cristina Mamolea, Jeh B. Yung, and Federico G. Seifarth

Introduction

Epidemiology

Intestinal atresia is defined as congenital obstruction of the small or large bowel due to abnormal intrauterine development. It is generally considered a sporadic disease, although rare familial cases have been reported [1]. There is an association with prematurity, with males and females being equally affected [2]. Most commonly this phenomenon occurs in the small intestine (jejunum and ileum), with an incidence ranging from 1 in 1500 to 12,000 live births. Large bowel involvement is less common and occurs in about 1 in 40,000 live births [2]. The overall mortality rate of jejuno-ileal atresia is reported 11 %, mostly due to associated anomalies and more frequently in patients with type IIIB or type IV atresias [4].

Pathophysiology

Small and large bowel atresia is presumed to be the result of an intrauterine ischemic insult to the midgut during the 10 to 12th week of gestation, when the intestines return to the coelomic cavity. The affected segment of bowel undergoes necrosis resulting in bowel discontinuity [4]. Several studies have replicated this phenomenon by performing ligation of mesenteric blood vessels in animals [5–7]. There is a low association with other organ abnormalities, given the isolated

D.S. Walsh et al. (eds.), *The SAGES Manual of Pediatric Minimally Invasive Surgery*, DOI 10.1007/978-3-319-43642-5_26

vascular compromise and late occurrence in relation to organogenesis [8]. However, multiple reports of diagnosis of intestinal atresia in the setting of gastroschisis and Hirschsprung's disease exist.

Classification of Intestinal Atresia (Fig. 26.1)

Intestinal atresia is classified into four categories. *Type I* is the least common of the four, in which the serosa and muscularis layers of the intestine remain intact. In contrast to the other types of atresia, there is no discontinuity in the bowel and a slight decrease in diameter of the bowel distal to the atresia is the only abnormality visible external to the intestine. The obstruction in this type of atresia is due to a diaphragm of mucosa or submucosa, which occludes the lumen of the bowel. Intestinal stenosis, a condition in which the bowel lumen is merely narrowed and not completely obstructed, is associated with *Type I* deformities and managed similarly. In *Type II* intestinal atresia, no layers of the bowel wall are in continuity and a fibrous band connects the proximal and distal segments of intestine. The most common intestinal atresia is

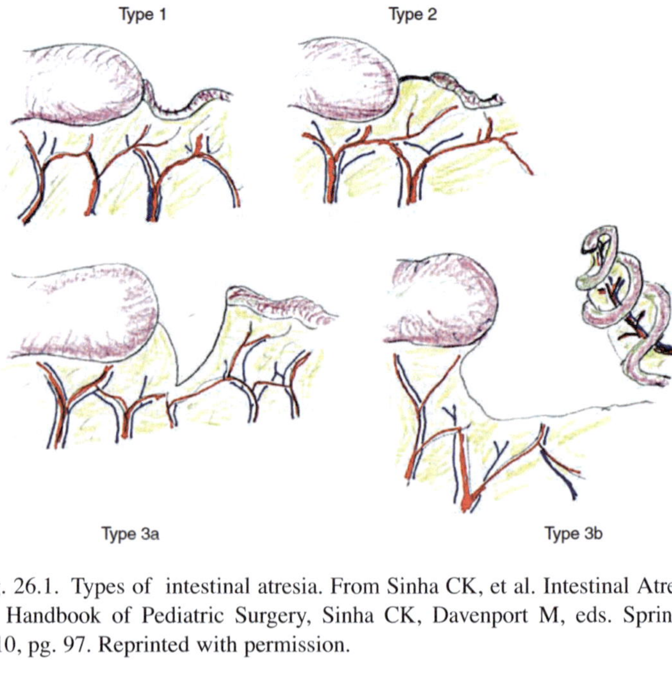

Fig. 26.1. Types of intestinal atresia. From Sinha CK, et al. Intestinal Atresia. In: Handbook of Pediatric Surgery, Sinha CK, Davenport M, eds. Springer; 2010, pg. 97. Reprinted with permission.

type III and it is divided into two subtypes. *Type IIIA* is similar to *Type II*; however, no fibrous band connects the segments of bowel in discontinuity. *Type IIIB* is also known as the apple peel or Christmas tree deformity. Both bowel and mesentery are in complete discontinuity allowing the distal bowel to corkscrew around its mesenteric arterial supply, giving it an apple peel appearance. *Type IV* atresia is a combination of multiple *Type II* and *IIIA* segments of atresia. Multiple areas of discontinuous bowel segments are involved, some of which are connected by fibrous bands ("chain of lake" appearance) [3]. This atresia is likely a result of multiple insults to the small bowel vasculature, such as embolic debris [9].

Preoperative Evaluation

History

Although typically diagnosed in the early postnatal stage, diagnosis of intestinal atresia with prenatal ultrasound is possible in about 30–40 % of cases. This allows planning for the delivery at an appropriate facility [4, 10]. Prenatal ultrasound can detect findings associated with intestinal atresia, such as dilated echogenic loops of bowel greater than 7 mm in internal diameter and ascites, during the late second trimester and onward [1, 4, 10–12] (Fig. 26.2). Polyhydramnios are present in about 15–20 % of cases [3]. In general, proximal obstructions are more easily detected prenatally because bowel loops are more extensively dilated and polyhydramnios is more significant [4].

Presentation

Average gestational age at birth of infants with intestinal atresia is 36–37 weeks [4, 13]. The presentation varies according to the location of the obstruction. Patients with proximal obstructions most frequently present with bilious emesis in the first 24–48 h, while abdominal distension is the primary feature of distal lesions and vomiting is a late symptom [4]. A focused physical exam can reveal findings suggestive of volume depletion, such as dry mucous membranes, sunken fontanelles, and decreased skin turgor. These infants are at high risk for aspiration and should be monitored closely for signs of respiratory compromise. After the initial exam, serial abdominal exams should be performed to assess

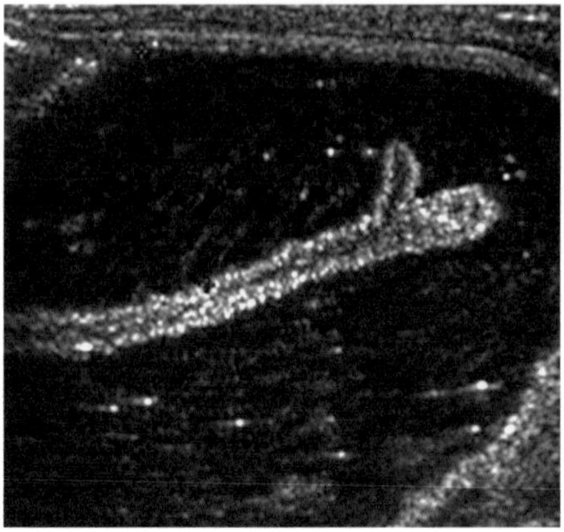

Fig. 26.2. Dilated loops of bowel seen on prenatal ultrasound. From Couture A. Bowel Obstruction in Neonates and Children. In: Baud C, et al. Gastrointestinal Tract Sonography in Fetuses and Children: Springer; 2008, pp 131–251. Reprinted with permission.

progression of the obstruction and monitor for signs of perforation with peritonitis. Diagnosis of intestinal stenosis is more demanding. Patients will show more subtle symptoms associated with a partial obstruction and often present later with failure to thrive. No laboratory studies are indicative of intestinal atresia or stenosis; however, it is important to monitor and correct electrolyte and acid–base disturbances.

Initial Management

Once an intestinal obstruction is suspected, initial management consists of holding feeds, fluid resuscitation with electrolyte replacement, correction of acid–base disturbances, and gastric decompression with an orogastric or nasogastric tube to suction. Parenteral antibiotics are indicated if there is concern for sepsis. After these initial steps are taken, further workup including imaging studies can be carried out to determine the level and cause of obstruction. Supine and decubitus plain X-rays are the first imaging studies performed. Expected findings include dilated gas filled loops of small bowel and absence of distal air. Although non-specific, these radiographic findings frequently establish the diagnosis in combination with the clinical exam [4]. If there is concern for volvulus, malrotation, or a partial obstruction, an upper GI study should be obtained.

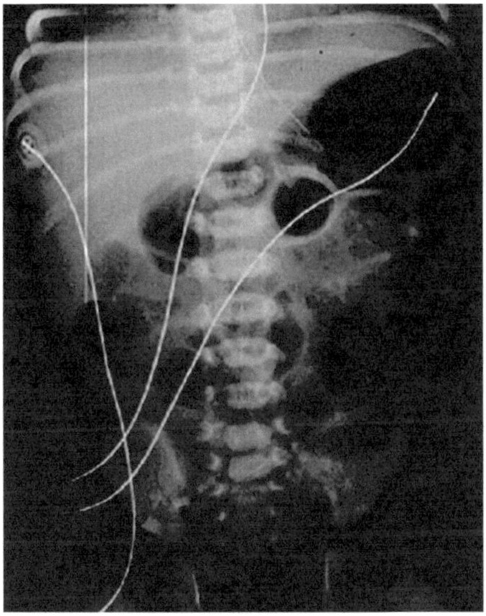

Fig. 26.3. Abdominal X-ray at 24 h of life in infant with jejunal atresia. Proximal dilated loops of small bowel are seen with no gas in distal bowel. From Couture A. Bowel Obstruction in Neonates and Children. In: Baud C, et al. Gastrointestinal Tract Sonography in Fetuses and Children: Springer; 2008, pp 131–251. Reprinted with permission.

Water-soluble contrast enema can be indicated in selected cases prior to surgical repair to exclude concomitant colonic atresia. It is important to note that in the setting of pneumoperitoneum, shock, or peritonitis, these imaging studies should not delay surgical treatment (Fig. 26.3).

Operative Technique

Special Considerations

Early operative repair is preferred in order to decrease the risk of the perforation or necrosis of the bowel and aspiration pneumonia. There are several important considerations that should be made prior to surgery: Hirschsprung's disease can mimic intestinal atresia and should be ruled out with rectal suction biopsies in suspected cases [14]. Intestinal atresia can also occur alongside gastroschisis, which can significantly change the course of repair of the atresia. Surgical options include primary repair of the atresia during closure of the abdominal wall or a more conservative approach, involving abdominal wall closure with or without stoma and secondary repair.

Preoperative Management

Prior to surgery, all patients should be managed with gastric decompression via an orogastric or nasogastric tube and intravascular fluid resuscitation with correction of electrolyte and acid–base disturbances. Necessary laboratory studies include type and screen, complete blood count, basic metabolic panel, and coagulation profiles. Water-soluble contrast enema should be considered to confirm patency of the colon [4]. Determining the appropriate timing of surgery requires balancing the advantages of optimization from a respiratory, cardiac, and metabolic perspective with the risks of delayed repair, such as vomiting, aspiration, sepsis, and parenteral nutrition [15].

Instruments

In the operating room, basic laparoscopic instruments, a bowel stapler, suction, and a suction biopsy kit will be necessary.

Steps

1. Position the infant in supine position at the lower end of the operating table (or in transverse position). An orogastric tube should have already been placed preoperatively to decompress the stomach.
2. The surgeon stands at the patient's feet with the assistant to his left and scrub nurse to his right. Monitors are placed on either side at the head of the table.
3. Using an intra- or infraumbilical incision, access the peritoneal cavity via the open Hassan technique. Place a 11-mm trocar and establish a pneumoperitoneum of 8–10 mmHg.
4. The authors use the 10-mm Storz Hopkins telescope with in-built 5-mm working channel to explore the peritoneal cavity and confirm the diagnosis. This telescope combines a 0-degree fiberoptic camera with a single working channel which allows single site exploration.

Place the patient in Trendelenburg or reverse Trendelenburg position to facilitate intra-abdominal exposure.

5. Once the atresia is identified, it can be exteriorized through the umbilical incision to complete the procedure in a standard open fashion. Proximal and distal small bowel should be marked with two antimesenteric stay sutures to maintain orientation. Alternatively, exploratory laparoscopy can be omitted and the procedure can be performed by exteriorizing small bowel through a limited inferior periumbilical incision. Run the bowel to evaluate for distal patency and rule out additional segments of atresia. Injection of normal saline allows to assess for distal patency of the small intestine [4] (Fig. 26.4).
6. Depending on location and level of the atresia, the proximal segment can be significantly dilated. Assess caliber discrepancy and consider resection (in cases of high jejunal atresia) or tapering of the proximal obstructed segment.
7. Using a GIA bowel stapler, resect the atretic portion(s) of bowel. Tapering enteroplasty can be achieved by antimesenteric longitudinal bowel resection using a 5 mm GIA stapler.
8. Reanastomose the bowel ends in a single-layer hand-sewn technique to create an end-to-oblique anastomosis using 4–0 or 5–0 absorbable suture (polyglactin or polydioxanone) in an interrupted seromuscular fashion. Alternatively, a stapled side-to-side, functional end-to-end

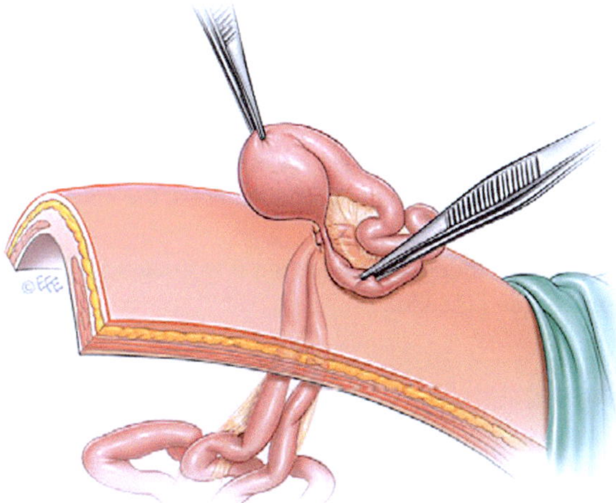

Fig. 26.4. Exteriorized loops of bowel. From Schier F, Turial S. Laparoscopy in children. 2nd ed. Heidelberg: Springer; 2013: 126–7. Reprinted with permission.

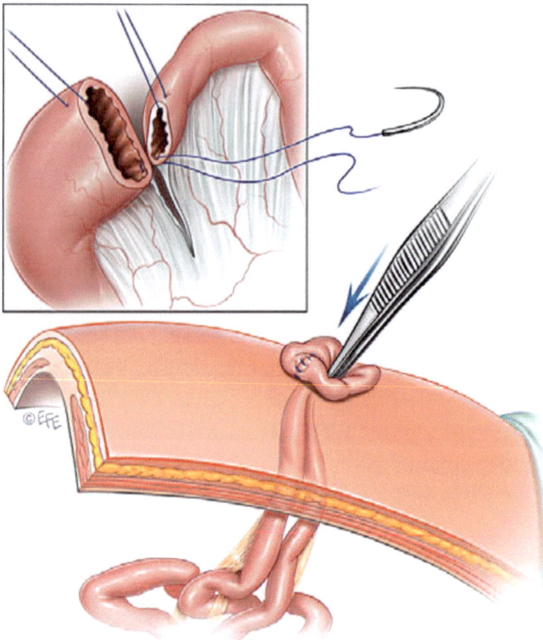

Fig. 26.5. Fashioning the anastomosis and return of the bowel to the abdominal cavity. From Schier F, Turial S. Laparoscopy in children. 2nd ed. Heidelberg: Springer; 2013: 126–7. Reprinted with permission.

anastomosis, using a 5 mm GIA stapler can be considered. Close the mesenteric defect with fast absorbable suture (Fig. 26.5).

9. Return the bowel to the abdominal cavity. Consider replacing the umbilical port and laparoscope for one final check.
10. Remove the trocar. Close the fascial defect at the umbilical port with absorbable suture.
11. Perform suction biopsy of the rectum if suspicion for Hirschsprung's disease is given [15, 16].

Pearls/Pitfalls

There are several principles to keep in mind when performing this procedure. When the bowel is exteriorized through the umbilical port, avoid exteriorizing more loops of bowel than are necessary. Bowel edema developing during the procedure can make reducing the bowel through the small umbilical incision difficult [17]. When the proximal segment of small bowel is severely dilated, resection or tapering of the dilated bowel may be necessary to reduce the risk of ineffective peristalsis. Resection is preferred to imbrication when tapering due to risk of recurrence and need for revision with plication. However, when multiple segments of atresia are present, care should be taken to preserve intestine length. Adequate bowel length is considered to be at least 30 cm of jejunum and ileum with an intact ileocecal sphincter, but ideally more than 75 cm [4].

Postoperative Care

Postoperative Management

Postoperative management is focused on nutritional support. Nasogastric decompression is continued until bowel function has returned. Once bowel function returns, oral feeding is begun. However, parenteral nutritional support is continued until goal calories are achieved with oral intake. Postoperative ileus can take as long as 9 days with most patients being discharged between postoperative days 9–16 [4, 15, 16].

Complications

Complications include anastomotic leak, adhesions, and small bowel obstruction in the first year of life, reoperation for bowel dilatation, prolonged parenteral nutrition, and malabsorptive syndromes, such as short bowel syndrome [13]. An anastomotic leak rate similar to that seen in laparotomy can be expected since the anastomosis is fashioned extracorporeally. Current studies suggest the rate of small bowel obstruction in the first year of life after laparotomy is about 12% [4]. This rate is expected to decrease in laparoscopic-assisted repair.

Outcomes

The procedure is well tolerated with laparoscopic repair averaging an operative time of 48 min and with incisions measuring approximately 1–2.5 cm. Patients are at no increased risk of bleeding and typically do not require transfusion of blood products. Compared to the conventional open approach the decreased size of the incision offers a marked cosmetic benefit while the extracorporeal portion of the procedure allows open anastomosis without the morbidity of a traditional laparotomy incision [15]. Laparoscopic-assisted repair may also have increased benefits by reducing the risk of small bowel obstructions in the first year of life due to decreased formation of adhesions [18].

Summary

- Intestinal atresia is one of the most common causes of intestinal obstruction in neonates.
- The ability to exteriorize the small bowel in infants makes laparoscopic-assisted repair a safe and feasible technique for surgeons trained in laparoscopy.
- Laparoscopic-assisted technique offers safe repair of intestinal atresia and appears to reduce discomfort, improve cosmesis, and reduce the risk of adhesive postoperative small bowel obstruction.

References

1. Kumaran N, Shankar KR, Lloyd DA, Losty PD. Trends in the management and outcome of jejuno-ileal atresia. Eur J Pediatr Surg. 2002;12:163.
2. Dalla Vecchia LK, Grosfeld JL, West KW, et al. Intestinal atresia and stenosis: a 25-year experience with 277 cases. Arch Surg. 1998;133:490–6.
3. Iacobelli, BD, Zaccara A, SpiydakisI, et al.. Prenatal counseling of small bowel atresia: watch the fluid! Prenat Diagn. 2006;26:214
4. Burjonrappa S, Crete E, Bouchard S. Comparative outcomes in intestinal atresia: a clinical outcome and pathophysiology analysis. Pediatr Surg Int. 2011;27(4):437–42.
5. Louw JH. Resection and end-to-end anastomosis in the management of atresia and stenosis of the small bowel. Surgery. 1967;62:940.
6. Tibboel D, van der Kamp AW, Molenaar JC. The effect of experimentally induced intestinal perforation at an early developmental stage. J Pediatr Surg. 1981;16:1017.
7. Grosfeld JL, Ballantine TV, Shoemaker R. Operative management of intestinal atresia and stenosis based on pathologic findings. J Pediatr Surg. 1979;14:368.
8. Sweeney B, Surana R, Puri P. Jejunoileal atresia and associated malformations: correlation with timing of in-utero insult. J Pediatr Surg. 2001;36:774–6.
9. Komuro H, Amagai T, Hori T, et al. Placental vascular compromise in jejunoileal atresia. J Pediatr Surg. 2004;39:1701–5.

10. Basu R, Burge DM. The effect of antenatal diagnosis on the management of small bowel atresia. Pediatr Surg Int. 2004;20:177–9.
11. Phelps S, Fisher R, Partington A, Dykes E. Prenatal ultrasound diagnosis of gastrointestinal malformations. J Pediatr Surg. 1997;32:438.
12. Ghose I, Mason GC, Martinez D, et al. Hyperechogenic fetal bowel: a prospective analysis of sixty consecutive cases. BJOG. 2000;107:426.
13. Burjonrappa SC, Crete E, Bouchard S. Prognostic factors in jejuno-ileal atresia. Pediatr Surg Int. 2009;25(9):795–8.
14. Seo T, Ando H, Watanabe Y, et al. Colonic atresia and Hirschsprung's disease: importance of histologic examination of the distal bowel. J Pediatr Surg. 2002;37, E19.
15. Li B, Chen W, Wang S, Liu S, Li L. Laparoscopic-assisted surgery for neonatal intesintal atresia and stenosis: a report of 35 cases. Pediatr Surg Int. 2012;28:1225–8.
16. Abhyankar A, Mukhtar Z. Laparoscopy-assisted surgery for neonatal intestinal atresia: single-center experience. Asian J Endosc Surg. 2011;4(2):90–3.
17. Schier F, Turial S. Laparoscopy in children. 2nd ed. Heidelberg: Springer; 2013. p. 126–7.
18. Holcomb GW, Georgeson K, Rothenberg S. Atlas of pediatric laparoscopy and thoracoscopy. Philadelphia: Saunders/Elsevier; 2008. p. 9–13, 49.

27. Laparoscopic Resection of Abdominal Cysts and Duplications

Aaron P. Garrison and William Taylor Walsh

Introduction

Cystic duplications of the alimentary tract are rare and occur in roughly 1 in 4500 births [1–9]. There are two types of intestinal duplications, cystic and tubular. Cystic duplications account for 80 % [1–10]. The majority of these duplications present within the first 2 years after birth. Gastrointestinal duplications can occur anywhere from mouth to anus, but the most common locations and approximate distribution of intestinal duplications are (Fig. 27.1):

- Jejunum/ileum 50 %
- Esophagus 19 %
- Stomach 9 %
- Colonic 7 %,
- Rectum 5 %,
- Duodenal 4 %,
- Thoracoabdominal 4 %,
- Oral 1 % [1, 2]

The underlying pathophysiology is unknown, and theories as to the development of duplication cysts are varied. These include formation as a result of persistent embryonic diverticulum, a defect in recanalization, partial twinning, or secondary to a split notochord and fetal hypoxia [1, 2, 8]. Importantly, intestinal duplications share the muscular wall and blood supply with the adjacent intestine and, therefore, often reside within the leaves of mesentery [1]. The lining of the duplication is often the same as the adjacent native tissue, but it can also have ectopic mucosa. The most common ectopic tissue found is gastric tissue, but there have been documented cases of exocrine and endocrine pancreatic tissue.

D.S. Walsh et al. (eds.), *The SAGES Manual of Pediatric Minimally Invasive Surgery*, DOI 10.1007/978-3-319-43642-5_27

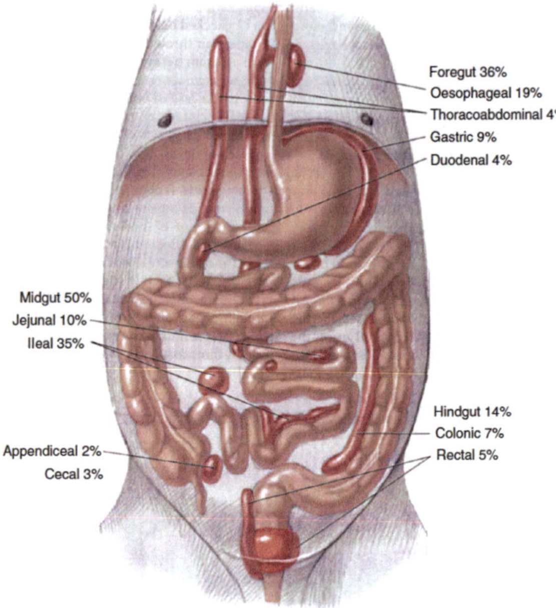

Fig. 27.1. Illustration with most common locations of alimentary duplications [2]. From Puri P, Mortell A. Duplications of the Alimentary Tract. In: Pediatric Surgery: Diagnosis and Management. Puri P, Hollwarth ME, eds. New York: Springer, 2009. 423–434. Reprinted with permission.

Ectopic tissue is more commonly found in cystic duplications than tubular duplications [1, 2, 8].

Ectopic gastric tissue can cause symptoms when the local anatomy is not able to handle the produced acid, which can result in bleeding or perforation. Infections of a duplication cyst can cause rapid enlargement, with complications including airway compromise or even meningitis in cases where there is a connection with the CNS.

Preoperative Evaluation

The history and clinical presentation is dependent upon the size, location, and tissue content of the duplication. Patients can present with obstructive symptoms, respiratory compromise, an asymptomatic but palpable mass, or with intussusception, bleeding, or perforation with peritonitis.

- Site specific findings include [1, 2]:
- Esophageal: can present with dysphagia or respiratory symptoms. Lesions are usually cystic and located in the posterior mediastinum.
- Gastric: can present with symptoms of peptic ulcer disease, if the cyst communicates with stomach.
- Duodenal: may present with jaundice, if obstructive.
- Intestinal: often present with symptoms of small bowel obstruction or intussusception.
- Colonic: can present with vague abdominal pain.
- Rectal: often present with a fistula or perineal mucosal swelling.
- Exam.
- Like clinical presentation, physical exam is dependent upon the location and clinical presentation of the duplication.
- Labs.
- Basic preoperative labs are recommended prior to surgery, including a complete blood count and a comprehensive metabolic panel.
- Imaging [1, 2, 8].
- Gold standard initial imaging for a cystic intestinal duplication is an abdominal ultrasound. Ultrasound will show an inner hyperechoic rim of mucosa–submucosa and an outer hypoechoic muscular layer.
- For suspected tubular duplications, a contrast enhanced CT scan is recommended to evaluate the extent of the duplication.
- A Technetium scan is recommended for tubular structures not amenable to resection for evaluation of ectopic gastric tissue.
- For thoracoabominal cases, a preoperative MRI is recommended to evaluate for vertebral abnormalities and to exclude a communication with spinal structures.

Technique

Patient Positioning

For esophageal duplications, it is recommended to place the patient in the lateral decubitus position with the affected side facing upward [10]. Often, cysts are more posterior than lateral, thus the patient is almost prone. For lesions in the right upper quadrant, it is recommend the patient lies in the supine position, at the end of the bed (frog-legged if patient is small, stirrups if they are larger) with the

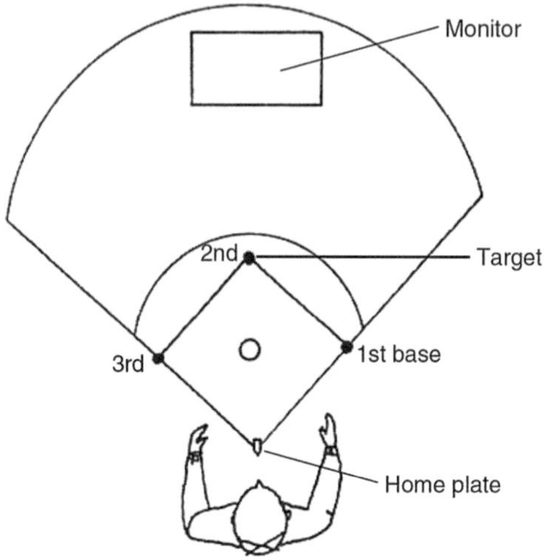

Fig. 27.2. Depiction of general laparoscopic technique, taken from SAGES manual [11]. From Meehan J. Pediatric Minimally Invasive Surgery: General Considerations. In: The SAGES Manual: Basic Laparoscopy and Endoscopy. 3rd edition. Soper N, Scott-Connor CEH, eds. New York: Springer, 2012. 443–447. Reprinted with permission.

surgeon positioned between the legs [3, 8]. For pelvic/rectal lesions, consideration should be given to positioning the patient at the end of the bed, with the surgeon standing above the patient's head (or to the patient's left side), so the target area is as shown in Fig. 27.2 [6]. The rectum may need to be irrigated with betadine if a combined transanal procedure is being considered.

Instruments

Rarely, the cyst can be enucleated and does not require a segmental resection. If no segmental resection is required, then all ports can be 3–5 mm. If segmental resection is required, then a 10 or 12 mm port may need to be used (typically as a camera port initially) to insert a stapler or exteriorize the bowel. Common instruments used include hook cautery, an energy device such as harmonic scalpel or Ligasure, blunt bowel graspers, and Maryland dissector. A newly developed 5 mm laparoscopic stapler may have some utility in these cases for smaller pediatric patients.

Port Positioning

The wide variety of location and presentation of alimentary tract duplications makes it difficult to standardize the operation. Preoperative planning, including relevant imaging, is key to successful laparoscopic excision of cysts. The patient should be placed in a position where the duplication can be triangulated.

The arrangement can be compared to the alignment of a baseball field as described in the SAGES manual [11].

1. The camera is placed at home plate.
   (a) umbilicus for abdominal cases
   (b) inferior tip of scapula [10] for thoracic cases
2. The target of interest is at second base.
3. The working ports are typically located at first and third bases.
4. Monitors should be placed in centerfield, directly behind the target at second base.
5. Accessory ports and assistants come in from the lateral fields, as necessary.
6. Liver retractor is commonly needed for stomach and distal esophageal cases.

Operative Details

Identify the cyst along the alimentary tract. Determine whether the cyst is tense. If the cyst appears under significant tension, or too large to exteriorize with a small incision, then the cyst may be drained using needle aspiration. The cyst should be dissected away from surrounding structures. Care should be taken when dissecting away from the shared muscular wall as this is the location of the shared blood supply.

Special Operative Considerations

Esophagus [7, 10, 11]

- In cervical duplications, care should be paid to the vagus and phrenic nerves and the thoracic duct.

- There are case reports of treating pediatric esophageal duplication cysts endoscopically by division of their common wall with a needle knife, allowing the duplication to drain internally [12].

Thoracoabdominal [1, 2]

- A combination of a thoracoscopic and laparoscopic approach should be considered.

Gastric [1–3, 5, 8]

- Laparoscopic segmental resection is recommended due to malignant potential.

Duodenal and pancreatic [1, 2]

- Consider fenestration of the cyst into duodenum
- Evaluate for drainage via ERCP/endoscopically.
- Roux-en-Y reconstruction might be necessary for proximal drainage.

Small bowel [1, 2, 6]

- Enucleation is usually difficult secondary to a shared blood supply.
- Simple resection and primary anastomosis is often the best surgical option.
- Resection is difficult in long tubular duplications due to bowel length that would be sacrificed. Management techniques include:
  - Wrenn method—Core out the mucosal line of long tubular duplications through multiple seromuscular incisions in the wall of the duplication.
  - Bowel lengthening—Separate the two sides (“leaves”) of blood vessels passing to each side of the small intestine. This excises the entire mucosa and almost the entire muscle wall. The remaining cuff should be over sewn.
  - A simple anastomosis between the distal end of the duplication and the normal bowel can allow for drainage.

Colonic [1, 2]

- Total colon duplications—Creation of an anastomosis between the two lumens can allow the two colons to drain through one anal orifice.
- If no colon reaches the perineum, a formal pull-through procedure is required.

Rectal

- Transanal or transcoccygeal (posterior sagittal) approaches are recommended, dependent upon location.

Postoperative Care

The postoperative course is dependent on the surgery performed. For esophageal duplications, the major concern is of iatrogenic injury to the native esophagus during dissection. A nasogastric tube is often left postoperatively. If a thoracic approach is used, then postoperative chest tube management should be considered. During the postoperative course, if there is suspicion of esophageal injury, then a contrast evaluation of the esophagus is recommended. For gastric, duodenal, small intestine, colonic, and rectal duplications, postoperative management mimics routine alimentary tract surgical management. The placement of nasogastric tube is necessary if there are signs of obstruction. Diet can be advanced as tolerated, depending on return of bowel function.

Summary

- The presentation, location, and treatment of cystic duplications of the alimentary tract is broad, thus the operative approach is individualized to the patient.
- Historically, the standard of care was open resection or enucleation, but with the use of minimally invasive techniques, sometimes a "hybrid" approach should be entertained.
- Minimally invasive approaches are most likely to be used for thoracic and cystic abdominal duplications.
- Given the variation in duplications, there is no single standard technique recommended for surgical resection.

References

1. Keckler SJ, Holcomb GW. Alimentary tract duplications. In: Holcomb GW, Murphy JP, editors. Ashcraft's pediatric surgery. 6th ed. Philadelphia: Sanders Elsevier; 2014. p. 539–53.
2. Puri P, Mortell A. Duplications of the alimentary tract. In: Puri P, Hollwarth ME, editors. Pediatric surgery: diagnosis and management. New York: Springer; 2009. p. 423–34.

3. Ford WD, Guelfan M, Lopez PJ, et al. Laparoscopic excision of a gastric duplication cyst detected on antenatal ultrasound. J Pediatr Surg. 2004;39(10):e8–10.
4. Hartin CW, Stanley TL, Escobar MA, et al. Laparoscopic excision of a newborn rectal duplication cyst. J Pediatr Surg. 2008;43(8):1572–4.
5. Pampal A, Yagmurlu A. Successful laparoscopic removal of mesenteric and omental cysts in toddlers: 3 cases with a literature review. J Pediatr Surg. 2012;47(8):E5–8.
6. Jancelewicz T, Simko J, Lee H. Obstructing ileal duplication cyst infected with Salmonella in a 2-year-old boy: a case report and review of the literature. J Pediatr Surg. 2007;42(5):E19–21.
7. Pujar VC, Kurbet S, Kaltari DK. Laparoscopic excision of intra-abdominal oesophageal duplication cyst in a child. J Min Access Surg. 2013;9(1):34–6.
8. Biebl M, Hechenleitner P, Renz O, et al. Laparoscopic resection of multiple gastric duplication cysts in an 8 year-old boy. J Pediatr Surg Case Rep. 2015;3(3):134–6.
9. Zahir I, Yusuf S, Zada F, et al. Duplication cysts in a new born. Int J Pathol. 2010;8:84–6.
10. Hirose S, Clifton MS, Bratton B, et al. Thoracoscopic resection of foregut duplication cysts. J Laparoendosc Adv Surg Tech A. 2006;16(5):526–9.
11. Meehan J. Pediatric minimally invasive surgery: general considerations. In: Soper N, Scott-Connor CEH, editors. The SAGES manual: basic laparoscopy and endoscopy. 3rd ed. New York: Springer; 2012. p. 443–7.
12. Walsh DS, Harris AS, Dokler ML, et al. Endolumenal management of tubular esophageal duplications. Society of American Gastrointestinal and Endoscopic Surgeons. 2012. Epublished at: http://thesagesmeeting.org/endolumenal-management-of-tubular-esophageal-duplications/.

28. Anomalies of Intestinal Rotation: Laparoscopic Ladd's Procedure

Eric J. Rellinger, Sarah T. Hua, and Gretchen Purcell Jackson

Introduction

Anomalies of intestinal rotation are congenital defects in the rotation and fixation of the midgut, which may remain asymptomatic throughout life, cause acute or chronic obstructive symptoms, or present with catastrophic midgut volvulus. Fetal intestinal elongation exceeds abdominal cavity growth at approximately 6 weeks of gestation, resulting in physiologic herniation of the intestine at the umbilical ring. At this point, the more proximal duodenojejunal limb is located cephalad to the superior mesenteric artery (SMA), while the more distal cecocolic limb lies caudal to this vascular pedicle (Fig. 28.1a). In normal development, both intestinal limbs will undergo a 270° counterclockwise rotation (as viewed by the observer; Fig. 28.1a–d) [1]. This process begins during the period of herniation and is completed as the intestines return to the abdominal cavity, beginning in week 10 of gestation. Specifically, the duodenojejunal limb rotates behind the SMA and fixates in the left upper quadrant at the ligament of Treitz, while the cecocolic limb rotates anterior to the SMA and ultimately becomes positioned in the right lower quadrant by 12 weeks of gestation (Fig. 28.1e). Wide fixation of the ligament of Treitz and cecum creates a broad mesenteric root that minimizes the risk of volvulus. Interruption of normal rotation at any point can give rise to anomalies of intestinal rotation, producing a heterogeneous spectrum of anatomic variations and clinical manifestations.

D.S. Walsh et al. (eds.), *The SAGES Manual of Pediatric Minimally Invasive Surgery*, DOI 10.1007/978-3-319-43642-5_28

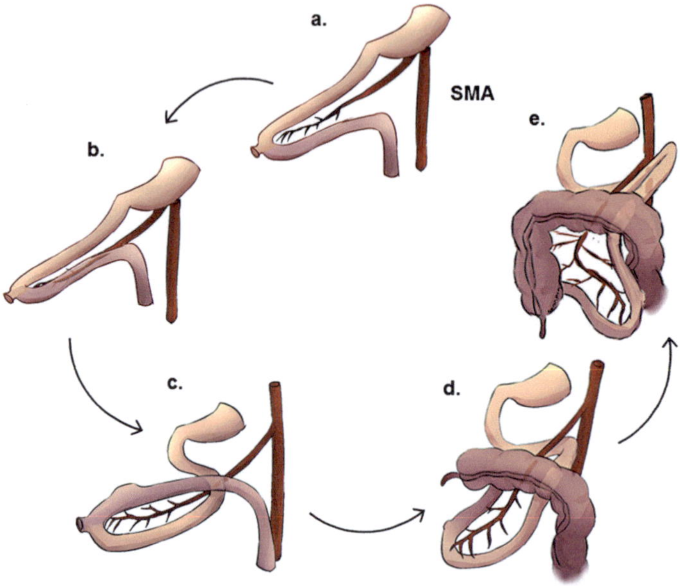

Fig. 28.1. Normal midgut herniation, rotation, and fixation occur from 6 to 12 weeks of gestation. (**a**) Physiologic herniation of the intestine occurs at 6 weeks with a cephalad duodenojejunal limb and a caudal cecocolic limb in relation to the superior mesenteric artery (SMA). (**b–e**) The midgut undergoes a 270° counterclockwise rotation (from the viewer's perspective) around the SMA, resulting in a left-sided ligament of Treitz and fixation of the cecum in the right lower quadrant.

Epidemiology

Malrotation occurs in approximately 1 out of every 500 births [2]. Symptomatic malrotation is estimated to be far less frequent, becoming clinically evident in only 1 out of every 6000 births [3]. The overarching concern with malrotation is the risk of midgut volvulus, wherein the narrow mesenteric pedicle becomes acutely torsed and may result in long-segment bowel ischemia from the jejunum to the distal transverse colon.

Pathophysiology

In classic malrotation, the duodenojejunal limb rotation arrests early and becomes positioned to the right of the midline. Partial rotation of the cecocolic limb displaces the cecum in the epigastrium in close approximation to the duodenojejunal junction, creating a narrow mesenteric pedicle that is susceptible to volvulus (Fig. 28.2a). This configuration also frequently results in congenital bands known as Ladd's bands, which extend from the cecum and terminal ileum over the surface of the second portion of the duodenum and can cause symptoms of duodenal obstruction by extrinsic compression. Atypical malrotation, also known as malrotation variant, duodenal malposition,

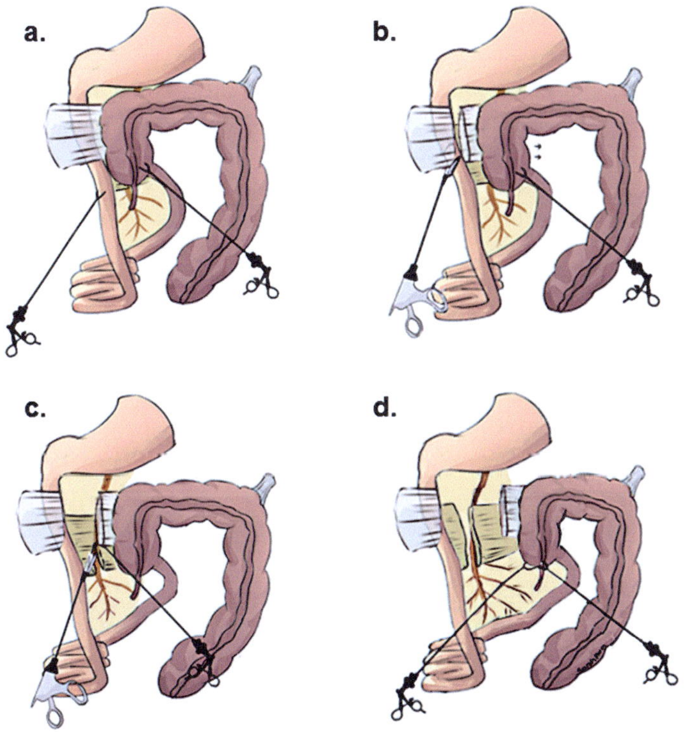

Fig. 28.2 Key components of the laparoscopic Ladd's procedure. (**a**) Upon entry into the abdominal cavity, the upper intestinal anatomy should be defined. Nonrotation featuring a right-sided ligament of Treitz is depicted in the illustration. (**b**) Paraduodenal Ladd's bands extending from the cecum are sharply divided. (**c**) The ileocecal mesentery is widened by incising the anterior mesenteric leaflet. (**d**) Intracorporeal or extracorporeal appendectomy may then be performed. The small intestine is positioned to the right of the abdomen and the colon positioned to the left

or low-lying ligament of Treitz, is a more recently recognized abnormality of intestinal rotation in which the ligament of Treitz lies to the left of the midline but remains suboptimally positioned. Patients with atypical malrotation have a lower risk of volvulus, and they are more likely to have persistent obstructive symptoms following operative intervention [4].

Preoperative Evaluation

History

Newborns and infants with malrotation most commonly present with new onset bilious emesis [2]. Somnolence, lethargy, hematemesis, melena, and hematochezia are symptoms that may portend underlying vascular compromise and should prompt rapid resuscitation and emergent open exploration without further radiographic evaluation. Volvulus is less common in older children, who have more variable symptoms with abdominal pain being the most common complaint [5]. Patients may also present with nonspecific findings including chronic abdominal pain, intermittent episodes of emesis, early satiety, weight loss, failure to thrive, malabsorption, and diarrhea [1].

Examination

Abdominal distension is the most common sign in neonates and infants with midgut volvulus, but a normal abdominal examination has been reported in up to 60 % of patients [6]. The onset of compromised intestinal blood flow may be heralded by the development of peritoneal signs.

Laboratory Findings

Laboratory values can be normal in asymptomatic malrotation and symptomatic disease with intermittent volvulus. Hypochloremia may be seen with severe dehydration. Leukocytosis or leukopenia and lactic acidosis suggest compromised intestinal blood flow.

Imaging

Only stable patients with concern for malrotation and no evidence of intestinal ischemia should undergo further radiographic evaluation. Abdominal radiographs may demonstrate proximal gastric or duodenal intestinal obstruction, but a nonspecific bowel gas pattern does not rule out rotational anomalies or volvulus. The upper gastrointestinal contrast study is the gold standard for diagnosis of malrotation. With malrotation, the key finding is an abnormal duodenojejunal junction, which is normally located to the left midline and at the level of the pylorus or gastric antrum. This may be demonstrated by a duodenum that does not cross the midline or a low-lying ligament of Treitz. The second and third portions of the duodenum may be positioned outside of their normal posterior and retroperitoneal locations, and with follow through, the small bowel can be noted to be predominately located to the right of the midline with the large bowel to the left. A corkscrew-shaped duodenum is a common sign of midgut volvulus, while a z-shaped configuration of the duodenum may be seen with obstructing Ladd's bands [7]. Ultrasonography, which can define the relationships of the SMA, superior mesenteric vein (SMV), and duodenum, has gained popularity in the evaluation of malrotation, but its role remains disputed. Left-sided or anterior SMV (in relation to the SMA) and absence of the duodenum behind the SMA are the predominant radiographic features of rotational anomalies. These findings are sometimes incidentally demonstrated on cross-sectional imaging, such as computed tomography [7].

Surgical Indications

Immediate operative exploration is the standard of care for the treatment of acute midgut volvulus [2]. Urgent or elective exploration is recommended for children with symptomatic obstructive symptoms and radiographic evidence of malrotation. Controversy exists regarding the optimal management of asymptomatic patients with radiographic evidence of rotational anomalies. Distended stomach and bowel may cause inferior displacement of the ligament of Treitz giving a false impression of atypical malrotation on the anteroposterior (AP) view. Repeat imaging may be warranted when the bowel is less dilated [8]. Exploration can be considered in asymptomatic patients who are younger in age, while observation may be appropriate in older children and adults with appropriate counseling and education concerning the potential risks and benefits [9].

Technique

The laparoscopic Ladd's procedure has a controversial, but increasingly recognized role in both the diagnosis and treatment of anomalies of intestinal rotation. Laparoscopic exploration permits direct visualization of the ligament of Treitz and cecum to verify or refute preoperative concern for malrotation and allows for correction of these defects without the need for formal laparotomy. Furthermore, internal hernias and congenital bands can be both identified and safely corrected by a laparoscopic approach. Laparoscopy is generally discouraged in the setting of midgut volvulus, as emergent abdominal decompression and intestinal detorsion are needed, and the risk of damage to edematous bowel likely outweighs the potential benefits of laparoscopy. As such, open Ladd's procedure is generally recommended in the setting of midgut volvulus.

Special Considerations

Young age and small size are relative contraindications for the laparoscopic Ladd's procedure. The reduced intra-abdominal domain and delicate tissues encountered in neonates should limit laparoscopic Ladd's procedures to experienced minimally invasive pediatric surgeons. Furthermore, laparoscopic exploration should be approached with caution in children with rotational anomalies associated with diaphragmatic hernia or abdominal wall defects as their postsurgical adhesions decrease the risk of volvulus and increase the risks of laparoscopic exploration.

Anatomy

Intestinal rotation may arrest at any stage of development, resulting in aberrant fixation of the ligament of Treitz and cecum. In normal intestinal development, the ligament of Treitz lies to the left of the midline, while the cecum ultimately fixates in the right lower quadrant. Early arrest of intestinal rotation after only 90° of rotation displaces the ligament of Treitz to the right of the midline and leaves the cecum in the epigastrium (Fig. 28.2a). This configuration, frequently referred to as nonrotation, features Ladd's bands that extend from the base of the cecum and terminal ileum to the right upper quadrant. The underlying duodenum may be extrinsically compressed by these bands resulting in symptoms of obstruction.

Positioning

After the induction of general anesthesia, the child is placed supine on the operating table with both arms tucked. Nasogastric and urinary decompression are recommended [10]. For smaller infants and neonates, the patient or bed may be rotated 90° to permit the surgeon to stand at the foot of the child. Lithotomy may be considered in older children. Once insufflation is achieved, the child is placed in reverse Trendelenburg. Visualization of the ligament of Treitz may be enhanced by tilting the patient left side up (~30°). Muscular relaxation optimizes intra-abdominal working space [11].

Instruments

Laparoscopic Ladd's procedure may be performed using a 5-, 10-, or 12-mm trocar for an umbilical or periumbilical camera port, depending upon the plan for intracorporeal or extracorporeal appendectomy. Two additional 5- or 3-mm ports are required for instrument access to triangulate the operative field, typically positioned in the right and left lower quadrants (Fig. 28.3). Atraumatic bowel graspers are used to orient the bowel and gain exposure, and scissors with monopolar energy, bipolar forceps, or an ultrasonic scalpel can be employed for division of paraduodenal Ladd's bands and widening of the mesentery. In small patients, monopolar energy sources should be used with caution in the division of paraduodenal bands given the increased risk of thermal spread. Additional laparoscopic instruments (e.g., endoscopic stapler) may be necessary if the surgeon elects to perform an intracorporeal appendectomy.

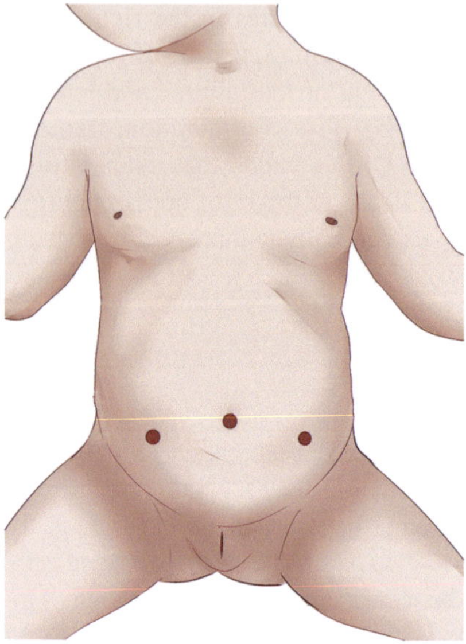

Fig. 28.3. Location of ports for a laparoscopic Ladd's procedure. A 5-, 10-, or 12-mm trocar is placed at the umbilicus or periumbilically, depending upon the plan for intracorporeal or extracorporeal appendectomy. Additional 5- or 3-mm trocars or stab incisions are then placed to permit appropriate triangulation, typically in the right lower and left lower quadrants.

Steps

Initially, a periumbilical incision is made for placement of a 5-, 10-, or 12-mm trocar for the camera, depending upon the plan for intracorporeal or extracorporeal appendectomy. Performing an extracorporeal appendectomy permits the use of a 5-mm infraumbilical trocar and is generally less expensive. Open (i.e., Hasson) or closed (Veress) techniques may be utilized to access the peritoneum. Pneumoperitoneum is achieved with 6–12 mmHg of carbon dioxide insufflation, depending upon the size of the patient. Additional 5- or 3-mm trocars or stab incisions are then employed in the right lower and left lower quadrants to permit appropriate triangulation.

The first step in the procedure is to verify whether or not the intestine is abnormally rotated. If the ligament of Treitz appears normally positioned to the left of the midline and the cecum is located in the right lower quadrant, the entire length of the bowel should be evaluated for another source of intra-abdominal pathology. In the presence of classic nonrotation featuring paraduodenal Ladd's bands, the adhesions should be grasped and sharply divided with scissors, bipolar forceps, or ultrasonic dissecting shears (Fig. 28.2b). Partial rotation anomalies may feature a tortuous duodenum that requires careful division of paraduodenal bands, which may be facilitated by placing leftward traction on the cecum. Formal kocherization of the duodenum is generally not recommended, but special care should be taken to ensure that all paraduodenal bands are divided. Attention may then be turned to widen the mesentery (Fig. 28.2c). Continued leftward traction on the cecum facilitates further division of the anterior peritoneal leaflet of the ileocecal mesentery. At this point, the cecum should be adequately mobile to reach the infraumbilical port site and perform an extracorporeal appendectomy. Alternatively, an intracorporeal appendectomy may be performed (Fig. 28.2d). At the completion of the appendectomy, the small bowel should be positioned to the right side of the abdomen and the colon positioned to the left. Hemostasis is confirmed, and the ports are removed under direct visualization. Absorbable sutures are used for closure of the infraumbilical fascial defect.

Pearls/Pitfalls

- Avoid direct handling of the intestine in small infants and neonates, as there is a greater risk of injury. Appropriate traction should be attainable by grasping congenital bands or the appendix.
- Paraduodenal bands should be divided sharply or using the ultrasonic scalpel or a bipolar vessel-sealing device to minimize risk of thermal injury. Ensuring complete division of paraduodenal bands is essential.
- Preoperative bowel preparation may be beneficial in the elective setting, as it minimizes the amount of colonic distension.

Postoperative Care

Evidence of volvulus, ischemia, and the need for bowel resection will prolong time to return of bowel function. Children with evidence of these findings are commonly managed with nasogastric decompression until evidence of return of bowel function. In the absence of significant obstruction or intestinal compromise, nasogastric decompression may be foregone.

Outcomes

The laparoscopic approach to Ladd's procedure, especially in infants, is relatively new procedure, and thus, the available literature is limited, especially with regard to long-term follow-up. Several retrospective case series suggest that the primary benefits of the laparoscopic Ladd's procedure are shorter time to full feeds (2 days vs. 6 days) and shorter hospital stay (3 days vs. 7 days) [12–14]. However, proponents of the open approach raise concern that the laparoscopic Ladd's procedure may have a heightened risk of recurrent volvulus, as compared to the standard open approach [1].

Summary

- Anomalies of intestinal rotation can have a myriad of clinical presentations, ranging from incidental imaging findings to acute volvulus requiring emergent surgical exploration and detorsion.
- Open exploration with Ladd's procedure is the recommended approach for the treatment of acute midgut volvulus.
- Laparoscopic Ladd's procedure is being increasingly used in the urgent and elective settings to diagnose and treat malrotation in older infants and children.
- Key components of the open Ladd's procedure must be preserved with the laparoscopic approach, including division of Ladd's bands, widening of the mesentery, appendectomy, and appropriate reorientation of the intestine.

References

1. Dassinger MS, Smith SD. Disorders of intestinal rotation and fixation. In: Coran AC, editor. Pediatric surgery. 7th ed. Philadelphia: Saunders; 2012. p. 1111–25.
2. Torres AM, Ziegler MM. Malrotation of the intestine. World J Surg. 1993;17(3):326–31.
3. Song C, Upperman JS, Niklas V. Structural anomalies of the gastrointestinal tract. In: Gleason C, editor. Avery's disease of the newborn. 9th ed. Philadelphia: Saunders; 2012. p. 979–93.

4. Mehall JR, Chandler JC, Mehall RL, Jackson RJ, Wagner CW, Smith SD. Management of typical and atypical intestinal malrotation. J Pediatr Surg. 2002;37(8):1169–72.
5. Nehra D, Goldstein AM. Intestinal malrotation: varied clinical presentation from infancy through adulthood. Surgery. 2011;149(3):386–93.
6. Bonadio WA, Clarkson T, Naus J. The clinical features of children with malrotation of the intestine. Pediatr Emerg Care. 1991;7(6):348–9.
7. Marine MB, Karmazyn B. Imaging of malrotation in the neonate. Semin Ultrasound CT MR. 2014;35(6):555–70.
8. Applegate KE, Anderson JM, Klatte EC. Intestinal malrotation in children: a problem-solving approach to the upper gastrointestinal series. RadioGraphics. 2006;26(5):1485–500.
9. Graziano K, Islam S, Dasgupta R, Lopez ME, Austin M, Chen LE, et al. Asymptomatic malrotation: Diagnosis and surgical management: An American Pediatric Surgical Association outcomes and evidence based practice committee systematic review. J Pediatr Surg. 2015. Epub 2015/07/25.
10. Bax NM, van der Zee DC. Laparoscopic treatment of intestinal malrotation in children. Surg Endosc. 1998;12(11):1314–6.
11. Little DC, Smith SD. Malrotation. In: Holcomb III GW, Murphy JP, editors. Ashcraft's pediatric surgery. 5th ed. Philadelphia: Elsevier; 2010. p. 424–32.
12. Fraser JD, Aguayo P, Sharp SW, Ostlie DJ, St Peter SD. The role of laparoscopy in the management of malrotation. J Surg Res. 2009;156(1):80–2.
13. Stanfill AB, Pearl RH, Kalvakuri K, Wallace LJ, Vegunta RK. Laparoscopic Ladd's procedure: treatment of choice for midgut malrotation in infants and children. J Laparoendosc Adv Surg Tech A. 2010;20(4):369–72.
14. Bass KD, Rothenberg SS, Chang JH. Laparoscopic Ladd's procedure in infants with malrotation. J Pediatr Surg. 1998;33(2):279–81.

29. Laparoscopic Exploration for Pediatric Chronic Abdominal Pain

Ian C. Glenn and Aaron P. Garrison

Introduction

Chronic abdominal pain (CAP) is known by many terms which are frequently used interchangeably, including "recurrent abdominal pain," "functional abdominal pain," "nonorganic abdominal pain," and "psychogenic abdominal pain." It should be made clear that these are not necessarily equivalent entities. A commonly accepted definition for chronic abdominal pain is abdominal pain which occurs at least weekly over a period of at least 2–3 months.

"Functional gastrointestinal disorder" (FGID) is an umbrella term encompassing the clinical symptoms of the GI tract which cannot be explained by an organic cause. The Rome criteria were first created in 1989 in an attempt to standardize diagnosis of FGID. The fourth iteration of these criteria are due to be released in 2016.

Irritable bowel syndrome (IBS) is often mentioned in conjunction with chronic abdominal pain and related diagnoses. IBS is characterized by abdominal pain and irregularity of bowel movements, alternating between constipation and diarrhea.

Epidemiology

The incidence of CAP has been reported as 10–25 % in school-aged children. There is a correlation between age and incidence among females, but an inverse correlation was noted in males. There is a slight female predominance overall for pediatric CAP. Presentation with CAP prior to age five is uncommon, and organic causes should be thoroughly ruled out prior to making a diagnosis of functional disease in this age group.

D.S. Walsh et al. (eds.), *The SAGES Manual of Pediatric Minimally Invasive Surgery*, DOI 10.1007/978-3-319-43642-5_29

Early studies investigating pediatric CAP found an organic etiology in approximately 5 % of cases. However, more recent studies, likely benefitting from advances in technology and better understanding of gastrointestinal pathophysiology, have found organic causes in up to 30 % of cases of CAP.

Pathophysiology

Causes of chronic abdominal pain are manifold, but etiologies which are often difficult to diagnose, yet must be excluded, include inflammatory bowel disease, celiac disease, carbohydrate malabsorption, peptic ulcer disease, gastroesophageal reflux disease (GERD), infection, gynecologic disorders, and pancreaticobiliary disease.

True chronic abdominal pain without another "organic" cause is incompletely understood and likely multifactorial in nature. However, research suggests that dysregulation within the enteric nervous system, particularly as relates to pain pathways, as well as abnormal signal transduction between the central and enteric nervous systems play strong contributory roles. The end result is visceral hypersensitivity and the interpretation of non-nociceptive stimuli as painful and/or an exaggerated pain response to noxious stimuli.

Differential Diagnoses for Organic Causes of Chronic Abdominal Pain

Inflammatory bowel disease
Celiac disease
Carbohydrate malabsorption
Peptic ulcer disease
Gastroesophageal reflux disease (GERD)
Infection
Gynecologic disorders
Urologic disorders
Pancreaticobiliary disease
Drug effect
Lead toxicity

Preoperative Evaluation

The most important consideration in evaluating chronic abdominal pain is to rule out organic disease, particularly those that may be life threatening. Concerning features include constitutional symptoms, recurrent vomiting, hematemesis, hematochezia or melena, failure to thrive, jaundice, and persistent leukocytosis.

History

A thorough history is the foundation of good medical practice. It is important for the patient to provide as much information in his/her own words as possible. Particular attention should be paid to the quality, location, duration, associated symptoms, and palliating or precipitating factors of the pain. Details regarding the patient's bowel habits should also be clarified. A dietary history, including weight changes and any food allergies or intolerances is especially important. A past medical history of psychiatric disorder also appears to be associated with CAP. Prior surgeries or procedures, as well as their indications, should be taken into consideration. Any medications or supplements, prescription or over-the-counter, taken by the patient should be clarified. The relationship between any medications and symptoms should be ascertained.

Perinatal difficulties, including pregnancy marked by excessive nausea, vomiting, pain, or fatigue; breech presentation or requirement for cesarean section; low birth weight; and neonatal disorders such as respiratory distress or colic, are all associated with CAP.

Given the association between psychosocial factors and CAP, a thorough social history should be obtained from the patient and any family members present. Family history of CAP, functional abdominal pain, or FGID, as well as migraine, psychiatric, and substance abuse disorders have shown to be associated with CAP. All of this strongly suggests that psychosocial factors play a strong role in pediatric chronic abdominal pain. As a surgeon, establishing trust and appropriate expectations is crucial.

Exam

A detailed physical examination is the pillar of sound medicine. The general appearance of the patient should be noted for gross signs of malnutrition, dysmorphia, lanugo, or abnormal development. A complete physical exam should be conducted with special attention given to the abdominal exam. Inspection, auscultation, percussion, and palpation should be performed, in that order. A thorough hernia exam should be conducted.

Interaction between the child and caregiver may give insight into any psychosocial contributors to the patient's symptoms. Growth charts and patterns should be documented and reviewed, as CAP of the functional variety is typically associated with normal growth.

Laboratory Studies

There is no set of blood tests which must be checked on every patient with abdominal pain. However, if recent studies are not available, it is reasonable to check a complete blood count with differential, liver function tests, and urinalysis. If there is concern for metabolic derangement, a basic metabolic panel may be drawn. Erythrocyte sedimentation rate and fecal studies for ova and parasites are at the discretion of the clinician. Amylase and lipase should be ordered if there is concern for pancreatitis. In order to evaluate for celiac disease, a serum test for anti-tissue transglutaminase immunoglobulin A may be ordered. Less commonly, testing for serum anti-endomysial immunoglobulin A may be sent. While screening for anti-gliadin antibodies was previously popular, it is no longer recommended.

Imaging

Historically, many practitioners consider plain film radiography, computed tomography (CT), and/or ultrasound as routine studies in evaluation of abdominal pain. There is no evidence to suggest that these imaging studies have any value unless they are indicated by history, physical exam, or laboratory findings.

Other Tests

There is no indication for routine endoscopy, pH probe study, *H. pylori* testing, or hydrogen breath testing. These should only be ordered as clinically indicated. However, if there is a suspicion of celiac disease, such as in patients who have positive antibodies to tissue transglutaminase or endomysium, upper endoscopy is warranted. It is important that the patient has been eating a gluten-containing diet at the time of biopsy. Multiple endoscopic biopsies should be obtained from multiple portions of the duodenum, including the bulb. Full-thickness biopsies are typically not required.

Surgical Indications

Diagnostic laparoscopy in the pediatric patient with chronic abdominal pain should be employed for diseases which are unable, or unlikely, to be diagnosed with less invasive means and for which treatment exists.

Pragmatically, the clinical situation is rarely this straightforward, and often a thorough laboratory and radiographic workup is negative. A reasonable guideline is to perform diagnostic laparoscopy in patients who have had symptoms for 3–6 months without relief from medical management and with no identifiable organic cause for their pain. We would recommend a few office visits to establish a relationship with the family and ensure appropriate expectations.

Technique

Special Considerations

Port placement, which is discussed below, should be amenable to examining all four quadrants of the abdomen as well as the pelvis and running the small bowel. Initial port placement should be compatible with performing appendectomy or cholecystectomy, as indicated.

Anatomy

When performing diagnostic laparoscopy, attention should be paid to anatomic features which may be contributing to symptoms of chronic abdominal pain. This includes malrotation, adhesive disease (which can be secondary to prior trauma or surgery), and Meckel's diverticulum.

Positioning

The patient is positioned on the operating table in the supine position. Following induction of anesthesia and intubation, larger patients should have arms tucked at their sides. When able, patients should be secured to the table such that the table position may be changed (e.g., head-up or head-down positions). Blankets and/or warmers should be employed to ensure normal body temperature, especially for smaller patients. More details on patient position during diagnostic laparoscopy are found in other sections of this book.

Instruments

A typical laparoscopic instrument tray is ideal. Atraumatic bowel graspers to run the bowel and hook cautery, or other energy device, for any adhesions encountered are frequently utilized.

Steps

Port position depends on clinical background and pre-op suspicion as to the etiology of the abdominal pain (Fig. 29.1). Pain located in the right lower quadrant is best evaluated with a setup similar to laparoscopic appendectomy. Most commonly this involves three 5-mm ports, at the

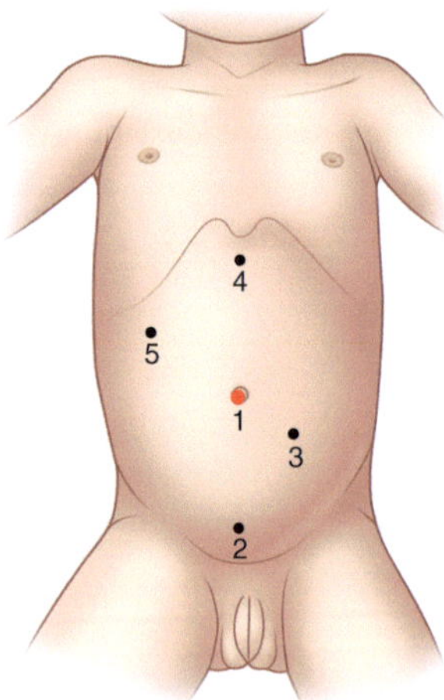

Fig. 29.1. Recommended port placement for laparoscopic surgery. A port is first placed at position 1 to accommodate the laparoscope. A 5-mm port is initially used. A 12-mm port may be utilized to accommodate the 10-mm laparoscope and, if needed, laparoscopic specimen pouch. All other ports should be 3–5 mm. Ports 1, 2, and 3 may be used to evaluate the length of the small bowel and to perform an appendectomy. Port 4 may be added to perform cholecystectomy, with the option of adding port number 5 to assist in surgery.

umbilicus, the left lower quadrant, and the suprapubic region. When the camera is placed in the left lower quadrant port, the surgeon is also set up to run the bowel. It is common to start at the ileocecal valve and work back proximally to the ligament of Treitz. An additional port or stab incision may be needed in the right upper quadrant if a cholecystectomy is planned or if additional retraction is needed to expose the ligament of Treitz.

Pearls/Pitfalls

It is the policy of some surgeons to always perform an appendectomy during diagnostic laparoscopy, even if the structure appears grossly normal. The clinical significance of a pathologic diagnosis of chronic appendicitis or a fibrotic appendix remains controversial. However, the gold standard for the procedure should be relief of symptoms, regardless of the ultimate diagnosis.

Postoperative Care

Outcomes

The incidence of identifying pathology via diagnostic laparoscopy ranges from 20 to 100 %, depending on the study. An interesting, yet controversial, entity is appendiceal colic. There is debate over whether this chronic right lower quadrant pain is a true disease process. These patients tend to be predominantly female and present with pain at McBurney's point, and many have associated nausea, vomiting, and postprandial worsening of pain. Laboratory examination is invariably normal, and imaging findings are not consistent with acute appendicitis. Historically, contrast studies may demonstrate irregular filling and/or emptying of the appendix. Some studies show success rates (resolution of symptoms) in up to 89–98 % of cases. Proper patient selection is the key.

Up to 50 % of all patients with chronic abdominal pain will ultimately have complete resolution of their symptoms. One-quarter of all children with CAP will continue to have some element of abdominal pain into adulthood. These patients do not typically benefit from additional surgery and should be referred to gastroenterology or pain management for long-term management of symptoms. Characteristics associated with positive long-term outcomes include female sex, later age of onset, good psychosocial support system and environment, and fewer operations.

Complications

Diagnostic laparoscopy is an overall safe and well-tolerated procedure in the pediatric population. The serious complication rate, which includes vascular, visceral, and bladder injuries, is 1 % or less and typically associated with port placement.

Summary

- Chronic abdominal pain is an incompletely understood entity which is roughly defined as abdominal pain which occurs at least weekly and persists for 2–3 months.
- Initial evaluation should be conducted by the patient's primary pediatrician with the possible involvement of a gastroenterologist.
- Pain without an identifiable cause which persists for 3–6 months should be investigated with diagnostic laparoscopy.
- Port position should be optimized to facilitate evaluation and removal of the appendix and gallbladder, and run the entire length of the small bowel.

Suggested Reading

Bax KNMA, Georgeson KE, Rothenberg SS, et al. Endoscopic surgery in infants and children. New York: Springer; 2008.

Liacouras C, Piccoli D. Pediatric gastroenterology. 1st ed. Philadelphia: Mosby; 2007.

Subcommittee on Chronic Abdominal Pain. Chronic abdominal pain in children, Pediatrics. Mar 2005; 115(3)812–815.

Wylie R, Hyams JS, Kay M. Pediatric gastrointestinal and liver disease. 5th ed. Toronto: Elsevier; 2015.

30. Laparoscopic Lysis of Adhesions for Pediatric Bowel Obstruction

Melody R. Saeman and Diana L. Diesen

Introduction

Epidemiology

Abdominal adhesions are associated with chronic pain, infertility, and bowel obstruction. Postoperative adhesions are estimated to form in 93 % of adults, but only a fraction become symptomatic [1]. The reported incidence of symptomatic adhesive small bowel obstruction (ASBO) in children after various abdominal operations ranges from 1 to 37 %. A 4-year Scottish population analysis of 1581 postsurgical children reported 8.3 % of readmissions possibly related and 1.1 % directly related to adhesions (5.3 %, excluding appendectomy) [2]. Meta-analysis had an overall ASBO incidence of 4.2 % [3], with procedure-specific reports vary from 0.7 % after appendectomy [4] to 37 % in neonates with gastroschisis at a 10-year median follow-up [5]. Higher rates of surgical adhesions have been observed in neonates although increased appendectomies in older children possibly skew the data [2]. A review found the ASBO aggregate incidence was 6.2 % in neonates and 4.7 % in infants and older children [6]. ASBO mean incidences by specific neonatal and pediatric procedures are reported in Tables 30.1 and 30.2. The majority of ASBOs reportedly occur in the first year, but the length of follow-up is limited. In a 30-year study period, van Eijck et al. reported a presentation range of ASBO from 8 days to 13 years after laparotomy for gastroschisis or omphalocele, with 85 % in the first year [5]. The majority of ASBO case series have a follow-up less than 5 years and report a 58–100 % presentation in the first year [6]. Festen found the majority (87 %) of ASBO after various abdominal surgeries occurred within 3 months [7].

D.S. Walsh et al. (eds.), *The SAGES Manual of Pediatric Minimally Invasive Surgery*, DOI 10.1007/978-3-319-43642-5_30

Table 30.1. Aggregate (mean) incidence of ASBO in specific neonatal laparotomy.

Condition	Total cases	Cases with adhesions (%)
Malrotation	196	28 (14.2)
Gastroschisis	252	32 (12.6)
Necrotizing enterocolitis	125	13 (10.4)
Exomphalos	185	16 (8.6)
Hirschsprung's disease	122	10 (8.1)
Congenital diaphragmatic hernia	394	25 (6.3)
Intestinal atresia	363	21 (5.7)

From Lakshminarayanan B, Hughes-Thomas AO, Grant HW. Epidemiology of adhesions in infants and children following open surgery. Seminars in pediatric surgery. 2014;23(6):344–8. Reprinted with permission from Elsevier.

Table 30.2. Aggregate (mean) incidence of ASBO in general surgery of childhood.

Condition	Total cases	Case with adhesions (%)
Colorectal surgery	248	35 (14)
Tumor surgery	2043	113 (5.5)
Fundoplication	473	39 (8.2)
Small bowel surgery	123	7 (5.7)
Choledochal cyst	63	2 (3.1)
Appendicectomy	477	7 (1.4)
Pyloromyotomy	901	1 (0.1)

From Lakshminarayanan B, Hughes-Thomas AO, Grant HW. Epidemiology of adhesions in infants and children following open surgery. Seminars in pediatric surgery. 2014;23(6):344–8. Reprinted with permission from Elsevier.

Pathophysiology

Intra-abdominal adhesions are the result of traumatic or congenital scar formation between two normally unattached peritoneal surfaces [8]. Operative techniques resulting in tissue trauma, intra-abdominal infections, inflammation, hemoperitoneum, foreign bodies, and exposure to radiation are risk factors for adhesion formation [9, 10].

Deposits of a fibrin matrix gel form between two injured surfaces. Insufficient fibrinolysis in the postoperative state inhibits reabsorption of these deposits. Adhesions form when the extracellular collagenous matrix of the fibrin bands is infiltrated with fibroblasts, smooth muscle cells, neovascularization, and occasionally nerve endings [9]. The presence of peritonitis or active inflammation at the initial operation has a higher rate of dense adhesions [6, 7, 11].

Preoperative Evaluation

Best practice guidelines for the diagnosis and clinical management of ASBO have only been published for the adult population [12]. However, the initial management in children is similar to adults [13]. Diagnosis of ASBO in children requires a thorough history and physical exam.

History

Crampy abdominal pain, nausea, vomiting, bloating, and obstipation are the most frequent symptoms of ASBO. The time course of symptoms and the quality of emesis should be clarified. It is important to have a clear understanding of prior operations, operative approach (i.e., open versus laparoscopic), and underlying pathology. History of constant abdominal pain and lethargy is concerning.

Exam

Abdominal distention and high-pitched or absent bowel sounds can be encountered; however, these signs may not be present with a higher level of obstruction or at an early presentation. It is important to examine healed surgical incisions and bilateral groins for hernias. Altered mental status, abdominal tenderness, distention, peritonitis, tachycardia, and fever are potential signs of bowel ischemia. Patients should be evaluated for signs of hypovolemia including poor capillary filling, mottling, cool skin with reduced turgor, dry mucus membranes, and sunken anterior fontanelle (infants). It is important to be aware that lethargy can prevent a reliable abdominal exam, especially in small children and infants [13].

Labs

Laboratory evaluation should include white blood cell count (WBC count), electrolytes, and BUN/creatinine. Elevation of WBC is a concerning for ischemia but may also be seen in dehydration.

Imaging

Upright and supine plain abdominal films are standard to detect the presence of air fluid levels, distended loops of small bowel, and paucity of gas in the colon [12]. The risks compared to benefits of CT scan utilization in the diagnosis of ASBO in children are not well understood [13]. A small retrospective review by Wang et al. of 47 surgically proven ASBO cases reported a 91.5 % sensitivity with 78 % correct identification of location and 68 % identification of cause of ASBO using multidetector CT scan in children [14]. It is important to note that CT utility is decreased in infants and small children with less fat and can be difficult to interpret. CT scan in obstructed adults has a 95 % sensitivity and specificity in high-grade obstructions with transition point localization and identification of ischemia [15]. While not recommended as routine in adults, CT can predict failure of nonoperative management by identifying free intraperitoneal fluid, paucity of gas in the colon, mesenteric edema, lack of the "small bowel feces sign," and evidence of devascularized bowel [12]. Children are more susceptible to the long-term consequences of radiation, and CT scan should only be judiciously used in obstructed children with a concern for a concurrent intra-abdominal abscess or diagnostic uncertainty [13].

Surgical Indications

Absolute indications for emergent surgery include patients in extremis, signs of bowel ischemia, peritonitis, or perforation [13]. Initial management of children with ASBO without indications for immediate surgical exploration is debated [16, 17]. It is established that adults with partial ASBO can safely undergo nonoperative management [12], but no trials exist to direct conservative management in children. Management of pediatric ASBO has traditionally been more aggressive. Review of the Kids' Inpatient Database (KID) data from 2003 to 2006 reported 85.5 % operative rate in children ages 2–20 admitted with ASBO [18].

Conservative management consists of nasogastric decompression, parenteral fluids, correction of electrolytes, and serial abdominal exams. Surgery is indicated if the patient's exam worsens; the patient develops signs of ischemia/perforation, or if the patient does not improve with medical management. A systematic review of conservative management in children with ASBO reported a range of success from 0 to 75 % [19]. Study variations, patient age, severity of presentation, and clinical resources (two studies reported limited capacity for parenteral fluids) likely account for the range. Conservative management in children less than 1 year of age has been noted to have a higher failure rate [20, 21]. Over half of studies report a success rate of conservative management in more than 50 % of patients. Patients successfully managed conservatively had a shorter hospitalization and time to feeding [19]. This review suggests that conservative management of ASBO can be effective in children.

Review of the KID data found a 1.67 odds ratio of small bowel resection with operative intervention delayed until hospital day 3–14, and no difference in small bowel resection between operating on day 1 versus day 2. It is recommended that stable patients without concerning signs of perforation, strangulation, or peritonitis can be safely managed conservatively for 48 h in children over 2 years and 24–48 h in children less than 2 years of age [18]. It is crucial that these patients are closely observed for signs of deterioration in either their physiology or abdominal exam and receive prompt operative management at recognition of these changes. If patients do not improve over the observation period, it is recommended that they also receive operative intervention [18].

An increasing body of literature supports the use of Gastrografin in adults with ASBO as an adjunct to conservative therapy. Visualization of contrast in the cecum 4–24 h after administration has a 96 % sensitivity and 98 % specificity for nonoperative resolution in adults [22]. It is currently controversial if Gastrografin is simply a diagnostic aid or is therapeutic in partial ASBO. It is possible that the high osmolarity shifts fluid into the obstructed bowel creating a pressure gradient to relieve the obstruction [23]. Two small observational pediatric studies reported 85 % and 75 % of children with ASBO successfully resolved nonoperatively with Gastrografin after failing 48 h of conservative therapy [24, 25]. While the evidence for the use of Gastrografin in pediatric ASBO is limited, it appears to be safe and should be further investigated.

Technique

Special Considerations

Bastug first reported laparoscopic adhesiolysis for ASBO in 1991 [26]. Decades later, evidence for laparoscopy in ASBO is limited in adults [27] and sparse in children with only observational studies [28–32]. Analysis of KID data found an increase in the rate of laparoscopic lysis of adhesions (LOA) for ASBO from 7.2 to 17.2 % between 1997 and 2009 [30]. This same analysis found a lower complication rate, shorter length of stay, lower total hospital cost, and lower puncture/laceration incidence with a conversion rate less than 2 % [30]. This suggests the laparoscopic approach is safe although current publications do not identify patient characteristics for successful laparoscopic use [28–32]. The incidence of postoperative adhesions is decreased with a laparoscopic technique in any surgery, further supporting this method [33]. Pooled analysis of laparoscopic adhesiolysis for adult ASBO found decreased mortality, morbidity, pneumonia, wound infections, and length of stay. While laparoscopic operative time was longer, there was no difference in the rates of bowel injury or reoperation [34].

The only absolute contraindications to laparoscopic adhesiolysis are patient intolerance of pneumoperitoneum or inability to safely place ports due to distention. Relative contraindications may include history of multiple procedures, peritonitis, free air, or stranulaged/gangrenous bowel though these case may be started laparoscopically and converted if needed. All other patients with surgical indications treated by an experienced laparoscopic surgeon may have an initial laparoscopic attempt after adequate resuscitation.

Anatomy

Single-band adhesions are present in 70 % of children with ASBO and have higher laparoscopic success rates [7]. Although, single bands are difficult to predict as the severity of adhesions is not correlated with the scale of the initial operation. Patients with a history of multiple procedures tend to have more adhesions, which should be taken into consideration before attempting a laparoscopic approach. Bowel distention over 4 cm and distal obstructions are associated with converstion to laparotomy.

Positioning

The patient is positioned supine with placement of a nasogastric tube and a urinary catheter. Decompression with nasogastric aspiration for several hours prior to the procedure can alleviate bowel distention in some cases and improve visualization. The ability to tilt the patient intra-operatively in various directions is important to allow visualization of certain areas of the abdomen depending on the location of the adhesions. For example, the use of reverse Trendelenburg in a patient with a prior upper abdominal surgery facilitates exposure to the upper abdomen.

Instruments/Port Placement

The prior scar should be avoided during trocar placement. The umbilicus is the preferred location for initial trocar placement using the open (Hasson) technique. However, an alternative location should be used if the scar is over the umbilicus. Palmer or Veress needle insufflation should be avoided in patients with significant distention. The initial port size should be selected appropriately based on patient and camera size. 3 mm and 5 mm cannulas are sufficient for the remaining two to three port sites. An angled telescope can be helpful for maximal visualization. Standard laparoscopy instruments, including scissors for sharp excision of bands as well as atraumatic graspers such as Babcock-type and DeBakey-type forceps, should be available.

Steps

When using the open technique, an umbilical incision is often the first choice. This can be an infraumbilical, transumbilical, or supraumbilical incision. The incision is carried down to the fascia, which is then incised under direct visualization. A trocar is positioned into the peritoneal cavity, and the abdomen is insufflated while monitoring initial pressures. Alternatively, if the umbilicus has previously been used to gain access to the abdomen, one may access the abdomen in alternate locations. For example, one may attempt supraumbilical access if the patient had previously had an infraumbilical incision. One can also use an open technique to gain access in the left upper quadrant as this area tends to have less adhesions in the case of a prior midline incision. A cut-down technique can be used to carefully dissect through the layers of the abdominal wall using a muscle-sparing technique. Once identified, the peritoneum is lifted off the intra-abdominal structures and sharply incised. A port is then placed and the abdomen inspected. Two to three additional 3-mm or 5-mm ports can be placed under direct visualization in appropriate working relation to triangulate the location of adhesions. Alternatively, triangulating ports to access the right lower quadrant allows exposure to run the bowel.

If visualization is inadequate for safe placement of the initial trocar or remaining trocars, blunt dissection can be performed with a finger through the initial port site or using the tip of the trocar with camera visualization. This maneuver can clear adhesions and allow visualization for safe placement of a second trocar though care must be taken to avoid enterotomies. If this is not successful, the fascia of the initial site can be closed, and an alternate site can be used. Conversion to an open procedure may be necessary if proper visualization is not obtained. If significant bowel distention is encountered, the pneumoperitoneum itself may allow for some bowel decompression when given time and combined with adequate nasogastric decompression and optimized positioning.

Only adhesions causing obstructive pathology or impaired visualization should be lysed. It is recommended to limit cautery use to prevent thermal tissue damage; scissors are preferred. Some adhesions will separate simply with tension. While three trocars are the minimum required for adhesiolysis and bowel manipulation, it is important to remember that extra trocars can be placed to allow lysis of adhesions and improve visualization. Once trocars are placed, the distal collapsed bowel should be identified to locate the site of obstruction. After lysis of adhesions, the bowel should be inspected for bleeding or perforation. The bowel should be run in a retrograde fashion from the cecum using the hand-to-hand technique with atraumatic graspers. It is essential that the bowel is manipulated gently. In the case of friable/distended bowel, it is recommended that only the mesentery is handled. If this cannot be done safely, conversion is appropriate. Manipulation of dilated and edematous bowel increases the risks of perforation, persistent obstruction, and formation of more adhesions. This is an argument for earlier surgical intervention. After confirmation that the obstruction has been relieved and the bowel has been inspected for injury, the ports should be removed under direct visualization. The fascia is closed to prevent future hernia formation.

Pearls/Pitfalls

- Moving the camera to different trocars can help expose difficult areas of the abdomen.
- Consider alternate site of entry into the abdomen.
- Understanding when to convert to an open procedure is essential for a safe operation. In the case of extensive adhesions requiring conversion to laparotomy, partial laparoscopic lysis of adhesions can be performed to limit the size and extent of the laparotomy. Conversion to open laparotomy should be considered if the patient cannot tolerate insufflation; visualization is limited from diffuse or dense adhesions; the bowel cannot be manipulated without injury; there is bowel perforation that cannot be approached laparoscopically; the etiology of the obstruction cannot be located; or bowel resection is necessary.
- In the case of bowel resection, a small abdominal incision can be made to exteriorize the bowel [12, 27, 29, 31, 35–37].

Postoperative Care

The nasogastric tube is typically kept in place for 24 h postoperatively. Feeding is initiated after the return of bowel function. Discharge criteria should include absence of fever, taking oral nutrition, and pain well controlled on oral pain medications [36].

Outcomes

A multicentric study reported an average of 24 h for return of bowel function, feeding initiated an average of 2.6 days postoperatively, and an average 4.6 day hospitalization after LOA [29]. The KID data analysis of the laparoscopic approach found longer operative times but lower complication rates, shorter lengths of stay, lower total hospital costs, and lower rates of bowel perforation [30]. It is not definitively known if LOA results in a decreased recurrence rate, although there is an overall decrease in ASBO with a laparoscopic approach to initial abdominal operations [33].

Complications

Overall postoperative LOA complications have been reported at 5.6 % and include postoperative shock, hemorrhage, hematoma, seroma, wound complications, infection, fistula, and pulmonary complications [30]. A laparoscopic case series of ASBO in children reported specific incidence of complications, including intra-abdominal abscess (4 %), anastomotic stricture (3 %), anastomotic leak (1 %), bowel obstruction (1 %), and respiratory failure (1 %) [28].

Summary

- Children with ASBO and no indications for emergent surgery should undergo nonoperative management (with or without Gastrografin) for 24 to 48 h in infants and children.
- A laparoscopic approach should be used in patients failing nonoperative management without peritonitis, concerns of ischemic bowel, or severe distention.
- Alternate access sites should be considered based on the child's surgical history.
- Surgeons should have a low threshold for conversion to open.

References

1. Menzies D, Ellis H. Intestinal obstruction from adhesions–how big is the problem? Ann R Coll Surg Engl. 1990;72(1):60–3.
2. Grant HW, Parker MC, Wilson MS, Menzies D, Sunderland G, Thompson JN, et al. Adhesions after abdominal surgery in children. J Pediatr Surg. 2008;43(1):152–6.
3. ten Broek RP, Issa Y, van Santbrink EJ, Bouvy ND, Kruitwagen RF, Jeekel J, et al. Burden of adhesions in abdominal and pelvic surgery: systematic review and met-analysis. BMJ. 2013;347:f5588.
4. Tsao KJ, St Peter SD, Valusek PA, Keckler SJ, Sharp S, Holcomb 3rd GW, et al. Adhesive small bowel obstruction after appendectomy in children: comparison between the laparoscopic and open approach. J Pediatr Surg. 2007;42(6):939–42. discussion 42.
5. van Eijck FC, Wijnen RM, van Goor H. The incidence and morbidity of adhesions after treatment of neonates with gastroschisis and omphalocele: a 30-year review. J Pediatr Surg. 2008;43(3):479–83.
6. Lakshminarayanan B, Hughes-Thomas AO, Grant HW. Epidemiology of adhesions in infants and children following open surgery. Semin Pediatr Surg. 2014;23(6):344–8.

7. Festen C. Postoperative small bowel obstruction in infants and children. Ann Surg. 1982;196(5):580–3.
8. Ouaissi M, Gaujoux S, Veyrie N, Deneve E, Brigand C, Castel B, et al. Post-operative adhesions after digestive surgery: their incidence and prevention: review of the literature. J Visc Surg. 2012;149(2):e104–14.
9. Duron JJ. Postoperative intraperitoneal adhesion pathophysiology. Colorectal Dis. 2007;9 Suppl 2:14–24.
10. Awonuga AO, Saed GM, Diamond MP. Laparoscopy in gynecologic surgery: adhesion development, prevention, and use of adjunctive therapies. Clin Obstet Gynecol. 2009;52(3):412–22.
11. Choudhry MS, Grant HW. Small bowel obstruction due to adhesions following neonatal laparotomy. Pediatr Surg Int. 2006;22(9):729–32.
12. Di Saverio S, Coccolini F, Galati M, Smerieri N, Biffl WL, Ansaloni L, et al. Bologna guidelines for diagnosis and management of adhesive small bowel obstruction (ASBO): 2013 update of the evidence-based guidelines from the world society of emergency surgery ASBO working group. World J Emerg Surg. 2013;8(1):42.
13. Lautz TB, Barsness KA. Adhesive small bowel obstruction–acute management and treatment in children. Semin Pediatr Surg. 2014;23(6):349–52.
14. Wang Q, Chavhan GB, Babyn PS, Tomlinson G, Langer JC. Utility of CT in the diagnosis and management of small-bowel obstruction in children. Pediatr Radiol. 2012;42(12):1441–8.
15. Paulson EK, Thompson WM. Review of small-bowel obstruction: the diagnosis and when to worry. Radiology. 2015;275(2):332–42.
16. Feigin E, Kravarusic D, Goldrat I, Steinberg R, Dlugy E, Baazov A, et al. The 16 golden hours for conservative treatment in children with postoperative small bowel obstruction. J Pediatr Surg. 2010;45(5):966–8.
17. Eeson GA, Wales P, Murphy JJ. Adhesive small bowel obstruction in children: should we still operate? J Pediatr Surg. 2010;45(5):969–74.
18. Lautz TB, Raval MV, Reynolds M, Barsness KA. Adhesive small bowel obstruction in children and adolescents: operative utilization and factors associated with bowel loss. J Am Chem Soc. 2011;212(5):855–61.
19. Lin LH, Lee CY, Hung MH, Chen DF. Conservative treatment of adhesive small bowel obstruction in children: a systematic review. BMJ Open. 2014;4(9), e005789.
20. Vijay K, Anindya C, Bhanu P, Mohan M, Rao PL. Adhesive small bowel obstruction (ASBO) in children-role of conservative management. Med J Malaysia. 2005;60(1):81–4.
21. Young JY, Kim DS, Muratore CS, Kurkchubasche AG, Tracy TF, Luks FI. High incidence of postoperative bowel obstruction in newborns and infants. J Pediatr Surg. 2007;42(6):962–5.
22. Branco BC, Barmparas G, Schnüriger B, Inaba K, Chan LS, Demetriades D. Systematic review and meta-analysis of the diagnostic and therapeutic role of water-soluble contrast agent in adhesive small bowel obstruction. Br J Surg. 2010;97:470–8.
23. Di Saverio S, Catena F, Ansaloni L, Gavioli M, Valentino M, Pinna AD. Water-soluble contrast medium (Gastrografin) value in adhesive small intestine obstruction (ASIO):

a prospective, randomized, controlled, clinical trial. World J Emerg Surg. 2008;32(10):2293–304.

24. Bonnard A, Kohaut J, Sieurin A, Belarbi N, El Ghoneimi A. Gastrografin for uncomplicated adhesive small bowel obstruction in children. Pediatr Surg Int. 2011;27(12):1277–81.
25. Lee CY, Hung MH, Lin LH, Chen DF. Evaluation of a water-soluble contrast agent for the conservative management of adhesive small bowel obstruction in pediatric patients. J Pediatr Surg. 2015;50(4):581–5.
26. Bastug DF, Trammell SW, Boland JP, Mantz EP, Tiley 3rd EH. Laparoscopic adhesiolysis for small bowel obstruction. Surg Laparosc Endosc. 1991;1(4):259–62.
27. Vettoretto N, Carrara A, Corradi A, De Vivo G, Lazzaro L, Ricciardelli L, et al. Laparoscopic adhesiolysis: consensus conference guidelines. Colorectal Dis. 2012;14(5):e208–15.
28. Alemayehu H, David B, Desai AA, Iqbal CW, St Peter SD. Laparoscopy for small bowel obstruction in children–an update. J Laparoendosc Adv Surg Tech A. 2015;25(1):73–6.
29. Becmeur F, Besson R. Treatment of small-bowel obstruction by laparoscopy in children multicentric study. GECI. Groupe d'Etude en Coeliochirurgie Infantile. Eur J Pediatr Surg. 1998;8(6):343–6.
30. Lee J, Tashjian DB, Moriarty KP. Surgical management of pediatric adhesive bowel obstruction. J Laparoendosc Adv Surg Tech A. 2012;22(9):917–20.
31. van der Zee DC, Bax NM. Management of adhesive bowel obstruction in children is changed by laparoscopy. Surg Endosc. 1999;13(9):925–7.
32. Aguayo P, Fraser JD, Ilyas S, St Peter SD, Holcomb 3rd GW, Ostlie DJ. Laparoscopic management of small bowel obstruction in children. J Laparoendosc Adv Surg Tech A. 2011;21(1):85–8.
33. Gutt CN, Oniu T, Schemmer P, Mehrabi A, Buchler MW. Fewer adhesions induced by laparoscopic surgery? Surg Endosc. 2004;18(6):898–906.
34. Wiggins T, Markar SR, Harris A. Laparoscopic adhesiolysis for acute small bowel obstruction: systematic review and pooled analysis. Surg Endosc. 2015.
35. Becmeur F. Laparoscopy and small bowel obstruction in children. Saudi Med J. 2003;24(Suppl):S15–7.
36. Sallinen V, Wikstrom H, Victorzon M, Salminen P, Koivukangas V, Haukijarvi E, et al. Laparoscopic versus open adhesiolysis for small bowel obstruction - a multicenter, prospective, randomized, controlled trial. BMC Surg. 2014;14:77.
37. Reissman P, Wexner SD. Laparoscopic surgery for intestinal obstruction. Surg Endosc. 1995;9(8):865–8.

31. Laparoscopic Meckel's Diverticulectomy

David Rodeberg and Sophia Abdulhai

Introduction

Epidemiology

Although Meckel's diverticulum (MD) is an infrequent finding, it is the most common congenital anomaly in the GI tract. It is found in approximately 2 % of the general population [1]. It was first documented in the late sixteenth century, but it was not described in detail until 1809 by the German anatomist, Johann Meckel [2]. The majority of MD are found incidentally; less than 5 % are symptomatic, and the risk of developing symptoms decreases with age [3, 4]. The incidence of MD is equal between males and females; however, males have been found to be twice as likely to develop symptoms. Also, in a multicentered epidemiologic study, Alemayehu et al. reported a higher incidence of symptomatic MD in Caucasians (63.4 % compared to 4.7 % in Black Americans, 16.4 % in Hispanics) [5].

Embryology

Meckel's diverticulum is caused by a failure of normal obliteration of the omphalomesenteric duct, also known as the vitelline duct. In early embryonic development, the omphalomesenteric duct provides the embryo nourishment from the yolk sac by serving as a channel between the yolk sac and the early midgut. With fetal growth, the yolk sac regresses as the placenta becomes the primary source of nourishment for the embryo; as a result, the omphalomesenteric duct also involutes and is obliterated by weeks 5–7.

D.S. Walsh et al. (eds.), *The SAGES Manual of Pediatric Minimally Invasive Surgery*, DOI 10.1007/978-3-319-43642-5_31

The omphalomesenteric duct is associated with the right and left vitelline vessels. The omphalomesenteric duct and vitelline vessels, along with the urachus and the umbilical vessels, combine to form the umbilical cord. At this time, the umbilical vessels become the dominant blood supply to the fetus, and the vitelline vessels start to regress. The right vitelline artery remnant gives rise to the superior mesenteric artery (SMA), and the left obliterates [6, 7].

Incomplete obliteration of the omphalomesenteric duct can lead to a range of anomalies (Fig. 31.1). If the proximal segment next to the small bowel fails to obliterate, it forms a MD, which is the most common anomaly. The majority of MD are free of attachments to the abdominal wall (75 %) although some may remain attached to the umbilicus, the ileal mesentery, or another segment of the abdominal wall by a fibrous band [7, 8]. If the entire duct fails to obliterate, then it will develop into a fistula between the ileum and the umbilicus. If the distal portion persists and the proximal portion obliterates, then this will become a sinus tract at the umbilicus. If the central portion remains, then it creates an

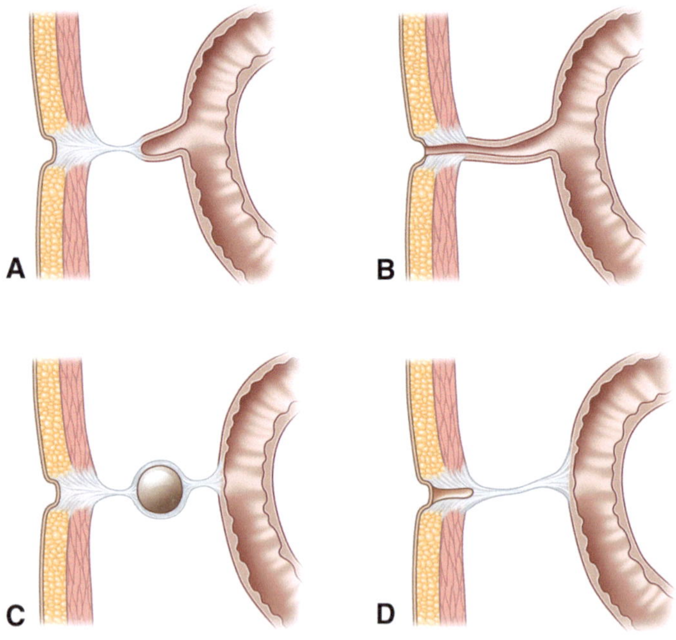

Fig. 31.1. (**a**) Meckel's diverticulum, (**b**) omphalomesenteric fistula, (**c**) omphalomesenteric cyst, and (**d**) remnant vitelline artery/fibrous cord.

omphalomesenteric cyst. The duct can also incompletely obliterate and leave a fibrous band without a MD [9, 10]. Some of these anomalies may subsequently result in bowel obstruction either by causing internal hernias or proving a fixation point for volvulus.

Pathophysiology

Meckel's diverticulum is located on the antimesenteric border of the ileum and contains all of the layers of the intestinal wall making it a true diverticulum. It is located within 20–100 cm (average 50 cm) proximal to the ileocecal valve [2, 8, 11]. The blood supply to the MD is the remnant vitelline artery, which now arises from a terminal branch of the superior mesenteric artery (SMA) [10]. The rules of 2s are frequently used to describe MD [7, 12].

Rules of 2s

2 % of the population.
Twice as common in males.
2 % are symptomatic.
Usually 2 cm in diameter.
Usually 2 in. long.
Located within 2 ft of the ileocecal valve.

As the cells of the omphalomesenteric duct are pluripotent, the MD may contain ectopic mucosa. It has been estimated that 12–50 % of MD contain heterotopic mucosa, most commonly gastric mucosa followed by pancreatic tissue [4, 13–15]. Less commonly, the diverticulum may contain colonic tissue, Brunner's glands, hepatobiliary tissue, and small bowel malignancies such as carcinoid, gastrointestinal stromal tumors, lymphoma, leiomyosarcoma, adenocarcinoma, and intraductal papillary mucinous neoplasm [5, 16].

Preoperative Evaluation

History

Most MD are asymptomatic and are usually found incidentally when undergoing surgical exploration for other intra-abdominal processes.

The most common presentations for symptomatic MD are bleeding, intestinal obstruction, and inflammation.

Episodic painless hematochezia occurs when MD contains ectopic gastric mucosa that secretes hydrochloric acid. This can cause ulceration on the adjacent ileum, leading to bleeding and perforation. Meckel's diverticulum is the most common etiology of intestinal bleeding in children. Bleeding can occur in MD containing malignancies, but this has been described predominantly in adults [17, 18].

Obstruction related to MD can be caused by intussusception, volvulus, or internal abdominal wall herniation. It is the second most common presentation of MD in children, but the most common presentation in adults. Intussusception can occur when the MD inverts into the lumen of the ileum, acting as a lead point. Volvulus most commonly occurs when a loop of small bowel twists around a fibrous band remnant or an incompletely obliterated omphalomesenteric duct connecting the small bowel to the umbilicus. Loops of bowel can also be obstructed through an internal herniation of bowel around a mesodiverticular band, which is the remnant vitelline artery from the diverticulum to the mesentery [13, 17]. Littre's hernia is the presence of a Meckel's diverticulum in a hernia sac, most commonly in an inguinal (50 % of cases), umbilical, or femoral hernia [7, 19].

Meckel's diverticulitis most commonly occurs secondary to an enterolith in the lumen, similar to the pathophysiology of acute appendicitis, and most commonly occurs in adult patients. Inflammation of the MD can also occur from peptic ulceration of the ileal mucosa or from a foreign body in the diverticular orifice (i.e., gallstones or ingested foreign objects such as bones or toothpicks) [17, 20].

If the omphalomesenteric duct is completely patent or if the distal portion is patent, then umbilical drainage can also be a presenting symptom.

Exam

In most studies, the most common presenting symptom of MD in children under the age of 5 years is episodic painless hematochezia. This bleeding is acute and can be massive, often requiring blood transfusions. The stool is often dark red or "currant jelly." These bleeding ulcers can also perforate and cause peritonitis. Obstruction is the second most common presentation and is more common in adults. These patients present with crampy abdominal pain, nausea, bilious emesis, and obstipation.

Patients presenting with diverticulitis have signs and symptoms that are similar to those of acute appendicitis [4, 13].

Laboratory Testing

If the patient is presenting with rectal bleeding, a hemoglobin, hematocrit, and type and cross are required. A white blood cell count is also helpful to delineate an inflammatory process such as diverticulitis. If the patient is presenting with obstructive symptoms, a metabolic panel is indicated to evaluate for electrolyte abnormalities.

Imaging

Abdominal X-Ray

Conventional X-rays may occasionally show an enterolith, evidence of a bowel obstruction, or a gas-/fluid-filled diverticulum. If a patient has a perforation, then free air could optimally be seen on upright chest X-ray or at left lateral decubitus film. Barium studies may show a blind-ending pouch in the distal ileum, but it has low sensitivity secondary to poor filling of the diverticulum from stenosis of the neck, obstructing intestinal contents, contraction of the tunica muscularis, and/or overlapping of small bowel [21].

Ultrasound

High-resolution ultrasonography has been utilized in diagnosing MD. It classically would show a fluid-filled structure in the mid-lower abdomen with a connection to a peristaltic small bowel loop [22]. During episodes of diverticulitis, it would have an appearance similar to appendicitis.

Computed Tomography (CT)

CT is currently the most widely used imaging modality to evaluate for abdominal pain, obstructive symptoms, or potential inflammation. In a study by Kawamoto et al., MD was detected in up to 47.5 % of all patients and 57 % of symptomatic patients [23]. It is the best modality for Meckel's diverticulitis and obstruction. An adjunctive imaging modality is CT enterography, where a large volume of oral contrast is ingested to achieve adequate small bowel distention to evaluate the small bowel [21].

Meckel's Scan

This is the most accurate diagnostic study (sensitivity and specificity >90 %) for detecting MD containing gastric mucosa. It is performed using technetium-99 m, which is taken up by the mucin-secreting cells of the ectopic gastric mucosa. It is a commonly used diagnostic test for rectal bleeding since it is noninvasive with a low radiation burden [21, 24].

Angiography

This is another useful imaging modality if the patient presents with active large volume bleeding. Meckel's diverticulum can be diagnosed by seeing a blush at the site of the persistent vitelline artery arising from the distal SMA. This has less sensitivity as it is only diagnostic if there is bleeding of at least >0.5 ml/min [21, 25]. This modality also allows the option of angiographic embolization that may control bleeding until operative resection.

Other Tests

Double Balloon Enteroscopy

This is a less commonly used modality for diagnosis. It is performed by transoral or transanal endoscopy. This diagnostic tool has also been described as an aid in surgical resection, where the endoscopic light is directed to the abdominal wall indicating the location of the diverticulum and allowing resection through a single small umbilical incision [9, 17, 26]. This modality has largely been replaced by laparoscopic evaluation.

Laparoscopy

Despite all of our imaging modalities, MD is still a difficult diagnosis to make, except in the setting of rectal bleeding with a positive Meckel's scan. In cases when the diagnosis is uncertain, laparoscopy is recommended as the definitive diagnostic and therapeutic intervention [27, 28].

Surgical Indications

There is clear consensus that surgical resection is indicated for all symptomatic MD; however, there is controversy regarding resection of incidentally found MD. In a retrospective study of MD, Cullen et al. described a 6.4 % cumulative lifetime risk of developing complications and found surgical resection of incidental MD had less morbidity compared to surgical resection of complicated MD; therefore, they recommend surgical resection of all MD [29]. Alternatively, Soltero et al. recommended against prophylactic resection as they found a 9 % risk of morbidity after MD resection in these patients and calculated that 800 asymptomatic diverticula had to be removed to prevent one death [3]. Between these two extreme positions, other studies, such as Park et al., found that certain characteristics may be predictive for the development of complications and recommended diverticulectomy of incidental diverticula that meet any of the following four criteria: (1) male sex, (2) age less than 50 years, (3) diverticular length greater than 2 cm, and (4) abnormal features of the diverticula such as thickened tissue or a palpable mass [14]. Other studies have also recommended prophylactic resection if there is a narrow diverticular base [30]. At this time, most pediatric surgeons will perform a resection of an incidentally identified MD if it does not significantly increase the risk of the primary procedure.

Technique

Special Considerations

If a patient is presenting with obstruction, then either laparotomy or laparoscopy (performed by a surgeon experienced in laparoscopic small bowel resection and lysis of adhesions) is the procedure of choice. If a Littre's hernia is present, then a MD resection should be performed first followed by herniorrhaphy [7, 31]. There are various new surgical techniques that are being published, such as hand-assisted laparoscopic resection and single-site surgery; however, these are beyond the scope of this chapter and will not be discussed further [32–34]. Instead, this chapter will focus on laparoscopic MD resection.

Anatomy

As described above, a MD is found on the antimesenteric border of the ileum within 2 ft of the ileocecal valve. It receives its own blood supply from the mesentery of the ileum, usually from the remnant vitelline artery.

Instruments

30° laparoscope, 10 or 12 mm trocar through the umbilicus for the laparoscope and subsequent endoscopic stapler, two additional 5 mm trocars as working ports, atraumatic bowel graspers, a laparoscopic electrocautery or other energy devices, or vascular clip can all prove useful for this procedure.

Steps

Standard general anesthesia and preoperative antibiotics are utilized. A preoperative time-out should be performed. For patients with hematochezia, blood products should be readily available. A Foley catheter should be placed for decompression of the bladder if the patient has not voided immediately before entering the OR suite. A chlorhexidine/alcohol skin preparation should be performed, and the patient should be draped to expose the entire abdomen.

- The first step is entrance into the abdomen. We recommend entrance using the Veress needle technique or the Hassan technique using a 10–12 mm trocar through the umbilicus into the peritoneum under direct visualization and subsequent insufflation.
- Insufflation is achieved using carbon dioxide pneumoperitoneum at 8–12 mmHg.
- A 30° laparoscope should then be introduced through the umbilical port.
- Two additional 5 mm trocars should then be inserted through the left lower quadrant and suprapubic region, similar to sites used for an appendectomy (Fig. 31.2).
- The cecum should first be identified, and this will be facilitated by moving the patient into a left lateral decubitus and Trendelenburg's position.
- A systematic exploration of the small intestine from the terminal ileum to the jejunum should then be performed in a retrograde fashion using blunt bowel graspers.

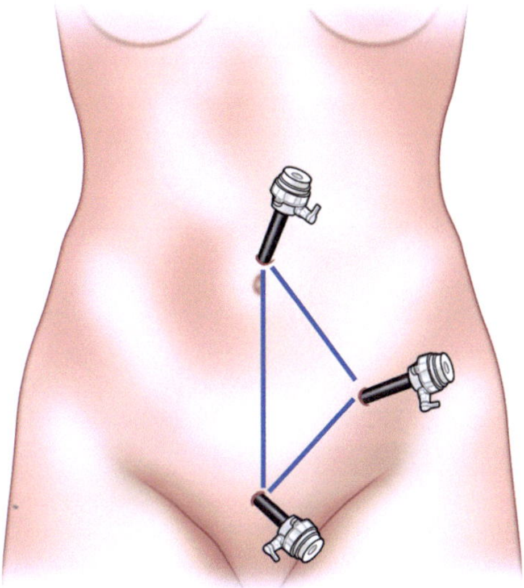

Fig. 31.2. Trocar locations.

- Once located, the diverticulum will need to be released from the mesentery by dividing the feeding vessel using an energy device or vascular clip.
- The MD should then be grasped and delivered through the umbilical port site under direct visualization by placement of the laparoscope through one of the other working ports. The umbilical incision may need to be extended.
- A segmental resection of the diverticulum and adjacent ileum should be performed if the patient is presenting with bleeding to ensure removal of all ectopic mucosa and the bleeding ileal ulcer (Fig. 31.3).
- Re-approximation of the small bowel may be performed using a hand-sewn anastomosis or a side-to-side functional end-to-end stapled anastomosis.
- In the case of an incidentally found MD or if the patient is not presenting with bleeding or perforation, then a diverticulectomy may be performed by either a wedge resection (Fig. 31.4) with a hand-sewn anastomosis or a tangential diverticulectomy using a stapler (Fig. 31.5), taking care not to narrow the lumen.
- Once the anastomosis is completed and hemostasis is achieved, the fascia and skin should be closed per the surgeon's preference.

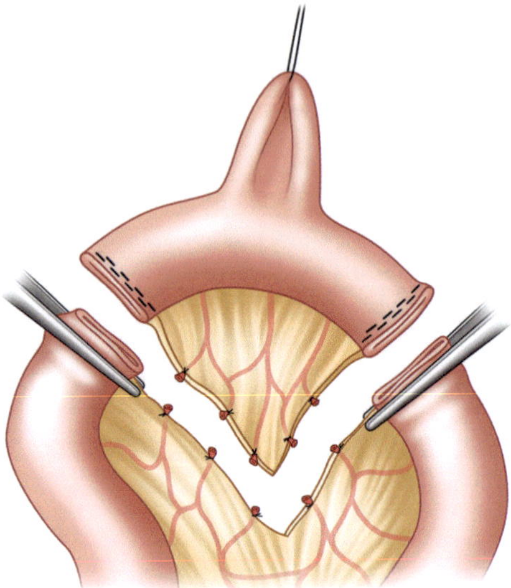

Fig. 31.3. Segmental resection of MD and adjacent small bowel.

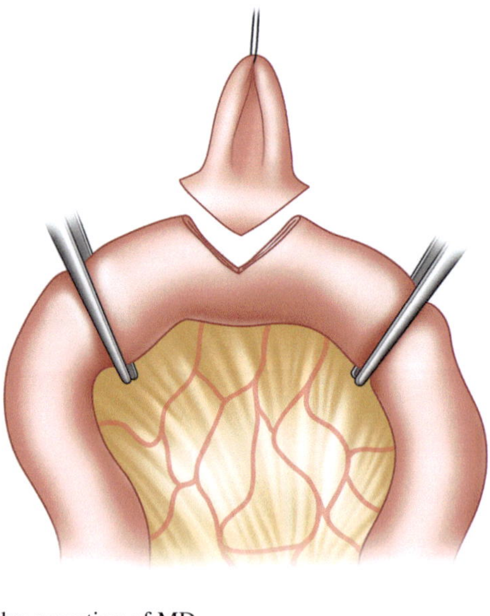

Fig. 31.4. Wedge resection of MD.

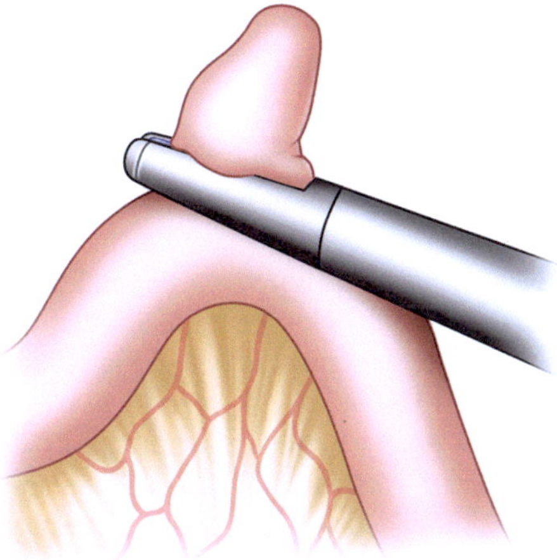

Fig. 31.5. Tangential diverticulectomy with stapler.

Pearls/Pitfalls

Although the majority of the ectopic mucosa is found at the tip of the diverticulum, there is the risk of potentially leaving remnant ectopic mucosa behind in the ileum when a tangential stapled resection is performed [35, 36]. This technique of MD resection is especially discouraged in patients presenting with bleeding or perforation and, therefore, a segmental resection of the MD and 2–3 cm of ileum to each side is frequently recommended [37, 38]. However, Palanivelu et al. report that a simple tangential diverticulectomy in complicated MD without evidence of base involvement is an acceptable alternative. He performed a tangential diverticulectomy in 10 patients with complicated MD and found that of the patients that were followed up (8 patients for 24 months), there was no evidence of disease recurrence [39].

Even in the cases of incidentally found MD, there is controversy as to the recommended surgical procedure. Sarli et al. recommend tangential resection if the MD is asymptomatic/uncomplicated and the diverticulum is not broad based or short, but suggest that all specimens should be inspected after removal to ensure there is no ectopic tissue at the resection margin [40]. A short diverticulum is defined as one that is less than twice the length of the base [37]. At this time, most surgeons will perform a tangential resection for uncomplicated MD.

Postoperative Care

Outcomes/Complications

The most common complication is bowel obstruction secondary to adhesions, occurring in up to 5–10 % of patients [29, 33, 41]. Other complications include bleeding, infection (wound infection and intra-abdominal abscess), wound dehiscence, anastomotic leak, and incisional hernia. Overall surgical morbidity and mortality in symptomatic MD are reported as 2–13 % and 0–2 %, respectively [8, 11, 14, 29, 42]. Park et al. reported a higher incidence of morbidity and mortality in incidental MD (20 % and 1 %) compared to symptomatic MD (13 % and 0 %); however, the complications could not be attributed to the actual diverticulectomy in the incidental patients [14]. A 1–2 % morbidity after an incidental diverticulectomy is more widely reported, although the majority of these studies do not describe the surgical techniques used in the patients [29]. In a 10-year retrospective review on outcomes after laparoscopic-assisted Meckel's diverticulectomy, Chan et al. reported one complication of a wound infection in a total of 18 patients but required conversion of two cases to laparotomy for ischemic bowel and intussusception [43]. Shalaby et al. had no reported complications after laparoscopic resection of incidental and symptomatic MD at 1 year based on a study of 30 patients, and only one patient required conversion to a laparotomy for intestinal duplication [28]. Additional studies also describe low morbidity of 7–12 % for laparoscopic resection of MD, similar to laparotomy [30, 35, 44].

The consensus in the current literature is that laparoscopy is a safe and feasible method of managing MD without evidence of increased morbidity or mortality compared to laparotomy. However, it is clear that laparoscopy has several advantages compared to laparotomy. Ruscher et al. performed a retrospective study comparing the length of hospital stay and cost of laparoscopic versus open Meckel's diverticulectomy [12]. Patients that underwent an open procedure had longer hospital lengths of stay and incurred higher hospital charges.

Summary

- Although a rare anomaly, MD is the most commonly found congenital defect in the gastrointestinal tract, and the majority are asymptomatic.

- The most common presenting symptoms are bleeding, obstruction, and inflammation.
- There are multiple imaging modalities available to evaluate for a MD, but the only imaging modality with high specificity and sensitivity is a Meckel's scan for bleeding secondary to ectopic gastric mucosa.
- Surgical resection is indicated for all symptomatic MD, but there is controversy in regard to resection of incidentally found MD.
- Most complication rates published are combined for open and laparoscopic diverticulectomy, but there is more recent data showing laparoscopic resection is a safe and cost-effective method for surgical management of a MD.

References

1. Haber JJ. Meckel's diverticulum. Am J Surg. 1947;73:468–85.
2. Janjua RM, Shultka R, Goebbel L, Pait TG, Shields CB. The legacy of Johann Friedrich Meckel the Elder (1724-1774): a 4-generation dynasty of anatomists. Neurosurgery. 2010;66(4):758–71.
3. Soltero M, Alexander B. The natural history of Meckel's diverticulum and its relation to incidental removal. A study of 202 cases of diseased Meckel's diverticulum found in King County, Washington, over a fifteen year period. Am J Surg. 1976;132(2): 168–73.
4. Chen JJ, Lee H, Yeng CY, Chan WT, Jiang CB, Sheu JC, Wang NL. Meckel's diverticulum: factors associated with clinical manifestations. ISRN Gastroenterol. 2014;2014:390869.
5. Alemayehu H, Hall M, Desai AA, St Peter SD, Snyder CL. Demographic disparities of children presenting with symptomatic Meckel's diverticulum in children's hospitals. Pediatr Surg Int. 2014;30(6):649–53.
6. Carlson B. Human embryology and developmental biology. 5th ed. Philadelphia: Saunders; 2012.
7. Skandalakis PN, Zoras O, Skandalakis JE, Mirilas P. Littre hernia: surgical anatomy, embryology, and technique of repair. Am Surg. 2006;72(3):238–43.
8. St-Vil D, Brandt ML, Panic S, Bensoussan AL, Blanchard H. Meckel's diverticulum in children: a 20-year review. J Pediatr Surg. 1991;26(11):1289–92.
9. Vane DW, West KW, Grosfeld JL. Vitelline duct anomalies. Experience with 217 childhood cases. Arch Surg. 1987;122(5):542–7.
10. Konvolinka CW. Patent omphalomesenteric duct. Surgery. 2012;131(6):689–90.
11. Matsagas M, Fatouras M, Koulouras B, Giannoukas AD. Incidence, complications and management of Meckel's diverticulum. Arch Surg. 1995;130:143–6.
12. Ruscher KA, Fisher JN, Hughes CD, Neff S, Lerer TJ, Hight DW, Bourque MD, Campbell BT. National trends in the surgical management of Meckel's diverticulum. J Pediatr Surg. 2011;46(5):893–6.

13. Turgeon DK, Barnett JJ. Meckel's diverticulum. Am J Gastroenterol. 1990;85(7):777–81.
14. Park JJ, Wolff BG, Tollefson MK, Walsh EE, Larson DR. Meckel diverticulum: the Mayo Clinic experience with 1476 patients (1950–2002). Ann Surg. 2005;241(3):529–33.
15. Sancar S, Demirci H, Sayan A, Arikan A, Candar A. Meckel's diverticulum: ten years' experience. Ulus Cerrahi Derg. 2015;31(2):65–7.
16. Jadloweic C, Bayron J, Marshall WT. Is an incidental Meckel's diverticulum truly benign? Case Rep Surg. 2015;10:679097.
17. Kharma R, Jain VK. Emergency surgery for Meckel's diverticulum. World J Emerg Surg. 2008;3:27.
18. Caracappa D, Gullà N, Lombardo F, Burini G, Castellani E, Boseli C, Gemini A, Burattini MF, Covarelli P, Noya G. Incidental finding of carcinoid tumor on Meckel's diverticulum: case literature review, should prophylactic resection be recommended? World J Surg Oncol. 2014;12:44.
19. Chan KW, Lee KH, Mou JW, Cheung ST, Tam YH. The use of laparoscopy in the management of Littre's hernia in children. Pediatr Surg Int. 2008;24(7):855–8.
20. Chan KW. Perforation of Meckel's diverticulum caused by a chicken bone: a case report. J Med Case Reports. 2009;3:48.
21. Elsayes KM, Menias CO, Harvin HJ, Francis IR. Imaging manifestations of Meckel's diverticulum. AJR Am J Roentgenol. 2007;189(1):81–8.
22. Mostbec GH, Liskutin J, Dorffner R, Bittmann B, Resinger M. Ultrasonographic diagnosis of a bleeding Meckel's diverticulum. Pediatr Radiol. 2000;30(6):382.
23. Kawamoto S, Raman SP, Blackford A, Hruban RH, Fishman EK. CT detection of symptomatic and asymptomatic Meckel diverticulum. AJR Am J Roentgenol. 2015;205(2):281–91.
24. Sinha CK, Pallewatte A, Easty M, Coppi P, Pierro A, Misra D, Biassoni L. Meckel's scan in children: a review of 183 cases referred to two paediatric surgery specialist centres over 18 years. Pediatr Surg Int. 2013;29(5):511–7.
25. Mahajan MS. An unusual appearance of Meckel's diverticulum as site of bleed on gastrointestinal bleeding scan. World J Nucl Med. 2013;12(3):111–5.
26. Fukushima M, Kawanami C, Inoue S, Okada A, Ima Y, Inokuma T. A case series of Meckel's diverticulum: usefulness of double-balloon enteroscopy for diagnosis. BMC Gastroenterol. 2014;14:155.
27. Sagar J, Kumar V, Shah DK. Meckel's diverticulum: a systematic review. J R Soc Med. 2006;99(10):501–5.
28. Shalaby RY, Soliman SM, Fawy M. Laparoscopic management of Meckel's diverticulum in children. J Pediatr Surg. 2005;40(3):562–7.
29. Cullen J, Kelly KA, Moir CR, Hodge DO, Zinsmeister AR, Melton LJ. Surgical management of Meckel's diverticulum. An epidemiologic, population-based study. Ann Surg. 1994;220(4):564–9.
30. Prasad S, Chui CH, Jacobsen AS. Laparoscopic-assisted resection of Meckel's diverticulum in children. JSLS. 2006;10(3):310–6.
31. Qin D, Liu G, Wang Z. Littre's hernia in a paediatric patient. Afr J Paediatr Surg. 2014;11(4):351–3.

32. Qi S, Huang H, Wei D, Lv C, Yang Y. Diagnosis and minimally invasive surgical treatment of bleeding Meckel's diverticulum in children using double-balloon enteroscopy. J Pediatr Surg. 2015;50(9):1610–2.
33. Duan X, Ye G, Bian H, Yang J, Zheng K, Liang C, Sun X, Yan X, Yang H, Wang X, Ma J. Laparoscopic vs. laparoscopically assisted management of Meckel's diverticulum in children. Int J Clin Exp Med. 2015;8(1):94–100.
34. Chan KW, Lee KH, Wong HY, Tsui SY, Wong YS, Pang KY, Mou JW, Tam YH. Laparoscopic excision of Meckel's diverticulum in children: what is the current evidence? World J Gastroenterol. 2014;20(41):15158–62.
35. Alemayehu H, Stringel G, Lo IJ, Golden J, Pandya S, McBride W, Muensterer O. Laparoscopy and complicated Meckel diverticulum in children. JSLS 2014;18(3). doi:10.4293/JSLS.2014.00015.
36. Mukai M, Takamatsu H, Noguchi H, Fukushige T, Tahara H, Kaji T. Does the external appearance of a Meckel's diverticulum assist in choice of laparoscopic procedure? Pediatr Surg Int. 2002;18:231–3.
37. Varcoe RL, Wong SW, Taylor CF, Newstead GL. Diverticulectomy is inadequate treatment for short Meckel's diverticulum with heterotopic mucosa. ANZ J Surg. 2004;74:869–72.
38. Schmid SW, Schafer M, Krahenbuhl L, Buchler MW. The role of laparoscopy in symptomatic Meckel's diverticulum. Surg Endosc. 1999;13:1047–9.
39. Palanivelu C, Rangarajan M, Senthilkumar R, Madankumar MV. Laparoscopic management of symptomatic Meckel's diverticula: a simple tangential stapler excision. JSLS. 2008;12(1):66–70.
40. Sarli L, Costi R. Laparoscopic resection of Meckel's diverticulum: report of two cases. Surg Today. 2001;31:823–5.
41. Lüdtke FE, Mende V, Köhler H, Lepsien G. Incidence and frequency or complications and management of Meckel's diverticulum. Surg Gynecol Obstet. 1989;169(6):537–42.
42. Piñero A, Martínez-Barba E, Canterast M, Rodriquez JM, Castellanos G, Parrilla P. Surgical management and complications of Meckel's diverticulum in 90 patients. Eur J Surg. 2002;168:8–12.
43. Chan KW, Lee KH, Mou JW, Cheung ST, Tam YH. Laparoscopic management of complicated Meckel's diverticulum in children: a 10 year review. Surg Endosc. 2008;22(6):1509–12.
44. Prasad TR, Chui CH, Singaporewalla FR, Ong CPC, Low Y, Yap TL. Meckel's diverticular complications in children: is laparoscopy the order of the day? Pediatr Surg Int. 2007;23:141–7.

32. Laparoscopic Management of Pediatric Inflammatory Bowel Disease

Kevin N. Johnson and James D. Geiger

Introduction

Inflammatory bowel disease (IBD) includes both Crohn's disease (CD) and ulcerative colitis (UC), which are separate disease processes that often have similar clinical presentations. Among all patients with IBD during their lifetime, 25 % will present before the age of 18, with an incidence of approximately five patients per 100,000 among pediatric patients [1]. Pediatric patients with IBD have a genetic predisposition to IBD in 11–42 % of cases, with a higher likelihood of a genetic component the younger the age at diagnosis [2]. Crohn's disease is twice as common as ulcerative colitis in children, although in patients less than 6 years of age, indeterminate colitis is the most common presentation, with the presentation of signs of CD in other parts of the bowel often not manifesting until the teenage years [1]. Additionally, the traditional presentations of IBD that are classic in adult patients are often not present in pediatric patients.

The use of laparoscopy is well established for the treatment of IBD in the adult population but is less well established in pediatric patients. The use of laparoscopy in adults with IBD has been associated with improved cosmesis, decreased adhesions, and lower risk of abdominal wall hernias postoperatively [3, 4]. While the limited body of literature has not been able to demonstrate the same benefits in the pediatric population, laparoscopic surgery has been shown to be a safe and effective approach to surgery for IBD in pediatric patients [5].

D.S. Walsh et al. (eds.), *The SAGES Manual of Pediatric Minimally Invasive Surgery*, DOI 10.1007/978-3-319-43642-5_32

Preoperative Evaluation

In all patients with IBD, a thorough history and physical exam are key in delineating if, when, and what type of surgical intervention is recommended. Depending on the length of illness, nutritional status may be compromised, due to chronic illness as well as symptoms, including abdominal pain, nausea, and frequent bowel movements causing food aversion. While studies have shown that poor nutritional status is associated with higher complication rates, current studies have not conclusively shown a benefit to administration of preoperative parenteral nutrition [6]. Additionally, adjuvant therapies that patients have undergone, or are on currently, may affect their immune function. Corticosteroids are a mainstay treatment of acute disease flares in IBD and have been shown to affect rates of wound infection and anastomotic leakage [7]. Additionally, immunotherapies increase risks of intra-abdominal infections as well as rates of anastomotic leaks postoperatively [8, 9].

An additional consideration is the significant risk of compromising future fertility in females, with pelvic operations leading to decreased fertility in 80–90 % patients with either UC or CD [10]. This is thought to be related to pelvic dissection or the presence of pelvic sepsis rather than the systemic disease state, although dyspareunia and fear of incontinence may contribute as well by decreasing the desire for intercourse. Most recent recommendations are for reperitonealizing the pelvis whenever possible following dissection to avoid entrapment of the fallopian tubes and ovaries to try and minimize this risk. Additionally, recent studies have shown that this decrease in fertility may be transient and gradually resolve over time [11].

Crohn's Disease

In pediatric patients, CD is more common than UC, with peak presentation in the teenage years in children. Among pediatric patients that present with CD during childhood, around 80 % will require surgical intervention for their disease during their lifetime [12]. Multiple medical therapies exist in the treatment of both chronic disease and acute disease flares, with the main medication classes being steroids and biologic agents.

Surgical treatment of Crohn's disease (CD) is varied and complex. There are a variety of presentations of CD, ranging from mildly symptomatic disease to bowel perforation and resultant sepsis, with obstructive symptoms related to ileocecal disease and abscess being the most common presentations in our practice. As most patients will have additional operations in the subsequent 15 years after their initial operation, choosing an operative approach that does not limit future surgical approaches should be considered [13]. Evaluation of all of the bowel is critical in the surgical treatment of CD, as evaluation for signature signs, including creeping fat and bowel inflammation, helping in determining the extent of disease, and making sure that any anastomoses are made with bowel that is grossly free of disease whenever possible. However, the presence of microscopically positive margins does not increase the rate of intra-abdominal sepsis in the postoperative period [14]. When strictures are known or suspected, preoperative assessment using capsule endoscopy, MR enterography, or a contrast study with small bowel follow-through, or intraoperative assessment is necessary to identify all areas of disease.

Described below is the laparoscopic technique for resection of ileocolonic disease, which is among the most common surgical interventions performed for CD (Fig. 32.1). Adaptations of this technique are viable for many other surgical interventions needed for the treatment of CD involving the small bowel.

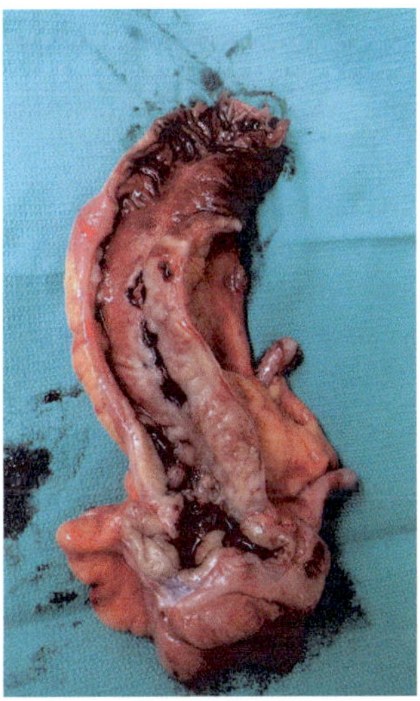

Fig. 32.1. Specimen following ileocecal resection for Crohn's disease.

Technique

1. The patient is positioned in the lithotomy position with both arms tucked. A Foley catheter and orogastric tube are placed for decompression of the bladder and stomach.
2. Trocars are introduced into the abdomen, with 5 mm trocars placed at the umbilicus, one in the left lower quadrant along the left mid-clavicular line, and one in the right upper quadrant along the right mid-clavicular line. This allows for access to all four quadrants of the abdomen.
3. The abdomen is explored to evaluate all of the small bowel and visible portions of the colon for evidence of disease, including creeping fat and bowel inflammation.
4. The diseased portion of the terminal ileum is identified and freed from surrounding structures using electrocautery and sharp dissection, taking care to identify and preserve the right ureter. The cecum is often taken as part of the resection if the diseased portion of small bowel is within 10 cm of the ileocecal valve.
5. Once the portion of small bowel and colon that will be resected is determined, the mesentery is divided using an energy-based device such as a harmonic scalpel just below the bowel. This facilitates exteriorization of the specimen later.
6. A linear cutting stapler is used to divide the bowel.
7. One of the trocar sites, usually the periumbilical site, is then extended to allow removal of the diseased portion of bowel. A wound protector is placed prior to removal (Fig. 32.2).
8. Silk stay sutures are used to approximate the anti-mesenteric borders of the two blind ends of bowel.
9. Enterotomies are created using electrocautery, and a linear cutting stapler is used to create a common channel.
10. Following inspection of the lumen for any evidence of bleeding, the common enterotomy is closed using either a linear cutting stapler or 3-0 PDS suture with a second layer of 3-0 silk sutures to imbricate the suture line.

Alternate Techniques

- A single-port technique can be used, with the port in the periumbilical position.
- The diseased segment of bowel can be exteriorized through the periumbilical incision following dissection for manual inspection and hand-sewn anastomosis if desired.

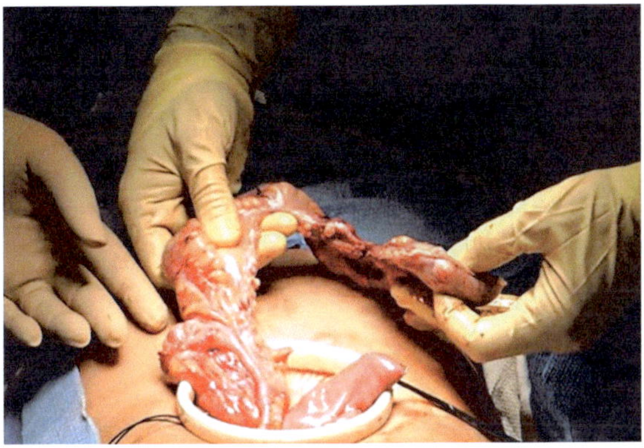

Fig. 32.2. Exteriorization of the terminal ileum through a wound protector following division of the mesentery.

- Multiple variations of this technique are outlined below.

Stricture

The use of laparoscopic or laparoscopic-assisted surgery in the treatment of stricture for Crohn's disease allows for evaluation of the small bowel, with resection or exteriorization of the involved portion if stricturoplasty is to be performed. Preservation of bowel length is a significant concern with any patient with CD, and stricturoplasty can be performed using a laparoscopic-assisted approach. In our experience, we prefer a single-port approach for this operation. This approach involves externalization of the involved segment of bowel through a small incision and subsequent stricturoplasty or bowel resection depending on the length and number of strictures and the length of remaining bowel. In the evaluation of diseased segments of bowel, instruments such as ball bearings can be used to locate and determine the severity of strictures intraoperatively.

Fistula

Treatment of fistulizing Crohn's disease is challenging with any approach. There exists a wide variety of fistulizing diseases, ranging from fistulas between loops of small bowel to enterocutaneous fistulas or entero-vesicular fistulas or entero-colonic fistulas. Additionally, there is often an associated phlegmon with fistulizing disease, which prompts preoperative drainage prior to any operative intervention. In these cases, dissection is often difficult, and a laparoscopic approach to these cases is challenging, with a low threshold to convert to an open operation depending on the degree of inflammation, the size of an associated phlegmon if present, and the degree of scarring that is present.

Abscess/Phlegmon

The presence of abscess or phlegmon without evidence of free perforation in patients with CD often indicates a contained perforation of the bowel. Often, a percutaneous drain will be placed in these collections, which will allow for resolution of the acute process and may result in the formation of a fistula tract when the drain is removed. In these cases, laparoscopy may be used for resection of the diseased segment of bowel in the future, once the acute process has resolved, if needed for recurrent abscess or fistula formation. In up to 30 % of patients, surgical intervention can be avoided following drain placement [15].

Perforation

The presence of free perforation, with the presence of free air, free fluid, and possibly peritoneal signs, does not preclude evaluation using laparoscopy. In many cases, identification of the involved segment of bowel, as well as evaluation of the remaining bowel, is possible laparoscopically if the perforation is found relatively early. Significant contamination and resultant inflammation may preclude complete laparoscopic exploration in some cases.

Postoperative

Data regarding the rates of disease recurrence of CD among pediatric patients is lacking due to the transition of pediatric patients to adult care. Data from the adult literature shows rates of disease recurrence requiring surgery were 25–35 % at 5 years and 40–70 % at 15 years [13]. With these high rates of recurrence, reducing scarring by performing laparoscopic surgery versus open may aid in easing future operations.

Ulcerative Colitis

In the pediatric population, ulcerative colitis often presents with crampy abdominal pain rather than rectal bleeding, as occurs in adults. Additionally, as many pediatric patients with CD will present with pancolitis, caution must be taken prior to determining the final diagnosis, as many patients with CD will present with pancolitis in this population. Incidence of UC is approximately 2–3 out of 100,000 children annually [16]. Treatment of the condition often begins with medical management, for which aminosalicylates and corticosteroids are first line therapy. Additionally, biologic agents, most commonly infliximab (Remicade) and adalimumab (Humira), are an option for patients that fail first line therapies and will often be given in addition to immune modulators such as azathioprine, mercaptopurine, and cyclosporine.

Surgical treatment of UC is based on a number of factors, including response to medical therapies, patient and family tolerance for cancer risk, and nutritional status with the disease. Acute indications for surgery include fulminant colitis, profuse gastrointestinal bleeding, and severe disease causing acute systemic illness. The most common approach to surgical intervention is for a two-stage approach, in which the colon and rectum are resected, a pouch is created and anastomosed to the anus, and a diverting ileostomy is created to be taken down subsequently given a period of recovery. The operative description of this technique is described below. Potential scenarios that may lead to different operative approaches will be outlined as well.

Technique

1. The patient is positioned in the lithotomy position with both arms tucked. A Foley catheter and orogastric tube are placed for decompression of the bladder and stomach.
2. Single-port technique can be used in which the port is inserted through a Pfannenstiel incision (Fig. 32.3). An additional 5 mm port can be added for the dissection if needed.
3. The patient is placed in the reverse Trendelenburg position.
4. The sigmoid colon is lifted anteriorly and medially, and the left ureter is identified and preserved. The inferior mesenteric artery is identified.
5. The retroperitoneum is opened at the sacral promontory, and dissection is carried out proximally to the inferior mesenteric artery, which is ligated using an energy device, stapler with a vascular load, or clips.

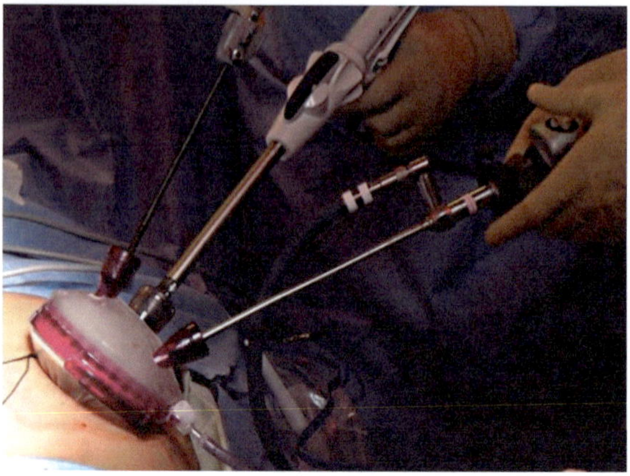

Fig. 32.3. Example of single-site port in place.

6. Lateral attachments are then taken starting on the left side of the colon, and the splenic flexure is mobilized as well.
7. The ascending colon is then mobilized in a similar fashion, taking care to identify and preserve the right ureter and to preserve the ileocolic pedicle, as this will be the vascular supply to the pouch.
8. Mesenteric windows are created on either side of the ileocolic pedicle, which is divided as distal as possible with an energy device, stapler with a vascular load, or clips.
9. The pelvic dissection is completed down to the levator muscles, taking care to preserve the presacral nerves.
10. The rectum is divided at the anorectal junction using a laparoscopic stapler.
11. The port is removed and a wound protector is introduced for externalization of the colon (Fig. 32.4).
12. The terminal ileum is divided using a linear stapler.
13. The terminal ileum is checked for length to make sure that it will reach the pelvis for the pouch.
14. An 8–10 cm j-pouch is created using a linear stapler. Sizing of the pouch is based on the judgment of the surgeon and is related to the size of the patient.
15. The anvil for the EEA stapler is introduced into the distal end of the j-pouch, a purse-string suture is used to secure it in place, and the pouch is placed back within the abdomen.
16. The mesentery of the pouch and distal small bowel is evaluated to make sure it is not twisted.

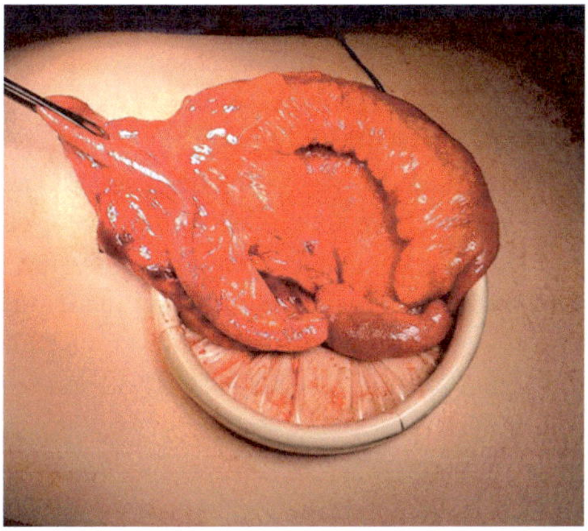

Fig. 32.4. Exteriorization of the colon through a wound protector.

17. The EEA stapler is used to create the ileoanal anastomosis. In the Trendelenburg position, saline is infused into the pelvis, and a leak test is performed on the pouch.
18. The ileum is run ~30–40 cm proximal to the pouch and brought through the abdominal wall for formation of a diverting ileostomy.

Endorectal Dissection

1. Alternatively, an endorectal dissection can be carried out through an abdominal approach from just above the peritoneal dissection down to 1.5 cm above the dentate line. This replaces step 10 above.
2. The mucosal and submucosal tube is then prolapsed into the peritoneum, and a TA stapler is used to transect the rectal tube externally.
3. Subsequently, an EEA stapler is used to anastomose the j-pouch, as outlined above.
4. Geiger et al. describe this alternate technique in detail [17].

Alternate Techniques

- A laparoscopic technique can be used, with one of the port sites being extended for exteriorization of the colon.
- For the single-stage technique, the diverting ileostomy is omitted.
- Hand-sewn ileoanal anastomosis can be performed instead of EEA-stapled anastomosis.

In pediatric patients undergoing colectomy for ulcerative colitis, multiple factors must be taken into account when deciding on the operative approach taken. Laparoscopic or laparoscopic-assisted colectomy is possible in the majority of cases.

A single-port technique, as described here, is technically challenging, and literature reviews have shown inconsistent but potential benefits to the technique [18]. A j-pouch is created at the time of colectomy, outside of cases in which an end ileostomy and three-stage reconstruction are undertaken, which is only used in patients with fulminant colitis and associated acute systemic illness. Alternative approaches are discussed below.

Single Stage

Single-stage colectomy with j-pouch and without diverting ileostomy is controversial but with proper patient selection and education can be effective. In patients with adequate nutritional status and minimal immunosuppression due to steroids or other immunomodulating therapies such as Remicade, single-stage repair can be appropriate. Frank discussion with patients and families is important in outlining the significant risks of leak from the pouch and resultant sepsis in patients considering undergoing a single-stage colectomy and reconstruction.

Three Stage

The three-stage resection and reconstruction are generally only performed in patients with fulminant colitis and associated acute systemic illness, in which minimizing the patient's operative time is of the utmost importance. Due to the need for a quick operation, the surgeon must decide whether a laparoscopic approach is the most efficient way to proceed, which will likely depend on the surgeon's experience with laparoscopic techniques.

Postoperative

Following colectomy for UC, multiple issues may arise in both the acute and long-term time periods, with morbidity rates around 30 % in the initial postoperative period [19]. Initial postoperative complications include anastomotic leak, infection, obstruction, and stricturing of the ileoanal anastomosis. Stricturing of the ileoanal anastomosis (IAA) can be treated with anal dilations, although this can be difficult for parents to perform at home, and some families will elect to have these performed under sedation in the hospital setting.

Pouchitis is among the most common complications following IAA, occurring in 26–47 % of children postoperatively [20]. Proper treatment with antibiotics should follow an appropriate work-up ruling out other causes, including retained rectal mucosa, stricturing of the ileoanal anastomosis, and CD. Known risk factors for pouchitis include smoking, caffeine use, stress, and NSAID use. Approximately 10 % of pouch procedures will fail relating to persistent and severe pouchitis that is refractory to treatment, requiring excision of the pouch and permanent ileostomy [21].

Functionality following pouch reconstruction has lower rates of incontinence and less frequent stooling than in adult studies. To date, studies have shown that the use of laparoscopy does not adversely affect long-term functionality when compared to open operations [5].

Indeterminate Colitis

In the evaluation of children, particularly children younger than 8 years old, indeterminate colitis is a common presentation for inflammatory bowel disease [2, 22]. Manifestations of extra-colonic disease may not occur for many years, making the distinction between CD and UC difficult in many cases. For obvious reasons, this influences the choices made when deciding the type and extent of surgery undertaken. In patients with medically refractory disease and pancolitis, total colectomy is often undertaken. Creation of a j-pouch may potentially be complicated by presentation of CD later in life, which leads to higher rates of morbidity in patients with indeterminate colitis following pouch creation [23].

Summary

- Pancolitis is a common presentation for children with inflammatory bowel disease. However, determining whether the patient has UC or CD may not be possible as extra-colonic manifestations of CD may not occur until the adolescent years.

- Benefits of laparoscopic surgery for IBD in adult patients include reduced scarring, improved cosmesis, and reduced risk of abdominal wall hernias. These benefits have not been proven in the limited literature for pediatric patients.
- As children with CD will likely require surgery for their disease during their lifetime, minimizing scarring and maintaining bowel length are of the utmost importance when performing surgery.

References

1. Sawczenko A, Sandhu BK, Logan RF, Jenkins H, Taylor CJ, Mian S, Lynn R. Prospective survey of childhood inflammatory bowel disease in the British Isles. Lancet. 2001;357:1093–4.
2. Bousvaros A, Sylvester F, Kugathasan S, et al. Challenges in pediatric inflammatory bowel disease. Inflamm Bowel Dis. 2006;12(9):885–913.
3. Wexner SD, Reissman P, Pfeifer J, et al. Laparoscopic colorectal surgery: analysis of 140 cases. Surg Endosc. 1996;10:133–6.
4. Dasari BV, McKay D, Gardiner K. Laparoscopic versus open surgery for small bowel Crohn's disease. Cochrane Database Syst Rev. 2011;1, CD006956.
5. Page AE, Sashittal SG, Chatzizacharias NA, et al. The role of laparoscopic surgery in the management of children and adolescents with inflammatory bowel disease. Medicine. 2015;94(21), e874.
6. Crowell K, Messaris E. Risk factors and implications of anastomotic complications after surgery for Crohn's disease. World J Gastrointest Surg. 2015;7(10):237–42.
7. Eriksen TF, Lassen CB, Gögenur I. Treatment with corticosteroids and the risk of anastomotic leakage following lower gastrointestinal surgery: a literature survey. Colorectal Dis. 2013;16:O154–60.
8. Serradori T, Germain A, Scherrer ML, et al. The effect of immune therapy on surgical site infection following Crohn's disease resection. Br J Surg. 2013;100:1089–93.
9. El-Hussuna A, Krag A, Olaison G, et al. The effect of anti-tumor necrosis factor alpha agents on postoperative anastomotic complications in Crohn's disease: a systematic review. Dis Colon Rectum. 2013;56:1423–33.
10. Bharadwaj S, Philpott JR, Barber MD, et al. Women's health issues after ileal pouch surgery. Inflamm Bowel Dis. 2014;20(12):2470–82.
11. Ban L, Tata LJ, Humes DJ, et al. Decreased fertility rates in 9639 women diagnosed with inflammatory bowel disease: a United Kingdom population-based cohort study. Aliment Pharmacol Ther. 2015;42:855–66.
12. Caprilli R, Gassull MA, Escher JC, et al. European evidence based consensus on the diagnosis and management of Crohn's disease: special situations. Gut. 2006;55 Suppl 1:i36–58.
13. Bernell O, Lapidus A, Hellers G. Risk factors for surgery and postoperative recurrence in Crohn's disease. Ann Surg. 2000;231:38–45.

14. Fazio VW, Floriano M, Church JM, et al. Effect of resection margins on the recurrence of Crohn's disease in the small bowel: a randomized controlled trial. Ann Surg. 1996;224(4):563–73.
15. Clancy C, Boland T, Deasy J, et al. A meta-analysis of percutaneous drainage versus surgery as the initial treatment of Crohn's disease-related intra-abdominal abscess. J Crohns Colitis. 2016;10(2):202–8. doi:10.1093/ecco-jcc/jjv198.
16. Jakobsen C, Paerregaard A, Munkholm P, et al. Pediatric inflammatory bowel disease: increasing incidence, decreasing surgery rate, and compromised nutritional status: a prospective population-based cohort study 2007–2009. Inflamm Bowel Dis. 2011;17:2541–50.
17. Geiger JD, Teitelbaum DH, Hirschl RB, Coran AG. A new operative technique for restorative proctocolectomy: the endorectal pull-through combined with a double-stapled ileo-anal anastomosis. Surgery. 2003;134(3):492–5.
18. Podda M, Saba A, Porru F, Pisanu A. Systematic review with meta-analysis of studies comparing single-incision laparoscopic colectomy and multiport laparoscopic colectomy. Surg Endosc. 2016. doi:10.1007/s00464-016-4812-2.
19. Patton D, Gupta N, Wojcicki JM, et al. Postoperative outcome of colectomy for pediatric patients with ulcerative colitis. J Pediatr Gastroenterol Nutr. 2010;51(2):151–4.
20. Ceriati E, De Peppo F, Rivosecchi M. Role of surgery in pediatric ulcerative colitis. Pediatr Surg Int. 2013;29:1231–41.
21. Meagher AP, Farouk R, Dozois RR, et al. J ileal pouch-anal anastomosis for chronic ulcerative colitis: complications and long-term outcome in 1,310 patients. Br J Surg. 1998;85:800–3.
22. Carvalho RS, Abadom V, Dilworth HP, et al. Indeterminate colitis: a significant subgroup of pediatric IBD. Inflamm Bowel Dis. 2006;12(4):258–62.
23. Odze RD. A contemporary and critical appraisal of 'indeterminate colitis'. Mod Pathol. 2015;28:S30–46.

33. Laparoscopic Management of Intussusception

Nicholas E. Bruns and Anthony L. DeRoss

Background

Ileocolic intussusception is a condition that affects children between 3 months and 5 years of age, with 85 % of patients being less than 3 years of age [1]. There is a slight male predominance with a male/female ratio of 3:2.

Patients most frequently present with abdominal pain, emesis, and/or bloody stools. Diagnosis is made with ultrasound, and the first line of treatment consists of pneumatic or hydrostatic reduction. In a recent meta-analysis, pneumatic reduction was found to be successful in 83 % of cases, compared to 70 % in hydrostatic reduction [2]. When nonoperative reduction fails, abdominal exploration should be pursued.

Approximately 90 % of ileocolic intussusceptions are idiopathic, thought to be due to lymphoid hyperplasia from a viral infection that serves as a lead point. The most common cause of a pathologic lead point is a Meckel's diverticulum. In children 4 years old or greater, approximately 50 % of patients have a pathologic lead point [3].

Indications and Contraindications

Laparoscopy should be considered in the child with a diagnosis of intussusception who has failed three attempts of nonoperative reduction or if it is unclear whether complete reduction has occurred [4, 5]. It may also be used in the patient with suspicion for a pathologic lead point, such as older children or those with recurrent intussusception. In the patient with high suspicion for a small bowel intussusception after an equivocal ultrasound and

D.S. Walsh et al. (eds.), *The SAGES Manual of Pediatric Minimally Invasive Surgery*, DOI 10.1007/978-3-319-43642-5_33

enema, laparoscopy may be diagnostic and therapeutic. The only absolute contraindication to laparoscopy is hemodynamic instability. Relative contraindications include perforation, peritonitis, and previous abdominal surgery.

Anatomy

The majority of cases occur at the ileocecal junction, although jejuno-jejunal, jejuno-ileal, and colocolic intussusceptions have been described. Pathologic lead points should be considered for small bowel intussusception, recurrent intussusception, or intussusception in older children (>5 years old). Small bowel intussusception is often a benign finding on imaging [6], but may also be encountered postoperatively after almost any other pediatric surgical procedures including such variety as circumcision, tonsillectomy, appendectomy, or Wilms' tumor resection [7].

Patient Positioning and Operating Room Setup

The patient is placed in the supine position in slight Trendelenburg with the left side rotated down. Positioning may be altered based on preoperative imaging if the intussusception is not identified in the right lower quadrant. The operating surgeon stands at the patient's left with the assistant on the patient's right (Fig. 33.1a). Laparoscopic monitors should be placed across the table in direct view of each participant.

Bowel preparation is unnecessary as patients are typically obstructed. Appropriate fluid resuscitation should be initiated. Intravenous antibiotics should be given preoperatively. A nasogastric tube should be placed to decompress the stomach. Patients may have swallowed a significant amount of air from crying during enema reduction attempts.

Trocar Position and Instrumentation

A 5-mm, 30-degree laparoscope should be placed in the umbilicus. The intussusception should be identified before placing additional ports. Most commonly, two 3-mm or 5-mm instruments will be placed under direct visualization through stab incisions in the left lower quadrant and suprapubic region to triangulate toward an ileocolic intussusception (Fig. 33.1b).

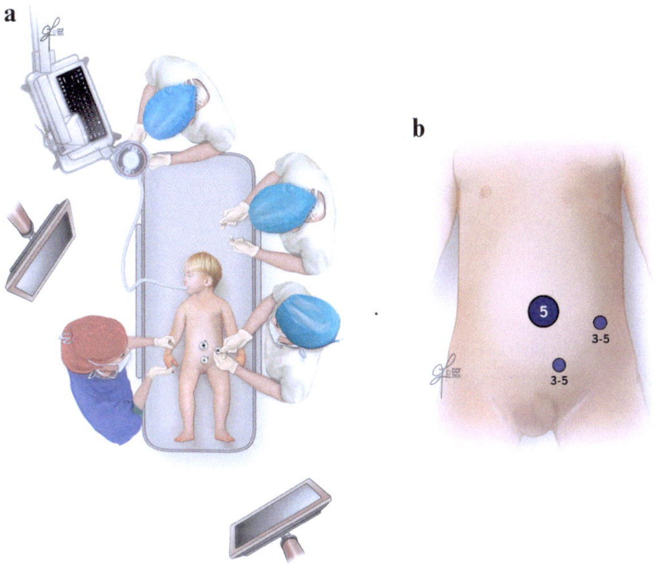

Fig. 33.1. Operating room setup (**a**) with standard trocar placement (**b**). Trocar placement may be altered based on location of the intussusception on air or contrast enema. Reprinted with permission, Cleveland Clinic Center for Medical Art & Photography © 2015. All rights reserved.

Instrument size should be chosen such that the instruments can grasp the entire diameter of the bowel to minimize injury from tangential grasps. In larger children, this may prohibit the use of 3-mm instruments. Port placement may be adapted based on the location of the intussusception on imaging, although the intussusception ultimately should reduce to the right lower quadrant. More extensive intussusceptions may require additional ports to improve ergonomics.

Technique

1. Assess the anatomy.
   a. Identify the intussusception. If no intussusception is present, it may have reduced spontaneously, and the procedure is complete.
   b. Look for pathologic lead points, such as a Meckel's diverticulum.

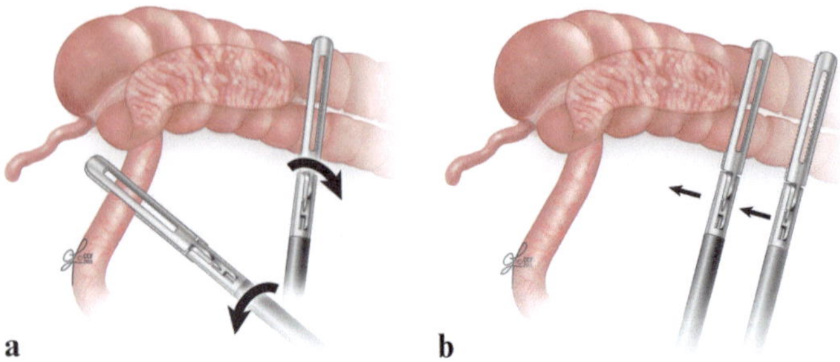

Fig. 33.2. Laparoscopic reduction technique. The standard laparoscopic reduction technique (**a**) is performed by applying steady traction to ileum with countertraction from the cecum. The traditional open technique (**b**) may be reproduced laparoscopically by applying pressure from distal to proximal in a sequential fashion. Reprinted with permission, Cleveland Clinic Center for Medical Art & Photography © 2015. All rights reserved.

c. Determine the feasibility of continuing laparoscopically based on bowel distention or ischemia.

2. Atraumatic graspers should be used to manipulate the bowel. Reduction may be attempted initially with one instrument by providing traction on the ilium, but this reduction using this method can be challenging. If reduction is not achieved, then an additional instrument may provide countertraction on the cecum (Fig. 33.2a). Pressure should be firm and steady for several minutes. The traditional open technique of applying pressure from distal to proximal in a sequential fashion may be attempted but can be difficult to reproduce laparoscopically (Fig. 33.2b).
3. If the intussusception is extensive, an on-table enema under fluoroscopy with simultaneous laparoscopic traction may be performed.
4. If still not reduced, consider conversion to a laparoscopic-assisted procedure through extension of a port site incision or placement of an incision over the lesion large enough to externalize the intussusception and perform open reduction. In cases series, the rate of conversion to an open procedure has been 10–30 % [8–10].
5. If the laparoscopic or laparoscopic-assisted approach is not successful, a formal laparotomy should be done. If open reduction is not possible, resection should be performed with an ileocecectomy or right hemicolectomy.

6. Once the intussusception is reduced, the bowel should be assessed for viability before closing the incisions. If a segment of bowel is necrotic or remains ischemic, a segmental resection is required. Any serosal tears or mesenteric rents should be repaired primarily (Fig. 33.3).
7. Because the incisions are similar to those done for an appendectomy, many surgeons recommend removing the appendix after reduction to minimize ambiguity regarding the presence of the appendix for that patient in the future. It is also believed that appendectomy will result in local operative adhesions, reducing the chance of recurrence. However, due to lack of randomized prospective trials studying appendectomy at the time of intussusception reduction, the option for appendectomy is at the discretion of the operating surgeon. The status of the appendix postoperatively should be documented clearly in the operative report.

Technical Pearls and Pitfalls

1. Steady traction should be applied for 15 min before converting to an open procedure.
2. Gentle compression of the colon at the distal edge of the intussusceptum for several minutes may aid in reduction by reducing edema.
3. In older patients, laparoscopic reduction may be unsuccessful more frequently due to the higher incidence of an anatomic lead point. Resection should be performed in this case.
4. Conversion to laparoscopic-assisted or open reduction should be done without hesitation in difficult cases as 10–30 % will not reduce laparoscopically. Delaying conversion places the patient at increased risk of iatrogenic injury and increased operative time.
5. The serosa can be torn easily! Injury may be minimized by using instruments that span the entire diameter of the small bowel.

Intraoperative Complications

In the case of iatrogenic or ischemic perforation, the perforation should be repaired either laparoscopically or open.

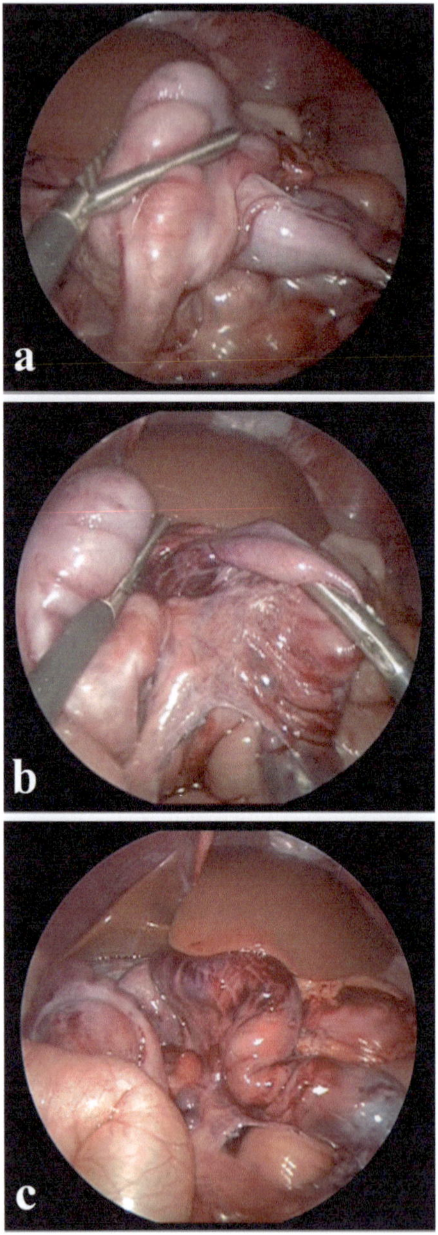

Fig. 33.3. Laparoscopic views of ileocecal intussusception before (**a**), during (**b**), and after (**c**) reduction.

Postoperative Management

It is the authors' practice to keep patients NPO overnight or for 12 h postoperatively, but this interval varies between clinicians and institutions. Diet may then be advanced as tolerated. Acetaminophen and/or ibuprofen is an adequate treatment for most patients' pain. Narcotics may be considered but should be minimized to prevent ileus, and prolonged need for narcotics should raise suspicion for an occult process.

In the case of recurrent intussusception, the initial treatment protocol should be repeated (hydrostatic or pneumatic reduction first, operative reduction second). Recurrence rates are approximately 3 % [5] after operative reduction and 5–12 % after nonoperative reduction based on the technique used [11]. Approximately half of the recurrences occur within the first 48 h. Recurrent intussusception after operative reduction should be assessed for a lead point. Most patients are discharged in 24–48 h to allow for observation during the highest risk period for recurrence.

Summary

- Laparoscopic exploration is a safe option for intussusception. Parents should be advised that conversion to an open procedure occurs commonly and should not be considered a complication
- Review preoperative radiographic studies to identify the location of the intussusception to plan optimal port placement.
- Atraumatic bowel graspers with jaws that span the entire diameter of the bowel should be used to minimize serosal tearing.
- For an intussusception that does not reduce laparoscopically, a fluoroscopic, laparoscopic-assisted enema may augment reduction.
- If there is difficulty with laparoscopic reduction, potential iatrogenic injury, or strong suspicion for a pathologic lead point, conversion to a laparoscopic-assisted or open procedure should be done in a timely fashion.

References

1. Mandeville K, Chien M, Willyerd FA, et al. Intussusception: clinical presentations and imaging characteristics. Pediatr Emerg Care. 2012;28:842–4. doi:10.1097/PEC.0b013e318267a75e.

2. Sadigh G, Zou KH, Razavi SA, et al. Meta-analysis of air versus liquid enema for intussusception reduction in children. AJR Am J Reoentgenol. 2015;205:W542–9. doi:10.2214/AJR.14.14060.
3. Ong NT, Beasley SW. The leadpoint in intussusception. J Pediatr Surg. 1990; 25:640–3.
4. Georgeson KE. Laparoscopic management of ileocolic intussusception. In: Rothenberg SS, Holcomb III GW, Georgeson KE, editors. Atlas of pediatric laparoscopy and thoracoscopy. Philadelphia, PA: Elsevier Health Sciences; 2008. p. 71–3.
5. Wei C-H, Fu Y-W, Wang N-L, et al. Laparoscopy versus open surgery for idiopathic intussusception in children. Surg Endosc. 2015;29:668–72. doi:10.1007/s00464-014-3717-1.
6. Doi O, Aoyama K, Hutson JM. Twenty-one cases of small bowel intussusception: the pathophysiology of idiopathic intussusception and the concept of benign small bowel intussusception. Pediatr Surg Int. 2004;20:140–3. doi:10.1007/s00383-003-1055-9.
7. Klein JD, Turner CG, Kamran SC, et al. Pediatric postoperative intussusception in the minimally invasive surgery era: a 13-year, single center experience. J Am Coll Surg. 2013;216:1089–93. doi:10.1016/j.jamcollsurg.2013.01.059.
8. Bonnard A, Demarche M, Dimitriu C, et al. Indications for laparoscopy in the management of intussusception: a multicenter retrospective study conducted by the French Study Group for Pediatric Laparoscopy (GECI). J Pediatr Surg. 2008;43:1249–53. doi:10.1016/j.jpedsurg.2007.11.022.
9. Fraser JD, Aguayo P, Ho B, et al. Laparoscopic management of intussusception in pediatric patients. J Laparoendosc Adv Surg Tech. 2009;19:563–5. doi:10.1089/lap.2009.0117.
10. Kia KF, Mony VK, Drongowski RA, et al. Laparoscopic vs open surgical approach for intussusception requiring operative intervention. J Pediatr Surg. 2005;40:281–4. doi:10.1016/j.jpedsurg.2004.09.026.
11. Gray MP, Li S-H, Hoffmann RG, Gorelick MH. Recurrence rates after intussusception enema reduction: a meta-analysis. Pediatrics. 2014;134:110–9. doi:10.1542/peds.2013-3102.

34. Laparoscopic Appendectomy

Harveen K. Lamba, Nicholas E. Bruns, and Todd A. Ponsky

Introduction

Acute appendicitis is the most common surgical emergency among children, and its incidence increases with age until adolescence. In the United States, approximately 70,000 children are affected each year, with peak incidence occurring at 12–18 years. Acute appendicitis can be either simple or complicated, with perforation and/or abscess formation occurring in the latter [1, 2].

In the case of simple acute appendicitis, appendectomy remains the generally accepted standard of care, although some centers now treat acute appendicitis with only medical management [3]. Timing of surgery for complicated appendicitis, on the other hand, remains controversial. Immediate operation in the face of a well-formed abscess may lead to an increased rate of postoperative complications, in particular, intra-abdominal abscess formation. In the case of complicated appendicitis, the surgeon may choose immediate surgical intervention or medical treatment with antibiotics and image-guided or surgical drainage. Medical management in the acute phase may then be followed by subsequent interval appendectomy in 2–3 months. Some surgeons may not even perform an interval appendectomy and only operate for recurrent symptoms. In a meta-analysis of 17 studies, conservative management with or without interval appendectomy was associated with better postoperative outcomes, fewer complications, fewer re-operations, and comparable hospital length of stay [4].

Surgical treatment of acute appendicitis has evolved over the past few decades. Prior to advances in minimally invasive surgery, right lower quadrant abdominal incisions were the gold standard surgical approach. In the past two decades, laparoscopic appendectomy has

D.S. Walsh et al. (eds.), *The SAGES Manual of Pediatric Minimally Invasive Surgery*, DOI 10.1007/978-3-319-43642-5_34

gained popularity and has been shown to improve patient outcomes. Advantages of laparoscopic appendectomy include shorter hospital stay, lower incidence of wound infection, reduced postoperative pain, and less conspicuous incision sites when compared to open appendectomy [5, 6]. In the case of complicated appendicitis, recent studies have shown no difference in the rate of abscess formation between laparoscopic and open appendectomy [7, 8]. Additionally, a laparoscopic approach confers the ability to completely visualize the abdominal cavity, enabling diagnosis and treatment of other abdominal pathologies.

The use of single-incision laparoscopic surgery may represent an improvement over conventional laparoscopic surgery. With the number of incisions reduced to one umbilical incision, the potential advantages are better cosmetic outcome, less postoperative pain due to non-penetration of the abdominal wall musculature, and avoidance of possible hemorrhagic complications from injury to the epigastric vessels. In recent years, an increasing number of articles have demonstrated the feasibility of this approach in different pathologies [9–16]. A recent randomized prospective study comparing single-incision appendectomy to the conventional laparoscopic approach found a longer operative time with the single-incision approach but, significantly, less postoperative pain and no difference between the two groups for early and late complications and length of hospital stay [17]. St. Peter et al. did a similar study in children and found that there was no clinical difference between single-port appendectomy and three-port appendectomy, except for a marginal increased operative time in the single-port group [18].

Technique

Other authors have already described several techniques for single-incision appendectomy. Below is one established technique.

Single-Incision Laparoscopic Appendectomy

Single-incision appendectomy is best suited for straightforward acute appendicitis cases and is easiest to perform when the appendix is freely mobile. This technique can essentially be divided into two techniques: extracorporeal and intracorporeal. The extracorporeal technique involves placing a laparoscopic grasper and camera through the umbilicus, exteriorizing the appendix, and performing an open, transumbilical appendectomy. The intracorporeal technique involves placing a camera and at least two other laparoscopic instruments (with or without trocars) through the umbilicus and performing the appendectomy inside the abdomen, removing the appendix at the end of the case. While the authors originally utilized the intracorporeal technique in the past, they have switched to the extracorporeal technique, as it seems to be easier, faster, less costly, and less painful. This technique was originally described using an operative laparoscope to exteriorize the appendix through the umbilicus and perform an extracorporeal appendectomy. Recently, alternatives to exteriorize the appendix without an operative laparoscope have been reported, and this technique is described here. The extracorporeal technique may be unique to children, as the thin abdominal wall and shorter distance from the cecum to the umbilicus allows the appendix to be easily exteriorized; however it can also be applied, although with more difficulty, in larger adolescents.

Extracorporeal, Single-Incision Technique

1. Make a 15-mm infraumbilical skin incision. A Veress needle is inserted to create 15 mmHg of pneumoperitoneum, and a 5-mm AnchorPort (Surgiquest, Inc., Orange, CT) is inserted into the umbilicus. This trocar has a low-profile, small-diameter head, and the phalange of the trocar allows re-insufflation at the end of the case even though the fascial incision is 10 mm.
2. Insert one 5-mm, 30-degree laparoscope into the abdominal cavity through the umbilical trocar. Place a 3-mm grasper, such as the MiniLap® Alligator Grasper (Teleflex Inc., Wayne, PA) within the same skin incision but through the fascia 2–4 mm inferior to the 5-mm trocar (Fig. 34.1).
3. Grab the appendix using the grasper. Aiming just below the tip ensures the appendix doesn't bend during removal and also allows for identification of the distal end of the appendix during extrication from the umbilicus (Fig. 34.2). Divide the abdominal wall fascial bridge between the 3-mm instrument and the 5-mm trocar. Extend this incision in larger patients (sometimes up to 15–20 mm is necessary). Bring the appendix to the abdominal wall surface through the fascial

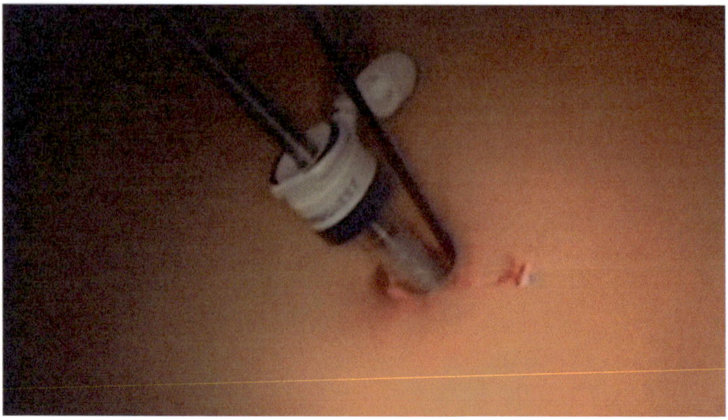

Fig. 34.1. Insertion of laparoscope and grasper through umbilical trocar.

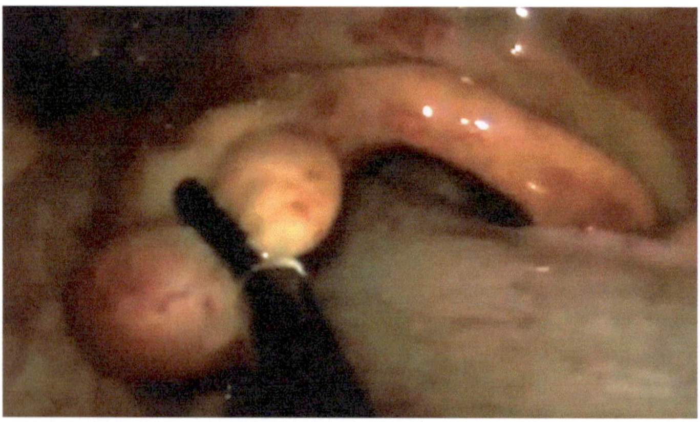

Fig. 34.2. Use grasper to grab distal end of appendix.

opening (Fig. 34.3). Divide the appendix and mesoappendix extracorporeally (Fig. 34.4). Ligate the appendix with two 3-0 Vicryl sutures and cauterize the mucosa (Figs. 34.5 and 34.6).

4. Because of the plastic anchor on the AnchorPort, the port can be reinserted into the new, larger fascial opening and still maintain insufflation. This allows for a brief insertion of the scope to assure no bleeding and ensures the presence of an adequately short appendiceal stump.

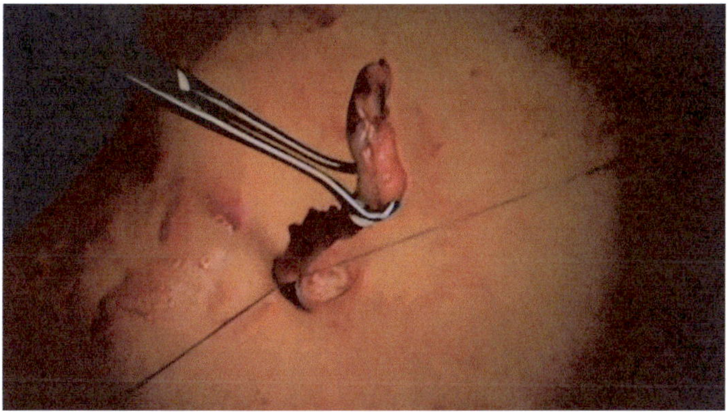

Fig. 34.3. Extracorporealization of appendix through umbilical incision.

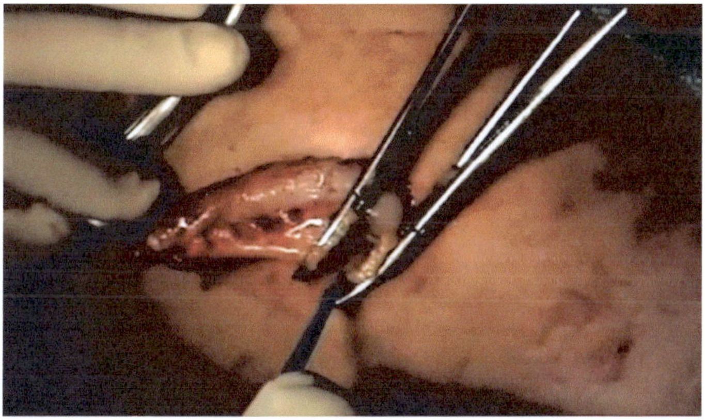

Fig. 34.4. Extracorporeal division of mesoappendix.

Intracorporeal, Single-Incision, Multiport Technique

1. Make a 2-cm infraumbilical or transumbilical incision.
2. If multiple, individual ports are utilized, insufflate with a Veress needle and then insert three AnchorPorts. Alternatively, one could insert 3-mm instruments through the fascia in the same skin incision as the trocar.

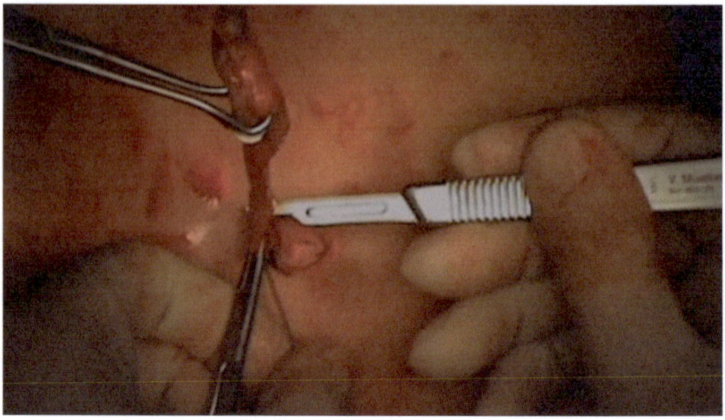

Fig. 34.5. Extracorporeal division of appendix.

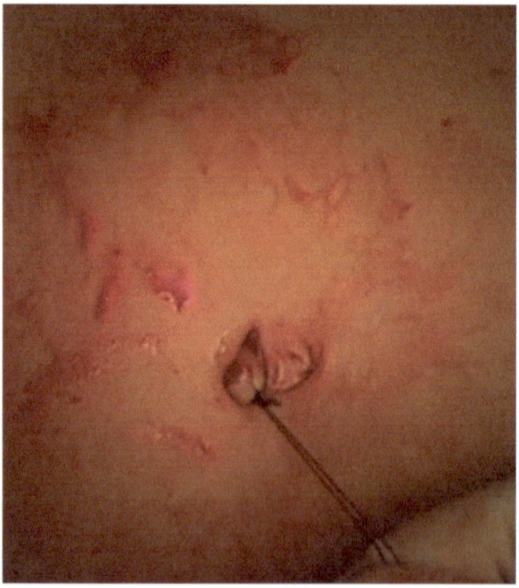

Fig. 34.6. Cauterization of appendix stump after division.

3. The use of a 2-cm Hasson incision and one multi-port trocar can alternatively be inserted in the umbilicus. The technique for intracorporeal appendectomy is discussed below in the three-port laparoscopic appendectomy section.

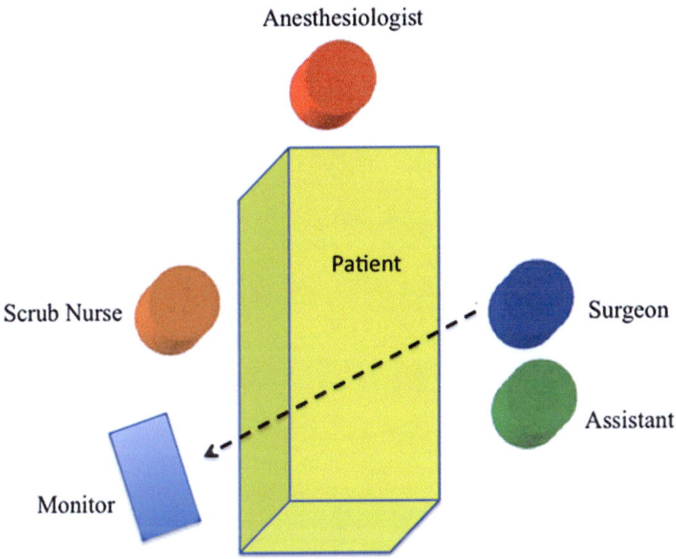

Fig. 34.7. Surgical team position. The surgeon and assistant stand on the left side. The scrub nurse is on the right side.

Traditional Three-Port Laparoscopic Appendectomy

Patient Position and Room Setup

1. Position the patient supine.
2. Although not mandatory, an orogastric tube can be placed to decompress the stomach and similarly a Foley catheter can be placed to decompress the bladder. If the patient urinates prior to surgery, a Foley catheter is rarely required. If placed, both catheters should be removed at the end of the case.
3. The surgeon and assistant stand on the patient's left side. The Mayo stand and scrub nurse are on the patient's right.
4. Place the monitor at the patient's hip on the right or directly below the feet (Fig. 34.7).

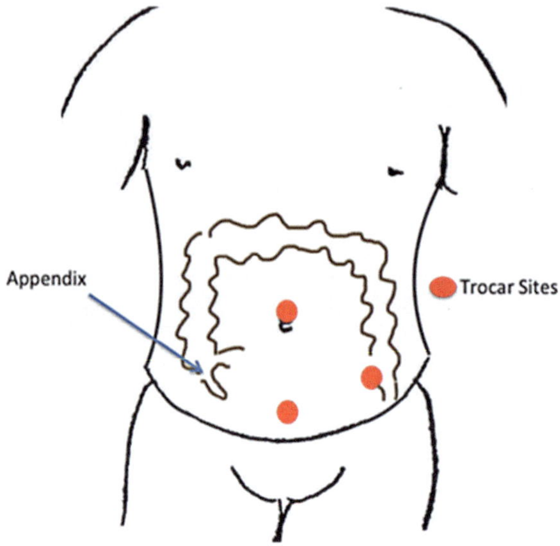

Fig. 34.8. Trocar placement.

Trocar Position and Choice of Laparoscope

1. Prep the abdominal wall from pubis to lower costal margin.
2. Place the initial 10–12 mm port at the umbilicus through open cut-down technique or Veress needle. Carbon dioxide pneumoperitoneum is established at a maximum pressure of 15 mmHg. Insert a 5-mm 30-degree telescope for visualization.
3. Place the second 3- or 5-mm port in the left lower quadrant.
4. The third 3 or 5-mm port is placed in the midline immediately over the pubis. Care is taken to avoid injury to the bladder (Fig. 34.8).

Performing the Appendectomy

1. Place the patient in Trendelenburg position and left side down to allow the intestines to slide out of the pelvis.
2. Perform a thorough exploration to confirm the diagnosis. If the appendix is normal, seek other sources for abdominal pain; run the small bowel to evaluate for a Meckel's diverticulum and in females, examine the ovary for torsion or cyst. If no other source is found, proceed with appendectomy.

3. Utilize two 5-mm atraumatic graspers through the midline suprapubic and left lower quadrant ports.
4. Follow the taenia coli down to their confluence at the base of the cecum and use the grasper through suprapubic port to grab the appendix 1 cm from the base, holding it up and toward the left upper quadrant. Prestige atraumatic graspers (Aesculap, Inc., Center Valley, PA) are an example of blunt graspers that are still sharp enough to get a strong, yet safe, hold of the appendix.
5. If the appendix is adherent to other bowel or abdominal wall, use of the suction as a dissection tool can gently break the adhesions. If the adhesions are not located close to the bowel, hook cautery can be used for dissection. Free the appendix from tip to base, progressing in the opposite direction, if necessary.
6. Intracorporeal division can be performed with the use of Endoloops (Ethicon, Somerville, NJ) or stapling devices.

Endoloop Technique

In many cases, especially when the appendix is very adherent to surrounding structure and a shortened mesoappendix makes it difficult to identify the base of the appendix, the mesoappendix is divided with electrocautery. This technique has proven safe in over 400 cases [19]. Some may prefer to divide the adhesions between the appendix and the surrounding mesentery using energy devices. Once the mesoappendix is divided, three sequential 0 Monofilament Endoloops are used to ligate the base of the appendix, and the appendix is divided sharply between the proximal two loops and the distal loop. Remove the appendix through the umbilical port using a specimen retrieval bag.

Stapling Technique

Create a window in the mesentery at the base of the appendix. A vascular stapler is used to transect the mesoappendix, and another load is used to transect the base of the appendix. Cut the appendix as close as possible to the cecum, leaving a very short stump. Examine the mesentery and base of the appendix for bleeding. Remove the appendix through the umbilical port using a specimen retrieval bag.

Technical Pearls and Pitfalls

- The extracorporeal single-site technique may be challenging in larger patients. However, this challenge can be mitigated by creating a generous infraumbilical incision of 1.5–2 cm.
- Do not waste time. If there is difficulty performing the single-incision technique, do not hesitate to convert to the three-port technique. Creating an iatrogenic perforation in a non-perforated appendix from an overly zealous attempt to extracorporealize may be harmful to the patient.
- Some have described the use of wound protectors or surgical gloves to prevent wound infection in the extracorporeal, single-port technique.
- During three-port laparoscopy with an appendix that is adherent to multiple structures and difficult to dissect, hook cautery may be used to separate the mesoappendix from the appendix.
- Use of endo-loops may be more cost-effective than stapling in the intracorporeal technique [19].
- Single-incision technique may allow for a higher tissue concentration of local anesthetic at the incision.

Postoperative Management

In patients with non-perforated appendicitis, the diet may be advanced as tolerated postoperatively. There is no need for additional antibiotics. Patients may be discharged home when they are tolerating a diet and are afebrile. In patients with perforated appendicitis, inpatient admission is required for broad spectrum intravenous antibiotics. The choice of antibiotics and duration differ based on institutional protocols. The authors prefer daily dosing of intravenous ceftriaxone (50 mg/kg) and metronidazole (30 mg/kg) as described by St. Peter et al. [20].

Complications

1. Bleeding from the epigastric vessels, ileac vessels, and appendicular artery are rare complications that may be avoided with careful port site placement and dissection.
2. Superficial wound infection for non-perforated appendicitis has been shown to be 3.3 % after single-incision appendectomy and 1.7 % after

three-port appendectomy in one series [18]. After laparoscopic appendectomy for perforated appendicitis, superficial wound infection occurred in 0–2 % of patients, but intra-abdominal abscess formation occurred in 16–20 % [20].

3. Intraperitoneal fluid collection or abscess is a common complication following perforated appendicitis. Historically, some surgeons have used irrigation and suction to minimize this risk. However, a recent prospective randomized study suggested no difference between irrigation versus suction alone during laparoscopic appendectomy for perforated appendicitis in a pediatric population [21]. In fact, in a prospective cohort analysis of 1817 adults undergoing laparoscopic appendectomy, peritoneal irrigation was identified as an independent risk factor for postoperative abscess formation [22]. The same study analyzed characteristics of antimicrobial treatment and the incidence of intra-abdominal abscess and found the length of postoperative antibiotic treatment and antimicrobial combination therapy did not affect the development of intra-abdominal abscess, and prolonged antibiotic treatment did not prevent abscess formation.
4. Wound infection from stump leak may occur from disintegration of the avascular appendix base, diathermy burn, or overly tight ligature.
5. Small bowel obstruction is a known complication of appendicitis and can be seen after laparoscopic or open appendectomy procedures, although it appears less commonly than after open appendectomy [23].

Summary

- Laparoscopic appendectomy is the preferred treatment for acute appendicitis.
- Single-incision techniques may be preferred for non-perforated appendicitis in normal-weight children.
- Given the frequency in which pediatric surgeons perform appendectomies, it is important to select surgical devices that are cost-effective.

References

1. John M, Kirkwood KS. Sabiston textbook of surgery. Biological basis of modern surgical practice. Philadelphia: Saunders Elsevier; 2008. p. 1333–47. Appendix.
2. Chaitan K, Eden J, Daniel S, Angela S, Francois I. Effect of delay in presentation on rate of perforation in children with appendicitis. Am J Emerg Med. 2011;7(8):890–3. doi:10.1016/j.ajem.2010.04.005.

3. Wilms IM, de Hoog DE, de Visser DC, Janzing HM. Appendectomy versus antibiotic treatment for acute appendicitis. Cochrane Database Syst Rev. 2011;11, CD008359.
4. Simillis C, Symeonides P, Shorthouse AJ, Tekkis PP. A meta-analysis comparing conservative treatment versus acute appendectomy for complicated appendicitis (abscess or phlegmon). Surgery. 2010;147:818–29.
5. Sauerland S, Jaschinski T, Neugebauer EA. Laparoscopic versus open surgery for suspected appendicitis. Cochrane Database Syst Rev. 2010;10, CD001546.
6. Bennett J, Boddy A, Rhodes M. Choice of approach for appendicectomy: a meta-analysis of open versus laparoscopic appendicectomy. Surg Laparosc Endosc Percutan Tech. 2007;17:245–55.
7. Asarias JR, Schlussel AT, Cafasso DE, Carlson TL, Kasprenski MC, Washington EN, et al. Incidence of postoperative intraabdominal abscesses in open versus laparoscopic appendectomies. Surg Endosc. 2011;25:2678–83.
8. Piskun G, Kozik D, Rajpal S, Shaftan G, Fogler R. Comparison of laparoscopic, open, and converted appendectomy for perforated appendicitis. Surg Endosc. 2001;15:660–2.
9. Merchant AM, Cook MW, White BC, Davis SS, Sweeney JF, Lin E. Transumbilical Gelport access technique for performing single incision laparoscopic surgery (SILS). J Gastrointest Surg. 2009;13:159–62.
10. Chouillard E, Dache A, Torcivia A, Helmy N, Ruseykin I, Gumbs A. Single-incision laparoscopic appendectomy for acute appendicitis: a preliminary experience. Surg Endosc. 2010;24:1861–5.
11. Dapri G, Casali L, Dumont H, Van der Goot L, Herrandou L, Pastijn E, et al. Single-access transumbilical laparoscopic appendectomy and cholecystectomy using new curved reusable instruments: a pilot feasibility study. Surg Endosc. 2011;25:1325–32.
12. Saber AA, Elgamal MH, El-Ghazaly TH, Dewoolkar AV, Akl A. Simple technique for single incision transumbilical laparoscopic appendectomy. Int J Surg. 2010;8:128–30.
13. Ponsky TA, Diluciano J, Chwals W, Parry R, Boulanger S. Early experience with single-port laparoscopic surgery in children. J Laparoendosc Adv Surg Tech A. 2009;19:551–3.
14. Garey CL, Laituri CA, Ostlie DJ, St Peter SD. Single-incision laparoscopic surgery and the necessity for prospective evidence. J Laparoendosc Adv Surg Tech A. 2010;20:503–6.
15. Dutta S. Early experience with single incision laparoscopic surgery: eliminating the scar from abdominal operations. J Pediatr Surg. 2009;44:1741–5.
16. de la Torre RA, Satgunam S, Morales MP, Dwyer CL, Scott JS. Transumbilical single-port laparoscopic adjustable gastric band placement with liver suture retractor. Obes Surg. 2009;19:1707–10.
17. Frutos MD, Abrisqueta J, Lujan J, Abellan I, Parrilla P. Randomized prospective study to compare laparoscopic appendectomy versus umbilical single-incision appendectomy. Ann Surg. 2013;257:413–8.
18. St Peter SD, Adibe OO, Juang D, Sharp SW, Garey CL, Laituri CA, et al. Single incision versus standard 3-port laparoscopic appendectomy: a prospective randomized trial. Ann Surg. 2011;254(4):586–90.

19. Ponsky TA, Rothenberg SS. Division of the mesoappendix with electrocautery in children is safe, effective, and cost-efficient. J Laparoendosc Adv Surg Tech A. 2009; 19(1):S11–3.
20. St Peter SD, Tsao K, Spilde TL, Holcomb GW, Sharp SW, Murphy JP, et al. Single daily dosing ceftriaxone and metronidazole vs standard triple antibiotic regimen for perforated appendicitis in children: a prospective randomized trial. J Pediatr Surg. 2008;43(6):981–5.
21. St Peter SD, Adibe OO, Iqbal CW, Fike FB, Sharp SW, Juang D, et al. Irrigation versus suction alone during laparoscopic appendectomy for perforated appendicitis: a prospective randomized trial. Ann Surg. 2012;256(4):581–5.
22. Cho J, Park I, Lee D, Sung K, Baek J, Lee J. Risk factors for postoperative intra-abdominal abscess after laparoscopic appendectomy: analysis for consecutive 1,817 experiences. Dig Surg. 2015;32:375–81.
23. Tsao KJ, St Peter SD, Valusek PA, Keckler SJ, Sharp S, Holcomb 3rd GW, et al. Adhesive small bowel obstruction after appendectomy in children: comparison between the laparoscopic and open approach. J Pediatr Surg. 2007;42(6):939–42. discussion 942.

35. Laparoscopic Approach to Enteral Access for Chronic Constipation

Andrew T. Strong and Federico G. Seifarth

Introduction

Chronic constipation is a common pediatric complaint, comprising as much as 25 % of a pediatric gastroenterology practice [1]. Surgical intervention with creation of enteral access for antegrade continence enema (ACE) delivery is generally restricted to the patient population with intractable constipation, defined as constipation not responsive to optimal medical treatment for at least 3 months [2]. Fecal impaction is a hard mass in the lower abdomen with excessive stool in a dilated rectum on rectal examination, seen as mass in the distal colon on abdominal radiography [2].

Constipation is associated with nonspecific symptoms, including infrequent and or painful defecation, abdominal pain, and fecal incontinence in some instances [2, 3]. In addition to physical discomfort associated with passing firm stools, chronic intractable constipation (CIC) can be associated with additional psychosocial stress to both children and their caregivers [2]. This is amplified if patients with CIC experience overflow pseudo-incontinence. Despite its high incidence, a strict definition of constipation has been elusive.

While a myriad of definitions of constipation exist in the literature, the various iterations of the Rome Diagnostic Criteria for functional gastrointestinal disorders, created by the Rome Foundation, are the most widespread. The Rome Foundation has defined chronic constipation, dividing the pediatric population using developmental age 4 years as a divider. The most recent definitions are found in the Rome III Guidelines (Table 35.1).

D.S. Walsh et al. (eds.), *The SAGES Manual of Pediatric Minimally Invasive Surgery*, DOI 10.1007/978-3-319-43642-5_35

Table 35.1 Rome III criteria for chronic constipation

In the absence of organic pathology, ≥2 of the following must occur for >1 month in a child with *developmental age < 4 years* [4]
1. ≤2 defecations per week
2. At least one episode of incontinence per week after the acquisition of toileting skills
3. History of excessive stool retention
4. History of painful or hard bowel movements
5. Presence of large fecal mass in the rectum
6. History of large diameter stools that may obstruct the toilet Accompanying symptoms may include irritability, decreased appetite, and early satiety, which may disappear immediately following the passage of a large stool
In the absence of organic pathology, ≥2 of the following must occur at least once per week for >2 months in a *child with developmental age ≥4 years* with insufficient criteria for irritable bowel syndrome [5]
1. ≤2 defecations in the toilet per week
2. At least one episode of fecal incontinence per week
3. History of retentive posturing or excessive volitional stool retention
4. History of painful or hard bowel movements
5. Presence of a large fecal mass in the rectum
6. History of large diameter stools that may obstruct the toilet

Data from Hyman et al. Gastroenterology. 2006; 130(5): 1519–26 and Rasquin et al. Gastroenterology. 2006; 130(5): 1527–37

Epidemiology

True prevalence of childhood constipation is unknown, owing to inconsistent reporting and inconsistent definitions in available literature. Moreover, constipation has often been considered a symptom rather than a primary syndrome or disease, which may lead to further underreporting. A recent systematic review found childhood constipation ranging from 0.7 to 29.6% [IQR 5.3–17.4%] [6]. Those authors additionally report an equal distribution between male and female sex. The peak incidence is 4–6 years of age [6]. Longitudinal data suggest that the prevalence of constipation is increasing. Since 1979, in the United States, the number of outpatient visits with a complaint of constipation has doubled. Children under 15 years of age have the greatest number of outpatient visits for constipation as a chief complaint [7]. Finally, 30% of these patients continue to have symptoms after puberty. Historically, it was thought that constipation was a disease of the developed world, but recent studies in the Asian subcontinent and in Africa have dispelled this myth [6]. Despite high prevalence, only a small proportion of pediatric patients with constipation suffer from intractable constipation requiring surgical intervention.

Pathophysiology

Approximately 95 % of all childhood CIC is a result of a functional disorder without anatomical or physiologic etiology, such as severe idiopathic constipation, psychologic/psychosomatic constipation, nutritional constipation, or colonic inertia. The remaining 5 % of cases have an organic, medical, or anatomic explanation. Hirschsprung disease is the most common of these [3]. Neurogenic causes include myelomeningocele, cerebral palsy, and dysmotility syndromes [3]. Additional neuromuscular disorders are chronic intestinal pseudo-obstruction and intestinal neuronal dysplasia. Anorectal malformations are important to distinguish from others, as the surgical management for these disorders will differ. Anatomic malformations giving rise to CIC include anal fissure, anal stenosis, or imperforate anus [3]. Various endocrine disorders have as a symptom, constipation, which is often corrected with medical management of the primary disorder. These include both hyper- and hypothyroidism, hyperparathyroidism, diabetes mellitus, and diabetes insipidus [3]. Cystic fibrosis (mucoviscidosis) is an example of a genetic disorder causing CIC.

Preoperative Evaluation

A thorough history and physical exam stands at the beginning of every workup, with attention to clinical findings associated with anatomic and neurogenic causes of constipation. Typically, a careful history and a focused physical examination are sufficient to make a diagnosis of a functional disorder giving rise to CIC. It is of highest importance to recognize that patients who present with diarrhea or fecal incontinence as a primary symptom may in fact be experiencing pseudo-incontinence caused by chronic constipation and overflow. There are no telltale physical exam findings associated with idiopathic constipation. Abdominal examination may reveal a firm mass in the abdomen, especially in the left lower quadrant or suprapubic region. A perineal examination is crucial to rule out an anorectal malformation. Digital rectal examination may reveal the presence of stool and give clues about rectal tone.

If there is suspicion of metabolic or endocrine cause for constipation, appropriate laboratory workup should be completed. There are no specific laboratory tests that are necessary for diagnosis of constipation. A recent review found insufficient evidence to support *routine* use of abdominal radiography or colonic transit time studies to diagnose functional constipation. Moreover, no studies investigating rectal ultrasound, anal manometry, suction biopsy, and barium enema met their inclusion criteria and are thus not recommended for diagnosis [2]. However, for the purposes of surgical planning, abdominal X-ray and/or contrast enema may prove to be particularly valuable and rectal biopsies are indicated in all patients with suggestive symptoms for Hirschsprung disease.

Medical Management

Medical management of CIC depends on the underlying etiology of the condition. A combination of laxatives, stool softeners, and enemas is used to achieve symptomatic relief and help to evacuate the colon and thereby maintain continence. Beginning in 2011, the North American Society for Pediatric Gastroenterology, Hepatology and Nutrition (NASPGHAN) joined the European Society for Pediatric Gastroenterology, Hepatology and Nutrition (ESPGHAN) to generate a consensus document regarding treatment of functional constipation [2]. Overall their recommendations favor polyethylene glycol (PEG) for maintenance therapy or lactulose if PEG-enemas are not available [2]. For functional constipation, enemas are not recommended as maintenance therapy in children.

Indications for Surgical Management of Chronic Intractable Constipation

Prior to addressing enteral access for ACE administration, it is important to note that chronic incomplete evacuation can lead to progressive dilation of the rectum and sigmoid which is surgically managed in a different fashion. Four groups of patients may present in this manner:

- The first are patients with spinal disorders.
- The second are patients with anorectal malformations who have undergone prior repair followed by insufficient postoperative bowel management. In these patients CIC related to colonic hypomotility

leads to progressive rectosigmoid dilatation, leading to fecal impaction and eventual overflow pseudo-incontinence. These patients may present with incontinence or diarrhea. This can be easily diagnosed on an abdominal plain film or contrast enema revealing megarectosigmoid colon.

- Patients with Hirschsprung disease are a third group, who due to impaired proprioception or inadequate rectal motility may present with CIC and subsequent rectosigmoid dilation.
- The final group of patients is those with CIC who have failed medical management.

Patients with status post repair of an anorectal malformation may be able to restore normal evacuation with frequent enemas and an aggressive regimen of stimulant laxatives. For patients with irreversible megarectosigmoid due to unaddressed constipation after anorectal malformation repair, Hirschsprung disease, or idiopathic CIC, segmental resection of the dilated sigmoid with a colo-colonic anastomosis is indicated before evaluating enteral access for ACE administration. Sigmoidectomy can be performed in a conventional open operation, laparoscopically, transanally, or in a hybrid technique [8]. In general, a great proportion of the rectum should be preserved in patients with prior repair of anorectal malformations to allow for a reservoir for stool to produce a feeling of fullness. Patients with idiopathic CIC may undergo more complete rectal resection, as sphincter function and proprioception tend to be intact. Patients who have true fecal incontinence are not well served with sigmoidal resection, as it may convert a tendency toward constipation to one toward softer stools, exacerbated by laxative therapy. Thus patients with CIC and true fecal incontinence are better served with enteral access for ACE administration.

When medical management fails to resolve constipation, patients with neurogenic or neuromuscular causes of chronic constipation, anorectal malformations, and patients with idiopathic CIC utilize daily enemas to achieve evacuation. Adherence to a regular bowel management program can achieve social continence for many of these patients, but as they grow older, it becomes more convenient for them to be able to manage enema administration independently. In these patients, ACE administration has been demonstrated to improve quality of life [9, 10]. Patients who have not demonstrated some degree of success with rectal enemas are unlikely to have additional benefit from antegrade enemas. A careful assessment and preparation of the patients is crucial for the success of an antegrade enema operation. At least a 3-month course of retrograde enemas to prove responsiveness and compliance should be completed prior to consideration of enteral access ACE administration. Moreover, ACE delivery may require a lifelong commitment from the patient. Diverting ostomies and colectomy, except as discussed above, are not discussed in this chapter, but in some cases may be alternative surgical options.

Technique for Surgical Enteral Access for Antegrade Enemas

Antegrade enemas have been shown to be effective, and a variety of enteral access surgeries have been devised based on a flap-valve continence mechanism popularized by Mitrofanoff [11, 12].

Malone Procedure

The Malone procedure for antegrade continence enema (MACE) and its laparoscopic equivalent, laparoscopic antegrade continence enema (LACE), are widely accepted surgical options first described in 1990. The appendix is used to create a catheterizable stoma, allowing access to the cecum [13, 14]. LACE is recommended if no additional procedure is needed to aid in urinary continence. In the classic MACE procedure, a muscle cutting right lower quadrant incision is made, and the stoma is customarily placed in the right lower quadrant. The stoma may be placed higher if the patient is wheelchair bound for ease of access. In recent years, most pediatric surgeons support the minimally invasive LACE approach. The resultant stoma from a LACE procedure is created in the umbilicus, preferably with a continence valve mechanism. LACE is performed under general anesthesia. The patient is positioned supine. A 5 mm port is placed in the umbilicus, and two additional 5 mm ports are placed either within the bilateral iliac fossae or in the left upper and lower quadrants. The cecum is mobilized such that the appendix can easily reach the umbilicus. Care must be taken to preserve the appendiceal vascular supply during mobilization. Creation of a continence valve using the cecum during a MACE or LACE procedure is recommended to prevent retrograde stool leakage. The cecum is mobilized more extensively and delivered extracorporeally, which may require a longer infraumbilical incision. A mesenteric window is fashioned to preserve the vascular supply the appendix. The appendix is folded along its base and the cecum is

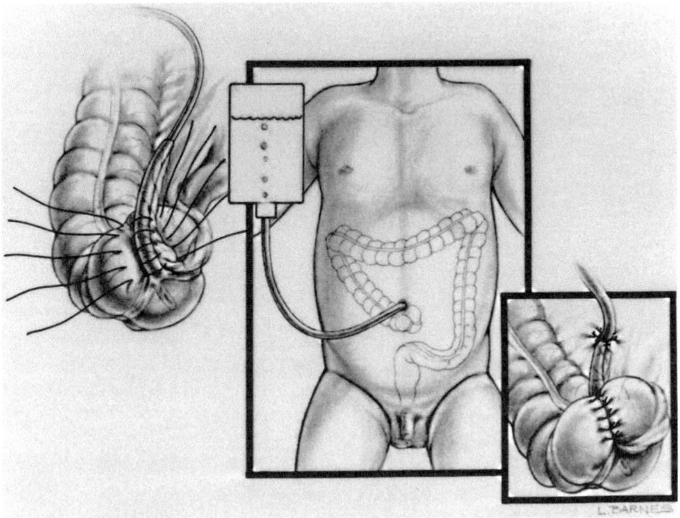

Fig. 35.1. Formation of continent appendicostomy. From left to right: plication of the cecum to create continence valve, final position of ostomy and colon with administration of antegrade enema, and final appearance of the suture continence valve. From Alberto Peña, Andrea Bischoff [15]. Reprinted with permission from Springer.

plicated around the base of the appendix (Fig. 35.1). The umbilical skin is incised in a V fashion for the appendix to skin V-Y anastomosis, which reduces the incidence of anastomotic strictures. To form the appendicostomy, the umbilicus is everted, and a V-shaped incision is made (vertex at the most distal portion of the umbilicus). The skin flap is then sutured around one half the circumference of the conduit and the remaining portion of the conduit is sutured to the umbilical rim V-Y technique) (Fig. 35.2). The stoma is created around a 10–12 French catheter, which should remain in situ for 4 weeks postoperatively.

In some cases the appendix is either surgically absent or has been used as a conduit to create an appendico-vesicostomy for bladder drainage during a simultaneous procedure (Mitrofanoff procedure). A neoappendix can be created from a tubularized cecal flap. A rectangular flap is fashioned from the anteromedial wall of the cecum. The flap is created with one or two mesenteric blood vessels for arterial inflow. The base of the flap must be fashioned such that once plicated, it is oriented toward the umbilicus. Typically the flap is 6–8 cm in length and must be of sufficient width to close around an 8–10 French catheter. Visualizing the flap can

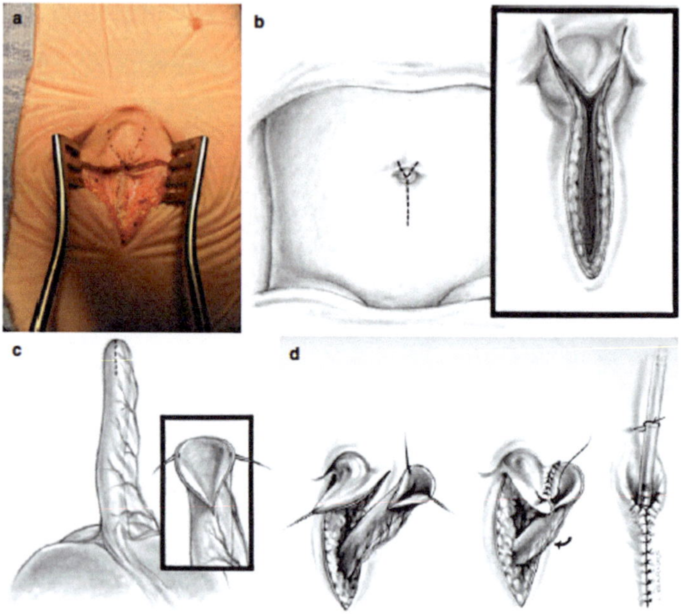

Fig. 35.2. Formation of the V-Y appendicostomy. (**a**) Intraoperative image. (**b**) Schematic of incision. (**c**) Appendiceal tip is cut to form an opening with an apex. (**d**) The triangular skin flap is sutured to the spatulated appendix, aligning the apex of the skin with the apex of the appendiceal opening. From Alberto Peña, Andrea Bischoff [15]. Reprinted with permission from Springer.

be thought of as two transverse cuts, parallel with the haustra, and a longitudinal cut connecting these two near the line of Toldt. The cecum is closed transversely and this suture line is continued, plicating the flap edges around a catheter. The cecum is then plicated around the neo-appendix to create a valve mechanism. The umbilical stoma is then fashioned in a similar V-Y fashion as described above

A final variation of the Malone technique involves utilizing the sigmoid to create a tubularized colonic flap to fashion a left-sided stoma that allows antegrade enemas into the proximal to mid sigmoid. This may result in more rapid evacuation and smaller enema doses.

Yang–Monti Procedure

A second variation to create a neo-appendix uses a segment of ileum (Yang–Monti procedure), in patients with absent appendix or patients status post Mitrofanoff procedure. The Yang–Monti procedure has been described with both a standard laparoscopic and robotic technique, though historically, it is more commonly performed as an open operation. The patient is in lithotomy and reverse Trendelenburg position to facilitate small bowel falling out of the pelvis. Four trocars are placed: a 5 mm or 10 mm camera port in the umbilicus, two 5 mm lateral working ports along the midclavicular line, and one 5 mm port between the umbilicus and pubis. Once intra-abdominal access is obtained and pneumoperitoneum established, a 2–3 cm ileal segment is isolated on a vascular pedicle. Intestinal continuity is restored with an end-to-end anastomosis. The pedicled ileal segment is opened longitudinally along its antimesenteric aspect and then tubularized around a 10–12 French catheter. One end of this conduit can be implanted to any easily reachable colonic segment, and the other used to create a stoma in the umbilicus or elsewhere in the abdominal wall.

Cecostomy Tube

A cecostomy tube is a viable alternative to an appendicostomy, ileal, or colonic conduit. In this technique a catheter is inserted directly into the cecum either with percutaneous techniques or with laparoscopic assistance. Certain tubes contain a continence valve to prevent retrograde leakage of stool (Fig. 35.3). Percutaneous cecostomy may be placed without (image-guided cecostomy) or with colonoscopic assistance for visualization. Depending upon local practice patterns, an image-guided percutaneous cecostomy tube may be placed by interventional radiology, gastroenterology, or the pediatric surgeon. All patients are given aggressive bowel preparation and asked to remain on a liquid diet for 1–2 days prior to the procedure. For an image-guided percutaneous procedure, the patient is brought to a room with C-arm capabilities. Either local or general anesthesia is used. The patient is positioned in a partial left lateral decubitus position (left side down) or full decubitus (left side down fetal position) with arms secured above the head. Ultrasound examination of the abdomen is preformed first to identify

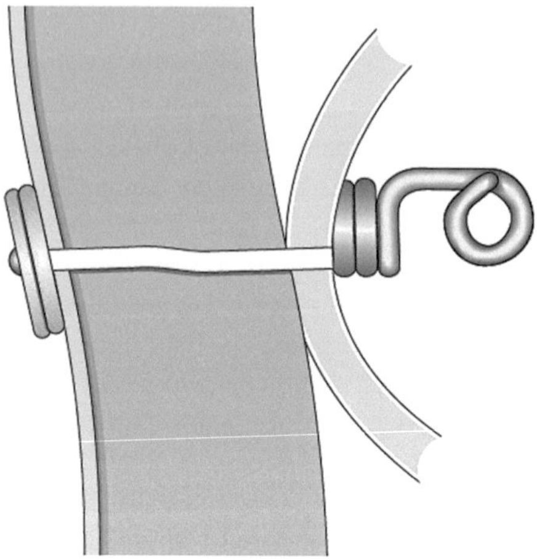

Fig. 35.3. Chait tube in situ. Image left is the skin. Pigtail is located within the cecum. From Yagmurlu A [16]. Reprinted with permission from Springer.

position of abdominal organs. A rectal Foley catheter is placed and used to insufflate the colon and cecum under fluoroscopic guidance. Generally the cecum is punctured under fluoroscopic guidance with a needle preloaded with retention sutures to oppose the cecum to the anterior abdominal wall. Using the Seldinger technique, the tract is dilated to accommodate an 8 French temporary catheter. Following placement, intraluminal position is confirmed with contrast injection and the tube is vented and secured [17, 18]. The colonoscopic corollary is placed in a manner identical to a percutaneous gastrostomy tube. A colonoscope is introduced and advanced to the cecum. Transillumination of the abdominal wall is used to aid in placement of a needle through which a guidewire is placed and grasped by a snare in the accessory port of the colonoscope. The entire scope is removed, and a bumpered tube is secured to the guidewire, which is pulled in a retrograde fashion to the cecum with the guidewire and secured [19]. Alternatively, cecostomy tube placement can be achieved similar to gastrostomy button placement using the push technique (see chapter: Minimally Invasive Gastrostomy).

The final variation of the cecostomy tube is a laparoscopic-assisted percutaneous endoscopic cecostomy (LAPEC), which extends the colonoscopic-assisted percutaneous cecostomy tube placement. In the operating room, general anesthesia is induced. A 5 mm umbilical trocar is placed and an additional two 5 mm ports are placed. The colonoscope is advanced, and the percutaneous tube is placed in the same manner as above with the exception of the initial retention sutures. The working laparoscopic ports may be used to assist in guiding the colon over the endoscope and holding the cecum to aid in needle insertion. Following tube placement, the cecum may be sutured to the anterior abdominal wall. Postoperative care is similar to the percutaneous cecostomy tube [20, 21].

Cecostomy tubes present several advantages over appendicostomy, colonic conduit, or ileal conduit. First, it is a relatively quick procedure that in some cases may even be able to be performed in the office setting. While there are similar issues with leakage, there is no risk of stomal stricture. Tube dislodgment is a risk and can be managed with repeat LAPEC or an open insertion technique. Relief of constipation and efficacy of ACE administration is as good or better than with the Malone or Yang–Monti procedures [21]. Moreover, prior to committing a patient to a stoma, a variation of the cecostomy tube can be used to create a percutaneous endoscopic colostomy tube in the sigmoid colon, which can be used as trial prior to formalization as a stoma depending upon response to treatment and patient preference.

Pearls and Pitfalls

Perhaps the most important pearls for ACE procedures relate to patient selection. All patients must both demonstrate successful emptying with retrograde enemas and compliance with regular administration prior to pursuing ACE. For obese patients, an umbilical appendicostomy is recommended, as it increases the likelihood of success in self-catheterization. Effective intraoperative positioning may aid in dissection and mobilization. Similar to performing a laparoscopic appendectomy, rotating the table such that the patient is right side up, and/or in Trendelenburg position may provide better visualization. This is true whether mobilizing the native appendix or creating a neo-appendix from a tubularized cecal flap with which to create the ostomy. When plicating the cecum around the appendix to form the continence valve, it is prudent to pass the feeding tube after each suture to verify unrestricted passage. In forming the ostomy, while spatulation may present a technically simpler technique, it is associated with a relatively high rate of stricture. The V-Y anastomosis avoids a circular suture line, which in turn proffers a decreased risk of stricture. Finally, cecostomy tubes can be viewed as either an end therapy or a trial of ACE, prior to committing the patient to a surgically formed catheterizable stoma.

Postoperative Care

Postoperative recovery is generally rapid. Enteral nutrition can begin on the first day or two postoperatively. Patients and/or caregivers must be given instruction in enema administration and be comfortable performing them prior to discharge. If the patient's native appendix is used, daily irrigations are begun after 24 h. The catheter or tube can be removed as early as 2 weeks after surgery. If a neo-appendix is created, the tube inserted at the time of stoma formation should be left in situ for 4 weeks postoperatively to allow full maturation of the stoma and reduce the risk of early stomal stenosis. Thereafter, twice daily catheterization should be performed, without regard to enema administration, which is typically once daily. In the case of a cecostomy tube, an oral diet is introduced over 1–2 days post op. The tube is irrigated twice daily with small volumes of saline. Enema administration typically begins after 10 days. The temporary catheter is exchanged for a more permanent Chait Trapdoor cecostomy tube 6–8 weeks after the initial procedure [17, 18].

Outcomes

The Malone procedure is associated with a high degree of success. A recent paper reviewed 203 consecutive ACE procedures by a single surgeon over 15 years with mean follow-up time of more than 5 years. Within the study group, 81 % had carried a preoperative diagnosis of chronic idiopathic constipation. All but six had an appendicostomy; the balance had a neo-appendix formed in one of the manners noted above. At follow-up, 93 % of patients regularly had a good result from enema administration, 6 % had a variable result, and one person had a poor outcome. There were 17 (9 %) that failed to reduce symptoms. There were 53 patients (26 %) who discontinued use due to resolution of constipation symptoms; 32 of these patients had their ACE enteral access reversed [22]. In a separate study of 117 patients with ACE, 69 % reported successful symptom resolution and an additional 20 % partial relief. Stomal stenosis developed in 38 % of patients, a leak in 35 % of all patients and stomal infection in 25 %. Stomal stenosis and/or leakage was generally an indication for revision, which occurred in 33 % of the patients [23]. Complication rates for formation of a neo-appendix have not been studied separately but are expected to follow trends of Malone-type appendicostomies. Studies of the Yang–Monti ileo-cecostomy have not been done; however, extrapolation from ileo-vesicostomy literature suggests that the majority of the patients achieved satisfactory symptom relief and cosmetic result [24].

Cecostomy tubes are generally well tolerated. A recent review of 290 patients with percutaneously placed cecostomy tubes found that while roughly 1/3 had complications, 85 % of early and 98 % of late complications were minor. Site pain, local inflammation, and nausea were the most common early complications. Late complications included tube dislodgement, leakage, and site pain [17].

Management of Complications

The two most common postoperative complications are stomal stenosis (~30 %) and leakage of enteric contents (~30 %). Stenosis may be managed with gentle dilation using soft catheters. In more severe stenosis, dilation with rigid dilators may be necessary in the operating room. Patients may require stomal revision. Leakage can be managed with local wound care and is generally self-limited. Persistent drainage can be managed in the operating room by either creating a continence valve if not formed at the index operation or complete revision of the conduit and stoma. In general, an easy-to-treat though high complication rate is a small price to pay for a continent stoma.

Summary

- Enteral access for ACE administration is indicated for patients with CIC who have failed other medical treatments but who are responsive to regular administration of retrograde enemas.
- Careful history and physical exam is necessary to identify certain correctable abnormalities leading to chronic constipation, including anatomic malformation.
- Several options exist to provide enteral access. Most surgeons favor laparoscopic or endoscopic techniques, which often offer a short hospital stay and low perioperative morbidity. Longer-term morbidity, while relatively common, is most often easily managed.
- In most cases there is an improvement in quality of life and relief of constipation symptoms for patients with surgical access for ACE; however, in many cases, establishing enteral access for ACE administration represents a lifelong commitment to that therapy, and as such preoperative education is of utmost importance.

References

1. Baker SS, Liptak GS, Colletti RB, Croffie JM, Di Lorenzo C, Ector W, et al. Constipation in infants and children: evaluation and treatment. A medical position statement of the North American Society for Pediatric Gastroenterology and Nutrition. J Pediatr Gastroenterol Nutr. 1999;29:612–26.
2. Tabbers MM, DiLorenzo C, Berger MY, Faure C, Langendam MW, Nurko S, et al. Evaluation and treatment of functional constipation in infants and children: evidence-based recommendations from ESPGHAN and NASPGHAN. J Pediatr Gastroenterol Nutr. 2014;58:258–74.
3. Pashankar DS. Childhood constipation: evaluation and management. Clin Colon Rectal Surg. 2005;18:120–7.
4. Hyman PE, Milla PJ, Benninga MA, Davidson GP, Fleisher DF, Taminiau J. Childhood functional gastrointestinal disorders: neonate/toddler. Gastroenterology. 2006;130: 1519–26.
5. Rasquin A, Di Lorenzo C, Forbes D, Guiraldes E, Hyams JS, Staiano A, et al. Childhood functional gastrointestinal disorders: child/adolescent. Gastroenterology. 2006;130:1527–37.
6. Van den Berg MM, Benninga MA, Di Lorenzo C. Epidemiology of childhood constipation: a systematic review. Am J Gastroenterol. 2006;101:2401–9.
7. Everhart JE, Ruhl CE. Burden of digestive diseases in the United States part II: lower gastrointestinal diseases. Gastroenterology. 2009;136:741–54.
8. Levitt MA, Pena A. Chapter 15: laparoscopy in the management of fecal incontinence and constipation. In: Holcomb III GW, Georgeson KE, Rothenberg SS, editors. Atlas of pediatric laparoscopy and thoracoscopy. Philadelphia: Saunders Elsevier; 2008. p. 81–9.
9. Har AF, Rescorla FJ, Croffie JM. Quality of life in pediatric patients with unremitting constipation pre and post Malone Antegrade Continence Enema (MACE) procedure. J Pediatr Surg. 2013;48:1733–7.
10. Mattix KD, Novotny NM, Shelley AA, Rescorla FJ. Malone antegrade continence enema (MACE) for fecal incontinence in imperforate anus improves quality of life. Pediatr Surg Int. 2007;23:1175–7.
11. Mitrofanoff P. Trans-appendicular continent cystostomy in the management of the neurogenic bladder. Chir Pediatr. 1980;21:297–305.
12. Malone P. Chapter 54: malone procedure for antegrade continence enemas. In: Spitz L, Coran AC, editors. Operative pediatric surgery. 6th ed. London: Hodder Arnold; 2006. p. 537–47.
13. Malone PS, Ransley PG, Kiely EM. Preliminary report: the antegrade continence enema. Lancet. 1990;336:1217–8.
14. Roberts JP, Moon S, Malone PS. Treatment of neuropathic urinary and faecal incontinence with synchronous bladder reconstruction and the antegrade continence enema procedure. Br J Urol. 1995;75:386–9.

15. Pena A, Bischoff A. Chapter 21: operations for the administration of antegrade enemas. In: Surgical treatment of colorectal problems in children. Switzerland: Springer International; 2015. p. 333–47.
16. Yagmurlu A. Laparoscopic cecostomy and sigmoidostomy button. In: Endoscopic surgery in infants and children. Berlin: Springer International; 2008. p. 335–8.
17. Khan WU, Satkunasingham J, Moineddin R, Jamal I, Afzal S, Chait P, et al. The percutaneous cecostomy tube in the management of fecal incontinence in children. J Vasc Interv Radiol. 2015;26:189–95.
18. Chait PG, Shlomovitz E, Connolly BL, Temple MJ, Restrepo R, Amaral JG, et al. Percutaneous cecostomy: updates in technique and patient care 1. Radiology. 2003;227:246–50.
19. Rivera MT, Kugathasan S, Berger W, Werlin SL. Percutaneous colonoscopic cecostomy for management of chronic constipation in children. Gastrointest Endosc. 2001; 53:225–8.
20. DeFreest L, Smith J, Whyte C. Laparoscopic-assisted percutaneous cecostomy for antegrade continence enema. J Laparoendosc Adv Surg Tech A. 2014;24:261–4.
21. Rodriguez L, Flores A, Gilchrist BF, Goldstein AM. Laparoscopic-assisted percutaneous endoscopic cecostomy in children with defecation disorders (with video). Gastrointest Endosc. 2011;73:98–102.
22. Randall J, Coyne P, Jaffray B. Follow up of children undergoing antegrade continent enema: experience of over two hundred cases. J Pediatr Surg. 2014;49:1405–8.
23. Siddiqui AA, Fishman SJ, Bauer SB, Nurko S. Long-term follow-up of patients after antegrade continence enema procedure. J Pediatr Gastroenterol Nutr. 2011;52: 574–80.
24. Boemers T, Schimke C, Ardelean M, Ludwikowski B. Evaluation of urinary and faecal continent stomas. J Pediatr Urol. 2005;1:85–8.

36. Laparoscopic-Assisted Pull-Through for Hirschsprung's Disease

Richard Cheek, Lauren Salesi, and Stefan Scholz

Etiology

Congenital aganglionic megacolon, or Hirschsprung's disease (HD), is a disorder characterized by an absence of ganglion cells in the distal intestine. It commonly presents as a functional obstruction in the newborn period. It affects up to 1 in 5000 live births [1, 2]. It occurs more commonly in males than females, with a ratio of 4:1, respectively [2, 3]. The median age of diagnosis is 2–6 months [4]. It is associated with other congenital anomalies in 18–20 % of cases, commonly involving the neurological, cardiovascular, urological, or gastrointestinal systems [5, 6].

Genetics

Hirschsprung's disease is known to have a genetic basis; however the inheritance pattern is complex. In addition to familial cases, it can occur in conjunction with a variety of other genetic diseases. Chromosomal anomalies are seen in 12 % of cases, and trisomy 21 is the most common (2–10 % of HD patients) [1, 2, 6–11]. Interestingly, an anomaly has been identified involving a locus on chromosome 10 that is associated with the *RET* oncogene [12]. Given this association it is not surprising that HD has been linked to familial medullary thyroid carcinoma, as well as multiple endocrine neoplasia type 2A [13–20]. Other conditions that have been associated with HD include Waardenburg syndrome, congenital central

D.S. Walsh et al. (eds.), *The SAGES Manual of Pediatric Minimally Invasive Surgery*, DOI 10.1007/978-3-319-43642-5_36

hypoventilation syndrome, Shprintzen–Goldberg syndrome, McKusick–Kaufman syndrome, Bardet–Biedl syndrome, Smith–Lemli–Opitz syndrome, cartilage–hair hypoplasia syndrome, and various limb anomalies and other isolated conditions [6].

Pathophysiology

During normal gestation, the enteric nervous system is formed by the migration of neural crest cells from proximal to distal along the gut. These pluripotent stem cells then differentiate into the ganglia of the submucosal (Meissner) and myenteric (Auerbach) plexuses. Hirschsprung's disease occurs when this process is incomplete. The result is an absence of normal innervation to the most distal portion of the GI tract. The aganglionic segment is unable to dilate and causes a functional obstruction, with normal bowel becoming distended proximally. The total length of the aganglionic segment is variable. Long-segment HD is defined as aganglionosis extending proximally beyond the splenic flexure. The anus is involved in all cases; the rectosigmoid colon is affected in 80 % of patients, the splenic flexure or transverse colon in 17 %, and the entire colon in 8 % [2].

Diagnosis

Over 90 % of patients present during the first 24–48 h of life with symptoms such as abdominal distention, bilious emesis, and failure to pass meconium [2, 21]. In other instances, the presentation may be more indolent, and the diagnosis may be delayed for months or years. These patients typically suffer from chronic constipation, bloating, abdominal pain, poor weight gain, and feeding intolerance. When HD is suspected, workup should include plain abdominal X-ray and barium enema. If a transition zone is seen on contrast enema between normal or dilated bowel and the constricted distal segment, this is generally considered pathognomonic for HD (Fig. 36.1) [22]. Furthermore, failure to evacuate the contrast completely within 24 h is suggestive of the disease. More commonly, these studies may support but not necessarily confirm the diagnosis. Confirmation of HD is based on histological evaluation of tissue samples. Suction rectal biopsy is the gold standard for making the diagnosis. There is a normal paucity of ganglia in the region of the internal sphincter; therefore the biopsy should be taken at least 1–2 cm above

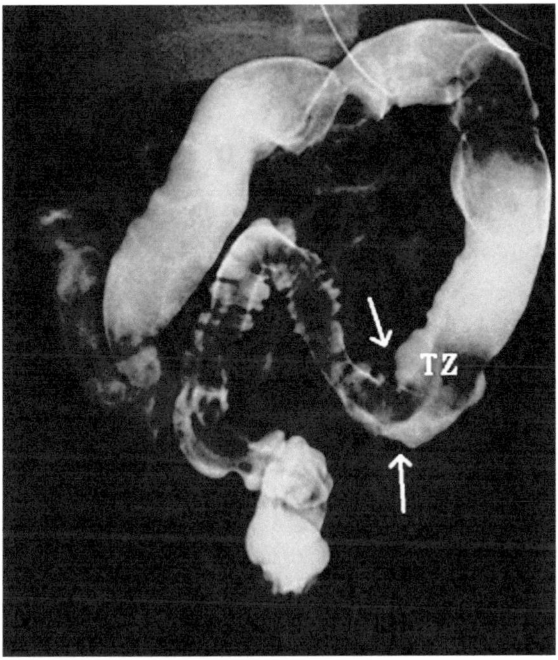

Fig. 36.1. Contrast enema post evacuation phase demonstrating the transition zone (*arrows*). The aganglionic Hirschsprung's bowel is distal to the transition zone (TZ—transition zone), which is less than 5 cm in length in most cases.

the dentate line. Acetylcholinesterase staining will demonstrate hypertrophied nerve trunks and a lack of normal ganglia in classical HD. Loss of calretinin immunostaining is also consistent with the diagnosis of HD [23].

Treatment

Traditionally, surgical treatment for Hirschsprung's disease was performed in two or even three stages. A leveling colostomy was done in the first stage, and this was subsequently reversed at a later time. Today, with advances in surgical techniques and perioperative management, surgery in uncomplicated cases is usually done as a single stage via minimally invasive approaches [24–27]. During the operation, frozen section seromuscular biopsies as well as the final doughnut are sent to determine the proximal margin of the resected segment. Care must be taken to resect all the abnormally innervated bowel including the transition zone bowel.

Surgical Techniques

Three surgical options were originally described to treat HD. The Swenson procedure involves excising the full-thickness aganglionic segment of bowel to the level just proximal to the internal sphincter and performing a colo-anal anastomosis. In the Soave procedure, the aganglionic segment is removed, but only the mucosa is resected from the aganglionic rectum. The normally ganglionated proximal bowel is then pulled through the split muscular cuff and a colo-anal anastomosis is created. The Soave procedure avoids any pelvic dissection and associated complications, such as pelvic nerve damage, seen with the Swenson. In the Duhamel procedure, the full-thickness rectal stump is left in place. The normal proximal bowel is pulled down posteriorly in the retrorectal space. A stapler placed through the anus is then used to create a side-to-side anastomosis. In this neorectum, the anterior wall is comprised of the aganglionic native rectum, and the posterior wall is normally innervated proximal bowel. This functional composition of the neorectal reservoir is intended to provide a more natural emptying mechanism, especially in cases of long-segment Hirschsprung's disease when the ileum may have to be pulled through. These original procedures have evolved into the modern era of surgery, and they are now frequently performed via transanal and/or laparoscopic approaches or a combination of both [2, 22].

Laparoscopic-Assisted Transanal Pull-Through (Georgeson/Soave Technique)

Appropriate Patient Selection

The diagnosis of HD must be confirmed by an experienced, reliable pathologist with a rectal biopsy. This technique is best suited for short-segment disease, and ideally the patient would have a barium enema study demonstrating a distal transition zone. Longer segment disease is a relative contraindication for this surgical option, and these patients may be better served by a Duhamel procedurel. Prematurity is a relative contraindication, as these patients may not have fully mature ganglion cells and histologic evaluation of biopsies may therefore not be reliable. The patients are managed with rectal stimulation and irrigation until term. Strict contraindications include significant malnutrition, active enterocolitis, or massively dilated proximal bowel; these patients should undergo a staged procedure, with an initial colostomy and a definitive operation once the contraindication has resolved.

Preparation

Preoperative antibiotics are given to cover gram-negative and anaerobic organisms. Surgical Care Improvement Project (SCIP) guidelines should be followed. Some surgeons recommend on-table colonic and rectal lavage with warm, diluted Betadine solution via a red rubber catheter. A formal preoperative bowel preparation is not recommended due to the presence of functional distal obstruction.

The procedure is performed with the patient under general anesthesia in the lithotomy position. A sterile circumferential lower body preparation is used. No IVs or lines should be in the lower extremities. After the prep, a urinary catheter is placed sterilely.

Laparoscopic-Assisted Leveling Biopsy

Prior to beginning the transanal portion of the operation, the exact location of the transition zone must be confirmed. Laparoscopy offers an efficient and minimally invasive approach to this step. One camera port and two working ports are placed on the right side of the abdomen and pneumoperitoneum is established (Fig. 36.2). The descending and sigmoid colon are visualized to identify the transition zone, which can be difficult to reliably see in neonates. A Hegar dilator placed transanally may facilitate elevation and manipulation of the sigmoid colon during this step.

A biopsy site is then chosen 2 cm proximal to the assumed transition zone, on the anti-mesenteric side of the colon. A "knuckle" of bowel is then grasped with Maryland forceps. Using scissors, a partial-thickness, seromuscular biopsy is taken (Fig. 36.3). Some surgeons prefer to take full-thickness biopsies on request of their pathologists; however, there currently is no definitive evidence that either of these strategies is superior. A stitch may be warranted to repair the defect at the biopsy site, in order to prevent contamination of the peritoneal cavity during the case. The biopsy is then sent for frozen section examination by the pathologist. While this is being done, the mesentery of the colon distal

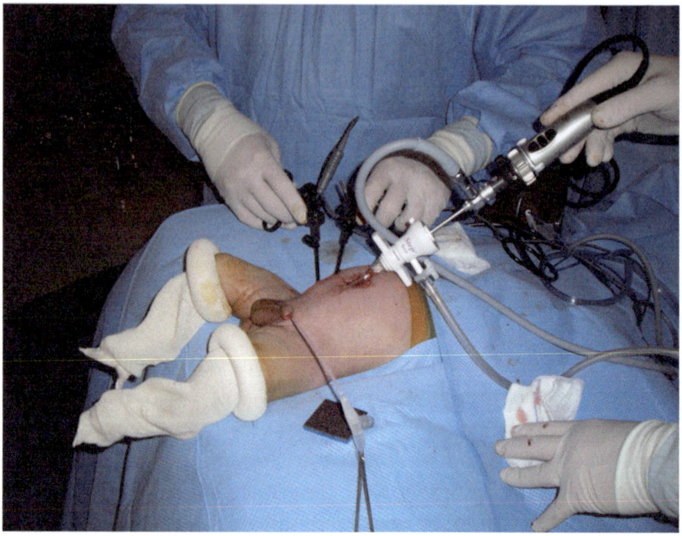

Fig. 36.2. Sterile lower body preparation with typical instrument position for laparoscopically assisted pull-through procedure. An additional 3 mm instrument may be placed transabdominally in the left upper quadrant for retraction if more extensive mesocolonic dissection for a longer segment of aganglionated colon becomes necessary (from http://www.clsnyder.com/WordPress/2008/05/19/hirschsprungs-disease-lap-assisted-transanal-pullthrough-tutorial/).

to the biopsy site can be taken down, staying close to the bowel (Fig. 36.4). If the pathologist cannot confirm normal ganglion cells and nerve fibers, additional biopsies will need to be taken, marching proximally until a normally ganglionated bowel with normal nerve fibers is found. Care must be taken to include transition zone bowel with some, but not all, completely normal ganglion cells into the pull-through. In most cases, the transition zone is less than 5 cm in length.

All mesenteric attachments are divided up to the confirmed normal colon. If there is concern that there is not enough length to reach the anus, the lateral peritoneal attachments to the colon along the white line of Toldt can be taken down laparoscopically, including the splenic flexure if necessary. While waiting for the frozen section of the biopsy specimen to confirm anatomically normal colon with ganglion cells and nerve fibers, the mesocolon can be dissected distal toward the rectum using the monopolar hook cautery or the JustRight bipolar dissector (JustRight Surgical, LLC, Louisville, CO). The mesenteric vessels should be divided proximal

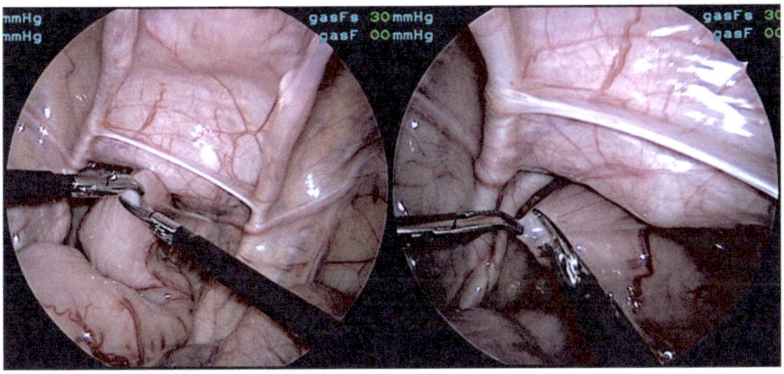

Fig. 36.3. Using scissors, one or two partial-thickness, seromuscular biopsies are taken. Some surgeons prefer to take full-thickness biopsies on request of their pathologists. The biopsy site should be closed with a figure-of-eight suture to prevent contamination and mark the area during the pull-through (Courtesy of Marcus D. Jarboe, MD, C.S. Mott Children's Hospital, University of Michigan, Ann Arbor, MI, USA).

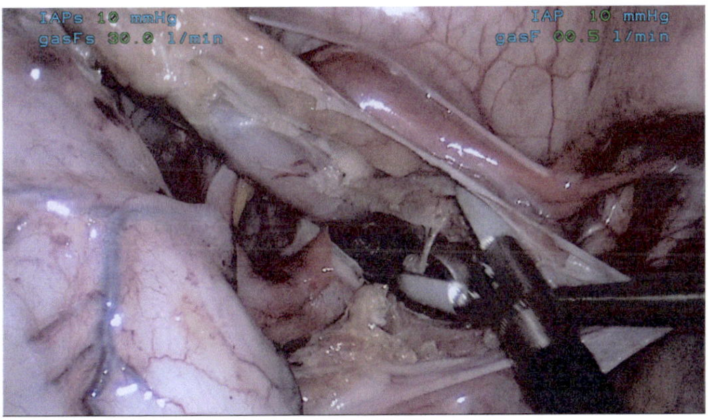

Fig. 36.4. Laparoscopic mesocolic dissection using the Maryland-shaped LigaSure device while awaiting the frozen section result of the colon biopsy. Alternatively, monopolar hook cautery works well for infants (Courtesy of Marcus D. Jarboe, MD, C.S. Mott Children's Hospital, University of Michigan, Ann Arbor, MI, USA).

to the marginal arteries, thereby gaining length while maintaining perfusion through this collateral arcade. The pelvic peritoneal reflection can be dissected to facilitate the transanal portion of the surgery. In some cases, when the biopsy specimen shows transition zone bowel, an additional, more proximal biopsy has to be taken. Once the leveling biopsy

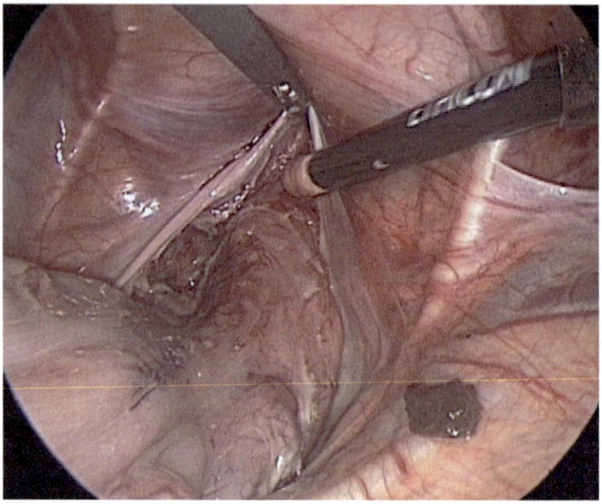

Fig. 36.5. After the laparoscopic mesocolic dissection has been performed, the pelvic peritoneal reflection can be divided. Some minimally invasive surgeons who prefer a Swenson-type full-thickness proctectomy perform part or most of the proctectomy laparoscopically instead of solely through the anus. Adapted from Technical modification of the Georgeson procedure for Hirschsprung's disease: a 12 Years experience with the laparoscopic-assisted mesocolon dissection. Ruggeri G, Randi B, Gargano T, Libri M, Maffi M, Lima M. JEMIS – Journal of Endoscopic, Minimally Invasive Surgery in Newborn, Children and Adolescent – ISSN 2283–7116 (DOI: http://dx.medra.org/10.1473/JEMIS14)).

site has established normal colon, the abdomen is desufflated and attention is turned to the perineum. Some surgeons prefer to continue with laparoscopic "full-thickness" proctectomy in the Swenson plane into the lower pelvis before turning to the transanal portion of the case (Fig. 36.5).

Transanal Pull-Through

The operating surgeon sits at the foot of the bed. Visualization may be augmented with Trendelenburg positioning and the use of a headlight. The anal canal is everted using either the Lone Star retractor or interrupted silk sutures, depending on surgeon preference. The squamocolumnar transitional epithelium, or dentate line, is identified. It is crucial that this transitional epithelium remains intact (Fig. 36.6). A nasal speculum is inserted into the anus to provide exposure. Using needle-tip electrocautery, a circumferential mucosal incision is made 0.5 cm above the dentate

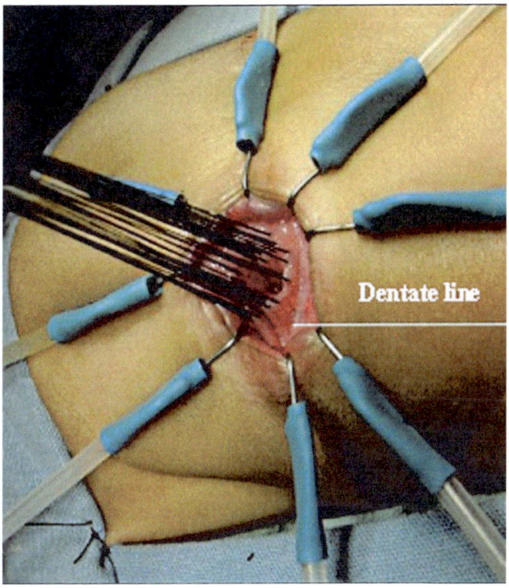

Fig. 36.6. Start of the transanal part of the minimally invasive pull-through procedure (Soave or Swenson). A Lone Star retractor is used to evert the anus and visualize the dentate line. Retraction sutures are placed in the rectal mucosa 1 cm above the dentate line. It is very important to make an incision with appropriate distance proximal to the dentate line since injury of the dentate line may lead to fecal incontinence later. Please note that this picture was taken from a completely transanal procedure without laparoscopic portion, and the patient is in a prone position (Courtesy of Luis de la Torre, MD, Pediatric Colorectal Surgery, Children's Hospital of Pittsburgh, Pittsburgh, PA, USA).

line in infants; for older children, a 1-cm margin is advised. The mucosal dissection is carried proximally for approximately 2 cm, staying within the relatively avascular submucosal plane (Fig. 36.7). Stay sutures placed in the mucosa may be helpful to aid with retraction during dissection. This step creates the mucosal resection within the muscular rectal cuff as described in the original Soave procedure. The dissection then proceeds toward proximal between mucosal and muscular plane of the rectal wall. Once the peritoneal reflection is reached, a circumferential incision is made through the outer muscular and serosal layers of the rectal wall into the abdominal cavity of the upper pelvis (Fig. 36.8). At this point, the rectal mucosal tube and the previously mobilized sigmoid colon are freely mobile. The entire colorectal specimen is then pulled through the rectal muscular cuff and out of the anus until the leveling biopsy site is reached, taking particular care to avoid rotation (Fig. 36.9).

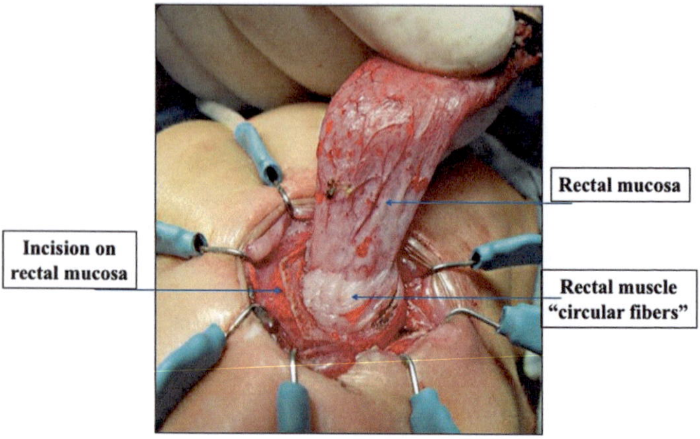

Fig. 36.7. Transanal rectal mucosectomy (Soave procedure) with dissection plane between rectal mucosa and submucosa/muscularis. Please note the hooks of the Lone Star retractor were advanced into the proximal aspect of the dentate line for exposure. The mucosal incision is well above the dentate line. For the Swenson procedure, the initial incision traverses the full-thickness rectal wall with the dissection plane just outside of the rectum (Courtesy of Luis de la Torre, MD, Pediatric Colorectal Surgery, Children's Hospital of Pittsburgh, Pittsburgh, PA, USA).

Before anastomosis, a posterior myotomy of the rectal muscular sleeve, which remains after the Soave procedure, must be performed. Some surgeons remove about one quarter of the muscular sleeve posteriorly to prevent re-scaring and recurrence of a tight muscular rectal cuff (Fig. 36.10). A final laparoscopic look can be performed before completion of the anastomosis to verify the correct non-rotated position of the pulled-through colon (Fig. 36.11).

It is advised to transect the distal bowel 2–3 cm proximal to the biopsy site in order to ensure that all aganglionic bowel is removed. Initial transection of the anterior half of the colon allows the posterior half to be used as a handle while the anastomosis is started. 4–0 Vicryl sutures are placed at 12, 3, and 9 o'clock. The remaining colon is transected and the anastomosis completed. The anastomotic stitches should include full-thickness bites of the colon on the proximal side; on the distal side, a sturdy bite of the distal end of the muscular cuff is taken and then a bite of the remaining rectal mucosa. The transitional epithelium of the dentate line should not be incorporated in these sutures (Fig. 36.12). Once the anastomosis is completed, a finger or Hegar dilator is used to check its patency.

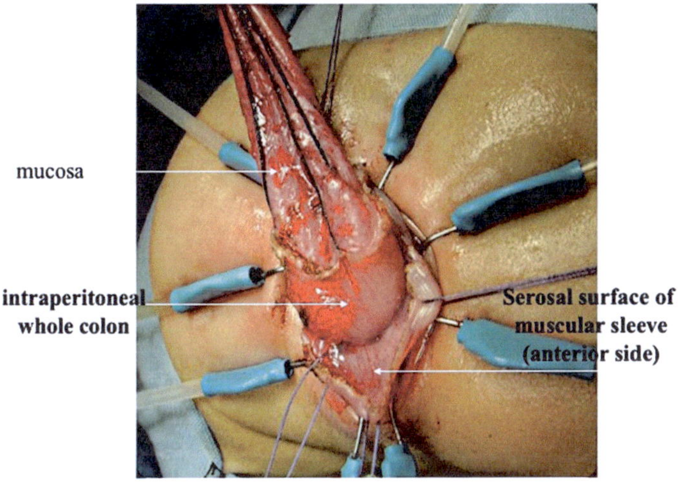

Fig. 36.8. Transanal dissection above the pelvic peritoneal reflection after division of the submucosal/seromuscular layer of the distal colon (Courtesy of Luis de la Torre, MD, Pediatric Colorectal Surgery, Children's Hospital of Pittsburgh, Pittsburgh, PA, USA).

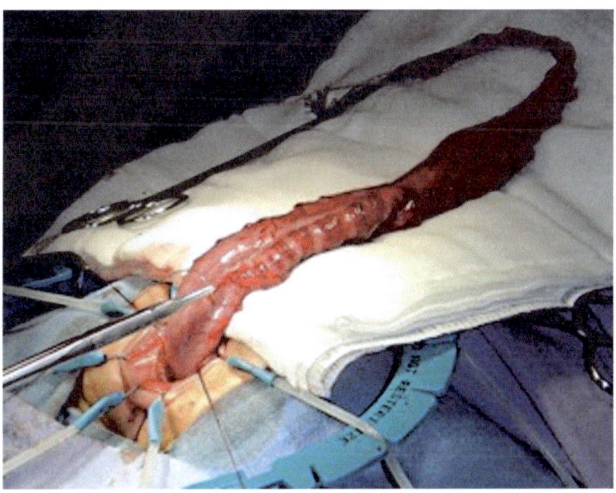

Fig. 36.9. The complete transanal specimen prior to colo-anal anastomosis. Before the anastomosis is fashioned, the proximal doughnut of the resected colon is given to the pathologist to evaluate for an anatomically normal bowel (Courtesy of Luis de la Torre, MD, Pediatric Colorectal Surgery, Children's Hospital of Pittsburgh, Pittsburgh, PA, USA).

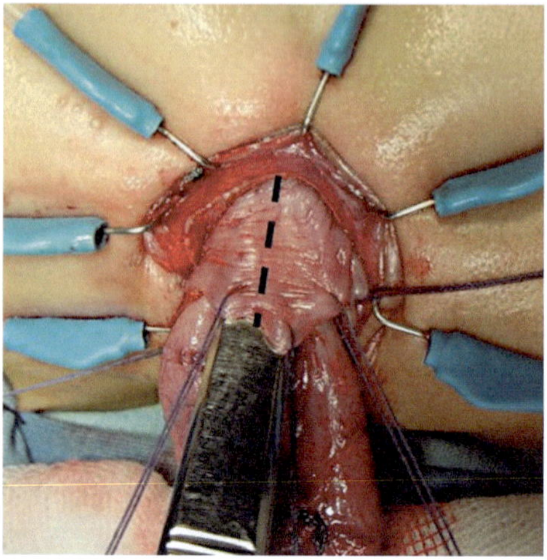

Fig. 36.10. Posterior myotomy of the rectal muscular sleeve remaining after the Soave procedure. Some surgeons remove about one quarter of the muscular sleeve posteriorly to prevent re-scaring and recurrence of a tight muscular rectal cuff (Courtesy of Luis de la Torre, MD, Pediatric Colorectal Surgery, Children's Hospital of Pittsburgh, Pittsburgh, PA, USA).

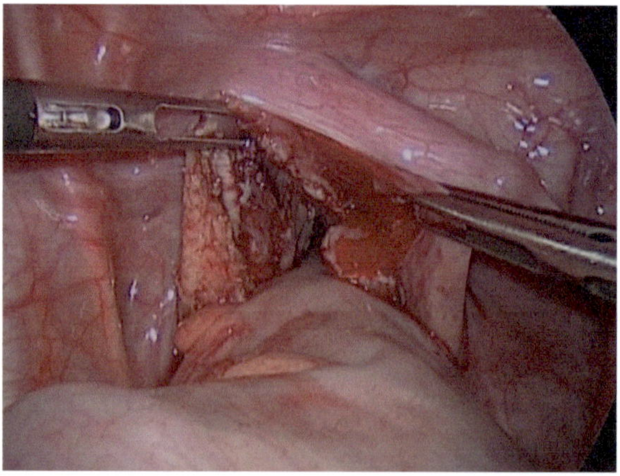

Fig. 36.11. Laparoscopic exploration to verify the non-rotated position of the colon, to check the absence of bleeding and appropriate tension of the bowel end (in this figure, the muscular rectal sleeve split medially in its anterior portion is also shown). Adapted from Technical modification of the Georgeson procedure for Hirschsprung's disease: a 12 years experience with the laparoscopic-assisted mesocolon dissection. Ruggeri G, Randi B, Gargano T, Libri M, Maffi M, Lima M. JEMIS – Journal of Endoscopic, Minimally Invasive Surgery in Newborn, Children and Adolescent – ISSN 2283–7116 (DOI: http://dx.medra.org/10.1473/JEMIS14).

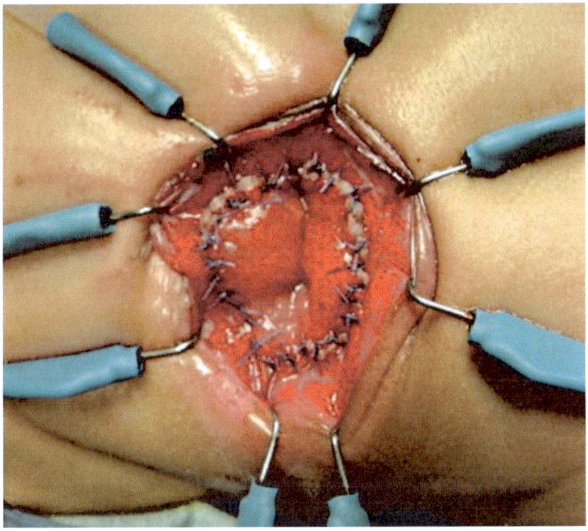

Fig. 36.12. Completed colo-anal anastomosis well proximal to the dentate line (Lone Star hooks at the dentate line) (Courtesy of Luis de la Torre, MD, Pediatric Colorectal Surgery, Children's Hospital of Pittsburgh, Pittsburgh, PA, USA).

The resected recto-colonic specimen is given to the pathologist with a clearly marked proximal margin for frozen section and confirmation of normal enteric anatomy of the transected full-circumference doughnut. Pathological routine includes evaluation of ganglion cell presence, number, and shape as well as size and anatomy of nerve fibers (<40 μm).

Gloves are then changed and the laparoscopy port sites closed, thus concluding the procedure.

If the surgeon prefers the Swenson approach, the rectum is dissected full thickness just proximal to the dentate line if the anal canal and the dissection plane snugly follows the rectal serosa. The Swenson procedure with full-thickness rectal dissection can also be performed completely laparoscopic before a transanal anastomosis is performed.

Postoperative Care

The nasogastric tube is removed with extubation. The Foley catheter is pulled directly after conclusion of the procedure or on the following morning. Oral nutrition can begin after the post-anesthesia recovery period several hours after the procedure, usually starting with clear liquids or breast milk, if available, and advancing as tolerated. Patients are discharged once there is evidence of bowel function and the patient is not "stooling out." Parents should be instructed on how to prevent perineal skin excoriation due to initially frequent bowel movements using barrier creams and powders. They should also be educated about the signs and symptoms of enterocolitis.

The first postoperative follow-up appointment is usually in 1–2 weeks. At this time the anastomosis is calibrated with Hegar dilators. Subsequently, the patient is brought back weekly for anastomotic dilation for the next 1–2 months. Some surgeons routinely have parents dilate the anastomosis on a daily basis, while others only dilate at the weekly checkups unless they feel the anastomosis is tight.

Postoperative Complications and Outcomes

Historically, the mortality rate in untreated cases of Hirschsprung's disease was as high as 88 % [28]. With advancements in surgical techniques and postoperative management, current mortality rates are less than 1 % [29]. Hirschsprung-associated enterocolitis is the most common cause of death. Primary surgical complications include anastomotic leak (5 %), stricture (5–10 %), bowel obstruction (5 %), pelvic abscess (5 %), and wound infection (10 %) [22]. Unfortunately, long-term outcomes are wrought with stooling problems.

Constipation and persistent obstructive symptoms are the most common long-term issues. Causes may be mechanical, such as anastomotic stricture, or functional, such as persistent or acquired aganglionosis, a colonic dysmotility disorder, or increased anal sphincter tone [30]. Many treatment options are available for these problems, and in most cases these symptoms improve in time [31].

Fecal incontinence and soiling are the second most common long-term issues. In the initial postoperative phase, diarrhea is common secondary to loss of colonic surface area for water absorption. In most patients, there is a sharp decline in the number of daily stools over the first 6 months, which subsequently tapers thereafter [32]. Eventually, 75–95 % of patients report no more than five stools per day [33–35]. Associated conditions such as Down syndrome increase the likelihood of having stooling and functional difficulties. Long-segment disease, especially total colonic aganglionosis, significantly increases these rates [33–38]. Despite the frequency of long-term issues, most patients report a good quality of life [31, 39–43].

Summary

- Hirschsprung's disease is a congenital disorder caused by incomplete neural crest cell migration to the distal intestine.
- Hirschsprung's disease can occur sporadically or in conjunction with various other genetic conditions.
- The diagnosis should be suspected in newborns presenting with lower GI obstructive symptoms. The standard workup includes abdominal X-ray and barium contrast enema. The definitive diagnosis is made by suction rectal biopsy.
- Treatment of Hirschsprung's disease is surgical, in order to remove the aganglionic segment of bowel. Subsequently, a variety of strategies have been described for restoring intestinal continuity and optimizing functional results.
- New surgical procedures have emerged to treat Hirschsprung's disease, such as the laparoscopic-assisted transanal pull-through, which utilize modern operative techniques to provide minimally invasive approaches. In the right patients, these procedures offer less morbidity and mortality, with similar or better long-term functional outcomes.

References

1. Bodian M, Carter C. A family study of Hirschsprung disease. Ann Hum Genet. 1963;26:261.
2. Townsend Jr CM, Beauchamp RD, Evers BM, Mattox KL. Sabiston textbook of surgery: the biological basis of modern surgical practice. 19th ed. Philadelphia: Saunders; 2012. ISBN-10: 1437715605.
3. Badner JA, Sieber WK, Garver KL, Chakravarti A. A genetic study of Hirschsprung disease. Am J Hum Genet. 1990;46:568–80.
4. Vorobyov GI, Achkasov SI, Biryukov OM. Clinical features diagnostics and treatment of Hirschsprung's disease in adults. Colorectal Dis. 2010;12(12):1242–8.
5. Ryan ET, Ecker JL, Christakis NA, et al. Hirschsprung's disease: associated abnormalities and demography. J Pediatr Surg. 1992;27(1):76–81.
6. Amiel J, Lyonnet S. Hirschsprung disease, associated syndromes, and genetics: a review. J Med Genet. 2001;38(11):729–39. doi:10.1136/jmg.38.11.729.
7. Goldberg EL. An epidemiological study of Hirschsprung's disease. Int J Epidemiol. 1984;13:479–85.
8. Garver KL, Law JC, Garver B. Hirschsprung disease: a genetic study. Clin Genet. 1985;28:503–8.
9. Spouge D, Baird PA. Hirschsprung disease in a large birth cohort. Teratology. 1985;32:171–7.

10. Brooks AS, Breuning MH, Meijers C. Spectrum of phenotypes associated with Hirschsprung disease: an evaluation of 239 patients from a single institution. The third international meeting: Hirschsprung disease and related neuro- cristopathies, Evian, France. 1998.
11. Torfs CP. An epidemiological study of Hirschsprung disease in a multiracial California population. The third international meeting: Hirschsprung disease and related neuro-cristopathies, Evian, France. 1998.
12. Sanchez-Mejias A, Fernandez RM, Lopez-Alonso M, et al. Contribution of RET, NTRK3 and EDN3 to the expression of Hirschsprung disease in a multiplex family. J Med Genet. 2009;46:862–4.
13. Verdy M, Weber AM, Roy CC, Morin CL, Cadotte M, Bro-chu P. Hirschsprung's disease in a family with multiple endocrine neoplasia type 2. J Pediatr Gastroenterol Nutr. 1982;1:603–7.
14. Mulligan LM, Eng C, Attie T, Lyonnet S, Marsh DJ, Hyland VJ, Robinson BG, Frilling A, Verellen-Dumoulin C, Safar A, Venter DJ, Munnich A, Ponder BAJ. Diverse phenotypes associated with exon 10 mutations of the RET proto-oncogene. Hum Mol Genet. 1994;3:2163–7.
15. Borst MJ, VanCamp JM, Peacock ML, Decker RA. Mutational analysis of multiple endocrine neoplasia type 2A associated with Hirschsprung's disease. Surgery. 1995; 117:386–91.
16. Caron P, Attie T, David D, Amiel J, Brousset F, Roger P, Munnich A, Lyonnet S. C618R mutation in exon 10 of the RET proto-oncogene in a kindred with multiple endocrine neoplasia type 2A and Hirschsprung's disease. J Clin Endocrinol Metab. 1996;81:2731–3.
17. Peretz H, Luboshitsky R, Baron E, Biton A, Gershoni R, Usher S, Grynberg E, Yakobson E, GraV E, Lapidot M. Cys 618 Arg mutation in the RET proto-oncogene associated with familial medullary thyroid carcinoma and maternally transmitted Hirschsprung's disease suggesting a role for imprinting. Hum Mutat. 1997;10:155–9.
18. Decker RA, Peacock ML, Watson P. Hirschsprung disease in MEN 2A: increased spectrum of RET exon 10 genotypes and strong genotype-phenotype correlation. Hum Mol Genet. 1998;7:129–34.
19. Romeo G, Ceccherini I, Celli J, Priolo M, Betsos N, Bonardi G, Seri M, Yin L, Lerone M, Jasonni V, Martucciello G. Association of multiple endocrine neoplasia type 2 and Hirschsprung disease. J Intern Med. 1998;243:515–20.
20. Borrego S, Eng C, Sanchez B, Saez ME, Navarro E, Antinolo G. Molecular analysis of the ret and GDNF genes in a family with multiple endocrine neoplasia type 2A and Hirschsprung disease. J Clin Endocrinol Metab. 1998;83:3361–4.
21. Lewis NA, Levitt MA, Zallen GS, et al. Diagnosing Hirschsprung's disease: increasing the odds of a positive rectal biopsy result. J Pediatr Surg. 2003;38:412–6. discussion 6.
22. http://www.sages.org/wiki/hirschsprung-disease/
23. Kapur RP, Reed RC, Finn LS. Calretinin immunohistochemistry versus acetylcholinesterase histochemistry in the evaluation of suction rectal biopsies for Hirschsprung disease. Pediatr Dev Pathol. 2009;12(1):6–15.
24. Langer JC, Fitzgerald PG, Winthrop AL, et al. One vs two stage Soave pull-through for Hirschsprung's disease in the first year of life. J Pediatr Surg. 1996;31:33–7.

25. Hackam DJ, Superina RA, Pearl RH. Single-stage repair of Hirschsprung's disease: a comparison of 109 patients over 5 years. J Pediatr Surg. 1997;32:1028–31.
26. Bufo AJ, Chen MK, Shah R, et al. Analysis of the costs of surgery for Hirschsprung's disease: one-stage laparoscopic pull-through versus two-stage Duhamel procedure. Clin Pediatr. 1999;38:593–6.
27. Keckler SJ, Yang JC, Fraser JD, et al. Contemporary practice patterns in the surgical management of Hirschsprung's disease. J Pediatr Surg. 2009;44:1257–60.
28. Burkardt DD, Graham JM, Short SS, Frykman PK. Advances in Hirschsprung disease genetics and treatment strategies: an update for the primary care pediatrician. Clin Pediatr (Phila). 2014;53:71–81.
29. Huang EY, Tolley EA, Blakely ML, Langham MR. Changes in hospital utilization and management of Hirschsprung disease: analysis using the kids' inpatient database. Ann Surg. 2013;257:371–5.
30. Langer JC. Persistent obstructive symptoms after surgery for Hirschsprung's disease: development of a diagnostic and therapeutic algorithm. J Pediatr Surg. 2004;39:1458.
31. Dasgupta R, Langer JC. Evaluation and management of persistent problems after surgery for Hirschsprung disease in a child. J Pediatr Gastroenterol Nutr. 2008;46:13.
32. Coran AG, Teitelbaum DH. Recent advances in the management of Hirschsprung's disease. Am J Surg. 2000;180:382.
33. Moore SW, Albertyn R, Cywes S. Clinical outcome and long-term quality of life after surgical correction of Hirschsprung's disease. J Pediatr Surg. 1996;31:1496.
34. Marty TL, Seo T, Matlak ME, et al. Gastrointestinal function after surgical correction of Hirschsprung's disease: long-term follow-up in 135 patients. J Pediatr Surg. 1995;30:655.
35. Sherman JO, Snyder ME, Weitzman JJ, et al. A 40-year multinational retrospective study of 880 Swenson procedures. J Pediatr Surg. 1989;24:833.
36. Neuvonen MI, Kyrklund K, Lindahl HG, et al. A population-based, complete follow-up of 146 consecutive patients after transanal mucosectomy for Hirschsprung disease. J Pediatr Surg. 2015;50(10):1653–8.
37. Ieiri S, Nakatsuji T, Akiyoshi J, et al. Long-term outcomes and the quality of life of Hirschsprung disease in adolescents who have reached 18 years or older—a 47-year single-institute experience. J Pediatr Surg. 2010;45:2398.
38. Menezes M, Puri P. Long-term outcome of patients with enterocolitis complicating Hirschsprung's disease. Pediatr Surg Int. 2006;22:316.
39. Yanchar NL, Soucy P. Long-term outcome after Hirschsprung's disease: patients' perspectives. J Pediatr Surg. 1999;34:1152.
40. Bai Y, Chen H, Hao J, et al. Long-term outcome and quality of life after the Swenson procedure for Hirschsprung's disease. J Pediatr Surg. 2002;37:639.
41. Ludman L, Spitz L, Tsuji H, Pierro A. Hirschsprung's disease: functional and psychological follow up comparing total colonic and rectosigmoid aganglionosis. Arch Dis Child. 2002;86:348.
42. Chumpitazi BP, Nurko S. Defecation disorders in children after surgery for Hirschsprung disease. J Pediatr Gastroenterol Nutr. 2011;53:75.
43. Hartman EE, Oort FJ, Aronson DC, et al. Explaining change in quality of life of children and adolescents with anorectal malformations or Hirschsprung disease. Pediatrics. 2007;119, e374.

37. Laparoscopic-Assisted Anorectal Pull-Through for Anorectal Malformations

Mohammad Ali Abbass and Federico G. Seifarth

Introduction

"Anorectal malformations" comprise a wide spectrum of anatomical malformations that have not yet been linked to any specific etiology. The incidence has been reported to be 1/4000–1/5000 births with a higher prevalence in males [1]. It has been strongly associated with certain familial associations [2] and also has been linked to multiple genetic disorders like Down syndrome [3].

In an attempt to unify the classification of anorectal malformations, an international committee agreed in 2005 on the Krickenbeck classification, which classifies the major types of anorectal malformations (ARM) into the following clinical groups: imperforate anus with perineal fistula, rectourethral fistula (bulbar or prostatic), rectovesical fistula, vestibular fistula, cloaca, imperforate anus without fistula, or anal stenosis.

Since the 1700s multiple approaches have been described by surgeons in an attempt to create a perineal orifice with or without temporary or permanent ostomies [4]. In 1982 Devries and Peña described the posterior sagittal anorectoplasty (PSARP) [4] which quickly became the standard for surgical correction of anorectal malformations. In 2000 Georgeson and colleagues introduced a laparoscopic approach for repair of high ARM [5]. Supporters of this laparoscopic procedure emphasize better visualization of the operative field with clear identification of high forms of recto-urinary fistulas. In addition, the laparoscopic technique prevents the sphincter complex from being divided, preserves the distal rectum, and allows accurate positioning in the center of the levator sling,

D.S. Walsh et al. (eds.), *The SAGES Manual of Pediatric Minimally Invasive Surgery*, DOI 10.1007/978-3-319-43642-5_37

which—according to some authors—improves anorectal resting and inhibitory pressure when compared to PSARP [6]. Laparoscopic-assisted anorectal pull-through aims to avoid weakening and destruction of the anal sphincter musculature and diminishing rectal scarring and has the potential of a one-stage procedure, saving the neonate from the morbidity of a colostomy [7].

Embryology

The exact embryology of the development of anorectal malformations is still unclear, and there are several possible explanations for development of these complex malformations. Prior fusion of the mesoderm at the dorsal aspect of the cloacal fold might be noted in some instances, and this will block the physiologic descent of the urogenital septum, resulting in an urorectal septal defect [8–10]. The anal canal forms after fusion of the ectoderm and hindgut endoderm, where they are separated by the perineal membrane. Disruption of this process can lead to fistulas. These fistulas historically were categorized into high or intermediate. High fistulas in male patients are defined by the hindgut blindly ending above the level of the anal sphincter with fistulation to the urethra or bladder. More complex disruption of the embryologic formation in females can lead to a single channel, unifying the urogenital tract and rectum—the cloaca.

In lower lesions, the fistula opening can frequently be identified at the perineum or scrotum in boys or the fourchette of the vagina in girls [11].

Perioperative Evaluation

History and Physical Exam

Anorectal malformations are rarely diagnosed prenatally and pediatric surgeons are consulted after neonates are found to have abnormal perineal or anal anatomy with a missing or "displaced" anus on initial examination or a failure to pass meconium. A thorough physical exam in patients with suspected anorectal malformations is crucial and allows early classification of many patients with ARM. A missing anal opening in the correct anatomical position and underdeveloped buttocks are frequent exam findings. It is important to identify a perineal orifice as fistula opening and not as a malpositioned anus. If the diagnosis cannot be made on initial presentation, reevaluation on the second day of life is advised. Frequently, cutaneous fistulas can be more easily visualized after rectal meconium pressure builds up after 24 h of life. Sacral X-rays and a radiographic invertogram in prone position help to distinguish high from low ARM. Associated anomalies of the VACTERL complex have to be ruled out, including examination of the heart, spine, and kidneys. Drooling or impossible passage of an NG tube are findings for an esophageal atresia [12].

Labs and Imaging

Standard perioperative labs should be obtained on all patients, including urinalysis to look for meconium in the urine. An echocardiogram rules out any cardiac malformations, and an abdominal ultrasound with focus on renal malformations is obtained. A spinal ultrasound to screen for tethered cord should also be performed. X-Rays include babygrams to assess the spine and the anatomy of the sacrum. If a neonate does not pass stool a cross table lateral X-ray film with the baby in prone position can help identifying the level of the anorectal malformation and guiding the surgeon regarding the next step in management.

In patients with a diverting colostomy and mucous fistula, a high-pressure distal colonography identifies the position of the rectum and the fistula tract before final corrective surgery [11].

Surgical Indications

Surgery is indicated for all patients with anorectal malformations. Laparoscopy is indicated for patients with recto-bladder neck fistulas and selected patients with rectal prostatic fistulas and occasionally for patients with cloacae. Conventional PSARP remains the gold standard in patients diagnosed with recto-perineal fistulas, rectourethral bulbar fistulas, rectovestibular fistulas, rectal atresia, most cloacae, and anorectal malformation without fistula [13].

Technique

Special Considerations

Performing a diverting colostomy prior to the definitive repair is advised in any patient with unclear level of the malformation or as bridging maneuver to transfer the patient's care to a center with experienced surgeons. It has multiple advantages: it buys time and a colostomy allows the surgeon to obtain a high-pressure colonography which offers detailed anatomical information about the type of the ARM and level of the fistula. Depending on the level of expertise of the surgeon, anorectal malformations diagnosed early after birth with perineal fistulas can be operated in one stage [14–16]. However, incomplete workup will increase the risk of injuring the urethra, the bladder neck, the vas deferens, or the seminal vesicle [17]. Colostomy takedown with definite repair should be attempted in the first 3 months of life to allow early adaptation to physiologic defecation [11].

Anatomy

The process of retaining and emptying stool is the result of a complex interaction between the sphincter musculature, the rectum, pelvic muscles, and the voluntary and involuntary nervous system. In opposition to the classic understanding of the anorectal and pelvic anatomy, sphincteric, rectal, and pelvic muscles need to be understood as continuum rather than anatomically and functionally independent muscles.

The muscle group that forms the sphincters and the levator ani sling are shaped like an inverted funnel. These muscles are innervated by the pudendal nerve. Stimulation of the upper end of the levator muscles will flex the rectum anteriorly and stimulation of the vertical muscle fibers elevates the anus, versus closing the anus when the parasagittal fibers are stimulated [7].

Positioning

The patient is placed transversely at the bottom part of the operating table and circumferentially prepped from nipples to toes. A Foley catheter should be placed under sterile conditions. The surgeon stands on the side of the head with the monitor on the opposite side, and the assistant stands at the end of the table to the patient's left. This position allows access to the patient for both laparoscopic and perineal portions of the procedure [7].

Technique Details

Dr. Georgeson's laparoscopic technique for repair of a high imperforate anus with high rectovesical/rectourethral fistula, as first presented at the surgical section meeting of the American Academy of Pediatrics in October of 1998 and subsequently published in 2000 [6], is described.

A proximal, divided sigmoid colostomy should be performed in the newborn period.

With the patient in transverse position on the operating room table, the abdomen is accessed via the umbilicus using a Veress needle or an open technique to place a 3 or 5 mm trocar. Pneumoperitoneum is established; caution should be taken not to cause bowel injury since proximal dilation can be present.

A 4 or 5 mm port is introduced below the right nipple at the inferior margin of the liver. The third port measures 3 or 5 mm and is placed in the right lower quadrant, forming a triangle with the previous two ports. The infrahepatic port is used for the camera, while the umbilical and right lower quadrant ports are used for 3 or 5 mm instruments (Fig. 37.1).

Suspending the bladder with a large monofilament U-stitch facilitates visualization of the pelvis. The initial step in the surgery is dissection of the peritoneal reflection at the distal rectum. It is crucial during this circumferential rectal dissection to stay close to the muscular wall to prevent inadvertent damage to ureters or the vas. Utilizing traction to the rectal wall, the dissection is continued distally until a fistula or the blind end of the rectum is reached. At the point of the rectovesical/urethral fistula, a clear tapering can be noted. The fistula is then divided and tied off with a pre-tied Endoloop. The divided rectal stump is closed in an identical fashion (Figs. 37.2, 37.3, and 37.4).

Once the rectum is mobilized, the other bowel loops should be retracted out of the pelvis. This will allow the surgeon to visualize the pelvic anatomy, including the prostate, levator muscles, and the pubococcygeus in the pelvic floor. The midline is easily identified and lies in the same plane as the distal end of the fistula and the urethra (Fig. 37.5).

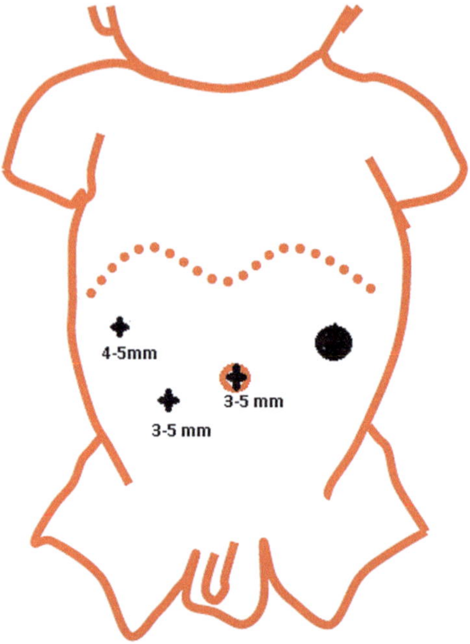

Fig. 37.1. Trocar sites [18]. From Lima M, Pull-through for high imperforate anus. In: Essentials of Pediatric Endoscopic Surgery. Saxena AK, Hollwarth ME, eds. Austria, Springer; 2009:281–288. Reprinted with permission.

The perineal dissection is the next step. The patient's knees are flexed and the feet are secured on an ether screen over the chest. This allows easy access to the perineum. The external anal area should be mapped using the transcutaneous electrostimulator. The area of maximal contraction should be marked with sutures and represents the site of the future anus.

A 1 cm vertical incision is created in the perineum and a plane strictly staying in the midline is identified by dividing muscular fibers of the muscle complex. Mostly blunt dissection is carried to a depth of approximately 2–2.5 cm. Under laparoscopic surveillance, a Veress needle on an expandable sheath is subsequently advanced through the perineal channel into the pelvis and guided behind the urethra, through the levator fascia, and into the space between urethra and the anterior aspect of the encircling levator ani muscles. Once in position, the needle is removed and replaced with a 10–12 mm cannula, radially expanding

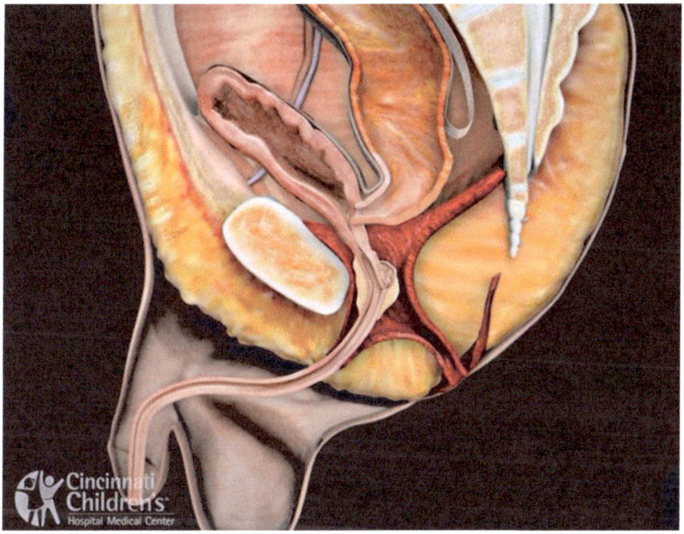

Fig. 37.2. Recto-bladder neck malformation. From Peña A, Bischoff A. Recto-bladder Neck Fistula. In: Surgical Treatment of Colorectal Problems in Children. 2015. Reprinted with permission from Springer.

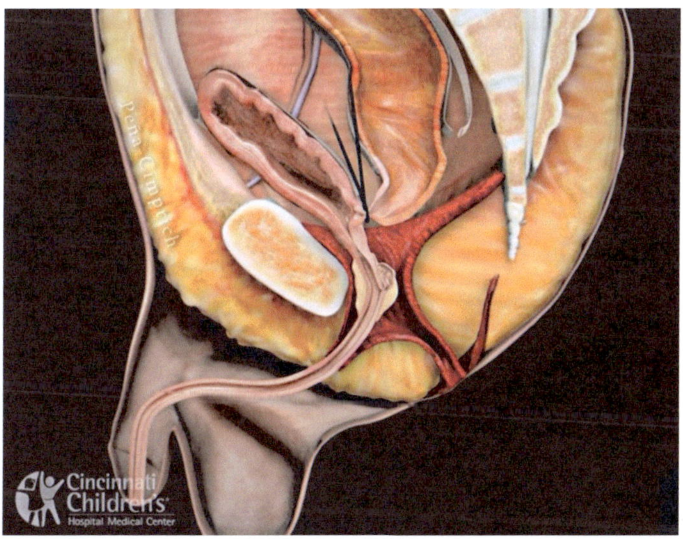

Fig. 37.3. Tying off recto-bladder fistula. From Peña A, Bischoff A. Recto-bladder Neck Fistula. In: Surgical Treatment of Colorectal Problems in Children. 2015. Reprinted with permission from Springer.

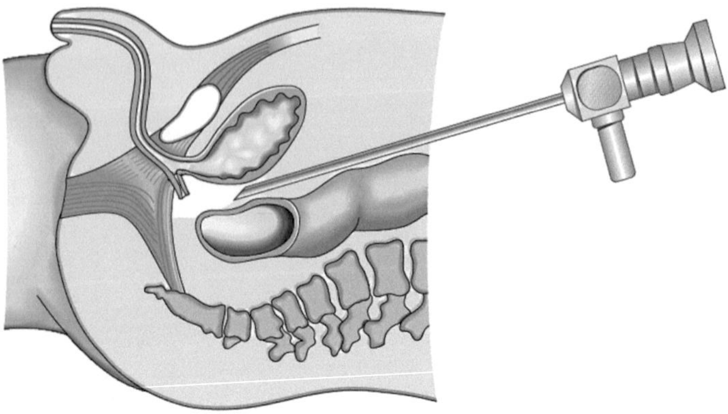

Fig. 37.4. Divided rectourethral fistula. From Inge TH. Georgeson's Procedure: Laparoscopically Assisted Anorectoplasty for High Anorectal Malformations. In: Endoscopic Surgery in Infants and Children. Klaas MA, et al. eds. 2008: 391–398. Reprinted with permission from Springer.

the pelvic floor. A blunt 5 mm clamp is advanced through this port, and the proximal end of the divided rectourethral fistula is exteriorized and secured to the perineal skin with absorbable sutures (Figs. 37.6 and 37.7).

The rectum should then be laparoscopically suspended to the presacral fascia to prevent future prolapse of the rectum. These sutures are also believed to pull the rectocutaneous junction in a cephalad direction and to sharpen the anorectal angle. Abdominal ports are removed after desufflation of the abdomen, and the three small incisions are closed with absorbable sutures [6].

Instruments

- Veress needle
- Three trocars (3–5 mm)
- Hook cautery
- 10–12 mm expandable port
- Laparoscopic dissection instruments

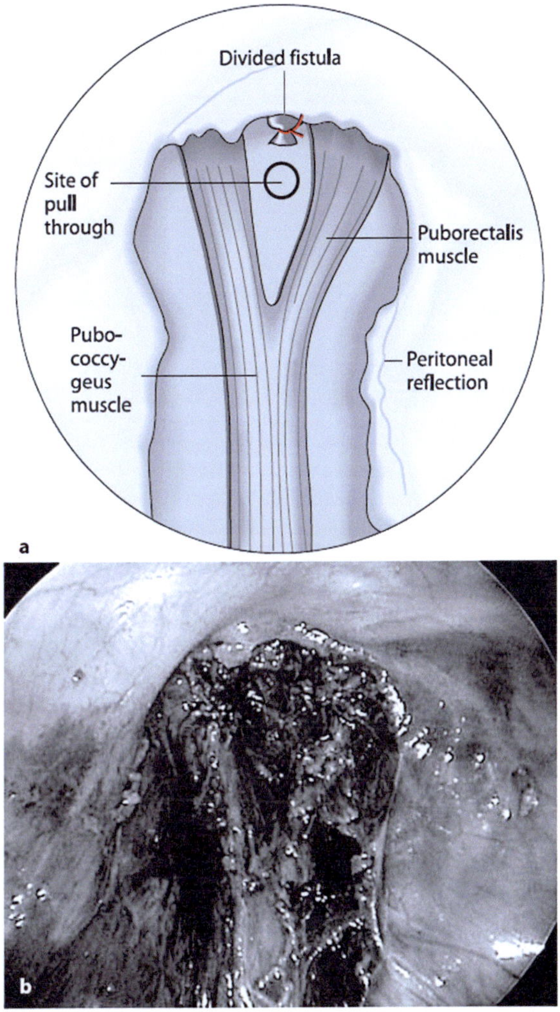

Fig. 37.5. Schematic and intraoperative view after division of rectourethral fistula. From Inge TH. Georgeson's Procedure: Laparoscopically Assisted Anorectoplasty for High Anorectal Malformations. In: Endoscopic Surgery in Infants and Children. Klaas MA, et al. eds. 2008: 391–398. Reprinted with permission from Springer.

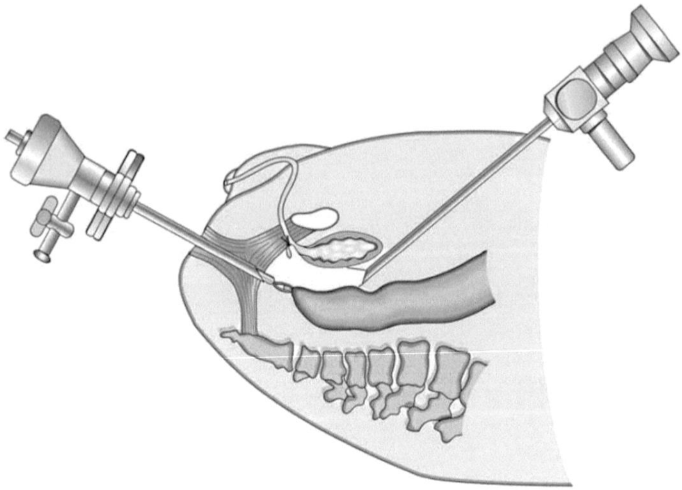

Fig. 37.6. Perineal pull-through of the distal rectum. From Inge TH. Georgeson's Procedure: Laparoscopically Assisted Anorectoplasty for High Anorectal Malformations. In: Endoscopic Surgery in Infants and Children. Klaas MA, et al. eds. 2008: 391–398. Reprinted with permission from Springer.

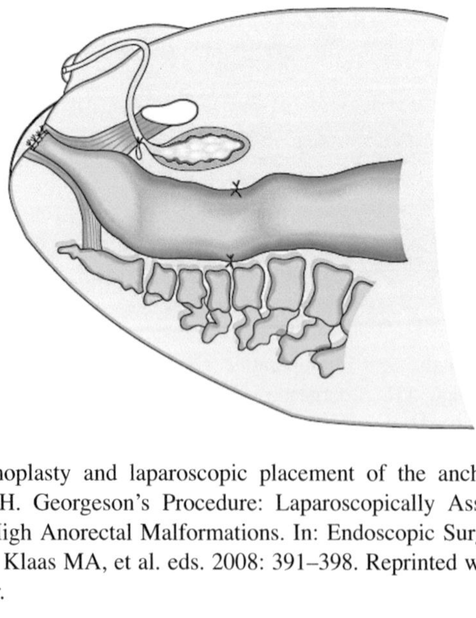

Fig. 37.7. Anoplasty and laparoscopic placement of the anchoring sutures. From Inge TH. Georgeson's Procedure: Laparoscopically Assisted Anorectoplasty for High Anorectal Malformations. In: Endoscopic Surgery in Infants and Children. Klaas MA, et al. eds. 2008: 391–398. Reprinted with permission from Springer.

Pearls/Pitfalls

- A high-pressure distal colostogram should be performed prior to this procedure to clearly identify the anatomy and the level of the rectal urethral fistula.
- Elevation of the bladder with a large transcutaneous stitch allows better visualization of the pelvic floor.
- Rectal dissection should be strictly performed at the outer muscular wall of the rectum to prevent damage to the vas and the urethra. Following the vas helps to identify the prostate.
- The anorectal angle changes when the knees are flexed onto the torso. Aiming the Veress needle too anteriorly carries the risk for urethral injury [7].
- Proper positioning of the divided colostomy is essential to perform a tension-free pull-through procedure. The initial sigmoid colostomy should be placed as proximal as possible. If placed too distally, takedown might be necessary to gain adequate length for the pull-through.

Postoperative Care

To prevent strictures, anorectal dilation starts 2–3 weeks after the pull-through procedure. Over an 8–12 week period, the anus and rectum are serially dilated with Hegar dilators from 8 to 14 mm diameter. The colostomy is reversed once the neo-rectum is consistently patent [7].

Outcomes

A systematic review of all studies reporting outcomes of laparoscopic-assisted anorectal pull-through (LAARP) was published in 2009. Out of four studies comparing PSARP vs. LAARP, LAARP was superior and had better outcomes with follow-up extending to 1 year postoperatively. The laparoscopic approach had better stool frequency, continence, anatomical positioning of the neo-rectum, and function of the anal sphincter (Table 37.1) [13, 19, 20].

One of the most recent reviews, published by Bischoff et al. in 2015, focused on describing all published data about the laparoscopic approach for repairing ARM. Contrary to most publications, this paper reinforced

Table 37.1 LAARP complications as reported by Al-Hozaim et al. [13]

Postoperative complication	No. of patients
Rectal prolapse	9 (7.2 %)
Vesicoureteral reflux	2 (1.6 %)
Incontinence	2 (1.6 %)
Irregular stooling pattern	1 (0.8 %)
Dysuria	1 (0.8 %)
Perineal infection	1 (0.8 %)
Residual diverticulum	1 (0.8 %)

From Al-Hozaim O et al. [13]. Reprinted with permission from Elsevier Limited

the lack of rigorous evidence to support a laparoscopic approach as superior to the open approach, largely due to the absence of standardized data characterizing the fistulas. According to this meta-analysis, most reviews are lacking objective classification of included malformations and apply inconsistent parameters for measuring the outcomes. This review included 622 patients and 68 published articles; clinical results were published including demographics, length of stay, and outcomes. Some reports used frequency of bowel movements after surgery, constipation, or perception of anal tones as objective outcome indicators; others used findings on rectal manometry, magnetic resonance imaging (MRI), or defecagrams and, still others, length of stay as outcomes. Bischoff's analysis concluded that laparoscopy was only justified in patients with recto-bladder neck fistulas and selected patients with rectoprostatic fistulas, cloaca with short common channel and high rectum, rectovestibular fistula, and anomalies with free floating rectum in the peritoneum. Laparoscopy was reported as never indicated in cases of recto-perineal, rectourethral bulbar and rectovestibular fistulas in addition to cases with rectal atresia and most cloaca and ARM without fistulas. No reported functional superiority of laparoscopy to posterior sagittal approach was recorded [21].

In his most recent text book, Peña et al. reviewed 41 publications which included 446 patients and reported that patients with perineal fistulas in both genders developed 100 % bowel control when operated with the open approach, with short operative time. The rationale for changing this highly successful, standard approach with laparoscopic repair is questionable by some. In cases with anorectal malformations without fistula, Peña advises against the laparoscopic approach since the open approach also has short operative time and length of stay. It is also noted that the laparoscopic approach for rectourethral bulbar fistulas in males is contraindicated since it is impossible to reach the fistula site laparoscopically. In rectourethral prostatic fistulas, Peña's analysis did not find any difference between either approach, but he emphasizes that the traditional approach renders a 66 % of bowel control by the age of three in males and 92 % have urinary control. In females, operative time to repair the most common vestibular fistula is short, and patients will tolerate a diet on the same day and can be discharged a day after [22].

Complications

In the same meta-analysis that discussed the outcomes of the LAARP vs. PSARP, nine studies reported overall outcomes after LAARP, with rectal prolapse being the most common complication, followed by vesicoureteral reflux and incontinence. Other complications reported included irregular stooling patterns, dysuria, perineal infection, and residual diverticulum (Table 37.1) [7].

Summary

- Since its introduction by Georgeson et al. in 2000, many centers have gained experience with the minimally invasive technique and have confirmed its merits. The main advantage of the laparoscopic technique lies in its exquisite visualization of the intrapelvic anatomy of the newborn.
- The laparoscopic approach is recommended in patients with imperforate anus and recto-bladder neck fistulas.
- Malformations with low fistulas are amenable to open repair, and laparoscopy is controversial.
- Unlike in the conventional open approach, laparoscopic visualization is internal, rather than external.
- Opponents of the laparoscopic approach criticize limited external visualization of the sphincter muscle complex and consequent missed ability to strictly dissect the tissue planes in the midline.
- Positioning the neo-rectum directly in the middle of the sphincter complex is crucial for future continence.

References

1. Brenner EC. Congenital defects of the anus and rectum. Surg Gynecol Obstet. 1915;20:579–88.
2. Pinsky L. The syndromology of anorectal malformation (atresia, stenosis, ectopia). Am J Med Genet. 1978;1(4):461–74.
3. Torres R, Levitt M, Tovilla J, et al. Anorectal malformations and Down's syndrome. J Pediatr Surg. 1998;33:194–7.
4. Peña A, Levitt M. Anorectal malformations. 6th ed. In: Pediatric surgery. London: BioMed Central Ltd; 2006. p. 1566. Chapter 101.
5. Stephens FD. Malformations of the anus. Aust N Z J Surg. 1953;23(1):9–24.
6. Georgeson KE, Inge TH, Albanese CT. Laparoscopically assisted anorectal pull through for high imperforate anus—a new technique. J Pediatr Surg. 2000;35(6):927–31.
7. Holcomb GW, Georgeson KE, Rothenberg SS. Atlas of pediatric laparoscopy and thoracoscopy. Philadelphia: Saunders; 2008. p. 115–9.
8. Haleblian G, Kraklau D, Wilcox D, et al. Y-type urethral duplication in the male. BJU Int. 2006;97:597–602.
9. Mauch TJ, Albertine KH. Urorectal septum malformation sequence: insights into pathogenesis. Anat Rec. 2002;268:405–10.
10. Fernbach SK. Urethral abnormalities in male neonates with VATER association. AJR Am J Roentgenol. 1991;156:137–40.
11. Coventery BL, editor. Pediatric surgery. Surgery: complications, risks and consequences. Adelaide: Springer; 2014. p. 25–116.
12. Coran AG. Pediatric surgery. 7th ed. Philadelphia: Elsevier Mosby; 2012. p. 1289–309.
13. Al-Hozaim O, Al-Maary J, AlQahtani A, Zamakhshary M. Laparoscopic-assisted anorectal pull-through for anorectal malformations: a systematic review and the need for standardization of outcome reporting. J Pediatr Surg. 2010;45(7):1500–4.
14. Albanese C, Jennings R, Lopoo J, et al. One-stage correction of high imperforate anus in the male neonate. J Pediatr Surg. 1999;34:834–6.
15. Goon H. Repair of anorectal anomalies in the neonatal period. Pediatr Surg Int. 1990;5:246–9.
16. Moore T. Advantages of performing the sagittal anoplasty operation for imperforate anus at birth. J Pediatr Surg. 1990;25:276–7.
17. Hong A, Acuna M, Peña A, et al. Urologic injuries associated with repair of anorectal malformations in male patients. J Pediatr Surg. 2002;37:339–44.
18. Bax K, Georgeson KE, Rothenberg SS, Valla JS, Yeung CK. Endoscopic surgery in infants and children. Berlin: Springer; 2008. p. 391–8.
19. Lin CL, Wong KKY, Lan CCL, et al. Earlier appearance and higher incidence of the rectoanal relaxation reflex in patient with imperforate anus repaired with laparoscopically assisted anorectoplasty. Surg Endosc. 2003;17:1646–9.
20. Wong KKY, Khong PL, Lin SCL, et al. Post-operative magnetic resonance evaluation of children after laparoscopic anorectoplasty for imperforate anus. Int J Colorectal Dis. 2004;20:33–7.

21. Bischoff A, Martinez-Leo B, Peña A. Laparoscopic approach in the management of anorectal malformations. Pediatr Surg Int. 2015;31(5):431–7.
22. Pena A, Bischoff A. Minimally invasive approach to anorectal malformation. In: Pena A, Bischoff A, editors. Surgical treatment of colorectal problems in children. Cham: Springer; 2015. p. 189–99.

38. Laparoscopic Pediatric Inguinal Hernia Repair

Nicholas E. Bruns and Todd A. Ponsky

Background

Inguinal hernia repair is the most commonly performed surgical procedure in infants and children. Inguinal hernias occur in 1–5 % newborns and 9–11 % of premature infants. The male/female ratio is approximately 4:1.

Over the last 20 years, numerous variations of minimally invasive techniques have been developed for pediatric inguinal hernia repair. As the overwhelming majority of pediatric inguinal hernias are indirect hernias due to a patent processus vaginalis, all commonly performed procedures are designed to close the internal ring, without the use of mesh. This chapter will describe in detail the authors' preferred technique which is a modification of the techniques described by Patkowski et al. [1] and Endo et al. [2]. As well, this chapter will review significant alternative procedures, but it is beyond the scope of this chapter to review all possible techniques. In addition to ligation of the internal ring, other techniques include resection of the hernia sac alone and destruction of the inverted hernia sac in girls.

When counseling patients and/or their family, it is important to make it clear that neither laparoscopic repair nor open repair is superior in terms of recurrence [3] or cosmetic result. However, some may find laparoscopy beneficial due to ability to assess the contralateral side, ease of repair in difficult settings such as incarceration or prematurity, and minimal manipulation of the cord structures and the inguinal floor.

D.S. Walsh et al. (eds.), *The SAGES Manual of Pediatric Minimally Invasive Surgery*, DOI 10.1007/978-3-319-43642-5_38

Indications and Contraindications

Once diagnosed, all reducible inguinal hernias should undergo elective repair. In the case of the premature infant with a reducible inguinal hernia, operative repair should be delayed until the patient is nearly ready for discharge home. However, the optimal timing of repair has not adequately been studied, and in fact, there is an ongoing multicenter trial comparing inpatient repair versus delayed repair for premature infants. Incarcerated inguinal hernias that do not reduce manually should undergo emergent operation. These may be approached laparoscopically so long as the patient is nontoxic appearing and does not have significant abdominal distention. The only absolute contraindication to laparoscopic repair is hemodynamic instability. A relative contraindication may be previous abdominal surgery.

Anatomy

The key structures of the laparoscopic repair include the vas deferens, spermatic vessels, inferior epigastric vessels, and internal ring. The pediatric inguinal hernia is an indirect hernia as a result of a patent processus vaginalis (Fig. 38.1).

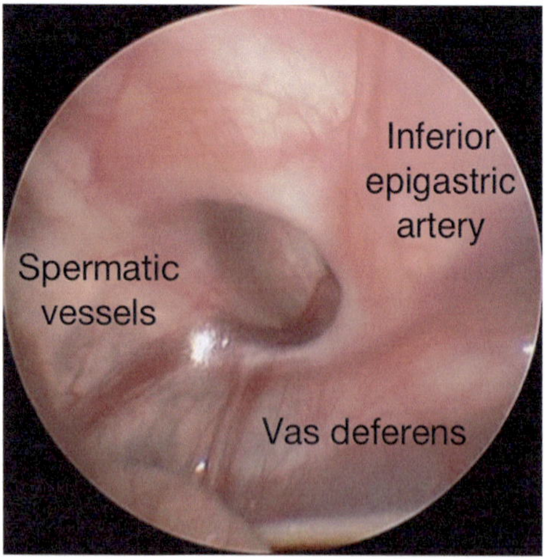

Fig. 38.1. Inguinal anatomy of a left-sided hernia as seen laparoscopically. Note the vas deferens medial to the internal ring, the spermatic vessels lateral to the internal ring, and the inferior epigastric artery superior.

Patient Positioning and Operating Room Setup

The patient is positioned supine with his or her legs spread slightly apart. The operating room table is typically kept flat, but Trendelenburg position may be used if the bowel is obscuring the view. The scrotum is prepped to allow for manual pressure to be applied to expel any air after the procedure. The patient should void before the procedure to eliminate the need for a urinary catheter. In younger patients, a Credé maneuver may be performed to empty the bladder.

The authors prefer to stand on the patient's left side, regardless of the side of the hernia, but some may find it easier to stand on the ipsilateral side of the hernia. The assistant stands on the same ipsilateral side, closer to the head of the patient. The laparoscopic monitor should be placed at the foot of the bed.

Trocar Position and Instrumentation

A 70-degree, 3-mm laparoscope is inserted infraumbilically. This may be substituted for a 5-mm, 30-degree laparoscope in larger children. A 3-mm Maryland dissector is placed through a stab incision. The location of this instrument is surgeon dependent; some place this on the left side, others prefer to place the instrument on the same side as the hernia, and still others place it in the umbilicus next to the camera. This instrument should have the capability to apply electrocautery to it (Fig. 38.2).

An 18-gauge spinal needle is used. The tip of the needle is bent slightly using a hemostat. This is loaded with a loop of 3-0 polypropylene suture such that the ends of suture are at the back of the needle and at the tip of the needle, a 1-mm loop of suture is exposed. The curve of the needle must be gentle or the suture will not pass through (Fig. 38.3).

Technique

1. After port placement and preparation of the spinal needle, the hernia is assessed and any contents are reduced laparoscopically with gentle tension.
2. The peritoneum is then thermally injured with electrocautery to stimulate scarring. This should be done on the medial, anterior, and lateral edges with caution to avoid the vas deferens and spermatic vessels. Aim to cauterize just inside the internal ring so the cautery line is not

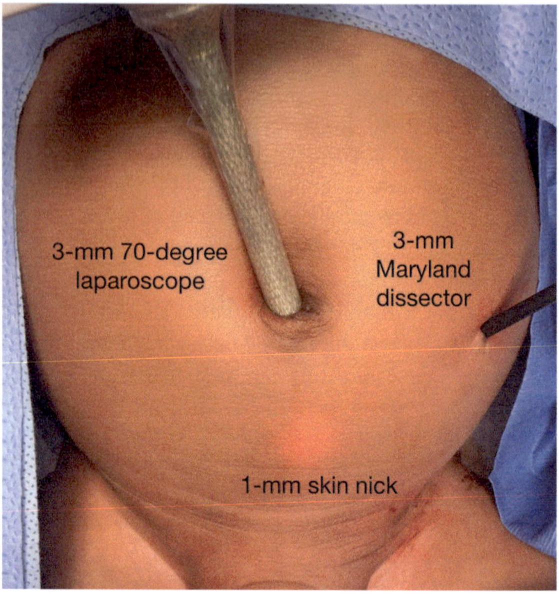

Fig. 38.2. Port placement for a left inguinal hernia.

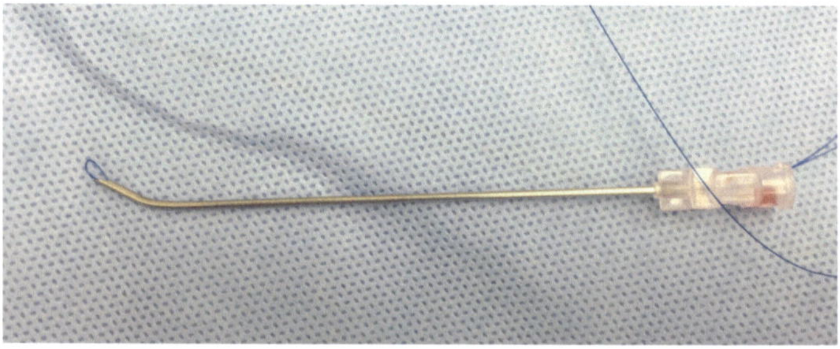

Fig. 38.3. Curved spinal needle with looped monofilament suture.

in the exact same location as the final resting spot of the suture. However, this may not be critical. This technique has been shown to significantly improve the durability of repair in rabbits [4]. In fact, Godoy has described treating small inguinal hernias in girls by inversion of the hernia sac and cauterization alone [5] (Fig. 38.4).

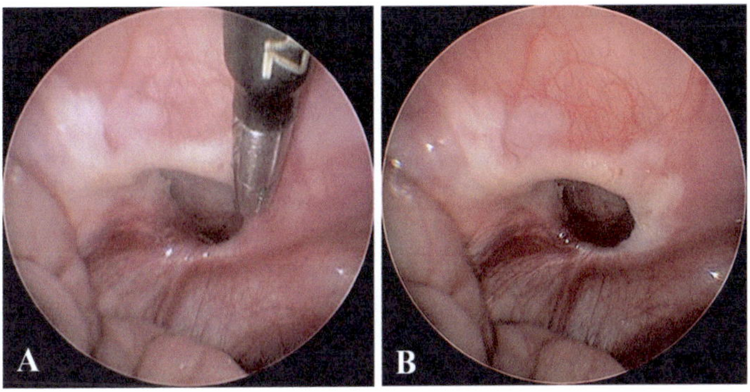

Fig. 38.4. (**a, b**) Cautery is applied to the anteromedial and anterolateral edges of the internal ring to stimulate scarring of the repair. Care should be used to avoid the spermatic vessels and vas deferens.

3. A 25-gauge finder needle is used to identify the 12 o'clock position of the internal ring (from the view of the laparoscope). The needle is inserted perpendicular to the abdominal wall. External palpation is used to determine the point of entry. An 11-blade scalpel is then used to make a 1-mm nick in the skin at this location. Insert the needle very far laterally on the patient, almost in the flank, so the needle traverses in a straight line, making it easy to advance the needle over the vas deferens and vessels. Next, hydrodissection is performed with 0.25 % bupivacaine or an alternative long-acting local anesthetic to separate the peritoneum off of the cord structures. In smaller patients, the local anesthetic may be diluted to remain beneath the maximum dosage. If a caudal block was performed by anesthesia, 5 mL of normal saline may be used. This is done on the lateral edge of the internal ring followed by the medial edge. It is critical to stay just under the peritoneum (between the peritoneum and the vessels), or the vessels may be lifted up with the peritoneum rather than separated away.
4. The previously prepared 18-gauge spinal needle is then directed through the 1-mm skin incision that was made at the 12 o'clock location overlying the internal ring and is directed along the lateral edge of the internal ring in the plane created by hydrodissection. From this lateral approach, pass the needle over the vessels and, if possible, over the vas deferens before piercing out of the peritoneum. However, sometimes it may be

necessary to pass over the vas deferens from the medial side. The tip of the needle should pierce through the peritoneum at the 6 o'clock position. The loop of polypropylene is the then advanced out of the needle and the needle is removed. The ends of the suture are then secured to the operating room drapes with a hemostat. A second curved needle is loaded with an additional polypropylene suture in similar fashion. The needle is inserted and directed medially around the internal ring such that it exits just lateral to the vas deferens at the location of the first suture. If it is difficult to pass over the vas deferens, a millimeter of tissue can be left between the needle and the first suture over the vas deferens. A Maryland dissector can aid in this process by providing counter-tension on the peritoneum. The needle is then directed through the first loop. The first loop is pulled snug, and then the second loop is pushed out of the needle. The needle is removed and then the first loop is pulled up, acting as a snare to bring the second loop around the defect (Fig. 38.5).

5. A 2-0 permanent braided suture is then exchanged through the loop of polypropylene and pulled around the defect. This is supported by animal research that showed improved durability of the repair when using braided suture, likely by increasing inflammation and scarring [6]. An animal study is currently underway comparing absorbable braided suture to permanent braided suture, but until the study completed, the authors recommend the use of permanent braided suture.
6. The looped end is cut, releasing the polypropylene suture. Pressure is applied externally to the scrotum to evacuate any remaining air. The four ends of the suture are tied to each other in two separate knots, resulting in double ligation. In infants, to improve the cosmesis and reduce the chance of suture granuloma, one strand of suture may be pulled out, and the remaining one may be tied for a single ligation (Fig. 38.6).
7. The ports are removed and the incisions are closed in standard fashion. The umbilical port site typically requires one interrupted fascial suture. After this, all incisions may be closed with surgical glue.

Technical Pearls and Pitfalls

- Hydrodissection greatly improves the ease of the procedure by creating a large extraperitoneal plane in which to pass suture around the internal ring while avoiding the vas deferens and spermatic vessels.

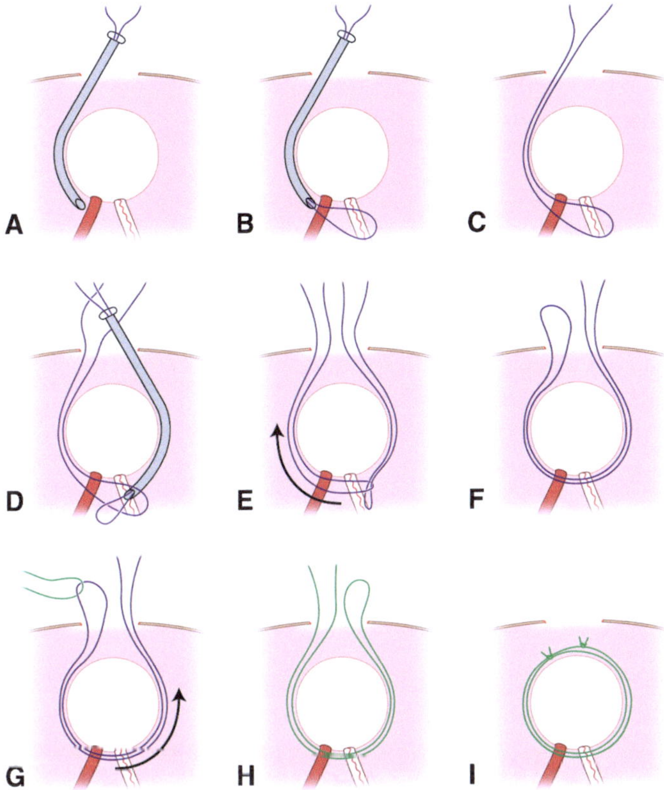

Fig. 38.5. Laparoscopic-assisted ligation of the left internal ring. The needle is passed lateral to the internal ring (**a**) and the suture is advanced (**b**). The needle is removed (**c**) and is then passed medially exiting the peritoneum through the loop of the existing suture (**d**). The first suture is pulled to snare the second suture (**e**) and bring it around the defect (**f**). A permanent braided suture is looped through the polypropylene and is pulled around the defect (**g, h**). The looped end is then cut and the ends are double ligated (**i**).

- Peritoneal injury (thermal or sharp) improves the durability of repair.
- In infants, single ligation, as opposed to double ligation, may reduce the rate of suture abscess.

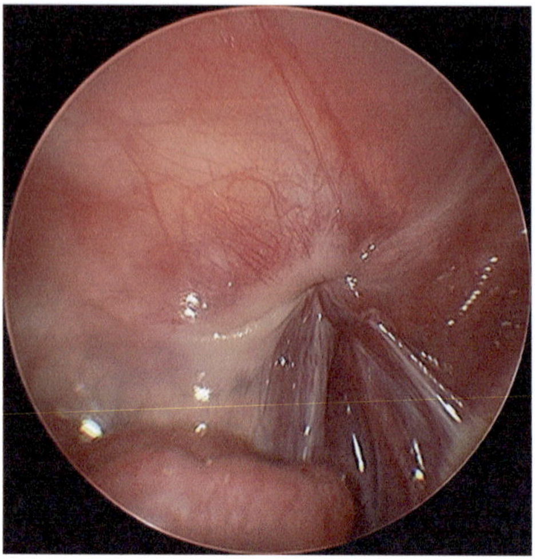

Fig. 38.6. Closed defect after repair.

Intraoperative Complications

An extraperitoneal hematoma may develop if a blood vessel is injured during the procedure. In the authors' experience, this has occurred one time and the hematoma was self-limited without the need for blood transfusion.

Alternative Techniques

1. As previously mentioned, there are several laparoscopic pediatric inguinal hernia techniques that have been developed. The first to be described laparoscopic closure of the internal ring was Schier in 1998 [7]. He described the use of a Z-stitch technique in which he intracorporeally used one or more sutures to ligate the internal ring. This technique was initially done in girls and then was later applied to boys. In an experience of 129 patients with approximately 6-month follow-up, there was one recurrence [8].
2. In 2007, Ozgediz et al. described subcutaneous endoscopically assisted ligation (SEAL) [9]. Under laparoscopic vision, a large needle is passed from outside the body, around the internal ring and out

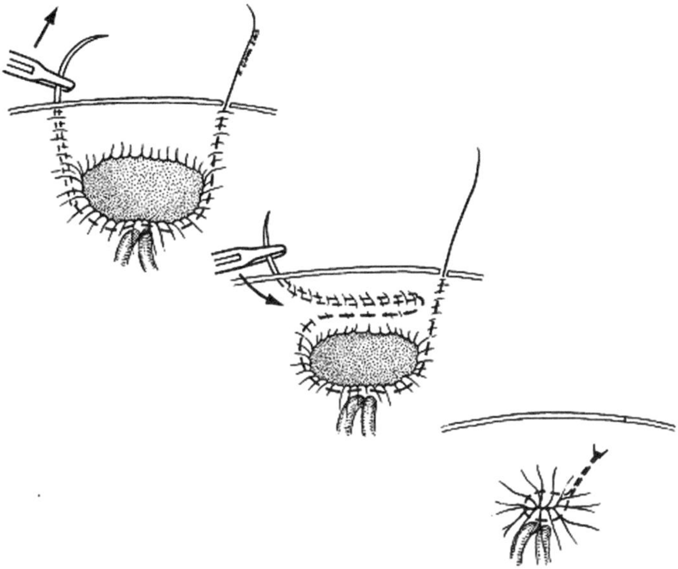

Fig. 38.7. Subcutaneous endoscopically assisted ligation (SEAL)) technique. From Ozgediz D et al. [9]. Reprinted with permission from Springer.

of the body, and the heel is backed out through the initial needle hole. The permanent braided suture is then ligated with the knot buried in the subcutaneous tissue. With this technique, there were 13 recurrences in 300 repairs, although there were only two recurrences in the last 100 repairs (Fig. 38.7).

3. An alternative approach to circumscribe the internal ring has been described by C. K. Yeung [10]. This technique utilizes a herniotomy hook to pass the suture lateral to the ring and through the peritoneum just above the vas deferens and spermatic vessels. The herniotomy hook is then passed on the medial edge of the internal ring and is used to retrieve the suture, circumscribing the patent processus vaginalis. With this technique, there were two recurrences in 298 repairs with mean follow-up of 21 months [10]. A similar technique is described by Spurbeck et al. in which they had one recurrence in 120 (0.8 %) with 2-week to 2-year follow-up [11] (Fig. 38.8).

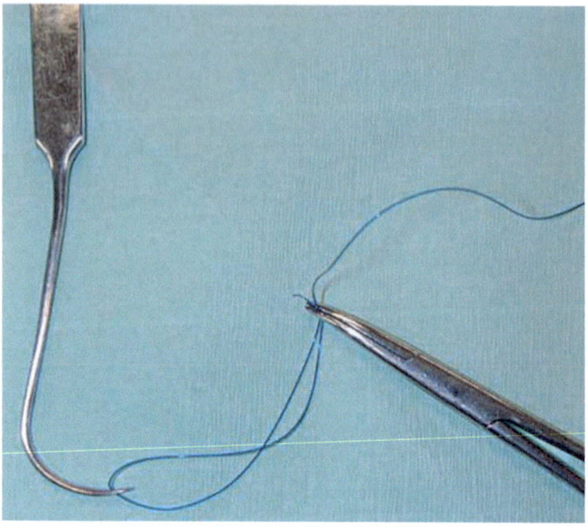

Fig. 38.8. Herniotomy hook as used by C. K. Yeung. From Yeung C. K. and Lee K. H. [10]. Reprinted with permission from Springer.

4. Becmeur described laparoscopic resection of the hernia sac with intracorporeal suture closure of the edges of the peritoneum with absorbable braided suture [12]. The initial experience published in 2004 included 96 inguinal hernia repairs. Of the 67 patients that had 6-month follow-up, there were no recurrences with this technique. A study by Boo et al. in 2012 supported these results with 202 patients with no recurrences with a mean follow-up time of 12 months [13].
5. In girls, laparoscopic inguinal hernia inversion and ligation (LIHIL) has been described using a pre-tied laparoscopic suture loop to ligate the inverted hernia sac. With this technique, they experienced 2 (0.8 %) recurrences in 241 repairs [14].
6. For internal rings of less than 10 mm, Riquelme et al. described resection of the patent processus vaginalis and parietal peritoneum surrounding the internal ring alone. There were no recurrences in 91 patients with follow-up ranging between 5 months and 4 years [15].

Postoperative Management

All patients with uncomplicated repairs go home the same day, if permitted by anesthesia. Premature infants (<50 weeks adjusted gestational age) or patients with comorbidities typically require overnight observation [16].

Suture abscess may occur, especially in younger patients with thin abdominal walls. In this case, the suture can be removed after several weeks. Anecdotally, this has not resulted in any recurrences. Postoperative hydroceles rarely occur and resolve spontaneously.

Summary

- The pediatric laparoscopic inguinal hernia repair is centered around the closure of the internal ring, most frequently by suture ligation.
- Hydrodissection greatly improves the ease of the technique by separating the peritoneum from the vas deferens and spermatic vessels.
- Braided permanent suture should be utilized based on animal studies.
- Peritoneal injury improves the durability of repair by stimulating scarring.

References

1. Patkowski D, Czernik J, Chrzan R, Jaworski W, Apoznański W. Percutaneous internal ring suturing: a simple minimally invasive technique for inguinal hernia repair in children. J Laparoendosc Adv Surg Tech A. 2006;16:513–7.
2. Endo M, Watanabe T, Nakano M, Yoshida F, Ukiyama E. Laparoscopic completely extraperitoneal repair of inguinal hernia in children: a single-institute experience with 1,257 repairs compared with cut-down herniorrhaphy. Surg Endosc. 2009;23:1706–12.
3. Alzahem A. Laparoscopic versus open inguinal herniotomy in infants and children: a meta-analysis. Pediatr Surg Int. 2011;27:605–12.
4. Blatnik JA, Harth KC, Krpata DM, Kelly KB, Schomisch SJ, Ponsky TA. Stitch versus scar—evaluation of laparoscopic pediatric inguinal hernia repair: a pilot study in a rabbit model. J Laparoendosc Adv Surg Tech A. 2012;22:848–51.
5. Godoy J. Una alternativa para el tratamiento laparoscopico de la hernia inguinal en ninas. Rev Ped Elec [en línea]. 2010;7(3). ISSN 0718–0918.
6. Kelly KB, Krpata DM, Blatnik JA, Ponsky TA. Suture choice matters in rabbit model of laparoscopic, preperitoneal, inguinal hernia repair. J Laparoendosc Adv Surg Tech A. 2014;24:428–31.
7. Schier F. Laparoscopic herniorrhaphy in girls. J Pediatr Surg. 1998;33:1495–7.
8. Schier F. Laparoscopic surgery of inguinal hernias in children—initial experience. J Pediatr Surg. 2000;35:1331–5.
9. Ozgediz D, Roayaie K, Lee H, Nobuhara KK, Farmer DL, Bratton B, Harrison MR. Subcutaneous endoscopically assisted ligation (SEAL) of the internal ring for repair of inguinal hernias in children: report of a new technique and early results. Surg Endosc. 2007;21:1327–31.

10. Yeung CK, Lee KH. Inguinal herniotomy: laparoscopic-assisted extraperitoneal technique. In: Bax KMA, Georgeson KE, Rothenberg SS, Valla JS, Yeung CK, editors. Endoscopic Surgery in Infants and Children. Berlin/Heidelberg: Springer; 2008;591–596.
11. Spurbeck WW, Prasad R, Lobe TE. Two-year experience with minimally invasive herniorrhaphy in children. Surg Endosc. 2005;19:551–3.
12. Becmeur F, Philippe P, Lemandat-Schultz A, Moog R, Grandadam S, Lieber A, Toledano D. A continuous series of 96 laparoscopic inguinal hernia repairs in children by a new technique. Surg Endosc. 2004;18:1738–41.
13. Boo Y-J, Han H-J, Ji W-B, Lee J-S. Laparoscopic hernia sac transection and intracorporeal ligation show very low recurrence rate in pediatric inguinal hernia. J Laparoendosc Adv Surg Tech A. 2012;22:720–3.
14. Lipskar AM, Soffer SZ, Glick RD, Rosen NG, Levitt MA, Hong AR. Laparoscopic inguinal hernia inversion and ligation in female children: a review of 173 consecutive cases at a single institution. J Pediatr Surg. 2010;45:1370–4.
15. Riquelme M, Aranda A, Riquelme-Q M. Laparoscopic pediatric inguinal hernia repair: no ligation, just resection. J Laparoendosc Adv Surg Tech A. 2010;20:77–80.
16. Coté CJ, Zaslavsky A, Downes JJ, Kurth CD, Welborn LG, Warner LO, Malviya SV. Postoperative apnea in former preterm infants after inguinal herniorrhaphy. A combined analysis. Anesthesiology. 1995;82:809–22.

39. Laparoscopic Epigastric Hernia Repair

Anne-Sophie Holler and Oliver J. Muensterer

Introduction

Epidemiology

Epigastric hernias account for 4 % [1] of all hernias in the pediatric population and 12.3 % of all epigastric hernias occur in children younger than 10 years [2]. In contrast to adults, there seems to be no male predominance of epigastric hernias in children [1]. Interestingly, familial history of surgically treated abdominal wall hernia has been found to be associated with an increased risk for surgical treatment of epigastric hernia [2].

Pathophysiology

Epigastric hernias are also known colloquially as fatty hernias of the linea alba. They result from a fascial defect in the upper abdominal midline fascia (the linea alba), through which preperitoneal fat, omentum, or peritoneum can herniate. Although herniation of bowel through an epigastric hernia with subsequent incarceration has been described [3], it is exceedingly rare. Therefore, epigastric hernias almost never present as an emergency.

There are several hypotheses concerning the etiology of epigastric hernias. In 1917, Moschcowitz first described the so-called vascular lacuna hypothesis, which postulates that the hernia is formed by vascular lacunae at the linea alba [4–6]. These lacunae result from small blood vessels that run from the transversalis fascia to the peritoneum and thereby perforate the linea alba. Over time, with periods of intermittent

D.S. Walsh et al. (eds.), *The SAGES Manual of Pediatric Minimally Invasive Surgery*, DOI 10.1007/978-3-319-43642-5_39

increase of abdominal pressure, the fascial defect enlarges and preperitoneal fat protrudes [4, 5, 7]. A second hypothesis involves the decussation hypothesis of Askar, which states that epigastric hernias occur only if a special abnormal midline pattern of fascial fiber decussation is present [6, 8, 9].

Preoperative Evaluation

History

Typically, children present with an epigastric mass somewhere midline between the umbilicus and the xiphoid process. This epigastric bulge may be either reducible or nonreducible. It is especially noticeable when the child is crying, stooling, or bearing down. Some children complain about pain or discomfort which can worsen during activity [1, 10].

Physical Examination

Epigastric hernias present as an either painful or indolent protrusion in the upper abdominal midline that often can be palpated, particularly when the patient contracts the abdominal musculature. In 13–20 % of the cases, epigastric hernias occur in multiple locations in the same patient [1, 6].

Laboratory Evaluation

There are no specific laboratory findings required. Whether preoperative laboratory evaluation is indicated prior to surgical repair depends on the individual patient, their previous medical history, as well as any significant comorbidities.

Imaging

Usually, the diagnosis can be made solely by physical examination. Ultrasound may help in uncertain cases or when discrimination between a subcutaneous lipoma, fibroma, or neurofibroma is not possible by physical examination [3, 6, 11, 12]. Magnetic resonance imaging can be helpful in obese individuals in which physical exam or ultrasound is compromised by soft tissue [11].

Surgical Indications

Epigastric hernias rarely, if ever, resolve spontaneously. Therefore, surgical repair is indicated at the time of diagnosis, especially if it is symptomatic [1, 6, 10].

Technique

Special Considerations

Classically, epigastric hernia repair has been performed by open surgical technique. A transverse incision is made over the site of the defect, incarcerated fat is removed, and the linea alba is closed by interrupted sutures. At the end of the surgery, a conspicuous scar is usually left in the epigastrium.

It is recommended to mark the location of the epigastric hernia on the skin preoperatively before the patient undergoes anesthesia, because it can be hard to detect the hernia once the patient is paralyzed under anesthesia with the abdominal musculature relaxed [10, 13, 14].

Anatomy

There is a small defect midline in the linea alba located in between the umbilicus and the xiphoid process. Most defects are small (0.7±0.6 cm), but may vary in size [1].

Patient Positioning

The child is placed in supine position. Some authors prefer to position the patient with their left side elevated to maximize the space between the left iliac spine and the ipsilateral costal margin when a left upper abdominal laparoscopic approach is planned [13]. For single-incision epigastric hernia repair, it is helpful to position a roll under the lumbar spine [10].

Instruments

To date, three different techniques for laparoscopic epigastric hernia repair have been described. The following equipment is used:

- Conventional (upper lateral) laparoscopic approach [13]: two or three 3-mm trocars, 2.7-mm 30° telescope, knot pusher, monopolar hook cautery, Maryland dissector, 3-mm needle holder, 3-mm hook scissor, and 2-0 braided polyester suture
- Conventional (lower abdominal) laparoscopic approach [14]: 5-mm trocar, 5-mm 30°-angle laparoscope, 3-mm dissector, 16-guage needle, and 2× 2-0 polyglactin suture
- SIPES (single-incision pediatric endosurgical) epigastric hernia repair [10]: 5-mm trocar, 5-mm 30° endoscope, 3-mm trocar, L-shaped electrocautery hook, 3-mm Maryland dissector, 16-gauge epidural (Tuohy) needle, and 2× 4-0 polypropylene suture

Operative Steps

Although all laparoscopic techniques include the identification of the midline fascial defect from the abdominal cavity, along with suturing the defect under laparoscopic vision, trocar positioning varies according to the technique used. In the conventional laparoscopic approach from the upper abdomen [13], the first trocar is inserted between the left iliac crest and costal margin at the level of the anterior to midaxillary line. A second port is inserted in approximately the midclavicular line at the level of the ninth intercostal space. If needed, a third trocar is placed in the suprapubic region. For the lower abdominal conventional approach [14], trocars are inserted in the umbilicus and the left lower flank, while all instruments and optics are inserted through the navel with the SIPES technique [10].

In all techniques, the peritoneum underlying the location of the epigastric hernia is incised and the fascial defect exposed by pulling the preperitoneal fat off the fascia bluntly (Fig. 39.1). Then, if present, the incarcerated preperitoneal fat is reduced into the abdominal cavity (Fig. 39.2). For a better exposure of the defect, it is helpful to gently push down the abdominal wall beyond the defect manually to create a more direct view onto the inside abdominal wall [10, 13, 14]. The defect can be closed by either suturing intracorporeally [13] or by a percutaneous suture technique [10, 14]. In the latter case, a 17-gauge Tuohy needle is inserted percutaneously

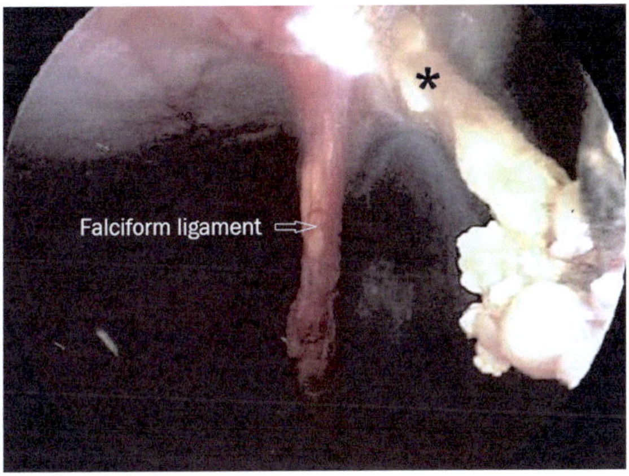

Fig. 39.1. The peritoneum is opened bluntly at the site of the epigastric hernia and incarcerated fat (*asterisk*) is removed by traction.

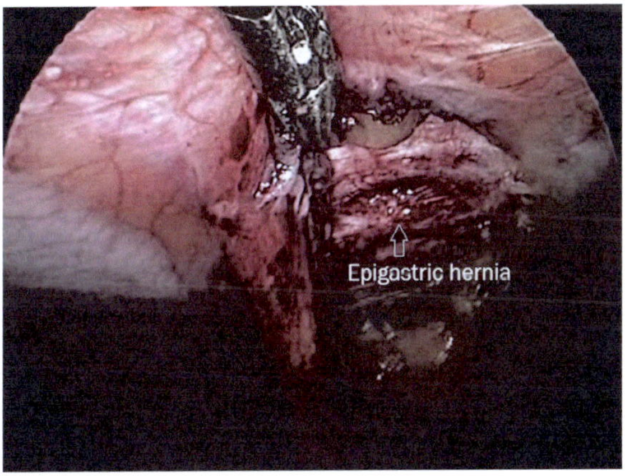

Fig. 39.2. Once the fat has been removed, the fascial midline defect is visible.

through one side of the defect (Figs. 39.3 and 39.4). A suture loop is passed through the needle into the abdomen. Through the same skin lesion, the needle and a second suture are inserted again on the contrary side of the fascial defect and into the loop. By pulling on the first suture, the second loop is "lassoed" around the defect. After that the suture is tied tightly down onto the fascia (Fig. 39.5), leaving the knot in the subcutaneous fat. Further stitches can be fashioned in the same manner, depending on the size of the defect [10, 14]. Alternatively, a Berci needle can be employed to pass the suture around the defect.

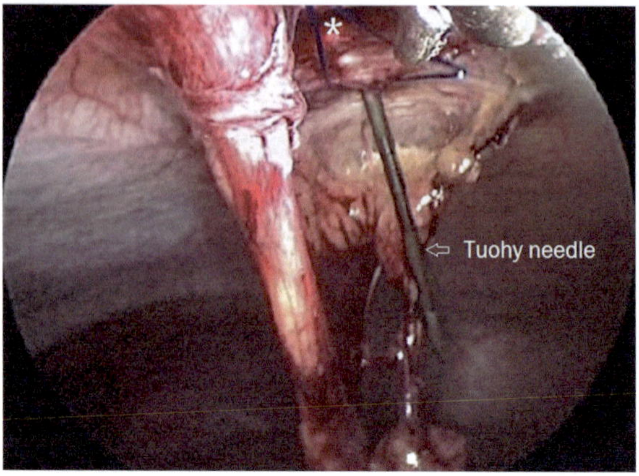

Fig. 39.3. Sutures are passed around the hernia defect (*asterisk*).

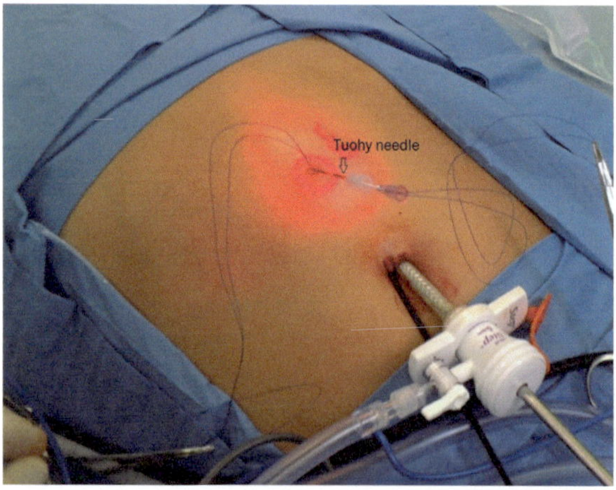

Fig. 39.4. In this case the procedure is performed in the lasso technique with the help of a percutaneous Tuohy needle at the site of the hernia.

Pearls/Pitfalls

In contrast to most other laparoscopic surgeries, the target area in epigastric hernias is the ventral abdominal wall. Therefore, the surgeon must learn to operate upward, which can be very challenging initially. In cases where the defect is located close to the umbilicus, the focus distance is short and the operating space small. Therefore, lesions that

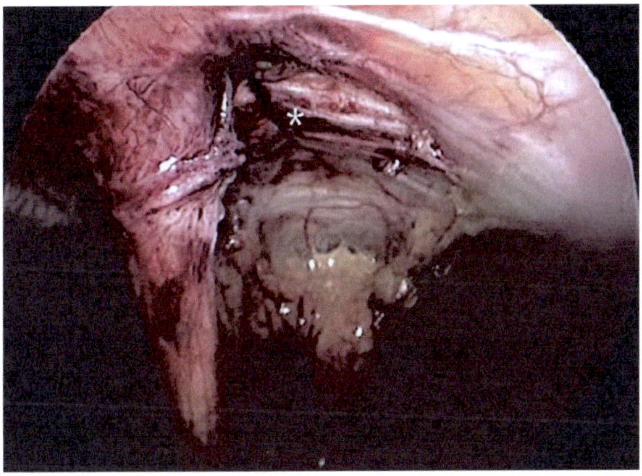

Fig. 39.5. After the suture is tied, closure of the epigastric hernia (*asterisk*) is confirmed by laparoscopy.

are closer than 4–5 cm from the umbilicus often are easier performed by the open technique through a small incision in the umbilicus and tunneling upward toward the defect from the outside [10]. As mentioned above, pushing down on the abdominal wall beyond the defect may increase maneuverability since it provides a more direct angle onto the defect [10, 13, 14].

Postoperative Care

Outcomes

There were no intraoperative or postoperative complications recorded in the published case studies. Particularly, no recurrent hernias were described [10, 13, 14]. Laparoscopic and particularly single-incision techniques purportedly provide excellent postoperative cosmesis.

Complications

General complications such as bleeding, wound infection, recurrence, and injury to intra-abdominal viscera and vessels are at least conceivable, but seem exceedingly rare [10, 13, 14].

Some adult publications classify epigastric hernias as ventral hernias. After laparoscopic ventral hernia repair, a recurrence rate of 4.7 % has been described. Risk factors were found to be a large defect, obesity, previous open repair, and perioperative complications [15, 16]. It must be noted, however, that these epigastric hernias are not the congenital type seen in the pediatric population or subject of this chapter.

Summary

- Epigastric hernias are defined as defects in the linea alba located between the umbilicus and the xiphoid process.
- Symptomatic hernias require surgical repair.
- Laparoscopic repair is a valid alternative to the conventional open technique since the laparoscopic complication and recurrence rate is at least as favorable with potentially better cosmesis.
- Laparoscopic epigastric hernia repair is technically challenging, however, since the working and viewing axis is oriented upward toward the abdominal wall.

References

1. Coats RD, Helikson MA, Burd RS. Presentation and management of epigastric hernias in children. J Pediatr Surg. 2000;35:1754–6.
2. Zöller B, Ji J, Sundquist J, Sundquist K. Shared and nonshared familial susceptibility to surgically treated inguinal hernia, femoral hernia, incisional hernia, epigastric hernia, and umbilical hernia. J Am Coll Surg. 2013;217:289–99. e1.
3. Harison CS. A case of strangulated epigastric hernia. S Afr Med J. 1965;39:679.
4. Moschowitz AV. Epigastric hernia without palpable swelling. Ann Surg. 1917;66: 300–7.
5. Lang B, Lau H, Lee F. Epigastric hernia and its etiology. Hernia. 2002;6:148–50.
6. Muschaweck U. Umbilical and epigastric hernia repair. Surg Clin North Am. 2003; 83:1207–21.
7. Gorganchian F, Santa Maria V, Dupuy Cash T, Mori I, Anania S. Topic: abdominal wall hernia—epigastric hernia: choice of approach, repair, results, follow up. Hernia. 2016;Suppl 1:S208–11.
8. Askar OM. A new concept of the aetiology and surgical repair of paraumbilical and epigastric hernias. Ann R Coll Surg Engl. 1978;60:42–8.
9. Askar OM. Aponeurotic hernias. Recent observations upon paraumbilical and epigastric hernias. Surg Clin North Am. 1984;64:315–33.

10. Babsail AA, Abelson JS, Liska D, Muensterer OJ. Single-incision pediatric endosurgical epigastric hernia repair. Hernia. 2014;18:357–60.
11. Graf JL, Caty MG, Martin DJ, Glick PL. Pediatric hernias. Semin Ultrasound CT MR. 2002;23:197–200.
12. Spangen L. Ultrasound as a diagnostic aid in ventral abdominal hernia. J Clin Ultrasound. 1975;3:211–3.
13. Albanese CT, Rengal S, Bermudez D. A novel laparoscopic technique for the repair of pediatric umbilical and epigastric hernias. J Pediatr Surg. 2006;41:859–62.
14. Moreira-Pinto J, Correia-Pinto J. Scarless laparoscopic repair of epigastric hernia in children. Hernia. 2015;19:623–6.
15. Heniford BT, Park A, Ramshaw BJ, Voeller G. Laparoscopic repair of ventral hernias: nine years' experience with 850 consecutive hernias. Ann Surg. 2003;238:391–9.
16. Earle DB, McLellan JA. Repair of umbilical and epigastric hernias. Surg Clin North Am. 2013;93:1057–89.

40. Minimally Invasive Approach to Pediatric Pancreatic Disorders

Meagan Elizabeth Evangelista and Danielle S. Walsh

Introduction

While pancreatic injury and illness are rare in the pediatric population, their treatment by minimally invasive techniques has dramatically altered management from prior eras. Following the development of both endoscopic and laparoscopic approaches to the pancreas in adults, these techniques were adapted to the pediatric population as instrumentation was refined and MIS skills in pediatric specialists advanced. Blunt trauma to the pancreas, pancreatic ductal obstruction from anomalies or stones, and mass lesions of the pancreas are the most likely etiologies necessitating intervention [1].

Traumatic injury is the most likely etiology of a pancreatic injury that subsequently requires surgical intervention in children. Blunt trauma to the mid-epigastrium can compress the soft pancreas between the external force and the spinal column, resulting in complete or partial transection of the organ. Management strategies differ based on early vs delayed presentation, the presence or absence of ductal transection, the presence or absence of concomitant injuries, and the clinical stability of the patient. When a complete pancreatic transection is diagnosed early in the stable patient, distal pancreatectomy via open or laparoscopic technique can lead to faster recovery and low morbidity [2]. However, when the diagnosis is delayed or the indication for distal pancreatectomy is less clear in the acute phase, the patient may go on to develop a pancreatic pseudocyst, named as such because they lack an epithelial lining [3]. Traumatic injury causes over 60 % of pancreatic pseudocyst formation and the majority are a result of abdominal impact with the handlebars of bicycles, followed secondly by falls [4].

D.S. Walsh et al. (eds.), *The SAGES Manual of Pediatric Minimally Invasive Surgery*, DOI 10.1007/978-3-319-43642-5_40

Inflammatory disorders of the pancreas can also result in ductal obstruction with subsequent pseudocyst formation requiring surgical therapy. Gallstone pancreatitis, familial pancreatic disorders, medication reactions, and ductal abnormalities, such as pancreatic divisum, can result in pancreatic pseudocysts or abscesses, though the origin of some pseudocysts is idiopathic [5, 6].

Neoplasms of the pancreas are rare in children, occurring in less than 1 in 500,000 children and consisting of solid pseudopapillary masses, pancreaticoblastoma, and pancreatic endocrine neoplasms [7]. Solid pseudopapillary masses of the pancreas occur most commonly in adolescent females, though they can occur in children. While more commonly in the head, and less amenable to laparoscopic resection in children, adolescent females may have them in the body and tail, permitting the use of laparoscopy for resection [8]. Both distal pancreatectomy and central pancreatectomy with implantation of the distal pancreas into the stomach have been described in children laparoscopically [9]. Pancreaticoblastoma occurs equally in the head and tail of the pancreas, and may be amenable to laparoscopic resection in selected cases, with or without neoadjuvant chemotherapy [10]. Pancreatic endocrine neoplasms are less common than in adults and may either produce a hormonally active product, such as is seen in insulinomas and gastrinomas, or be nonfunctional [10]. While there are reports of successful laparoscopic resection of these lesions, particularly with the assistance of intraoperative ultrasound, others caution that endocrine neoplasms can be multicentric, and the loss of manual palpation may result in a retained secondary lesion [11, 12]. Similarly, congenital hyperinsulinism refractory to medical control has been successfully treated with laparoscopic pancreatectomy, though outcomes in the largest reported series demonstrate a significantly higher percentage of patients still requiring medication for management than is reported in open series [13, 14].

Preoperative Evaluation

History and Physical Exam

A history of epigastric trauma accompanied by upper abdominal pain, tenderness, anorexia, emesis, and sometimes bruising of the epigastrium is a common presentation. Unfortunately, the trauma may have been felt mild initially, resulting in a delayed presentation when edema in the area of the injury is more severe. Much later, an epigastric mass due to a pseudocyst may be present on the exam. Pancreatic ascites or a pancreatic pleural effusion is rare but can result in a presentation of respiratory distress and more diffuse abdominal discomfort [15]. Other potential findings related to pancreatic injury include infection, necrosis, bleeding, and pseudoaneurysm formation [3].

The symptoms of hypoglycemia are commonly neurologic and may include irritability, confusion, seizures, vision changes, and, if left untreated, coma or death. The hallmark of insulinomas consists of hypoglycemic hyperinsulinemia, or Whipple's triad of fasting hypoglycemia, symptoms of hypoglycemia, and resolution of symptoms with administration of glucose. Gastrinomas can manifest as Zollinger–Ellison syndrome with gastroesophageal reflux and ulcers [10]. Inflammatory disorders may present as upper abdominal pain with or without radiation to the back, anorexia, pain with eating, nausea, and emesis. If infected, lesions may also be accompanied by fever and chills. Non-endocrine-producing tumors may present with pain or as an incidental finding.

Labs

Pediatric pancreatic trauma and inflammation can be suggested by elevated serum amylase and/or lipase. Following pancreatic trauma, a maximum serum amylase >1100 U/L is predictive of pseudocyst development or another complication and may warrant closer radiographic follow-up [16]. Measurements of hepatobiliary function may prove helpful adjuncts to assessment. Serum chemistry panels with calcium can assist with management of fluid balance, while calcium, lactate dehydrogenase, and white blood cell count can assist with predicting severity of illness as part of Ranson's criteria. The assessment of various metabolic disorders amenable to pancreatic resection is beyond the scope of this chapter. However, once diagnosed, glycemic control, in particular, should be frequently reassessed in the perioperative period. Conventional pancreatic tumor markers are generally unremarkable in this population, though some pancreaticoblastomas may test positive for alpha-fetoprotein [17].

Imaging

Due to the absence of radiation, ultrasound is the tool of choice for imaging pediatric pancreatic disorders. On ultrasound images, pseudocysts are usually well-defined, smooth-walled, anechoic, or hypoechoic masses. Some are multilocular with internal septations. If hemorrhage or infection is present, internal echoes or a fluid–fluid level may be seen. Pancreatitis may manifest as inflammation, and gallstones with or without biliary tree dilation can be perceived. However, contrast-enhanced CT scans, ideally with a pancreatic protocol, are common for diagnosis of traumatic pancreatic injury and are often used for planning surgical intervention. On CT, the capsule of the pseudocyst should appear well defined with a central area of low attenuation and an attenuation coefficient within a range relative to that of water [6, 18]. Incidental masses of the pancreas are commonly identified by CT. Magnetic resonance cholangiopancreatography (MRCP) is valued not only for reduction in radiation exposure to children but also for its ability to more thoroughly evaluate the hepatic, biliary, and pancreatic ductal system and tissue pathology [19]. In many centers, MRCP has largely replaced endoscopic retrograde cholangiopancreatography, though this remains a helpful adjunct for diagnosis, especially when combined with therapeutic interventions [20]. Endoscopic and laparoscopic ultrasound can also prove helpful for pancreatic surgery in children when available and the child is of an appropriate size [21].

Surgical Indications

Not all pancreatic lesions, particularity pseudocysts, require surgical treatment. Pseudocysts measuring less than 5 cm can sometimes resolve non-operatively. Medical therapies can reduce pancreatic stimulation and promote spontaneous resolution of the pseudocyst, and medical management is often the first-line therapy for hyperinsulinism [14, 22, 23]. Treatment options for inflammatory disorders and trauma include: bowel rest with total parenteral nutrition, post-pancreatic tube feedings, and octreotide acetate [24, 25]. In a review of pediatric pancreatic pseudocysts resulting from blunt abdominal trauma, six of ten patients recovered using total parenteral nutrition. The authors indicate that in these cases, all pseudocysts were diagnosed early via ultrasound and promptly treated with gut rest [26].

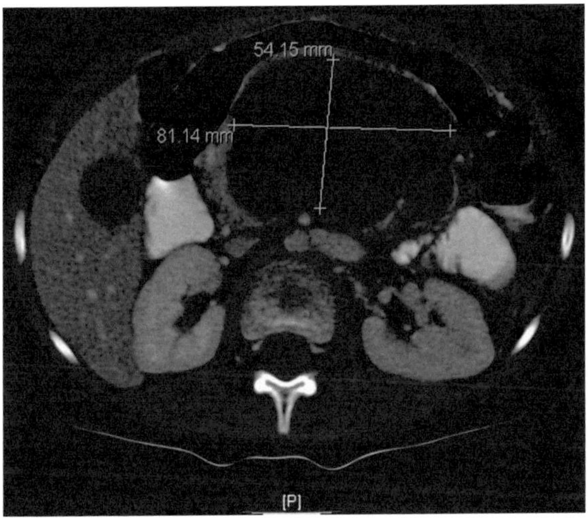

Fig. 40.1. A pancreatic pseudocyst 5 weeks after complete pancreatic transection. Note the apposition of the pseudocyst wall to the posterior stomach, making the lesion now amenable to cystogastrostomy.

In patients unresponsive to medical therapy or deemed candidates for resection or drainage, there are multiple techniques available. For pancreatic pseudocysts, internal and external drainage through surgery via open or laparoscopic technique, endoscopy, and interventional radiology have been described. While the majority are amenable to cystogastrostomy, a small percentage fail to approximate the posterior gastric wall and are better treated with a cystojejunostomy, which can also be performed laparoscopically [27]. With imaging advancements, endoscopic internal drainage was developed and has been used in the pediatric population since 1996 [23]. Surgical intervention for pseudocysts is typically delayed for 4–6 weeks from the initial insult to permit time for smaller lesions to resolve and larger lesions to adhere to the posterior gastric wall with a fibrous capsule [4] (Fig. 40.1). For mass lesions, surgical resection is indicated and is the mainstay of treatment, though in the case of locally advanced pancreaticoblastomas, neoadjuvant chemotherapy may be indicated.

Technique

Regardless of the indication for surgery, this chapter will focus on the techniques used in the most common indication for intervention, pseudocyst, and the most common operation for non-pseudocyst lesions, distal pancreatectomy.

Anatomy

The pancreas in divided into a head, body, and tail, with the body overlying the L1 vertebrae. This largely retroperitoneal structure sits with the head in the curve of the duodenum and the body and tail behind the stomach. The splenic artery follows the superior aspect of the gland from midline laterally, supplying short arterial branches along its length. Additional arterial supply arises from the inferior pancreatic artery, also a branch off the splenic artery. The splenic vein courses across the lower aspect of the tail as it heads more superiorly before merging with the superior mesenteric vein and entering the portal vein posterior to the pancreatic head. It drains the body and tail of the pancreas.

The duct of Wirsung, or main pancreatic duct, drains the length of the pancreas, emptying into the duodenum at the ampulla of Vater in conjunction with the common bile duct. The accessory duct of Santorini drains the dorsal bud and can have its own minor papilla for drainage. Pancreatic divisum occurs after failure of the embryonic ventral and dorsal pancreatic buds to properly fuse.

Positioning

Patients are typically positioned supine or in a partial right decubitus position with a roll behind the left lower rib cage.

Instruments

A standard 5-mm laparoscopic instrument tray, three to four 5-mm ports, a 12-mm port for a stapler, a 30-degree 5-mm laparoscope, a 5-mm clip applier, and an energy device, such as ultrasonic shears or other tissue-sealing device, are necessary. A laparoscopic biopsy needle for aspiration may be required for pseudocyst localization. One or more

45-cm vascular staple loads for a laparoscopic stapler are needed for either creation of the cystogastrostomy or transecting the pancreas. An endoscope, pediatric or adult, can be used for hybrid cystogastrostomy approaches, while an adult endoscope with a larger working channel is needed for purely endoscopic approaches.

Laparoscopic Internal Drainage of Pseudocysts

Laparoscopic cystogastrostomy for the treatment of pancreatic pseudocysts in the pediatric population has been done for nearly a decade [28]. A transumbilical laparoscope allows visualization of the anterior gastric wall with pneumoperitoneum. Following this, two trocars are inserted through the abdominal wall and anterior gastric wall such that they access the gastric lumen. This can be facilitated by the placement of stay sutures or T fasteners through the abdominal and anterior gastric walls for apposition of the two layers as well as insufflation of the stomach with gas through an NG tube. The pneumoperitoneum can then be released and a small amount of insufflation at a low pressure be placed intragastric for visualization through the ports. The posterior gastric wall will commonly have a protrusion identifying the site of the pseudocyst. After confirmation of pseudocyst location through needle aspiration with a laparoscopic device, cautery or an alternative energy device is used to create a posterior gastrotomy and enter the pseudocyst. Clear pancreatic fluid typically drains. For a hybrid approach, one of the transgastric trocars can be replaced by the endoscope for visualization, insufflation is accomplished through the endoscopic port, and an endoscopic needle knife can be used for aspiration and gastrotomy. A stapled anastomosis is performed to widen the opening and one or more firings can be utilized. The gastric distension is then relieved and pneumoperitoneum reestablished. The anterior gastrotomies can be closed by pulling the transgastric trocars back to an intraperitoneal location and either stapling the holes closed or hand suturing them. Laparoscopic drainage of pediatric pancreatic pseudocysts is proving to be a beneficial minimally invasive procedure providing definitive drainage. A nasogastric tube may or may not be left overnight and a contrast study prior to oral intake is not typically required in the absence of clinical concern for a leak. Oral intake can be initiated in less than 24 h or upon resolution of any ileus. The postoperative recovery time is significantly shorter than other treatment options, a notable benefit [28, 29]. The most common complications are anastomotic bleeding, leak, pancreatitis, infection, and premature closure.

Endoscopic Internal Drainage

The first case of pediatric pancreatic pseudocyst endoscopic drainage was reported by Wiersema et al. in 1996 [30]. There are two approaches to endoscopic drainage of pancreatic pseudocysts: transmural drainage or transpapillary drainage. Transmural drainage is indicated if the pseudocyst is in direct opposition to the stomach or duodenum. The pseudocyst must visibly bulge into the gastric or duodenal wall [31]. Transpapillary drainage is indicated if endoscopic retrograde cholangiopancreatography shows pseudocyst connection with the main pancreatic duct, and internal stenting is technically feasible [32]. However, cysts suspected to contain thick material or debris may be best managed by alternate techniques.

Endoscopic transmural drainage is accomplished with a flexible endoscope and a diathermy needle knife to puncture the pseudocyst through the posterior wall of the stomach. Over guidewire dilation enlarges the communication between the stomach and the pseudocyst. Both double J stents and double pigtail stents are used to maintain patency while the pseudocyst resolves [31] (Fig. 40.2). The AXIOS Stent and Electrocautery Enhanced Delivery System (Boston Scientific) was approved by the FDA in 2013 specifically for transgastric endoscopic drainage of pancreatic pseudocysts. Diet can be resumed post procedure after concern for procedural complications has passed. There are associated complications with internal endoscopic drainage. Bleeding, infection leading to abscess formation, stent dysfunction, pancreatitis, and pseudocyst recurrence are the main concerns. Most stents remain in place for 3–8 weeks before endoscopic removal.

Laparoscopic Distal Pancreatectomy

A 5-mm port is placed in the umbilicus and pneumoperitoneum is established. The remaining trocar positions are variable based on the patient size, but should allow access to the left upper quadrant, similar to a laparoscopic splenectomy. Port placement may vary depending on whether the surgeon elects to stand the patient's right side or between the legs. Generally, one port in the left upper quadrant and one in the medial

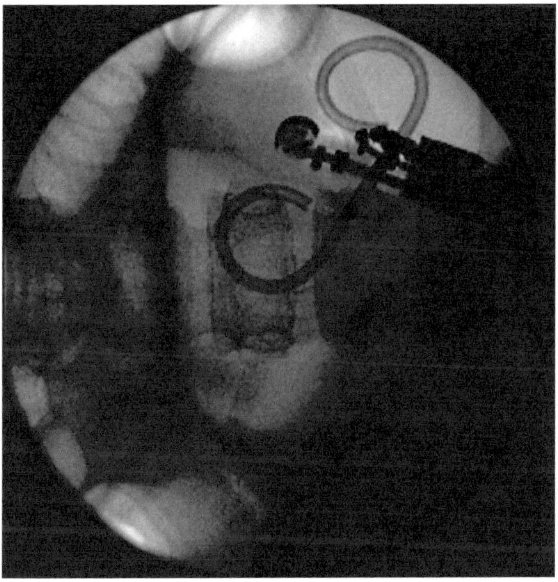

Fig. 40.2. Fluoroscopic image of a stent placed endoscopically for treatment of a pancreatic pseudocyst in a 9-year-old boy following trauma.

right upper quadrant can complement an optional epigastric port. All can be 5-mm in size until time for transection of the pancreas with an endoscopic stapler, at which point either the epigastric or a left upper quadrant port needs to be transitioned to a 12-mm port to accommodate the device. The gastrocolic ligament is opened, taking care to spare the gastroepiploic and short gastric vessels. A retractor in the epigastric port or transabdominal sutures to elevate the inferior aspect of the stomach permits visualization of the distal pancreas. In the setting of inflammation, some dissection may be required along the posterior wall of the stomach to elevate it off of the pancreas. If available, endoscopic ultrasound can be used at this time to either identify the lesion and a negative margin and/or assess the location of the vessels and their relationship to the mass. Dissection continues at the inferior aspect of the tail of the pancreas. Elevating the pancreas superiorly allows clearing of the relatively avascular posterior wall pancreas from inferior to superior. When the tail of the pancreas can be clearly identified, the splenic vein can similarly be seen posteriorly. The pancreatic tail can then be retracted superomedially to allow division of branches between the vein and the pancreas to be divided with an energy device. As the vein is left behind, small arterial branches from the splenic artery may

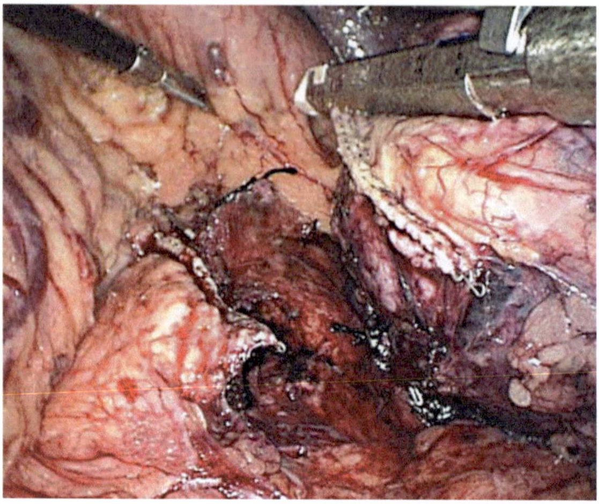

Fig. 40.3. The pancreatic body has been transected medial to the mass and dissection will now proceed laterally to the tail. From Palavivelu C, Shety R, Jani K, et al. Laparoscopic distal pancreatectomy. Results of a prospective non-randomized study from a tertiary center. Surg Endoscopy 2007 Mar:21(3):373–77. Reprinted with permission from Springer.

become visible and be similarly divided. If the pancreas has been divided due to trauma, the distal remnant will often be free now. If the pancreatic duct is visible at the transection site, suture closure of the duct and/or nearby tissue can minimize subsequent leak [33].

If the distal pancreatectomy is for a mass lesion located in the tail, it can be helpful to carefully create a window around the pancreas medial to the mass and pass a ¼-in. penrose drain around the body of the pancreas for retraction. This can make careful separation of the pancreas and/or mass from the splenic vessels easier through a medial to lateral approach when splenic preservation is intended. Alternatively, once the vessels are safely away, an endoscopic stapler with vascular loads can be used to transect the pancreatic parenchyma before proceeding laterally (Fig. 40.3).

A closed suction drain is commonly placed in the pancreatic bed and some surgeons place fibrin glue over the cut edge of the residual pancreas. The resected pancreas can be placed in a laparoscopic bag and withdrawn through an enlarged port site, with or without morcellation, or through a Pfannenstiel incision for malignancy. While splenic artery and vein preservation are ideal, this is significantly more technically difficult than division of these vessels at the proximal and distal aspects of the pancreas. For malignant lesions with adherence to the splenic vessels, splenic vessel preservation should be avoided, though the spleen may remain in situ and viable based on the short gastrics. In addition to energy devices, judicious use of clips can help control the vasculature. The spleen, if preserved, should be inspected for viability, with consideration given to performing a splenectomy if lacking perfusion. Even if the spleen is successfully preserved at the time of surgery, splenic vein thrombosis can complicate the postoperative period. Additionally, in the adult population, if the splenic vein is ligated, the splenic artery is also ligated to prevent segmental portal hypertension [34]. Uncontrolled bleeding, inability to identify the pathology, inadequate margins, and inadequate exposure are all indications for conversion to open techniques.

Outcomes

A five institution review of laparoscopic treatment of pediatric pancreatic pseudocysts showed 92% resulted in no complications and required no further operative intervention. Eight percent, one patient, had recurrence of the pseudocyst and required a distal pancreatectomy, following which the patient recovered [29]. Overall, laparoscopic techniques have proven to be successful with early oral nutrition and short postoperative hospital stays.

While there is limited outcome data on pediatric patients undergoing distal pancreatectomy, a large meta-analysis comparing open to laparoscopic resection in 1814 patients found laparoscopy led to lower complication rates (33.9% vs 44.2%), shorter hospital stays (by 4 days), and decreased blood loss [35]. One pediatric study reviewed the literature of patients who underwent laparoscopic resection of pseudopapillary tumors and reported excellent outcomes [36].

Pearls/Pitfalls

- In patients who develop pancreatic pseudocysts, intervention is ideally delayed 4–6 weeks to permit for both spontaneous resolution and maturity of the cyst wall.
- Laparoscopic cystogastrostomy can be performed with transgastric techniques, but the small size of the stomach with small working

space led this author to favor hybrid techniques in children under 15 kg, utilizing the endoscope for visualization.
- Endoscopic drainage is a rewarding procedure for children without debris in the cyst on preoperative imaging, if they are large enough for the adult endoscope. However, a second procedure to remove the stents is required.
- Distal pancreatectomy immediately after pancreatic transection can result in expeditious return to normal function with low complication rates; however, performing a spleen-sparing technique can prove more technically challenging.
- In pancreatic tail masses, creating a window around the pancreas medial to the tumor and working from medial to lateral can be easier than working from the tail toward tumor.

Summary

- While nonoperative management may allow some pseudocysts to resolve, minimally invasive techniques such as laparoscopic and endoscopic cystogastrostomy should be considered, are technically feasible, and are highly efficacious.
- Laparoscopic distal pancreatectomy is also a well-established procedure for both acute pancreatic transection and mass lesions of the pancreas.
- In comparison to open drainage procedures, the recovery time in laparoscopic procedures is shorter with decreased complication rates.
- Taken as a whole, laparoscopic and endoscopic approaches are advancing as the management strategy of choice for pediatric pancreatic disorders.

References

1. Vane DW, Grosfeld JL, West KW, et al. Pancreatic disorders in infancy and childhood: experience with 92 cases. J Pediatr Surg. 1989;24(8):771–6.
2. Igbal CW, St Peter SD, Tsao K, et al. Operative vs nonoperative management for blunt pancreatic transection in children: multi-institutional outcomes. J Am Coll Surg. 2014;218(2):157–62.
3. Stringer MD. Pancreatitis and pancreatic trauma. Semin Pediatr Surg. 2005;14:239–46.
4. Ford EG, Hardin WD, Mahour GH, et al. Pseudocysts of the pancreas in children. Am Surg. 1990;56(6):384–7.

5. Buntain WL, Wood JB, Woolley MM. Pancreatitis in childhood. J Pediatr Surg. 1978;13:143–9.
6. Nijs E, Callahan MJ, Taylor GA. Disorders of the pediatric pancreas: imaging features. Pediatr Radiol. 2005;35:358–73.
7. Perez EA, Gutierrez JC, Koniaris LG, et al. Malignant pancreatic tumors: incidence and outcome in 58 pediatric patients. J Pediatr Surg. 2009;44:197–203.
8. Alvise C, Giovanni B, Despoina D, et al. Laparoscopic pancreatectomy for solid pseudo-papillary tumors of the pancreas is a suitable technique: our experience with long-term follow-up and review of the literature. Ann Surg Oncol. 2011;18(2): 352–7.
9. Sokolov YY, Stonogin SV, Donskoy DV, et al. Laparoscopic pancreatic resections for solid pseudopapillary tumor in children. Eur J Pediatr Surg. 2009;19(6):399–401.
10. Tucker SM. Pediatric neoplasms of the pancreas: a review. Ann Clin Pathol. 2014;2(2):1017. 1–5.
11. Peranteau WH, Palladino AA, Bhatti TR, et al. The surgical management of insulinomas in children. J Pediatr Surg. 2013;48(12):2517–24.
12. Strong VE, Shifrin A, Inabnet WB. Rapid intraoperative insulin assay: a novel method to differentiate insulinoma from nesidioblastosis in the pediatric patient. Ann Surg Innov Res. 2007;1(6). doi:10.1186/1750-1164-1-6.
13. Al-Shanafey S. Laparoscopic vs open pancreatectomy for persistent hyperinsulinemic hypoglycemia of infancy. J Pediatr Surg. 2009;44(5):957–61.
14. Adzick NS, Thornton PA, Stanley CA, et al. A multidisciplinary approach to the focal form of congenital hyperinsulinism leads to successful treatment by partial pancreatectomy. J Pediatr Surg. 2004;39(3):270–5.
15. Ahearne PM. Pancreatic pseudocysts. In: Sabiston DC, Lyerly HK, editors. Sabiston essentials of surgery, 2nd ed. Philadelphia: W.B. Saunders. 1994;419–22.
16. Herman R, Guire KE, Burd RS, et al. Utility of amylase and lipase as predictors of grade of injury or outcomes in pediatric patients with pancreatic trauma. J Pediatr Surg. 2011;46:923–6.
17. Ohaki Y, Misugi K, Fukuda J, et al. Immunohistochemical study of pancreatoblastoma. Acta Pathol Jpn. 1987;37(10):1581–90.
18. Ros PR, Hamrick-Turner JE, Chiechi MV, et al. Cystic masses of the pancreas. Radiographics. 1992;12:673–86.
19. Rescorla FJ, Plumley DA, Sherman S, et al. The efficacy of early ERCP in pediatric pancreatic trauma. J Pediatr Surg. 1995;30:336–40.
20. Houben CH, Ade-Ajayi N, Patel S, et al. Traumatic pancreatic duct injury in children: minimally invasive approach to management. J Pediatr Surg. 2007;42:629–35.
21. Nadler EP, Novikov A, Landzberg BR, et al. The use of endoscopic ultrasound in the diagnosis of solid pseudopapillary tumors of the pancreas in children. J Pediatr Surg. 2002;37(9):1370–3.
22. de Blaauw I, Winkelhorst JT, Rieu PN, et al. Pancreatic injury in children: good outcome of nonoperative treatment. J Pediatr Surg. 2008;43:1640–3.
23. Paul MD, Mooney DP. The management of pancreatic injuries in children: operate or observe. J Pediatr Surg. 2011;46:1140–3.

24. Grant JP, James S, Grabowski V, et al. Total parenteral nutrition in pancreatic disease. Ann Surg. 1984;200:627–31.
25. Wensil AM, Balasubramanian SA, Bell TL. Resolution of a posttraumatic pancreatic pseudocyst with octreotide acetate in a pediatric patient. Pharmacotherapy. 2011;31(9):924.
26. Gorenstein A, O'Halpin D, Wesson DE, et al. Blunt injury to the pancreas in children: selective management based on ultrasound. J Pediatr Surg. 1987;22(12):1110–6.
27. Seitz G, Warmann SW, Kirschner HJ, et al. Laparoscopic cystojejunostomy as a treatment option for pancreatic pseudocysts in children—a care report. J Pediatr Surg. 2006;41:E33–5.
28. Saad DF, Gow KW, Cabbabe S, et al. Laparoscopic cystogastrostomy for the treatment of pancreatic pseudocysts in children. J Pediatr Surg. 2005;40:E13–7.
29. Yoder SM, Rothenberg S, Tsao K, et al. Laparoscopic treatment of pancreatic pseudocysts in children. J Laparoendosc Adv Surg Tech A. 2009;19 Suppl 1:S37–40.
30. Wiersema MJ. Endosonography-guided cystoduodenostomy with a therapeutic ultrasound endoscope. Gastrointest Endosc. 1996;44(5):614–7.
31. Kimble RM, Cohen R, Williams S. Successful endoscopic drainage of a posttraumatic pancreatic pseudocyst in a child. J Pediatr Surg. 1999;34(10):1518–20.
32. Haluszka O, Campbell A, Horvath K. Endoscopic management of pancreatic pseudocyst in children. Gastrointest Endosc. 2002;55:128–31.
33. Rutkoski JD, Segura BJ, Kane TD. Experience with totally laparoscopic distal pancreatectomy with splenic preservation for pediatric trauma—2 techniques. J Pediatr Surg. 2011;46(3):588–93.
34. Mohkam K, Farges O, Pruvot FR, et al. Towards a standard technique for laparoscopic distal pancreatectomy? Synthesis of the 2013 ACHBT Spring workshop. J Visc Surg. 2015;152(3):167–78.
35. Venkat R, Edil BH, Schulick RD, et al. Laparoscopic distal pancreatectomy is associated with significantly less overall morbidity compared to the open technique: a systematic review and meta-analysis. Ann Surg. 2012;255(6):1048–59.
36. Petrosyan M, Franklin AL, Jackson HT, et al. Solid pancreatic pseudopapillary tumor managed laparoscopically in adolescents: a case series and review of the literature. J Laproendosc Adv Surg Tech. 2014;24(6):440–4.

41. Laparoscopic Cholecystectomy for Biliary Dyskinesia, Cholelithiasis, and Cholecystitis

Moriah M. Hagopian and Diana L. Diesen

Introduction

Epidemiology

The prevalence of gallstones in children varies by country and is not commonly reported, with published rates ranging from 0.13 to 1.9 % [1]. Despite the relative infrequency of gallstone formation in children, reported rates of symptomatic gallbladder disease have been rising and can largely be attributed to an increase in nonhemolytic (cholesterol) stones and biliary dyskinesia [2]. There is a bimodal incidence occurring in infancy (often related to TPN use) and adolescence, with a propensity for the female gender after adolescence [1, 3]. Though a large percentage of stones can be attributed to hemolytic disease, gallstones in children have also been shown to strongly correlate with Hispanic heritage, obesity, and increased age [4, 5].

Pathophysiology

Gallstones form when there is an imbalance in the main components of bile (cholesterol, bile salts, and bilirubin) that leads to precipitation of crystals that can enlarge over time. There are four main types. The most common type of stone in children has historically been black stones, which comprise 20–40 % of gallstones, and these are associated with hemolytic (sickle cell disease, thalassemia, hereditary spherocytosis) and ileal disease [1]. However, cholesterol stones are becoming much more prominent and are thought to correlate with a rise in the rate of

D.S. Walsh et al. (eds.), *The SAGES Manual of Pediatric Minimally Invasive Surgery*, DOI 10.1007/978-3-319-43642-5_41

obesity in children. Notably, 17–50 % of gallstones may remain asymptomatic, and resolution has been reported to occur in 34 % of infants and 16 % of children [1, 6].

Cholecystitis occurs with obstruction of the cystic duct that leads to distension and/or necrosis of the gallbladder wall. This may occur in the setting of gallstones or secondary to bile stasis without gallstone formation in the case of acalculous cholecystitis.

Biliary dyskinesia is defined by having symptoms typically attributed to biliary colic in the setting of no gallstones and an ejection fraction (EF) <35 % on a cholecystokinin-hepatobiliary iminodiacetic acid (CCK-HIDA) scan, though the exact pathophysiology of the disorder remains unclear.

Preoperative Evaluation

History and Physical Exam

Children with biliary colic usually present with typical symptoms of right upper quadrant (85–94 %) or midepigastric (34 %) pain associated with nausea and vomiting (60 %) [1, 6, 7]. Older children may describe the pain as a postprandial, stabbing pain or as an episodic pain that occurs mostly at night. Children <5 years of age and those with hemolytic disease may present with nonspecific abdominal pain and irritability (24–46 %) [1, 6, 7]. Persistent pain associated with fever and expiratory arrest on palpation of the right upper quadrant (Murphy's sign) should raise concern for acute cholecystitis, while associated fever and jaundice should raise concern for cholangitis, choledocholithiasis, or pancreatitis (7–20 %) [1, 6, 7].

Labs

A basic hepatic biochemical profile that includes transaminases, alkaline phosphatase, gamma-glutamyltransferase, and an indirect and direct bilirubin level should be obtained. If there is concern for infection or obstruction, a CBC and lipase level may also be obtained.

Imaging

The most important imaging study to obtain is a transabdominal ultrasound (US). An echogenic gallstone in an otherwise normal exam is consistent with symptomatic cholelithiasis, while a thickened gallbladder wall and pericholecystic fluid may be seen in the setting of acute cholecystitis. Intrahepatic/extrahepatic ductal dilation may be seen in the setting of biliary obstruction such as in choledocholithiasis or biliary pancreatitis.

A CCK-HIDA study may be obtained in children who present with typical symptoms of biliary colic, but with a normal ultrasound examination. In adults, an EF <35 % at 30 min suggests poor contractile function and incomplete emptying of the gallbladder and is consistent with biliary dyskinesia, while an EF >65–80 % is consistent with biliary hyperkinesia. These values have been extrapolated to children; however, differences that may exist between young children and adults have been poorly studied and are not clearly understood. No filling of the gallbladder at one hour, especially after administration of intravenous (IV) morphine sulfate, is consistent with acute cholecystitis [8].

Other Tests

In cases where there is concern for hepatobiliary obstruction, magnetic resonance cholangiopancreatography (MRCP) or endoscopic retrograde cholangiopancreatography (ERCP) may help delineate the anatomy of the extrahepatic and intrahepatic biliary tract and identify the presence of ductal stones [9]. ERCP can also be therapeutic when an obstruction is identified.

Surgical Indications

Common indications for laparoscopic cholecystectomy include symptomatic cholelithiasis, acute cholecystitis, biliary pancreatitis and biliary dyskinesia, though some controversy exists over the latter. Patients with hemoglobinopathies who develop stones should also be considered for laparoscopic cholecystectomy, and safety has been demonstrated in sickle cell disease [10]. Less commonly, it has been suggested that patients with recurrent right upper quadrant pain and undetectable gallbladders on repeat ultrasonography undergo a laparoscopic cholecystectomy, as well as patients who have biliary hyperkinesia [11–13].

No absolute contraindications for performing a laparoscopic cholecystectomy exist. However, severe acute cardiopulmonary disease that precludes patients from undergoing abdominal insufflation, dense adhesions in the right upper quadrant, portal hypertension, coagulopathy, a cholecystoenteric fistula, and advanced acute cholecystitis may be considered relative contraindications and may be associated with a higher conversion rate [14].

Technique

Special Considerations

Several modifications to traditional laparoscopic cholecystectomy have been suggested when operating in children. These include placing trocars widely to allow for adequate working distance between ports, placement of the epigastric cannula at the left midclavicular line in small children <30 kg, and placement of the right lower quadrant cannula more inferiorly near the inguinal crease to improve cosmesis [15, 16] (Fig. 41.1). Additionally, extra caution should be exercised when placing trocars in children, as the abdominal wall is more pliable and elastic than in adults [15]. An open technique is recommended for initial trocar placement in an effort to decrease the risk of associated intra-abdominal injury in small children. However, the literature has been somewhat controversial in this regard, with some reports showing only less failed attempts, extraperitoneal insufflation, and omental injury with an open technique [17, 18]. Lastly, it is recommended that small children do not undergo single-incision laparoscopic surgery (SILS) cholecystectomy secondary to difficulties that may arise from operating in a restricted space [19]. The use of intraoperative cholangiography (IOC) varies by surgeon and institution, and selective IOC has been shown to be acceptable and safe, with most common bile duct stones passing spontaneously in children [20].

Anatomy

The borders of the hepatocystic triangle, also known as Calot's triangle, include the common hepaticduct medially, the cystic duct laterally/inferiorly, and the inferior border of the liver superiorly. Its contents include the cystic artery and the cystic lymph node. The right hepatic artery is located posterior to these structure but its proximity should be

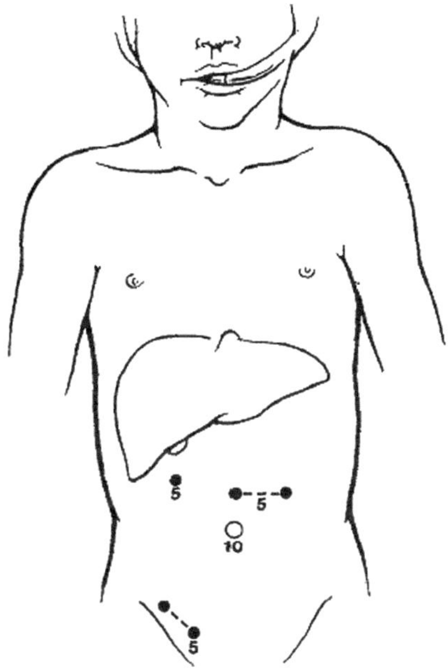

Fig. 41.1. Orientation of the four ports used for laparoscopic cholecystectomy in children. The midepigastric port should be positioned according to the patient's size; the smaller the child, the closer to the left midclavicular line. The right lateral port may also be placed more inferiorly in the right lower quadrant in smaller children. From Holcomb GW 3rd, et al. Laparoscopic cholecystectomy in infants and children: modifications and cost analysis. Journal of pediatric surgery. 1994;29(7):900–4. Reprinted with permission from Elsevier Limited.

kept in mind [21] (Fig. 41.2). Accessory hepatic ducts and arteries may also be found in this space. Careful dissection in this triangle must be performed during laparoscopic cholecystectomy in order to obtain the critical view of safety, which consists of clearly visualizing the cystic duct entering the gallbladder, with an empty space between the gallbladder and liver except for the cystic artery which traverses the space to enter the gallbladder [21] (Fig. 41.3).

Positioning

Depending on the size of the child, it may be helpful to have a foot board in place to prevent sliding when in reverse Trendelenburg position. Two monitors should be positioned at the 10 o'clock and 2 o'clock

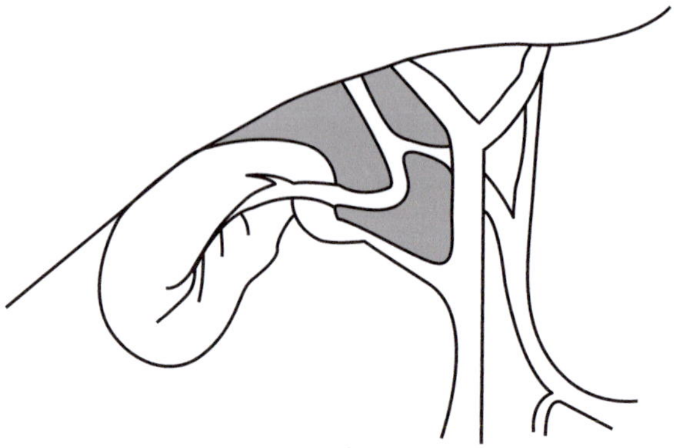

Fig. 41.2. Calot's triangle (*shaded area*). Bordered by the common hepaticduct medially, the cystic duct laterally/inferiorly, and the inferior border of the liver superiorly. Its contents include the cystic artery and the lymph node. The right hepatic artery is posterior to these structure but its proximity should be kept in mind during dissection. From Nagral S. Anatomy relevant to cholecystectomy. J Minim Access Surg. 2005;1(2):53–8. Copyright © Journal of Minimal Access Surgery (Open Access).

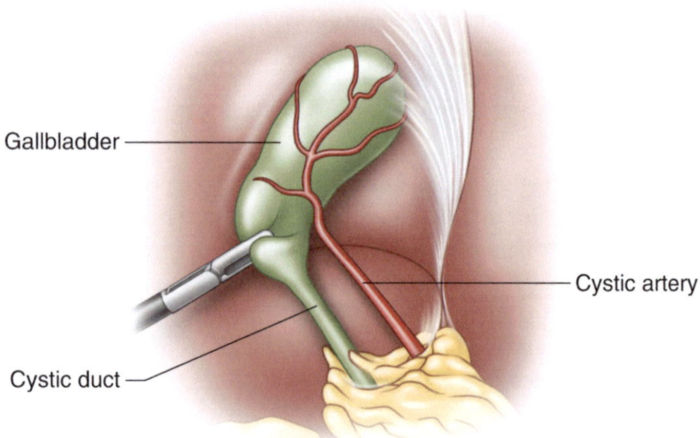

Fig. 41.3. Critical view of safety. The cystic duct is visualized entering the gallbladder with an empty space between the gallbladder and liver except for the cystic artery which traverses the space to enter the gallbladder.

position in direct line of vision for both the surgeon and first assistant [14]. After initial trocar placement, the bed should be positioned in reverse Trendelenburg with slight rotation to the child's left. In performing a SILS cholecystectomy, the child should be in the split-legged (French) position with the surgeon between the legs and the assistant to the child's left [19] (Fig. 41.4).

Instruments

A basic laparoscopic setup consisting of a high-quality videolaparoscope, two high-resolution monitors, and a high-flow carbon dioxide insufflator is needed [14]. The laparoscope may be 3 mm or 5 mm in size and may be either a 0° or 30° lens. Depending on the desired mode of entry, a Veress needle or Hassan cannula can be used, with placement of four trocars (three 3 mm or 5 mm and one 10 mm). Commonly used instruments include: a fine-tipped dissector, two graspers, endoshears, a monopolar L-hook, a suction irrigator, a 5 mm clip applier, and an endobag. Additionally, a stone retrieval grasper is helpful when there is spillage of gallstones [20]. In performing a SILS cholecystectomy, a right-angle light adapter is used in addition to the basic laparoscopic setup. Single-incision trocars include a SurgiQuest AnchorPort® trocar (SurgiQuest, Inc., Milford, Connecticut) and two 5 mm trocars versus a multiple access port such as a SILS™ Port (Medtronic, Minneapolis, Minnesota); instruments include a MiniLap alligator grasper (Stryker, Kalamazoo, Michigan), a reticulating gallbladder grasper, and another reticulating instrument [19].

Steps

An oral gastric tube may be placed to decompress the stomach. An open Hassan technique is recommended for initial trocar placement in small children, whereas either an open Hassan or a Veress needle may be used for bigger children. The abdomen is insufflated, and trocars are placed in the following positions: 10 mm umbilical, and 3 mm or 5 mm epigastric to the right of the falciform at the level of the inferior edge of the liver in bigger children (versus the left midclavicular line in small children), right subcostal midclavicular, and right subcostal lateral in bigger children (versus right lower quadrant in small children) [16]. The fundus of the gallbladder is grasped from the right

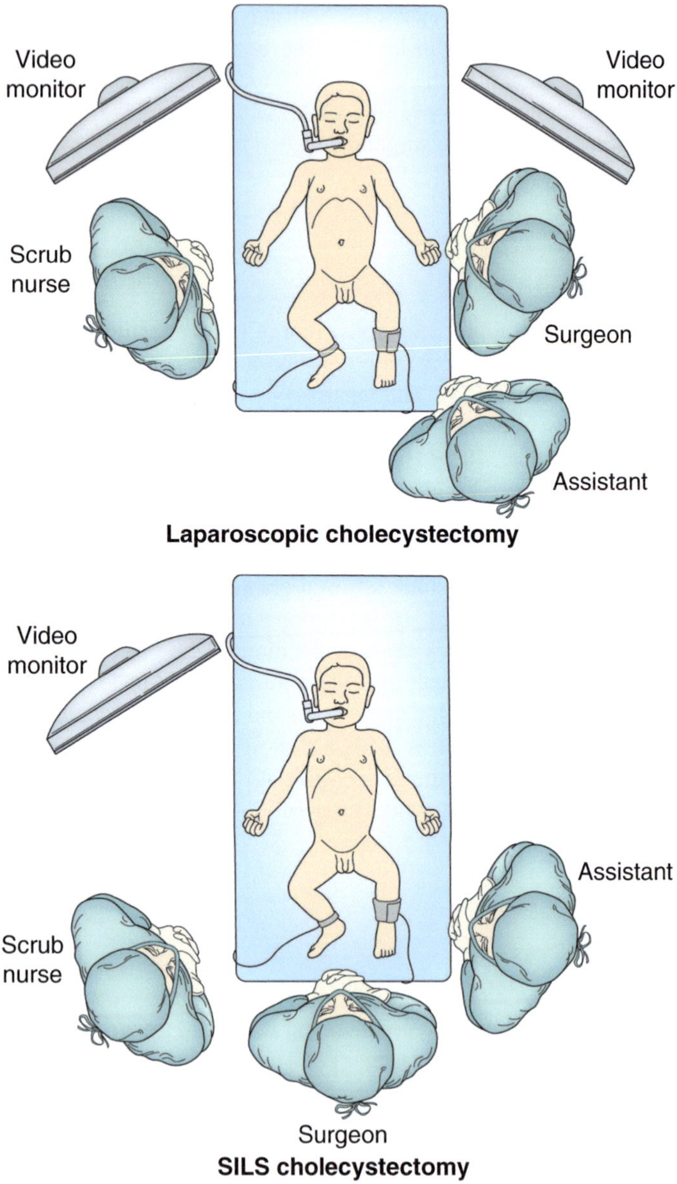

Fig. 41.4. Positioning of patient and operative team during: (*top*) laparoscopic cholecystectomy and (*bottom*) SILS cholecystectomy.

lateral/lower quadrant port and elevated to expose the porta hepatis. The infundibulum of the gallbladder is grasped through the right midclavicular trocar and retracted laterally and inferiorly to open the hepatocystic triangle. The visceral peritoneum overlying the area of the gallbladder/cystic duct junction is opened by grasping and gently pulling opposite of the infundibulum retraction on both the anterior and posterior sides until the cystic duct and artery and lymph node of Calot are identifiable. Gentle dissection around the cystic duct and artery is performed until the structures can be clearly traced onto the gallbladder. It is not necessary to dissect the cystic duct to its junction with the common duct, as this increases the risk of a common duct injury. However, it is necessary to dissect the triangle of Calot free of all tissue except for the cystic duct and artery in order to expose the base of the liver and obtain a critical view of safety. The cystic duct and artery are clipped and divided individually. The gallbladder is mobilized off the hepatic fossa using cautery or scissors; this dissection is helped by retracting the gallbladder away from the liver using the left hand and by flipping the gallbladder over the liver [14]. The gallbladder can be removed from the peritoneal cavity with or without the use of an endobag depending on the integrity of the gallbladder wall. Any bile that was spilled is suctioned, and any gallstones that were spilled are retrieved. All trocars are removed under direct visualization, the abdomen is desufflated, and the fascia is closed using either figure-of-eight and/or interrupted stitchs. The skin incisions for all port sites are closed with subcuticular suture.

The technique for a SILS cholecystectomy differs only slightly from the above described technique. An initial 15 mm horizontal infraumbilical skin incision is made. The abdomen is insufflated, three 3 mm or 5 mm trocars are placed in a horizontal fashion at the 10 o'clock, 5 o'clock, and 2 o'clock positions, and the laparoscope is inserted at the 5 o'clock position. In larger children, a multiport trocar may be placed via an open technique and rotated so that the trocars are in the above positions [19]. A MiniLap alligator grasper is inserted along the trocars at the 7 o'clock position and used to retract the fundus of the gallbladder cephalad prior to being clamped down to the drapes [19]. An alternative to using a MiniLap alligator grasper is to place a percutaneous stay suture in order to suspend the gallbladder cephalad. A reticulating grasper is used to retract the infundibulum of the gallbladder to the right and slightly cephalad before the handle is moved to the surgeon's right, away from the other instruments [19]. A dissector is placed through the 10 o'clock position and is used to proceed with the operation as usual. The three 5 mm fascial incisions are connected with electrocautery, the gallbladder is removed, and the incision is closed.

Two main techniques exist for IOC in children. In the first, a small lateral incision is made in the cystic duct, and a cholangiocatheter or small urethral catheter is inserted into the cystic duct and held/clipped in place while cholangiography is performed [16]. An alternative to this approach is to insert a Kumar clamp through a 5 mm trocar and position it across the infundibulum of the gallbladder. A small (23G) needle is introduced through the side arm in the clamp, contrast is instilled into the proximal gallbladder, and cholangiography is performed [15]. This technique avoids difficult cannulation of a small cystic duct, but cannot be performed in the setting of a cystic duct obstruction [15].

Pearls/Pitfalls

Fifteen to 20 % of people have variations in their biliary anatomy, the most relevant of which is a short cystic duct which can be associated with mistaking the common duct for the cystic duct [8]. If there is unclear anatomy, conversion to an open procedure should be performed. An IOC may also be performed; however, this has not been shown to decrease injury to the common bile duct, only to lead to faster identification of an injury. Several techniques may be employed in the setting of significant inflammation to aid in safe dissection: gallbladder decompression with needle aspiration, lateral to medial approach for lysis of adhesions, and a dome-down approach to dissection. A 30 mm or similar size endoscopic stapling device can also be used to divide the infundibulum of the gallbladder for a partial cholecystectomy [8]. In this situation, placement of a drain may be considered. Bleeding in the hepatocystic triangle is usually related to injury to the cystic artery or a branch of the right hepatic artery, and blind clipping in this area should be avoided; tamponade can often be achieved by applying gentle pressure with the gallbladder against the liver [14].

Postoperative Care

Outcomes

Laparoscopic cholecystectomy is associated with a decreased length of stay, analgesia use, and overall cost when compared to open cholecystectomy [16, 22, 23]. Same-day discharge has also been shown to be safe and may be better facilitated by the use of total IV anesthesia and a light diet for 72 h following surgery [24, 25]. SILS cholecystectomy follows the same course as laparoscopic cholecystectomy and offers no advantage over the latter except for with regard to cosmesis [19, 26]. Laparoscopic cholecystectomy with IOC has been shown to increase operative time without decreasing the rate of retained common bile duct stones or injury [27]. However, selective use of IOC may be beneficial given that 10–15 % of patients with biliary pancreatitis will have common bile duct stones on ERCP. Laparoscopic cholecystectomy with ERCP is often the treatment of choice for patients with bile duct stones, though some groups have performed laparoscopic cholecystectomy with common bile duct exploration. Though technically difficult and associated with a risk for stricture in small children, in experienced hands, it has been shown to be associated with decreased length of stay and cost, with similar morbidity when compared to laparoscopic cholecystectomy and ERCP [28].

Despite its wide use, controversy exists with regard to whether or not laparoscopic cholecystectomy should be offered for biliary dyskinesia, with one study showing only 44 % symptom resolution at long-term follow-up (>1 year) and other long-term studies demonstrating comparable benefit of operative and conservative therapy [1, 29, 30]. Factors associated with symptom improvement after laparoscopic cholecystectomy for biliary dyskinesia include a shorter duration of pain, a history of vomiting and epigastric pain, a low body mass index (BMI), and an EF <15 % [1, 31].

Complications

Major complications for laparoscopic cholecystectomy in children have been reported to occur in <0.5 % of cases, with a 30-day readmission rate of 7 % [32, 33]. Conversion to an open procedure occurs in 3 %

of cases; however, this should not be considered to be a complication [32]. Reported rates of common bile duct injury range from 0.36 to 0.44 % and occur more commonly in younger children [32, 34]. Other common complications include: injuries from trocar placement (<1 %), bile leak/biloma (4.5 %), bile spillage (5.9 %), stone spillage (30 %), retained stones, hematoma, intra-abdominal abscess, incisional hernia, damage to nearby structures, pancreatitis, and superficial wound infection [34]. If stones are spilled, attempts should be made to remove them in order to prevent abscess formation which can occur anywhere from 1.5 weeks to years later. Increased stool frequency, which may be seen in up to 25 % of adults, usually does not occur in children.

Summary

- Rates of symptomatic cholelithiasis related to cholesterol stones and biliary dyskinesia in children are rising and correlate with a rise in obesity.
- Laparoscopic cholecystectomy in children is safe and effective and can be performed as a same-day discharge procedure. The rate of major complications is low at <0.5 %.
- SILS cholecystectomy results in improved cosmesis, but it is otherwise similar to standard laparoscopic cholecystectomy.
- Careful dissection in the hepatocystic triangle should be performed staying away from the common bile duct.
- A critical view of safety should be obtained prior to clipping and dividing the cystic duct and artery. Avoid blind clipping in the hepatocystic triangle; if major bleeding occurs, convert to an open procedure.
- Selective use of IOC is safe.
- While not routine, laparoscopic cholecystectomy with CBD exploration results in decreased LOS and costs when compared to laparoscopic cholecystectomy with ERCP.

References

1. Svensson J, Makin E. Gallstone disease in children. Semin Pediatr Surg. 2012;21(3):255–65.
2. Walker SK, Maki AC, Cannon RM, Foley DS, Wilson KM, Galganski LA, et al. Etiology and incidence of pediatric gallbladder disease. Surgery. 2013;154(4):927–31. discussion 31–3.

3. Hebra A, Lesher A. Cholecystitis. In: Mattei P, editor. Fundamentals of pediatric surgery. New York: Springer; 2011. p. 579–85.
4. Mehta S, Lopez ME, Chumpitazi BP, Mazziotti MV, Brandt ML, Fishman DS. Clinical characteristics and risk factors for symptomatic pediatric gallbladder disease. Pediatrics. 2012;129(1):e82–8.
5. St Peter SD, Keckler SJ, Nair A, Andrews WS, Sharp RJ, Snyder CL, et al. Laparoscopic cholecystectomy in the pediatric population. J Laparoendosc Adv Surg Tech A. 2008;18(1):127–30.
6. Bogue CO, Murphy AJ, Gerstle JT, Moineddin R, Daneman A. Risk factors, complications and outcomes of gallstones in children: a single-center review. J Pediatr Gastroenterol Nutr. 2010;50(3):303–8.
7. Wesdorp I, Bosman D, de Graaff A, Aronson D, van der Blij F, Taminiau J. Clinical presentations and predisposing factors of cholelithiasis and sludge in children. J Pediatr Gastroenterol Nutr. 2000;31(4):411–7.
8. Khashab M, Giday SA, Van Arendonk KJ, Duncan MD. Gallbladder and biliary tree: asymptomatic (silent) gallstones and acute cholecystitis. In: Cameron AM, Cameron JL, editors. Current surgical therapy. 10th ed. Philadelphia: Elsevier Saunders; 2011. p. 335–41.
9. Dalton SJ, Balupuri S, Guest J. Routine magnetic resonance cholangiopancreatography and intra-operative cholangiogram in the evaluation of common bile duct stones. Ann R Coll Surg Engl. 2005;87(6):469–70.
10. Sandoval C, Stringel G, Ozkaynak MF, Tugal O, Jayabose S. Perioperative management in children with sickle cell disease undergoing laparoscopic surgery. JSLS. 2002; 6(1):29–33.
11. Adams SD, Blackburn SC, Adewole VA, Mahomed AA. Chronically symptomatic patients with undetectable gall bladder on ultrasonography could benefit from early cholecystectomy. Minim Invasive Surg. 2013;2013:630–753.
12. Lindholm EB, Alberty JB, Hansbourgh F, Upp JR, Lopoo J. Hyperkinetic gallbladder: an indication for cholecystectomy? Am Surg. 2013;79(9):882–4.
13. Huckaby L, Timmapuri S, Prasad R. Biliary hyperkinesia: a potentially surgically correctable disorder in adolescents. J Pediatr Surg Case Rep. 2013;1(9):314–6.
14. Hunter JG, Pham TH. Laparoscopic cholecystectomy, intraoperative cholangiography, and common bile duct exploration. In: Fischer JE, editor. Mastery of surgery, vol. 1. 6th ed. Philadelphia: Lippincott Williams and Wilkins; 2012. p. 1265–76.
15. Holcomb 3rd GW, Morgan 3rd WM, Neblett 3rd WW, Pietsch JB, O'Neill Jr JA, Shyr Y. Laparoscopic cholecystectomy in children: lessons learned from the first 100 patients. J Pediatr Surg. 1999;34(8):1236–40.
16. Holcomb 3rd GW, Sharp KW, Neblett 3rd WW, Morgan 3rd WM, Pietsch JB. Laparoscopic cholecystectomy in infants and children: modifications and cost analysis. J Pediatr Surg. 1994;29(7):900–4.
17. Ahmad G, O'Flynn H, Duffy JM, Phillips K, Watson A. Laparoscopic entry techniques. Cochrane Database Syst Rev. 2012;2, CD006583.
18. Ponsky TA, Krpata DM. Single-port laparoscopy: considerations in children. J Minim Access Surg. 2011;7(1):96–8.

19. Holcomb 3rd GW. Single-site umbilical laparoscopic cholecystectomy. Semin Pediatr Surg. 2011;20(4):201–7.
20. Mah D, Wales P, Njere I, Kortan P, Masiakos P, Kim PC. Management of suspected common bile duct stones in children: role of selective intraoperative cholangiogram and endoscopic retrograde cholangiopancreatography. J Pediatr Surg. 2004;39(6):808–12. discussion 12.
21. Nagral S. Anatomy relevant to cholecystectomy. J Minim Access Surg. 2005;1(2):53–8.
22. Kim PC, Wesson D, Superina R, Filler R. Laparoscopic cholecystectomy versus open cholecystectomy in children: which is better? J Pediatr Surg. 1995;30(7):971–3.
23. Jawad AJ, Kurban K, el-Bakry A, al-Rabeeah A, Seraj M, Ammar A. Laparoscopic cholecystectomy for cholelithiasis during infancy and childhood: cost analysis and review of current indications. World J Surg. 1998;22(1):69–73. discussion 4.
24. Jawaheer G, Evans K, Marcus R. Day-case laparoscopic cholecystectomy in childhood: outcomes from a clinical care pathway. Eur J Pediatr Surg. 2013;23(1):57–62.
25. Dalton BGA, Gonzalez KW, Knott EM, St Peter SD, Aguayo P. Same day discharge after laparoscopic cholecystectomy in children. J Surg Res. 2015;195(2):418–21.
26. Ostlie DJ, Juang OO, Iqbal CW, Sharp SW, Snyder CL, Andrews WS, et al. Single incision versus standard 4-port laparoscopic cholecystectomy: a prospective randomized trial. J Pediatr Surg. 2013;48(1):209–14.
27. Ding G-Q, Cai W, Qin M-F. Is intraoperative cholangiography necessary during laparoscopic cholecystectomy for cholelithiasis? World J Gastroenterol. 2015;21(7):2147–51.
28. Short SS, Frykman PK, Nguyen N, Liu Q, Berel D, Wang KS. Laparoscopic common bile duct exploration in children is associated with decreased cost and length of stay: results of a two-center analysis. J Pediatr Surg. 2013;48(1):215–20.
29. Srinath A, Saps M, Bielefeldt K. Biliary dyskinesia in pediatrics. Pediatr Ann. 2014;43(4):e83–8.
30. Gurusamy KS Junnarkar S Farouk M Davidson BR. Cholecystectomy for suspected gallbladder dyskinesia. Cochrane Database Syst Rev. 2009;(1). doi:10.1002/14651858.CD007086
31. Carney DE, Kokoska ER, Grosfeld JL, Engum SA, Rouse TM, West KM, et al. Predictors of successful outcome after cholecystectomy for biliary dyskinesia. J Pediatr Surg. 2004;39(6):813–6. discussion 6.
32. Kelley-Quon LI, Dokey A, Jen HC, Shew SB. Complications of pediatric cholecystectomy: impact from hospital experience and use of cholangiography. J Am Coll Surg. 2014;218(1):73–81.
33. Holcomb III GW, Andrews W. Gallbladder disease and hepatic infections. In: Coran AG, Caldamone A, Adzick NS, Krummel TM, Laberge JM, Shamberger R, editors. Pediatric surgery. 7th ed. Philadelphia: Elsevier Saunders; 2012. p. 1341–53.
34. Zeidan MM, Pandian TK, Ibrahim KA, Moir CR, Ishitani MB, Zarroug AE. Laparoscopic cholecystectomy in the pediatric population: a single-center experience. Surg Laparosc Endosc Percutan Tech. 2014;24(3):248–50.

42. Laparoscopic Treatment of Biliary Atresia

Dominic Papandria and Stefan Scholz

Introduction

Biliary atresia (BA) affects one in 10,000–16,700 live births [1, 2] and is the leading cause of pathologic jaundice in the neonatal period as well as the leading indication for liver transplantation under the age of 12 months [3]. Incidence is higher among females and among Asian populations.

Early attempts at surgical management of BA were met with poor outcomes and high rates of postoperative mortality and progressive liver failure [4, 5]. The introduction of portoenterostomy (PE) by Kasai in 1959 greatly improved outcomes, with biliary drainage achieved in 46 %, recovery from jaundice in 39 %, and 1-year survival rates of 30 % for initial patient cohorts that were previously considered to be "non-correctable" [6]. Technical refinements, improved medical management, and success in pediatric liver transplantation have together contributed to further advances in effective primary drainage of the liver, with transplant-free survival rates remaining as high as 70 % into adolescence, though only 30 % will avoid long-term progression to cirrhosis requiring transplant [7, 8].

Pathogenesis

Although previous attempts to describe the pathogenesis of BA focused on defects in the process of recanalization of the bile ducts at approximately 4 weeks gestation, more recent theories have proposed

D.S. Walsh et al. (eds.), *The SAGES Manual of Pediatric Minimally Invasive Surgery*, DOI 10.1007/978-3-319-43642-5_42

a multifactorial process. There are multiple reports citing epidemiologic data and animal models that appear to implicate genetic [9–12], viral [13–15], inflammatory [16], environmental, ischemic, and metabolic risk factors [17, 18], but the precise mechanism remains elusive. The frequent finding of pigmented stools that precede onset of clinical jaundice further suggests that postnatal exposures may serve to augment or attenuate the disease process [19].

Clinical Presentation

There appears to be no predilection for prematurity or decreased birth weight among infants diagnosed with BA. Approximately 15–30 % of patients will have associated congenital anomalies, including intestinal malrotation, preduodenal portal vein, polysplenia, interrupted inferior vena cava with or without azygous continuation, and various cardiac malformations. The onset of jaundice may occur at birth or up to 6 weeks thereafter and is typically progressive and eventually accompanied by acholic stools and dark urine. Physical exam may reveal firm hepatomegaly and laboratory studies will exhibit direct hyperbilirubinemia. Advanced disease may present with splenomegaly, ascites, and malnutrition [20].

Diagnosis

A multimodal approach is frequently necessary to establish a definitive diagnosis in suspected cases. In reviewing the complete metabolic profile, the aforementioned direct hyperbilirubinemia is nonspecific and is accompanied by variable alterations in serum transaminases, with a disproportionate increase in gamma-glutamyl transferase. In early disease, coagulopathy is rarely present, and only secondary to malabsorption of vitamin K, as hepatic synthetic capacity is typically preserved. An appropriate workup should exclude toxoplasmosis, syphilis, varicella, parvovirus, rubella, cytomegalovirus, and herpesvirus (TORCH) infections as well as infectious hepatitides. Normal serum alpha-1 antitrypsin should also be confirmed. There are three described anatomic variants of BA (Fig. 42.1), some of which make radiologic diagnosis challenging. Fasting ultrasound provides a noninvasive, well-tolerated assessment of the liver and biliary tree without exposure to ionizing radiation [21]. This may demonstrate an absent gallbladder or a triangular echogenic density

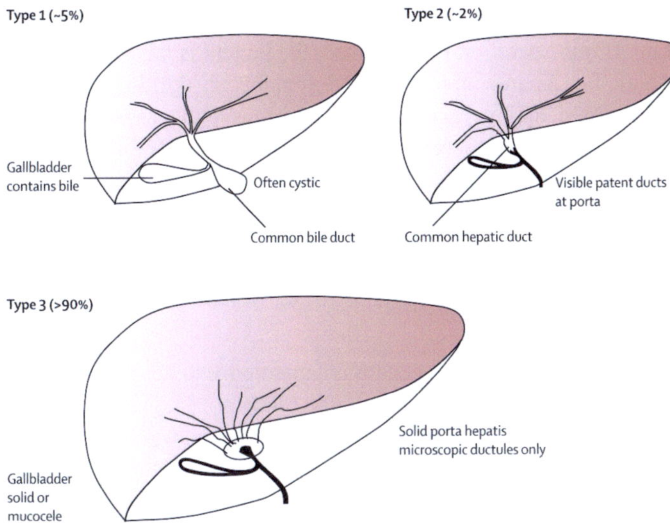

Fig. 42.1. Types of biliary atresia. From Hartley JL, Davenport M, Kelly DA. Biliary atresia. Lancet 2009 Nov 14;374(9702):1704–1713. Reprinted with permission from Elsevier Limited.

cephalad to the porta hepatis (the so-called triangular cord sign), both of which are suggestive of BA [22]. Hepatic scintigraphy (HIDA scan) demonstrating relatively good hepatic uptake with the absence of excretion of technetium-labeled compounds from the liver into the duodenum is diagnostic of biliary obstruction, but may be less reliable in cases of severe jaundice. Prior to HIDA scan, patients are routinely pretreated with phenobarbital (5 mg/kg/day) for 5 days to increase biliary secretion by stimulating hepatic enzymes to minimize false-positive studies. Other imaging modalities to image the bile ducts, such as endoscopic retrograde cholangiopancreatography and magnetic resonance cholangiopancreatography, are difficult to perform and interpret in an infant and are only used in selected centers. Percutaneous core biopsy of the liver is the most accurate diagnostic test, but also the most invasive, short of surgical exploration [23, 24]. Pathology characteristically reveals inflammation with ductular proliferation, with or without bile stasis, duct plugging, and giant cells. Indeterminate or false-negative results may reflect specimens acquired too early in the disease process to reflect the characteristic pathologic changes of duct proliferation.

In our institution, we advocate HIDA scan after completed medical workup. If non-secretion is confirmed, the patient is taken to the operating room for laparoscopic-guided percutaneous transhepatic or open cholangiogram and percutaneous liver biopsy. In cases of a microgallbladder, the cholangiogram is performed through a minilaparotomy. If biliary atresia is confirmed, a generous wedge liver biopsy is taken and a Kasai procedure is performed.

Operative Management

The open PE requires a generous laparotomy to access two or more quadrants to permit mobilization of the bilateral triangular hepatic ligaments to prolapse the liver anterior to the abdominal wall while using the corners of the incision as retractors. Excision of the remnant gallbladder and bile duct as well as fibrous plate at the porta hepatis is performed, followed by Roux-en-Y reconstruction for bilioenteric drainage via the portoenterostomy. The key of the procedure is dissection of the cone-shaped fibrous remnant at the level of the liver surface, just anterior to the portal vein bifurcation. For best long-term results, the bilious scar tissue must be removed directly on the liver surface without injuring the actual liver. The dissection must be carried as much lateral as possible with typical limitations of right and left portal venous and hepatic artery branches as well as below the portal vein bifurcation. The completely exposed liver surface at the porta hepatis is then covered by the Roux limb as a quasi-"sewer" to catch dripping bile from the area.

Laparoscopic Cholangiography

In many situations, the preoperative workup does not yield a definitive diagnosis. In other instances, the gallbladder or bile ducts may appear morphologically normal (as in type II BA) or found to contain pigmented bile on laparoscopic examination and aspiration. Contrast images of the biliary tree may provide valuable evidence when faced with equivocal evidence [20]. Confirmatory cholangiography can be performed laparoscopically in combination with open or laparoscopic PE under the same anesthetic.

The patient is positioned with the operating table level and trocars are placed as for laparoscopic Kasai (see below). Following inspection of the peritoneum and biliary structures, a purse-string suture is placed around the planned cholecystostomy either at the gallbladder infundibulum or at the fundus, depending on the degree of fibrotic change. If an initial percutaneous aspiration is attempted and yields clear fluid, further interrogation of the biliary tree is not indicated. Otherwise, the gallbladder is then opened using laparoscopic shears or the monopolar hook. An existing port site or percutaneous 14-gauge angiocath placed the right subcostal space can be used to deploy a cholangiogram catheter or rigid cannula, which is then navigated into the gallbladder lumen and secured with the purse-string suture. A second outer purse-string may be necessary following catheter placement if extravasation is noted with a test bolus of saline. Contrast is diluted to half-strength with normal saline and injection proceeds slowly under fluoroscopy. If the common bile duct is observed overlying the spine, rotation of the C-arm or the operating table can produce off-axis images. Trendelenburg positioning may also augment contrast delivery to the intrahepatic bile ducts if initial images are equivocal, and administration of intravenous glucagon may improve drainage of contrast into the duodenum if such flow is not initially evident [25]. Alternatively, an angiocath may be guided percutaneously transhepatically under direct vision with the laparoscope into the gallbladder to prevent leakage of contrast into the peritoneum, obscuring the cholangiogram. If one is versed with abdominal ultrasound, this technique could be employed entirely percutaneously without laparoscopic guidance. In typical cases of BA with a microgallbladder, all minimally invasive techniques may be technically difficult, and unroofing of the gallbladder to reveal a drop of white bile may be diagnostic.

Laparoscopic Portoenterostomy

Since first described by Esteves et al. in 2002 [26], the laparoscopic approach to PE has been subject to significant discussion and refinement. During the 16th Meeting of the International Pediatric Endosurgery Group (IPEG) in 2007 in Argentina, several international presenters reported poor short- and middle-term results after the minimally invasive Kasai procedure, which led to the recommendation by that group to abandon the laparoscopic approach until further evidence could be gathered. Several high-volume centers, predominantly in Asia and Argentina, have continued and refined the minimally invasive approach to date and report good mid- and long-term results.

Operative Technique

The infant is positioned at the foot of the operating table on a forced-air warming blanket, followed by placement of a nasogastric tube and urinary catheter. The surgeon is positioned at the patient's feet, with an assistant to the surgeon's right. A 12-mm trocar is placed either supra-umbilically or transumbilically using a Veress needle and Step™ dilating sheath (Medtronic Minimally Invasive Therapies, Minneapolis, MN) or via open placement with Hasson technique. A 30° 5-mm laparoscope is used to inspect the peritoneal contents and to facilitate placement of three additional 5-mm radially dilating trocars under laparoscopic vision: two ports are placed, each on either side of the umbilical port, for the surgeon's right and left hands, slightly above the umbilical level, just lateral to the rectus abdominis. The third 5-mm port is placed between the umbilical port and the left upper quadrant port, slightly below the umbilicus for use by the assistant (Fig. 42.2).

Liver retraction provides critical exposure of the porta hepatis, and various means have been described to attain adequate visualization. The transabdominal placement of a subxiphoid retention suture allows the surgeon to suspend the liver by the falciform ligament, and additional sutures can then be placed to retract the right and left lobes. Alternately, a 5-mm Nathanson retractor (Mediflex Surgical Products, Islandia, NY) may be placed through an epigastric incision through a

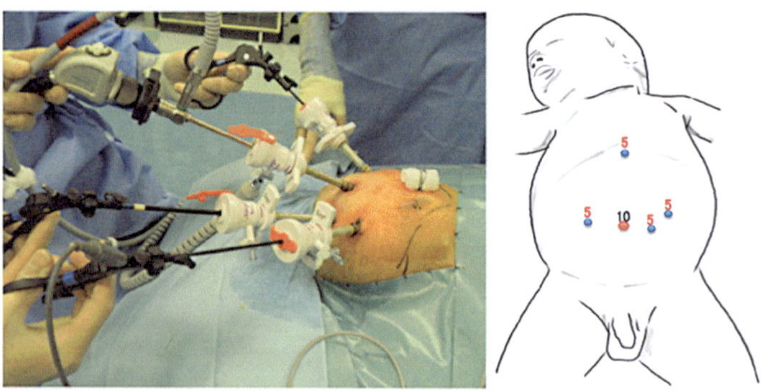

Fig. 42.2. Trocar positions during laparoscopic portoenterostomy. Note the 5-mm trocar in the epigastrium, specifically for the LigaSure device. Numbers indicate trocar size (mm). From Yamataka A, Lane GJ, Koga H, Cazares J, Nakamura H. Role of laparoscopy during surgery at the porta hepatis. S Afr Med J 2014;104(11):820–824. Doi:10.7196/SAMJ.8921.

dilating trocar sheath. The retractor is then affixed in place with a flexible table-mounted retractor clamp.

Monopolar electrocautery with a laparoscopic hook is then used in combination with blunt dissection with atraumatic graspers to expose the cystic duct and trace it to the biliary remnant. If cholangiography is indicated, the gallbladder may then be accessed as described in the section above. Liver core biopsies may also be obtained at this time, if needed. The biliary remnant is then divided at the level of the duodenum and elevated as dissection is carefully continued to skeletonize the distal remnant until the fibrous cone is visualized (Fig. 42.3). Dissection may be accomplished with monopolar cautery using hook or scissor, 5-mm ultrasonic shears (Ethicon, Somerville, NJ), depending on the surgeon preference. The JustRight Vessel Sealing System (JustRight Surgical, LLC, Louisville, CO), which utilizes a 3-mm instrument shaped like a Maryland dissector, can also be used. Excision of the fibrous cone (Fig. 42.4) exposes bile ductules, the microscopic structures that are the basis of biliary drainage following PE. It is therefore extremely important that thermal spread and related injury are minimized with the use of sharp dissection and judicious application from energy sources to control portal venous tributaries as they are encountered. Following completion of the distal remnant excision, the specimen is sent to pathology for histologic examination of the resected ductules and the PE is fashioned.

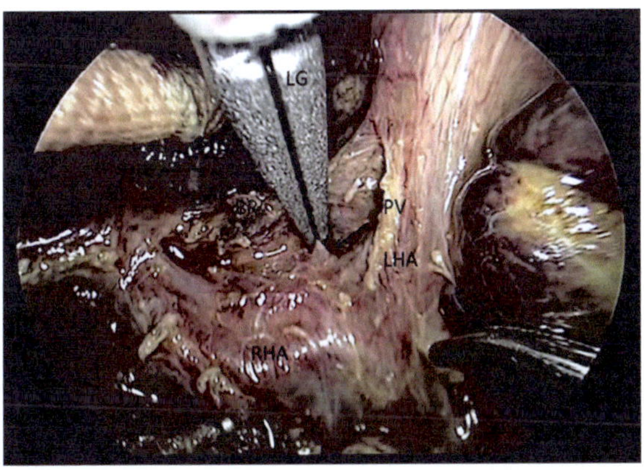

Fig. 42.3. A bipolar dissector isolates the biliary remnant and divides portal vein branches at the porta hepatis draining into the caudate lobe (*PV* portal vein, *BR* biliary remnant, *RHA* right hepatic artery, *LHA* left hepatic artery). From Yamataka A, Lane GJ, Koga H, Cazares J, Nakamura H. Role of laparoscopy during surgery at the porta hepatis. S Afr Med J 2014;104(11):820–824. Doi:10.7196/SAMJ.8921.

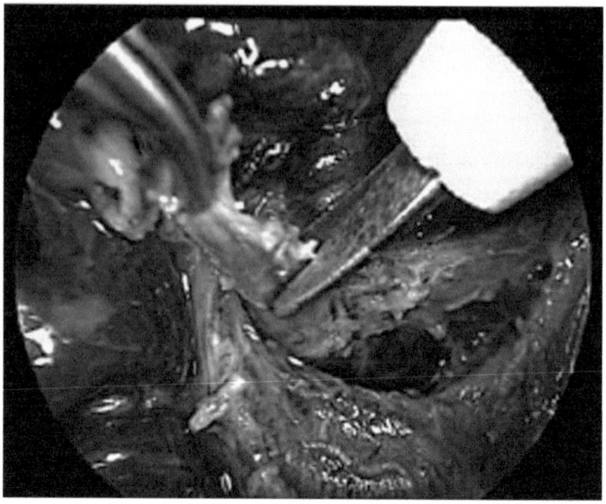

Fig. 42.4. Shallow transection of the biliary remnant being performed with laparoscopic shears. Adapted from Yamataka A. Laparoscopic Kasai portoenterostomy for biliary atresia. J Hepatobiliary Pancreat Sci 2013 Jun;20(5):481–486.

A pancreatico-enteric jejunal limb is measured out to 10–15 cm distal to the ligament of Treitz, and the bowel at this point is delivered per the umbilical incision following removal of the trocar. The bowel is then divided using a stapling device or electrocautery and oversewing of the distal enterotomy. The distal limb is then measured either intracorporeally or using the xiphoid as an external landmark to ensure that no tension will be imposed by the jejuno-jejunostomy. The standard length of the Roux limb is between 35 and 45 cm which is thought to prevent ascending cholangitis. The anastomosis is completed in hand-sewn end-to-side extracorporeal fashion (Fig. 42.5), and seromuscular tacking sutures are applied to affix the proximal limbs longitudinally to promote antegrade flow through the alimentary limb. A 1-cm longitudinal enterotomy is created using electrocautery on the antimesenteric aspect of the proximal Roux limb, and the bowel is inspected for perfusion and orientation prior to returning it into the abdomen. The 12-mm trocar is then replaced and laparoscopy resumes.

The transverse colon is elevated and a retrocolic mesenteric defect is carefully fashioned with electrocautery, through which the Roux limb is passed to lie at the porta hepatis. The PE is constructed using interrupted absorbable 5-0 monofilament suture, incorporating full-thickness bites

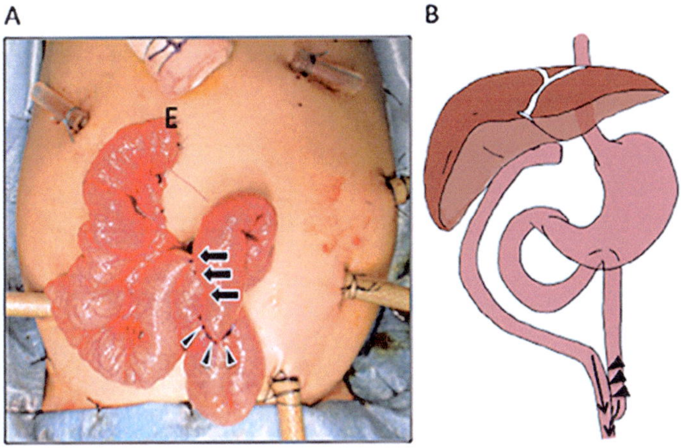

Fig. 42.5. Customizing the Roux-en-Y limb. (**a**) The jejunal loop is placed at the umbilicus and the distal end (E) of the limb is brought up to the xiphoid process. (**b**) The customized Roux-en-Y limb is approximated to the native jejunum for 8 cm cranially (*triangles*) to streamline flow into the distal jejunum (*arrows*), eliminate reflux into the Roux-en-Y limb, and prevent stasis in the Roux-en-Y limb. From Yamataka A, Lane GJ, Koga H, Cazares J, Nakamura H. Role of laparoscopy during surgery at the porta hepatis. S Afr Med J 2014;104(11):820–824. Doi:10.7196/SAMJ.8921.

of the bowel wall and small bites of hepatic parenchyma posterior to the portal plate along the back wall (Fig. 42.6). Anteriorly, suture placement should avoid any identifiable remnant of the left and right bile ducts to preserve these structures, which are typically found at two o'clock and ten o'clock. It is most important to extend the PE as far laterally as possible to include the highest possible number of bile ductules. The investing perivascular connective tissue of the hepatic arteries may be used to bolster closure at these positions [27]. Upon completion of the procedure, closed-suction drains may be placed at the porta hepatis and adjacent to the jejuno-jejunostomy using the existing 5-mm trocar sites prior to termination of laparoscopy. However, most operators avoid the postoperative use of drains and the risk of related complications may outweigh that of an occult anastomotic leak. The umbilical port site is closed in layers, and fascial defects at 5-mm trocar sites are separately closed at the surgeon's discretion, taking into account the patient's size and the presence of ascites.

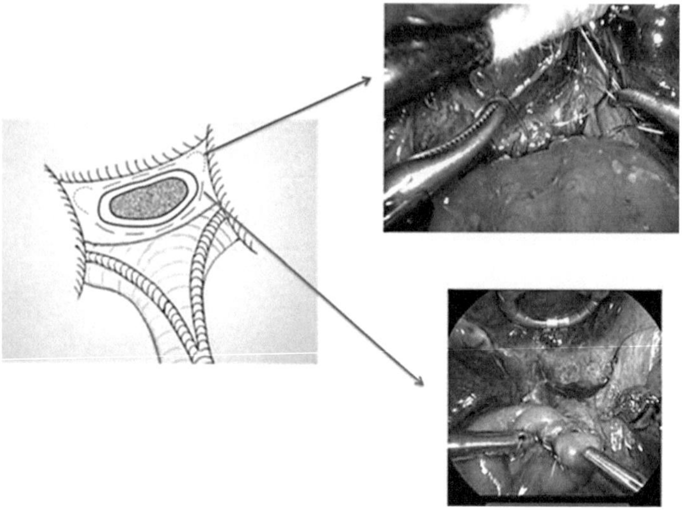

Fig. 42.6. Very shallow suture to the connective tissue at 2 o'clock and a shallow suture to the liver parenchyma at 4 o'clock. From Yamataka A. Laparoscopic Kasai portoenterostomy for biliary atresia. J Hepatobiliary Pancreat Sci 2013 Jun;20(5):481–486.

Robotic-Assisted Portoenterostomy

Very limited surgeon experience has been reported with respect to a robotic approach to the Kasai operation. Two separate case series were reported in 2007. Dutta and colleagues describe three such cases, of which two were performed using the da Vinci robotic surgical system (Intuitive Surgical, Inc., Sunnyvale, CA) for portal dissection and PE, while a third was performed as a "hybrid procedure," utilizing the robotic approach only for PE [28]. Meehan et al. present two robotic Kasai procedures in which the dissection and PE were performed with the da Vinci system without prior experience in laparoscopic Kasai [29]. Notably, both groups of investigators opted to perform construction of the Roux limb extracorporeally. Patient positioning, robot docking, movement arcs of wristed 5-mm instruments, instrument size proportional to an infant, and absent haptics feedback when manipulating the liver were cited as factors increasing the difficulty of robotic Kasai. Advantages described included improved endoscope image quality, three-dimensional visualization, surgeon comfort, movement downscaling, and degrees of freedom in movement for greater precision in instrument placement and manipulation. Little can be said regarding long-term outcomes in patient cohorts of this size, but no immediate major complications were reported, though one patient proceeded to transplant within the first postoperative year. Although it presents technical challenges and may not greatly improve the performance of the early stages of the operation, robotic-assisted laparoscopic PE may provide distinct advantages and merits further study.

Complications

Complications following PE include malabsorption of fat-soluble vitamins that may progress to overt malnutrition despite supplementation and growth retardation [30]. Cholangitis is a relatively common complication, occurring most frequently within months to a few years postoperatively. It is generally believed to result from reflux of enteric contents and bacteria up the Roux limb, although other mechanisms, such as bacterial translocation into the portal system and periportal lymphedema, have been suggested. The microorganisms in question are typically enteric flora [31], and repeated infections place the patient at risk for progressive cirrhosis. For this reason, perioperative corticosteroids and choleretics (ursodeoxycholic acid) [32] and routine prophylaxis with oral antibiotics [33] are used to decrease the frequency of such attacks. As mentioned above, some patients will not achieve adequate biliary drainage following PE, with progressive decline in liver function. Children that suffer recurrent jaundice and cholangitis that cannot be successfully medically managed are generally not helped by surgical revision [34–36], and most authors would refer such children for liver transplantation. Portal hypertension is also a common postoperative finding, and can evolve to ascites and variceal bleeding. Esophageal varices can be monitored and treated with flexible upper endoscopy. Endoscopic sclerotherapy can effectively address episodes of bleeding [37] or be undertaken prophylactically for asymptomatic lesions [38]. Other treatments for bleeding varices include endoscopic ligation [39] and placement of percutaneous transjugular intrahepatic [40] or surgical portosystemic shunts [41]. Transplantation is generally indicated for primary failure of PE, developmental failure secondary to progressive hepatic dysfunction, and recurrent episodes of cholangitis or complications of portal hypertension that are refractory to medical or endoscopic management. Five-year survival following liver transplantation for biliary atresia exceeds 90 % [42, 43].

Outcomes

Results of prospective studies comparing laparoscopic to open PE have been mixed, and to date only one trial has been registered with the US National Institutes of Health by Petersen et al. [44], the results of which were subsequently reported by Ure and colleagues. Investigators compared 12 consecutive patients managed with laparoscopic Kasai procedure with 28 historical controls. The study was halted following an interim analysis of postoperative outcomes at 6 months, which indicated that the rate of transplant-free survival following the laparoscopic operation was roughly half that following an open approach (42 % and 82 %, respectively) [45]. A post hoc analysis reported by Oetzmann and colleagues of complications following transplantation showed no advantage for operations performed after laparoscopic versus after open PE [46].

Sun and colleagues reported the results of a prospective examination of 95 procedures performed by a single surgeon between 2009 and 2011. In this study, patients were allocated to laparoscopic or open treatment arms by stratified randomization ($N=44$ and $N=47$ respectively following exclusion of four patients converted to open Kasai secondary to hemorrhage). Patients in the laparoscopic arm were reported to have longer operating times, lower blood loss volumes, and shorter time to full feeds compared to the open cohort, although the absolute differences for the latter two outcomes were modest. There were no significant differences between the groups when examining survival with native liver at 6 and 12 months, cholangitis, jaundice clearance, or other morbidity [47].

A recent meta-analysis examined published data from 11 studies comparing outcomes following laparoscopic and open Kasai procedures. The investigators performed statistical analyses of postoperative outcomes, including duration of operative time and hospital stay, volume of blood loss and rates of early jaundice clearance, cholangitis, variceal bleeding, and overall survival with native liver intact. The pooled comparison favored laparoscopy only for blood loss and for survival, with the differences in values for the remaining variables being statistically nonsignificant (Table 42.1) [48].

Summary

- Biliary atresia is a rare disease of infancy that is presently the most common indication for liver transplant during infancy.
- Surgical technique to address drainage of the biliary system has undergone significant refinement during the twentieth century, with

Table 42.1. Outcomes following laparoscopic versus open portoenterostomy.

Outcome	Lap	Open	Mean difference	[95 % CI]
Operative time (min)	134	190	16.57	[−11.67, 44.81]
Hospital stay (days)	83	124	−0.76	[−1.80, 0.28]
Blood loss (mL)	93	104	−7.05	[−13.59, −0.52][a]
Outcome (% of patients)	Lap	Open	Odds ratio	[95 % CI]
Early clearance of jaundice	58.1	66.3	0.70	[0.33, 1.48]
Cholangitis	43.8	38.9	1.01	[0.64, 1.60]
Variceal bleeding	12.6	7.4	1.90	[0.46, 7.92]
Survival	53.5	67.7	0.39	[0.21, 0.74][a]

Adapted from *Pediatr Surg Int* (2015) 31:261–269 (PMID: 25627699)
Lap laparoscopic, *Survival* two-year survival with native liver; 95 % CI—95 % confidence interval
[a]Statistically significant, comparison favors laparoscopic

long-term survival greatly improved following the introduction of the hepatic PE and advances in liver transplantation.

- Minimally access surgical techniques in the management of BA can be safely employed for performing the cholangiogram or liver biopsy and may offer typical advantages.
- The most important step during open or laparoscopic Kasai procedure alike is the depth and the width of the portal plate dissection, which may directly determine the success of the procedure.
- Outcomes following laparoscopic PE have not consistently been favorable in comparison to traditional open surgery.
- The laparoscopic or robotic Kasai procedure is currently only performed in selected high-volume Asian centers, and results should be reported in controlled studies with long-term follow-up.

References

1. Karrer FM, Lilly JR, Stewart BA, Hall RJ. Biliary atresia registry, 1976 to 1989. J Pediatr Surg. 1990;25(10):1076–80. discussion 1081.
2. McKiernan PJ, Baker AJ, Kelly DA. The frequency and outcome of biliary atresia in the UK and Ireland. Lancet. 2000;355(9197):25–9.
3. McDiarmid SV, Anand R, Lindblad AS, SPLIT Research Group. Studies of pediatric liver transplantation: 2002 update. An overview of demographics, indications, timing, and immunosuppressive practices in pediatric liver transplantation in the United States and Canada. Pediatr Transplant. 2004;8(3):284–94.
4. Thaler MM, Gellis SS. Studies in neonatal hepatitis and biliary atresia. I. Long-term prognosis of neonatal hepatitis. Am J Dis Child. 1968;116(3):257–61.

5. Thaler MM, Gellis SS. Studies in neonatal hepatitis and biliary atresia. II. The effect of diagnostic laparotomy on long-term prognosis of neonatal hepatitis. Am J Dis Child. 1968;116(3):262–70.
6. Kasai M. Treatment of biliary atresia with special reference to hepatic porto-enterostomy and its modifications. Prog Pediatr Surg. 1974;6:5–52.
7. Kuroda T, Saeki M, Morikawa N, Fuchimoto Y. Biliary atresia and pregnancy: puberty may be an important point for predicting the outcome. J Pediatr Surg. 2005;40(12):1852–5.
8. Hartley JL, Davenport M, Kelly DA. Biliary atresia. Lancet. 2009;374(9702):1704–13.
9. Nio M, Ohi R, Miyano T, Saeki M, Shiraki K, Tanaka K, et al. Five- and 10-year survival rates after surgery for biliary atresia: a report from the Japanese Biliary Atresia Registry. J Pediatr Surg. 2003;38(7):997–1000.
10. Leyva-Vega M, Gerfen J, Thiel BD, Jurkiewicz D, Rand EB, Pawlowska J, et al. Genomic alterations in biliary atresia suggest region of potential disease susceptibility in 2q37.3. Am J Med Genet A. 2010;152A(4):886–95.
11. Kohsaka T, Yuan ZR, Guo SX, Tagawa M, Nakamura A, Nakano M, et al. The significance of human jagged 1 mutations detected in severe cases of extrahepatic biliary atresia. Hepatology. 2002;36(4 Pt 1):904–12.
12. Cui S, Leyva-Vega M, Tsai EA, EauClaire SF, Glessner JT, Hakonarson H, et al. Evidence from human and zebrafish that GPC1 is a biliary atresia susceptibility gene. Gastroenterology. 2013;144(5):1107–15. e3.
13. Riepenhoff-Talty M, Gouvea V, Evans MJ, Svensson L, Hoffenberg E, Sokol RJ, et al. Detection of group C rotavirus in infants with extrahepatic biliary atresia. J Infect Dis. 1996;174(1):8–15.
14. Tyler KL, Sokol RJ, Oberhaus SM, Le M, Karrer FM, Narkewicz MR, et al. Detection of reovirus RNA in hepatobiliary tissues from patients with extrahepatic biliary atresia and choledochal cysts. Hepatology. 1998;27(6):1475–82.
15. Petersen C, Biermanns D, Kuske M, Schakel K, Meyer-Junghanel L, Mildenberger H. New aspects in a murine model for extrahepatic biliary atresia. J Pediatr Surg. 1997;32(8):1190–5.
16. Muraji T, Hosaka N, Irie N, Yoshida M, Imai Y, Tanaka K, et al. Maternal microchimerism in underlying pathogenesis of biliary atresia: quantification and phenotypes of maternal cells in the liver. Pediatrics. 2008;121(3):517–21.
17. Caton AR, Druschel CM, McNutt LA. The epidemiology of extrahepatic biliary atresia in New York State, 1983–98. Paediatr Perinat Epidemiol. 2004;18(2):97–105.
18. Harper P, Plant JW, Unger DB. Congenital biliary atresia and jaundice in lambs and calves. Aust Vet J. 1990;67(1):18–22.
19. Brent RL. Persistent jaundice in infancy. J Pediatr. 1962;61:111–44.
20. Cowles RA. The jaundiced infant: biliary atresia. In: Coran AG, Adzick NS, Krummel TM, Laberge J, Shamberger RC, Caldamone AA, editors. Pediatric surgery. 7th ed. Philadelphia: Elsevier Mosby; 2012. p. 1321–9.
21. Altman RP, Abramson S. Potential errors in the diagnosis and surgical management of neonatal jaundice. J Pediatr Surg. 1985;20(5):529–34.
22. Choi SO, Park WH, Lee HJ, Woo SK. 'Triangular cord': a sonographic finding applicable in the diagnosis of biliary atresia. J Pediatr Surg. 1996;31(3):363–6.

23. Balistreri WF. Neonatal cholestasis. J Pediatr. 1985;106(2):171–84.
24. Lefkowitch JH. Biliary atresia. Mayo Clin Proc. 1998;73(1):90–5.
25. Berci G. Patient positioning and logistics in the operating room during laparoscopic biliary surgery. In: Whelan RL, Fleshman J, Fowler DL, editors. The SAGES manual. 1st ed. New York, NY: Springer Science+Business Media, Inc.; 2006. p. 63–8.
26. Esteves E, Clemente Neto E, Ottaiano Neto M, Devanir Jr J, Esteves Pereira R. Laparoscopic Kasai portoenterostomy for biliary atresia. Pediatr Surg Int. 2002;18(8):737–40.
27. Yamataka A. Laparoscopic Kasai portoenterostomy for biliary atresia. J Hepatobiliary Pancreat Sci. 2013;20(5):481–6.
28. Dutta S, Woo R, Albanese CT. Minimal access portoenterostomy: advantages and disadvantages of standard laparoscopic and robotic techniques. J Laparoendosc Adv Surg Tech A. 2007;17(2):258–64.
29. Meehan JJ, Elliott S, Sandler A. The robotic approach to complex hepatobiliary anomalies in children: preliminary report. J Pediatr Surg. 2007;42(12):2110–4.
30. Andrews WS, Pau CM, Chase HP, Foley LC, Lilly JR. Fat soluble vitamin deficiency in biliary atresia. J Pediatr Surg. 1981;16(3):284–90.
31. Wu ET, Chen HL, Ni YH, Lee PI, Hsu HY, Lai HS, et al. Bacterial cholangitis in patients with biliary atresia: impact on short-term outcome. Pediatr Surg Int. 2001;17(5–6):390–5.
32. Meyers RL, Book LS, O'Gorman MA, Jackson WD, Black RE, Johnson DG, et al. High-dose steroids, ursodeoxycholic acid, and chronic intravenous antibiotics improve bile flow after Kasai procedure in infants with biliary atresia. J Pediatr Surg. 2003;38(3):406–11.
33. Bu LN, Chen HL, Chang CJ, Ni YH, Hsu HY, Lai HS, et al. Prophylactic oral antibiotics in prevention of recurrent cholangitis after the Kasai portoenterostomy. J Pediatr Surg. 2003;38(4):590–3.
34. Hasegawa T, Kimura T, Sasaki T, Okada A, Mushiake S. Indication for redo hepatic portoenterostomy for insufficient bile drainage in biliary atresia: re-evaluation in the era of liver transplantation. Pediatr Surg Int. 2003;19(4):256–9.
35. Muraji T, Tsugawa C, Nishijima E, Satoh S, Takamizawa S, Ise K, et al. Surgical management for intractable cholangitis in biliary atresia. J Pediatr Surg. 2002;37(12):1713–5.
36. Altman RP. Results of re-operations for correction of extrahepatic biliary atresia. J Pediatr Surg. 1979;14(3):305–9.
37. Shneider BL, Brown MB, Haber B, Whitington PF, Schwarz K, Squires R, et al. A multicenter study of the outcome of biliary atresia in the United States, 1997 to 2000. J Pediatr. 2006;148(4):467–74.
38. Goncalves ME, Cardoso SR, Maksoud JG. Prophylactic sclerotherapy in children with esophageal varices: long-term results of a controlled prospective randomized trial. J Pediatr Surg. 2000;35(3):401–5.
39. McKiernan P, Abdel-Hady M. Advances in the management of childhood portal hypertension. Expert Rev Gastroenterol Hepatol. 2015;9(5):575–83.
40. Huppert PE, Goffette P, Astfalk W, Sokal EM, Brambs HJ, Schott U, et al. Transjugular intrahepatic portosystemic shunts in children with biliary atresia. Cardiovasc Intervent Radiol. 2002;25(6):484–93.

41. Botha JF, Campos BD, Grant WJ, Horslen SP, Sudan DL, Shaw Jr BW, et al. Portosystemic shunts in children: a 15-year experience. J Am Coll Surg. 2004;199(2):179–85.
42. Vacanti JP, Shamberger RC, Eraklis A, Lillehei CW. The therapy of biliary atresia combining the Kasai portoenterostomy with liver transplantation: a single center experience. J Pediatr Surg. 1990;25(1):149–52.
43. Cowles RA, Lobritto SJ, Ventura KA, Harren PA, Gelbard R, Emond JC, et al. Timing of liver transplantation in biliary atresia-results in 71 children managed by a multidisciplinary team. J Pediatr Surg. 2008;43(9):1605–9.
44. National Library of Medicine—ClinicalTrials.org. Survival With Own Liver of Conventional Versus Laparoscopic Kasai for Biliary Atresia (NCT01063699). 2010. https://www.clinicaltrials.gov/ct2/show/NCT01063699. Accessed 3 Mar 2016.
45. Ure BM, Kuebler JF, Schukfeh N, Engelmann C, Dingemann J, Petersen C. Survival with the native liver after laparoscopic versus conventional Kasai portoenterostomy in infants with biliary atresia: a prospective trial. Ann Surg. 2011;253(4):826–30.
46. Oetzmann von Sochaczewski C, Petersen C, Ure BM, Osthaus A, Schubert KP, Becker T, et al. Laparoscopic versus conventional Kasai portoenterostomy does not facilitate subsequent liver transplantation in infants with biliary atresia. J Laparoendosc Adv Surg Tech A. 2012;22(4):408–11.
47. Sun X, Diao M, Wu X, Cheng W, Ye M, Li L. A prospective study comparing laparoscopic and conventional Kasai portoenterostomy in children with biliary atresia. J Pediatr Surg. 2016;51:374–8.
48. Lishuang M, Zhen C, Guoliang Q, Zhen Z, Chen W, Long L, et al. Laparoscopic portoenterostomy versus open portoenterostomy for the treatment of biliary atresia: a systematic review and meta-analysis of comparative studies. Pediatr Surg Int. 2015;31(3):261–9.

43. Laparoscopic Treatment of Choledochal Cysts

Bethany J. Slater and Steven S. Rothenberg

Introduction

Choledochal cysts (CDC) are congenital anomalies involving cystic dilation of the biliary tree. The incidence is approximately 1:100,000–1:150,000 in the United States. However, choledochal cysts are significantly more common in Asia. There is a significant female predominance (3–4:1) [1]. There are five different classifications of CDC, although type I, fusiform dilation of the common bile duct, is the most common type accounting for approximately 85 % of cases.

Etiology

The etiology remains unknown but is likely multifactorial. One of the main theories of the cause of CDCs is the presence of an underlying anomalous pancreatico-biliary ductal junction leading to reflux of pancreatic enzymes and thus damage to the common bile duct wall. In addition, distal obstruction of the common bile duct is an additional factor theorized to produce injury to the wall and subsequent dilation [2].

Preoperative Evaluation

History/Physical Exam

The classic presentation of patients with choledochal cysts is abdominal pain, jaundice, and a palpable right upper quadrant abdominal mass on exam. However, this triad of findings is only reported in a minority

D.S. Walsh et al. (eds.), *The SAGES Manual of Pediatric Minimally Invasive Surgery*, DOI 10.1007/978-3-319-43642-5_43

of patients. In infancy, painless jaundice is the most common presentation, while older children often present with intermittent abdominal pain and/or complications from stone or sludge obstruction. The majority of patients become symptomatic in the first decade of life.

Labs

Laboratory values are often normal in patients with CDC. However, liver function tests may reveal a conjugated hyperbilirubinemia in patients with obstruction of the common bile duct (CBD). Additionally, patients with evidence of liver injury may have a prolonged coagulation profile.

Imaging

Choledochal cysts are becoming more frequently diagnosed prenatally on anatomic ultrasounds in the second and third trimester, in which a cyst is identified in the porta hepatis. In infants and children, ultrasound is usually the initial imaging test obtained. It reveals a cystic mass in the right upper quadrant in continuity with the biliary tree. Magnetic resonance cholangiopancreatography (MRCP) is commonly performed to evaluate the type and extent of the CDC. In addition, hepatobiliary scintigraphy (HIDA) and endoscopic retrograde cholangiopancreatography (ERCP) are also occasionally used to determine patency of the biliary tract and to help delineate the anatomy, if unclear.

Surgical Indications

Complete cyst excision with reconstruction of the biliary system with a bilio-enteric anastomosis is indicated to prevent malignant transformation, cholangitis, and pancreatitis. In asymptomatic patients with prenatally diagnosed CDC, the timing of surgical resection has been controversial. Some authors recommend early surgical intervention (within the first month of life) to avoid cholangitis and liver damage [3, 4]. Early operation minimizes the risk of inflammation and adhesions around the cyst decreasing the difficulty of dissection and risk of injury. Most surgeons recommend surgical excision of asymptomatic infants within the first 6 months to a year.

Preoperative Preparation

If patients present with cholangitis, infection should be adequately treated prior to resection. Any coagulopathy should be corrected as well before surgical intervention.

Technique

Positioning

Patients are positioned supine at the foot of the bed in either a frog leg position or in stirrups depending on the size of the patient. The head of the bed should be slightly elevated during the procedure. The surgeon stands between the legs with the monitor placed by the patient's head (Fig. 43.1).

Ports

Three or four ports are typically used. A 4 or 5 mm port is placed at the umbilicus for the camera. The right-hand port (3–5 mm) is inserted in the midclavicular line slightly above the umbilicus. The left hand port

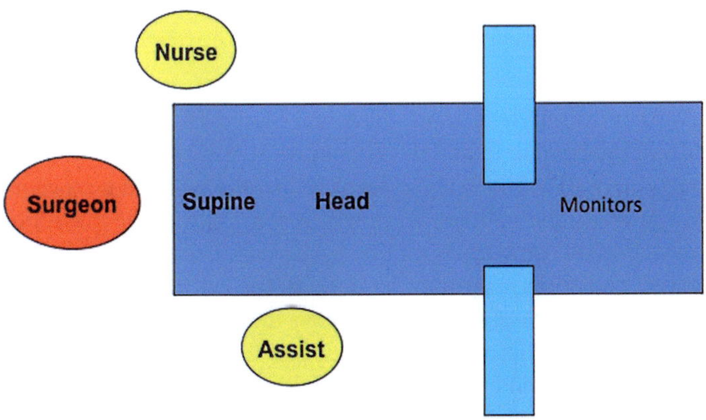

Fig. 43.1. Demonstrates patient positioning supine at the end of the bed with the surgeon between the legs and the monitor by the patient's head.

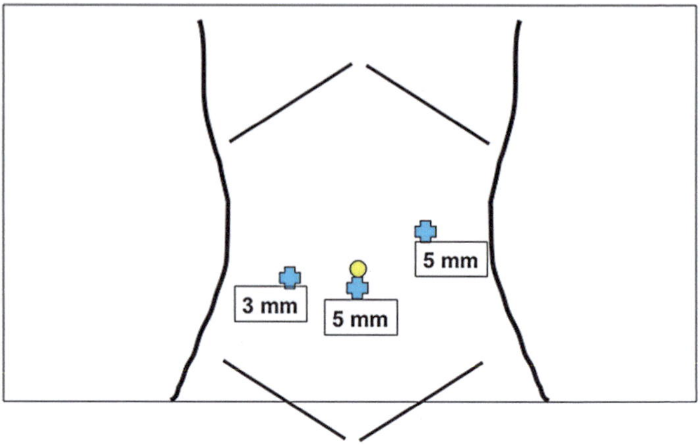

Fig. 43.2 Demonstrates port placement with a 4 or 5 mm port for the camera at the umbilicus, 3–5 mm port for the right hand in the midclavicular line slightly above the umbilicus, and a 3–5 mm port for the left hand slightly below the umbilicus

(3–5 mm) is inserted in the midclavicular line slightly below the umbilicus. This allows for an operating angle of approximately 90° toward the porta hepatis. If necessary, an additional port may be placed in the anterior axillary line in the right upper quadrant for a liver retractor or an assistant instrument (Fig. 43.2).

Steps

A #0 polypropylene transabdominal suture is placed through the falciform ligament to retract the liver upward. A similar suture is placed through the wall of the gallbladder to retract the gallbladder toward the right shoulder. The gallbladder is left in place during the dissection of the cyst to allow for retraction. The cystic duct is isolated and an intraoperative cholangiogram may be done if needed to further define the anatomy. This is rarely necessary given the accuracy of preoperative imaging. The cystic artery and duct are then clipped and divided. The cyst is dissected close to its wall with a combination of blunt dissection and electrocautery with care not to damage the portal vein and hepatic arteries (Fig. 43.3). Dissection should be continued to the bifurcation of the right and left common bile duct, and the common hepatic duct is divided just distal to the bifurcation (Fig. 43.4). Next, distal

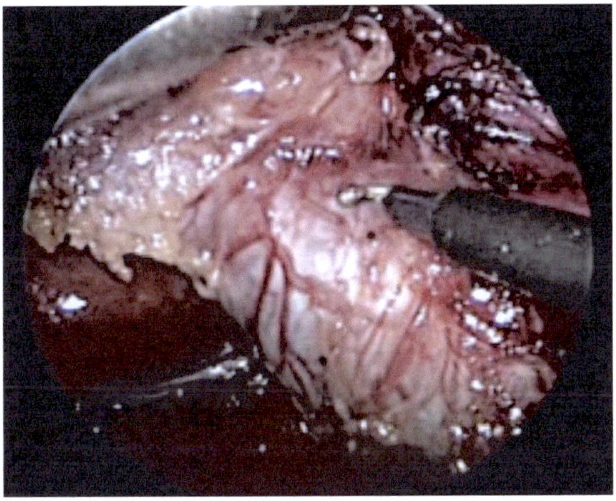

Fig. 43.3 Intraoperative picture demonstrating dissection of the cyst close to its wall

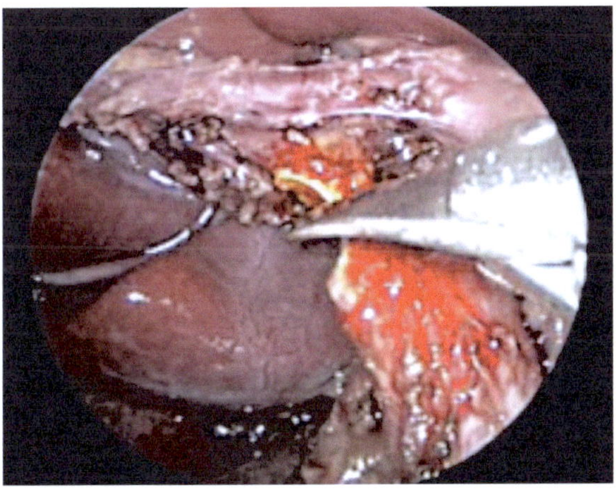

Fig. 43.4 Intraoperative picture demonstrating division of the cyst just distal to the bifurcation of the right and left common bile ducts

dissection is performed, and the duct is ligated behind the duodenum into the head of the pancreas so as to remove all biliary epithelial tissue. Ligation is done with a #0 polydioxanone loop (Fig. 43.5). Some advocate not ligating the distal stump, particularly in patients with a stenotic common bile duct radiographically [5]. In patients with repeated

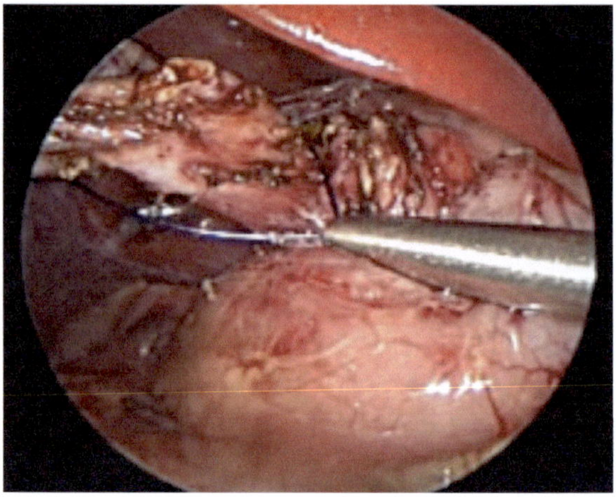

Fig. 43.5 Intraoperative picture demonstrating ligation of the distal cyst behind the duodenum into the head of the pancreas with an endoloop

cholangitis and significant pericystic inflammation, the anterior wall of the cyst can be opened and a mucosectomy performed. This leaves the posterior aspect of the cyst wall intact to avoid damage to the portal vein while removing the biliary epithelium which would be at risk for transformation to cholangiocarcinoma in the future [6].

Reconstruction

The most common types of reconstruction are the Roux-en-Y hepaticojejunostomy (HJ) and the hepaticoduodenostomy (HD). HD is technically easier given the proximity of the duodenum to the hepatic confluence, more physiologic, avoids complications associated with the Roux-en-Y, and allows for postoperative access to the anastomosis if required [7]. In a meta-analysis, the two types of reconstructions had similar postoperative complications. The HD group showed shorter operative times, decreased length of stay, and a higher rate of gastric reflux [8].

For the HD technique, the duodenum is completely Kocherized to prevent tension on the duodenum and anastomosis. A longitudinal duodenostomy is created at least 2 cm distal to the pylorus, on the antimesenteric side of the second portion of the duodenum (Fig. 43.6). The anastomosis is then performed using interrupted 4–0 polydioxanone sutures. The back wall is sutured first with the knots intraluminally (Fig. 43.7). At the corners, the knots are placed extraluminal, and then

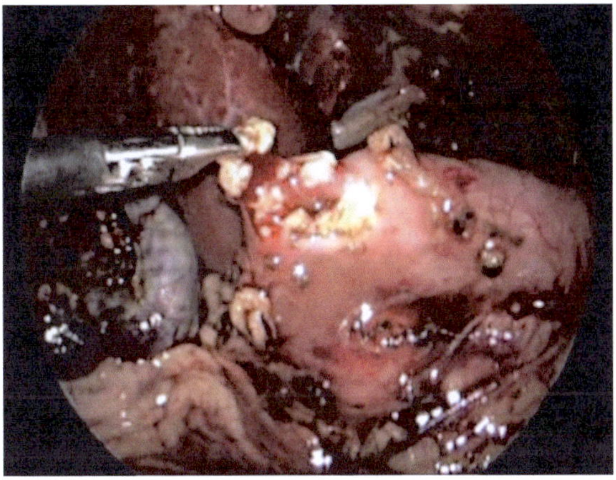

Fig. 43.6 Intraoperative picture of the creation of a longitudinal duodenotomy at least 2 cm distal to the pylorus on the antimesenteric side

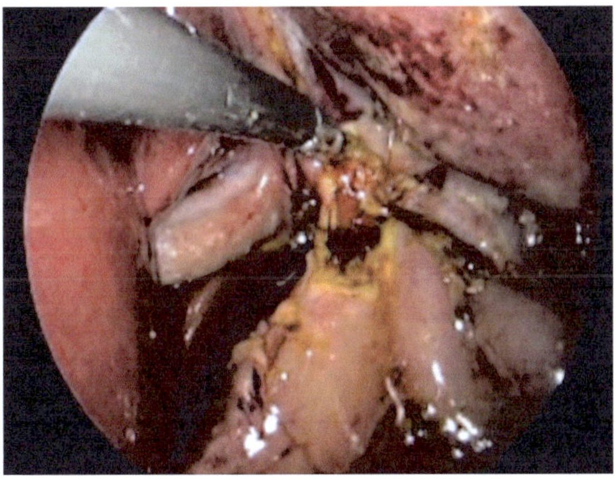

Fig. 43.7 Intraoperative picture demonstrating creation of the anastomosis with interrupted PDS sutures and the posterior wall with intraluminal knots

the anterior portion of the anastomosis is completed (Fig. 43.8). Finally, the gallbladder is freed from the liver, and the gallbladder along with the cyst is placed in a specimen bag and removed through the umbilical port site. A closed suction drain is usually left behind the anastomosis. There are reports supporting avoidance of drains after CDC excision, arguing that it is unnecessary in the majority of patients and minimizes postoperative pain and drain complications [9].

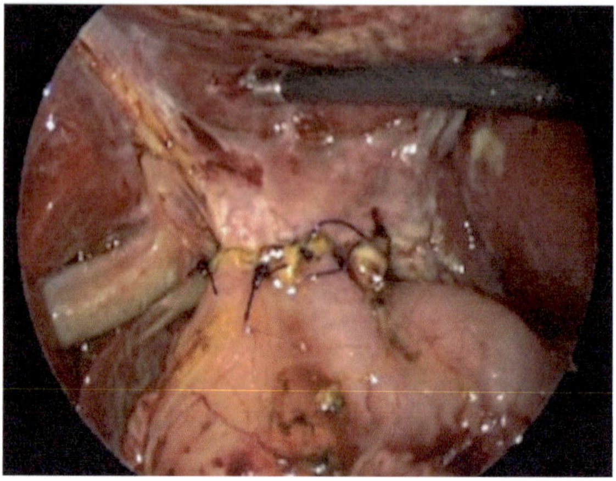

Fig. 43.8 Intraoperative picture demonstrating completion of the anastomosis and extraluminal knots for the anterior row

Pearls/Pitfalls

- Place a transabdominal suture through the falciform ligament and gallbladder to provide retraction and exposure.
- Leave the gallbladder in place initially to allow for retraction and assure that it does not obscure the view during dissection of the cyst.
- Dissect the cyst close to the wall to avoid injury to the portal vein and hepatic artery.
- Divide the proximal CBD just distal to the bifurcation. If the bifurcation is unclear, it can be visualized internally before transection to avoid division of the right and left hepatic ducts.
- Divide the distal CBD behind the duodenum at the level of the pancreatic head.
- Performing a hepaticoduodenostomy as the reconstruction method is technically easier than a hepaticojejunostomy and provides other advantages.
- An extensive Kocher maneuver of duodenum should be performed to prevent tension on the anastomosis.
- HD should be performed at least 2 cm distal to the pylorus to minimize bilious reflux.

Postoperative Care

Postoperative care is similar to other minimally invasive procedures involving the biliary or gastrointestinal tract. Diet is advanced as return of bowel function is evidenced. If a drain was left intraoperatively, it should be removed when drainage is clear and minimal. Patients also require long-term follow-up usually with an ultrasound and laboratory values annually for approximately 5 years and later if becomes symptomatic.

Outcomes

The first published case of laparoscopic CDC excision was by Farello et al. in 1995 [10]. Since that time there have been a number of reported series using the minimally invasive technique with good success and complication rates comparable or lower than that of open series [11–15]. The laparoscope affords magnification and aids in dissection of the cyst and creation of the anastomosis in addition to the other well-known advantages of minimally invasive surgery.

Complications

Complications of CDC resection include bleeding, bile duct leak, cholangitis, intrahepatic duct stone formation, pancreatitis, anastomotic stricture, and small bowel obstruction. Rates of bile duct leakage have been reported to be 0–20 % and often improve with nonoperative treatment [16]. Anastomotic strictures and intrahepatic calculi can be treated with endoscopic maneuvers or reoperation if necessary. Bowel obstruction appears to be minimized both with the laparoscopic technique and the HD anastomosis due to reduced bowel manipulation and avoidance of a roux limb and mesenteric defects.

Summary

- CDC is a relatively rare congenital disorder involving cystic dilation of the biliary tree.
- Manifestations consist of jaundice, abdominal pain, cholangitis, pancreatitis, and an abdominal mass.

- Due to the potential complications and development of carcinoma of the CDC, complete resection of the cyst with hepatico-enteric anastomosis is the standard treatment. Traditionally this has been performed with a large subcostal incision.
- More recently, minimally invasive techniques have become increasingly utilized.
- Laparoscopic CDC excision has shown good success with minimal complication rates.

References

1. de Vries JS, de Vries S, Aronson DC, Bosman DK, Rauws EA, Bosma A, et al. Choledochal cysts: age of presentation, symptoms, and late complications related to Todani's classification. J Pediatr Surg. 2002;37(11):1568–73.
2. Gonzales K, Lee H. Choledochal cyst. In: Coran A, Caldamone A, Adzick S, et al., editors. Pediatric surgery. 7th ed. Philadelphia: Elsevier; 2012.
3. Diao M, Li L, Cheng W. Timing of surgery for prenatally diagnosed asymptomatic choledochal cysts: a prospective randomized study. J Pediatr Surg. 2012;47(3):506–12.
4. Lugo-Vicente HL. Prenatally diagnosed choledochal cysts: observation or early surgery? J Pediatr Surg. 1995;30(9):1288–90.
5. Diao M, Li L, Cheng W. Is it necessary to ligate distal common bile duct stumps after excising choledochal cysts? Pediatr Surg Int. 2011;27(8):829–32.
6. Hay SA. Laparoscopic mucosectomy for large choledochal cyst. J Laparoendosc Adv Surg Tech A. 2008;18(5):783–4.
7. Santore MT, Behar BJ, Blinman TA, Doolin EJ, Hedrick HL, Mattei P, et al. Hepaticoduodenostomy vs hepaticojejunostomy for reconstruction after resection of choledochal cyst. J Pediatr Surg. 2011;46(1):209–13.
8. Narayanan SK, Chen Y, Narasimhan KL, Cohen RC. Hepaticoduodenostomy versus hepaticojejunostomy after resection of choledochal cyst: a systematic review and meta-analysis. J Pediatr Surg. 2013;48(11):2336–42.
9. Diao M, Li L, Cheng W. To drain or not to drain in Roux-en-Y hepatojejunostomy for children with choledochal cysts in the laparoscopic era: a prospective randomized study. J Pediatr Surg. 2012;47(8):1485–9.
10. Farello GA, Cerofolini A, Rebonato M, Bergamaschi G, Ferrari C, Chiappetta A. Congenital choledochal cyst: video-guided laparoscopic treatment. Surg Laparosc Endosc. 1995;5(5):354–8.
11. Gander JW, Cowles RA, Gross ER, Reichstein AR, Chin A, Zitsman JL, et al. Laparoscopic excision of choledochal cysts with total intracorporeal reconstruction. J Laparoendosc Adv Surg Tech A. 2010;20(10):877–81.
12. Liem NT, le Dung A, Son TN. Laparoscopic complete cyst excision and hepaticoduodenostomy for choledochal cyst: early results in 74 cases. J Laparoendosc Adv Surg Tech A. 2009;19(1):S87–90.

13. Liem NT, Pham HD, le Dung A, Son TN, Vu HM. Early and intermediate outcomes of laparoscopic surgery for choledochal cysts with 400 patients. J Laparoendosc Adv Surg Tech A. 2012;22(6):599–603.
14. Wang B, Feng Q, Mao JX, Liu L, Wong KK. Early experience with laparoscopic excision of choledochal cyst in 41 children. J Pediatr Surg. 2012;47(12):2175–8.
15. Liuming H, Hongwu Z, Gang L, Jun J, Wenying H, Wong KK, et al. The effect of laparoscopic excision vs open excision in children with choledochal cyst: a midterm follow-up study. J Pediatr Surg. 2011;46(4):662–5.
16. Chokshi NK, Guner YS, Aranda A, Shin CE, Ford HR, Nguyen NX. Laparoscopic choledochal cyst excision: lessons learned in our experience. J Laparoendosc Adv Surg Tech A. 2009;19(1):87–91.

44. Laparoscopic Splenectomy

Alessandra Landmann, Juan L. Calisto, and Stefan Scholz

Introduction

The laparoscopic approach to splenectomy has become the gold standard for most children. Minimally invasive techniques allow for decreased pain and minimal postoperative ileus leading to shorter hospital stay, earlier return to full activity, and improved cosmesis [1].

Indications for Splenectomy

Indications for splenectomy comprise a wide spectrum of pathological conditions. The acronym **SPLEEN** describes etiologies that may lead to splenomegaly necessitating splenectomy: sequestration (spherocytosis, sickle cell sequestration crisis), proliferation (rheumatoid arthritis, systemic lupus erythematosus), lipid deposition (Gaucher, Niemann-Pick), endowment (hemangioma, cysts, hamartoma, abscess), engorgement (trauma, sickle cell disease, portal hypertension, splenic vein thrombosis), and invasion (lymphoproliferative or malignant diseases) [2]. The most common indications in children are hereditary spherocytosis, immune thrombocytopenia purpura (ITP), and sickle cell disease [1, 3, 4].

The spleen is the most commonly injured abdominal organ in children (45 %) [5]. Treatment of pediatric trauma to the spleen depends on physiologic parameters and is overwhelmingly nonoperative, relying on close inpatient monitoring in combination with serial laboratory and physical exams. Some patients will require an intervention, with 10 % of

D.S. Walsh et al. (eds.), *The SAGES Manual of Pediatric Minimally Invasive Surgery*, DOI 10.1007/978-3-319-43642-5_44

those requiring a treatment necessitating splenectomy [4]. Laparoscopic splenectomy or splenorrhaphy may be an option, especially for hemodynamically stable children, but both are only infrequently utilized in the setting of trauma (<1 %). Other treatment modalities include angiography with splenic artery embolization (7 %) [4].

Splenectomy is chosen over splenorrhaphy in situations where there are concomitant abdominal injuries, hypotension, and traumatic brain injury [6]. Pediatric splenic tissue has a thicker capsule, and the presence of a compliant chest wall more resistant to rib fractures results in frequent splenic injuries that may be amenable to splenorrhaphy or partial splenectomy [7]. However, studies have shown that splenic preservation through partial splenectomy does not guarantee immunologic function and patients are still at risk for overwhelming postsplenectomy sepsis [8].

Splenic Sequestration Crisis

Defined as a sudden onset of splenomegaly associated with a decrease in hemoglobin of 2 g/dL and elevated reticulocyte count [9, 10], this disease usually occurs in sickle cell patients younger than 2 years old [9]. It represents a major cause of mortality [10] and the earliest life-threatening complication in this disease process [11]. Occurring in 10–30 % of children less than 6 years old, mortality for the first episode is up to 12 % [10]. Greater than 50 % will recur and overall mortality reaches 20 % [10].

Treatment involves correcting the hypovolemic shock through restoration of blood volume. In patients older than 2 years old, splenectomy is recommended [10], whereas those younger than 2 years old are placed on a monthly transfusion strategy until the second birthday [10, 11]. Patients will also frequently (66 %) have fever or active infection at the time of development of splenic sequestration [11] complicating the operative plan and postoperative care. Mortality has declined in recent years due to neonatal screening for sickle cell disease and parental education strategies [11], allowing for earlier diagnosis and treatment.

Anatomy

Key anatomic landmarks include (Fig. 44.1):

- *Splenorenal ligament*: this ligament contains the splenic vessels and the tail of the pancreas.

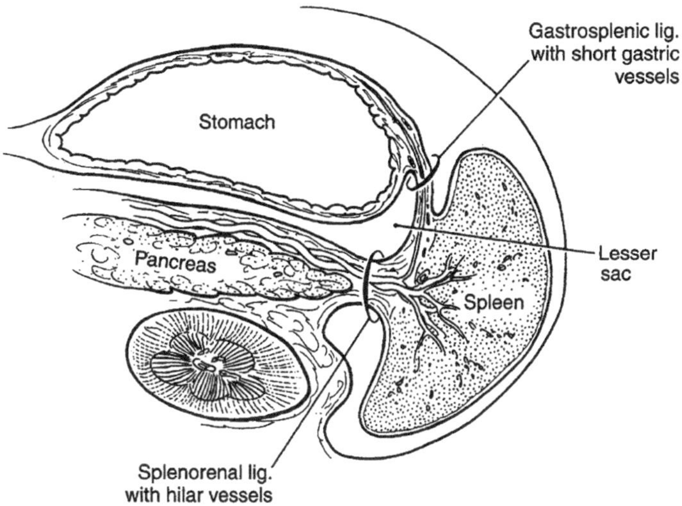

Fig. 44.1. Key anatomic landmarks for laparoscopic splenectomy. From Kathouda N. Laparoscopic Splenectomy. In: The SAGES Manual Volume 2: Advanced Laparoscopy and Endoscopy, Third Edition. Nguyen NT, Scott-Conner CEH, eds. Springer Science+Business Media. 2012. Reprinted with permission.

- *Gastrosplenic ligament*: this ligament contains the short gastric vessels and the left gastroepiploic artery.
- *Splenocolic ligament*: this ligament is avascular and attaches the spleen to the splenic flexure of the colon.

An accessory spleen can be found in 15–30 % of patients [3]. A small amount of residual splenic tissue may grow and can preserve immunologic function in the case of traumatic splenectomy or sickle cell autoinfarction. However, a meticulous search for superfluous tissue is a key operative step when immune-mediated disorders are present, such as ITP, as any remaining splenic tissue will cause failure of the operative treatment. Although initially thought to be a limitation of the laparoscopic approach, meticulous search for accessory spleens may be increased with improved visualization of intra-abdominal organs and increased identification of accessory spleens in laparoscopy (28 %) versus open (11 %) approach [12].

Wandering spleens are an uncommon cause of abdominal pain in pediatric patients [3]. In this situation, the spleen is not fixated with its normal ligamentous attachments, which may be lax or absent, and splenic torsion can occur with intermittent or permanent vascular occlusion. Patients may present with acute abdominal pain due to ischemia or a history of chronic, waxing, and waning abdominal pain.

Preoperative Assessment

A thorough history and physical exam should be performed in the office, with attention to splenic size and normal variants for age. Imaging is warranted in the setting of massive splenomegaly as surrounding anatomy may be severely distorted by the enlarged spleen [5]. If the spleen reaches into the pelvis, a laparoscopic approach may not be possible due to the sheer size of the spleen and the inability to visualize and divide the splenic vessels in a safe fashion.

Immunization should ideally occur 2 weeks prior to the operation and must include vaccines for *Haemophilus influenzae*, *Neisseria meningitidis*, and *Streptococcus pneumoniae* [9–11, 13, 14]. In the case of emergency splenectomy, immunization should occur 2 weeks after surgery. Pediatricians and primary care physicians should be aware of asplenic state to ensure compliance with vaccination schedules and need for booster immunizations as needed. In addition, careful family education is paramount to ensure that patients receive appropriate medical attention for lifelong risk of bacteremia.

Blood products should be available in the operating room, and an updated complete blood count with attention to platelet count should be reviewed prior to surgery. Platelet transfusion may be required for severe thrombocytopenia due to ITP, and patients may require transfusion prior to operation or during the operation.

Absolute contraindications to laparoscopic approach include inability to tolerate general anesthesia, portal hypertension with underlying liver cirrhosis, and severe uncorrected coagulopathy. Massive splenomegaly reaching into the pelvis [15–17] is a relative contraindication, although many cases of successful laparoscopic approach have been reported [16]. Dissection of the splenic hilum, whether through an anterior or lateral approach, is the most important step [18], and laparoscopic manipulation of a massively enlarged spleen may be difficult due to limited working space, increasing risk of injury to surrounding organs [18].

Operative Technique

Lateral Approach

After the induction of anesthesia, a Foley catheter and a nasogastric tube are placed. The patient is then placed in right lateral decubitus position and a beanbag may be utilized (Fig. 44.2). The ideal position is a 45–75° elevation of the left side, with additional padding beneath the right flank or operative table break to allow maximization of the distance between the left flank and the left anterior superior iliac spine.

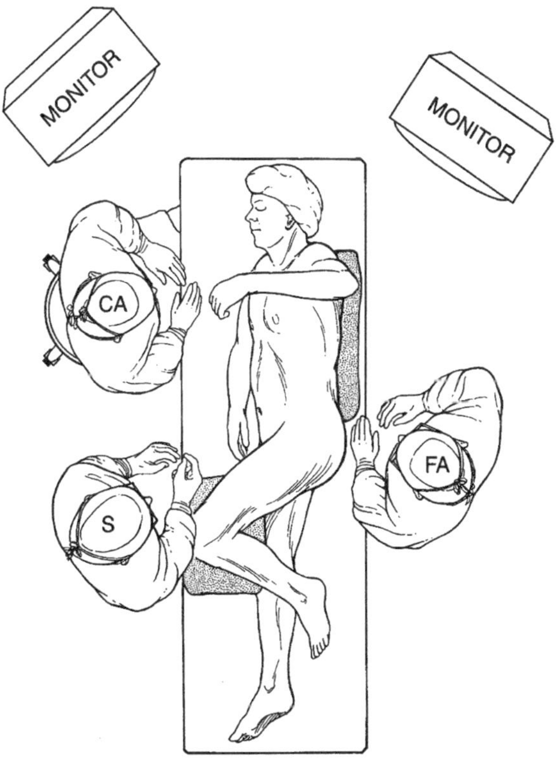

Fig. 44.2. Patient and surgeon positioning for laparoscopic splenectomy. From Kathouda N. Laparoscopic Splenectomy. In: The SAGES Manual Volume 2: Advanced Laparoscopy and Endoscopy, Third Edition. Nguyen NT, Scott-Conner CEH, eds. Springer Science+Business Media. 2012. Reprinted with permission.

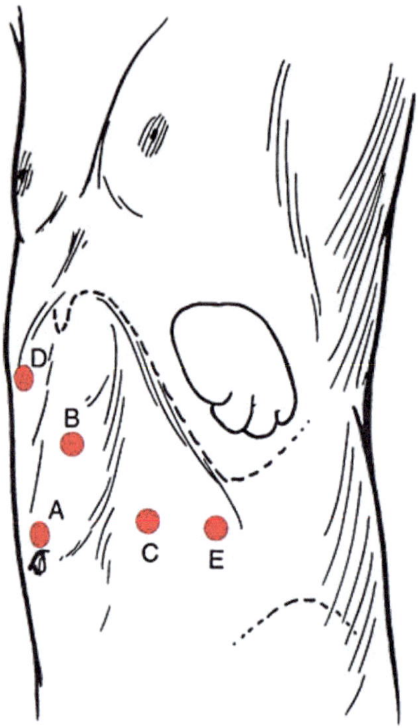

Fig. 44.3. Port placement for laparoscopic splenectomy. From Kathouda N. Laparoscopic Splenectomy. In: The SAGES Manual Volume 2: Advanced Laparoscopy and Endoscopy, Third Edition. Nguyen NT, Scott-Conner CEH, eds. Springer Science+Business Media. 2012. Reprinted with permission.

The surgeon then gains access to the peritoneal cavity either with a spring-loaded (Veress) needle or by open technique (Hasson). The umbilical port should be typically 12–15 mm to accommodate a 12 mm endoscopic stapler and a 10 mm or 15 mm endoscopic retrieval bag. Additional working ports are then placed under direct visualization; we recommend two 5 mm working ports in the left upper quadrant to facilitate traction and dissection and one additional working port in the left lower quadrant which will serve as the principle working port through which the endoscopic dissection device will be used, either an ultrasonic scalpel (Harmonic) or vessel sealer (LigaSure) (Fig. 44.3).

An initial search for accessory spleens, especially in the splenic hilum, is undertaken. The operative bed is then positioned to allow the

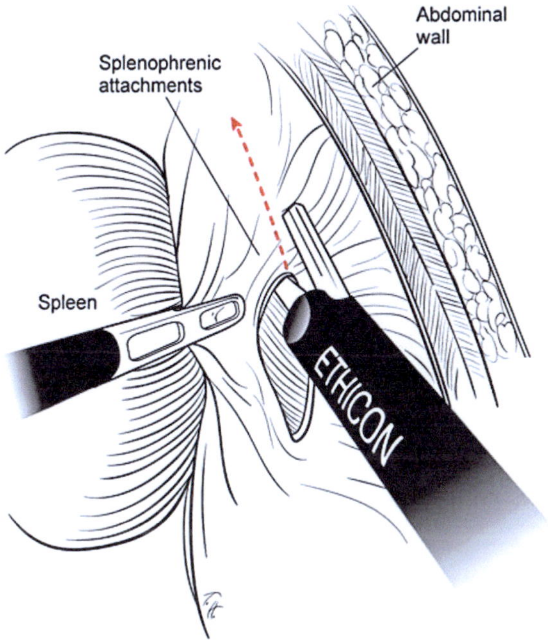

Fig. 44.4. Lateral dissection. From Kathouda N. Laparoscopic Splenectomy. In: The SAGES Manual Volume 2: Advanced Laparoscopy and Endoscopy, Third Edition. Nguyen NT, Scott-Conner CEH, eds. Springer Science+Business Media. 2012. Reprinted with permission.

left flank to be elevated, thus allowing the spleen to "hang" from its lateral attachments.

The splenocolic ligament is divided, followed by the gastrosplenic ligament (Fig. 44.4). Attention should be paid to adequate hemostasis of the short gastric vessels, which are in close proximity to the stomach. Medial traction is then placed on the spleen to allow division of the splenorenal ligament. The hilar splenic vessels can be divided using clips, vascular staplers or energy devices (LigaSure), or a combination of these. Many surgeons staple the splenic artery and the splenic vein separately to minimize the risk of an arteriovenous fistula between those vessels, although this may not be evidenced based (Figs. 44.5 and 44.6).

The spleen is then placed in an endoscopic retrieval bag (Fig. 44.7). In the case of massive splenomegaly, removal of the spleen may be challenging. Large enforced retrieval bags, which can be placed through a

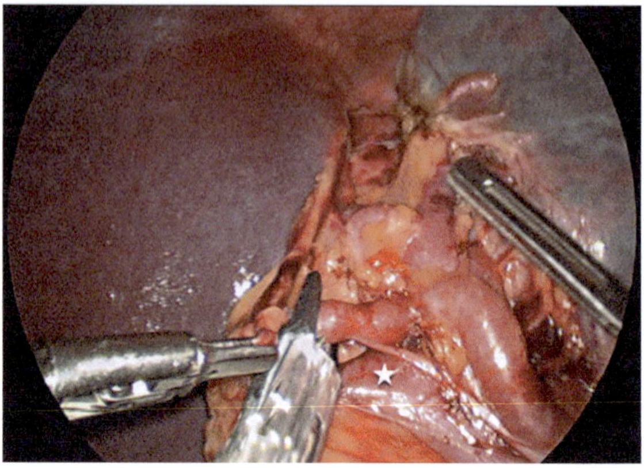

Fig. 44.5. View of the vasculature of the splenic hilum during laparoscopic splenectomy. The splenic artery is clipped proximal to its bifurcation. The *star* marks the splenic vein bifurcation.

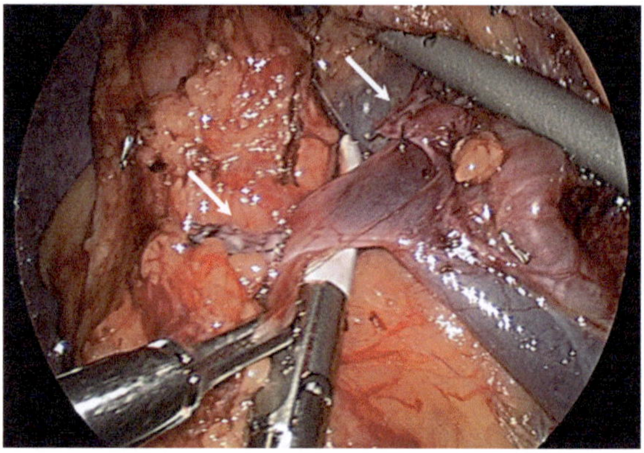

Fig. 44.6. Dissection of the splenic artery just proximal to its bifurcation with the Maryland-shaped LigaSure device. The vein is then clipped proximally and divided with a vascular-load stapler. The two *white arrows* point to the staple lines of the already divided splenic artery.

15 mm trocar, are available. Additional techniques for removal include careful finger fracturing or morcellation with a ringed forceps. Occasionally, a minilaparotomy or Pfannenstiel incision may be required. Care must be taken to avoid spillage of splenic fragments within the abdomen, which may lead to splenosis. The abdomen is

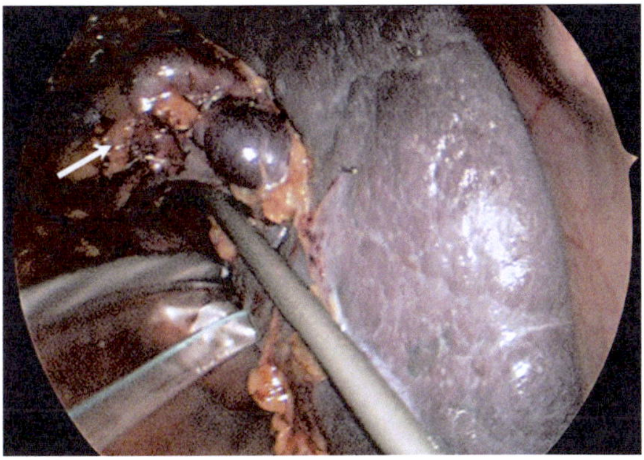

Fig. 44.7. After complete dissection of its attachments, the large spleen is then placed in an extra-large laparoscopic specimen bag introduced through the 15 mm umbilical port. Note the divided vasculature at the splenic hilum (*arrow*).

inspected for hemostasis and an additional cautious search for accessory splenic tissue is completed. Port sites are closed in a standard fashion. The patient is awoken from anesthesia and admitted for observation.

Benefits of the lateral approach to splenectomy include improved exposure due to dissection technique, thus less need to grasp and manipulate the spleen, leading to faster dissection and less risk of injury to the splenic capsule [17, 19]. This results in decreased operative time compared to the anterior approach [12] and, therefore, decreased operative cost and general anesthetic time.

Anterior Approach

The anterior approach may be beneficial in situations where a concomitant laparoscopic cholecystectomy will be performed. In contrast to the lateral approach, this technique involves initial control of the vascular pedicle [20] and may provide a benefit of reduced arteriovenous fistula formation when the vessels are individually ligated [20]. After induction of general anesthesia, a Foley catheter and a nasogastric tube are placed. Pneumoperitoneum is established at the umbilicus via similar techniques as mentioned above. Additional ports are placed under direct visualization along the left costal margin medially and laterally and an additional port site at the xiphoid process. Modification in port site placement may be necessary for concomitant procedures.

Dissection is begun and initial control of the vascular pedicle is established [20]. The gastrosplenic ligament is opened and the short gastric vessels are divided. The stomach is retracted medially and superiorly allowing exposure of the splenic hilum. The splenic artery and vein are divided. This may be accomplished with suture ligation, surgical clips, or an endoscopic stapler. The tail of the pancreas lies in direct contact with the splenic hilum or within 1 cm of the spleen in 70 % of cases, so care should be taken prior to firing a stapler across the hilar vessels [21]. The pancreatic tail is dissected off the spleen with the use of a laparoscopic hook cautery [20]. The splenocolic and splenorenal ligaments are divided; any splenic attachments to the diaphragm are taken down allowing complete mobilization. The spleen is placed in an endoscopic retrieval bag and removed from the abdomen. Careful hemostasis is established and the port sites are closed.

Partial Splenectomy

Laparoscopic partial splenectomy may be indicated for epidermoid and posttraumatic splenic cysts, intraoperative lacerations not amenable to splenorrhaphy, hematologic diseases, and splenomegaly of unknown etiology [22, 23]. All symptomatic splenic cysts and any cysts greater than 5 cm should be excised [24]. Preoperative planning is similar to total splenectomy, including vaccinations and availability of blood products, as not all children will have vascular anatomy amenable to partial splenectomy [25]. The goal is to maintain 20–30 % of the splenic volume to allow for maintenance of normal immune function, which can be verified by normal immunoglobulin levels [26]. Splenic regrowth may occur, although this is often not associated with recurrent hematologic symptoms [26]. When children require a salvage splenectomy, however, they benefit from the delay to loss of the immune function, as the child will inevitably be older with a more mature immune system [25] at repeat operation.

Patient positioning and port placement are similar to laparoscopic total splenectomy. The splenocolic ligament is divided. The splenorenal and gastrosplenic ligament are divided either superiorly or inferiorly, depending on which segment will be preserved. After ligating the vascular supply to the specimen being removed, a demarcation zone will develop (Fig. 44.8). The spleen is then transected 1 cm into the demarcation zone with staplers, ultrasonic scalpel (Harmonic), or endoscopic vessel sealing device (LigaSure) [23]. Control of hemorrhage is key [22] and, by maintaining transection within the zone of demarcation, can be more readily controlled. Splenic regrowth will occur during the

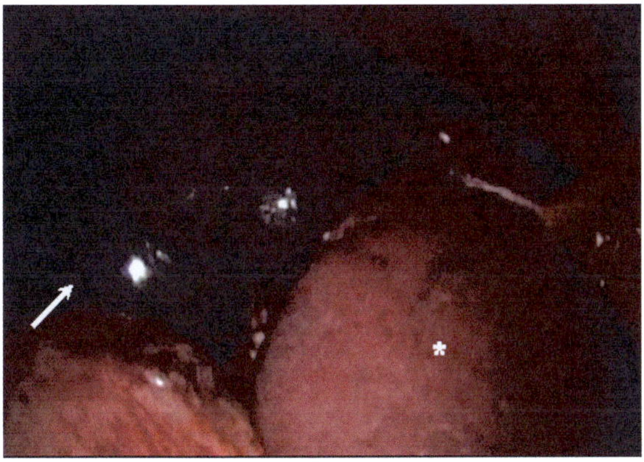

Fig. 44.8. Laparoscopic partial splenectomy for a 10 cm upper pole splenic cyst (*arrow*). The upper pole splenic vessels were divided as well as the short gastric vessels. The spleen has demarcated with the vital well perfused remaining part on the bottom of the picture (*star*) (Picture courtesy of Avraham Schlager, MD, Akron Children's Hospital, Akron, OH, USA).

first year after surgery and may be significant [22]. Partial splenectomy should be avoided if there is concern for parasitic cyst, as spillage of cyst contents may have significant hemodynamic consequences [23]. Concern for malignancy or any pathology at the splenic hilum would also warrant a conversion to total splenectomy [23].

Postoperative Care

Nasogastric tubes may be left for gastric decompression in case of varicose or large short gastric vessels. Diet can be advanced as tolerated by postoperative nausea. Patients are suitable for discharge postoperative day one or two once adequate oral pain control is obtained.

Complications

Intraoperative bleeding is higher in the laparoscopic versus an open control group and is the primary indication for conversion to an open procedure [5]. Other indications for conversion are massive splenomegaly and hollow viscus injury [5] with conversion rates up to 25 % in some case series [27].

Complications occurring after laparoscopic splenectomy include hemorrhage, pancreatitis, subphrenic abscess, wound infection, perforation of a hollow viscus, thrombocytosis, pleural effusion, pneumonia, pneumothorax (due to occult diaphragmatic injury), deep vein thrombosis, and portal vein thrombosis [5].

Residual splenic tissue can be problematic in immune-mediated diseases, especially ITP, with persistence of thrombocytopenia. To facilitate identification of residual splenic tissue, a damaged red blood cell scan can facilitate preoperative planning by localizing remaining splenic implants [27].

Overwhelming Postsplenectomy Sepsis

Overwhelming postsplenectomy sepsis (OPSI) is a rare but serious complication of splenectomy, most commonly occurring in children younger than five [5]. The incidence has been reported as about 4.4 % in children younger than 16 compared with 0.9 % in adults, although much of this data predates routine vaccination [26]. Typical organisms include encapsulated bacteria, such as *Streptococcus pneumoniae*, *Haemophilus influenzae*, and *Neisseria meningitidis*, due to the loss of the opsonization function of the spleen [28], although sepsis may occur in asplenic children by any bacterial, viral, fungal, or protozoan organism [13]. Rare sepsis can also occur due to *Capnocytophaga canimorsus* due to contact with dogs and babesiosis, a tick-borne illness [28]. Mortality from sepsis is reported at 38–70 % [13, 14], and risk of overwhelming postsplenectomy sepsis is 0.23 % per year or 5 % over lifetime [13]. In many occasions, a source is not identified and is thought to be occult colonization of the nasopharyngeal tract [14].

Vaccination against encapsulated bacteria should occur ideally 2 weeks prior to surgery or 2 weeks after surgery. If vaccines are administered prior to discharge, repeat vaccination should occur at 8 weeks [28]. A prophylactic antibiotic, typically daily penicillin, is administered until age five or for at least 1 year postsplenectomy [28]. However, many pediatricians and pediatric hematologists treat children up to age 18 with a prophylactic antibiotic.

Patients are given strict instructions regarding early signs of bacteremia, such as high fevers and rigors and the importance of urgent presentation for medical attention. Early prodrome may be followed by quick progression to septic shock [14]. Patients are given prophylactic high-dose antibiotics for these situations and should be started on empiric intravenous antibiotics once admitted to the hospital while awaiting blood culture results [28]. The clinical course mirrors Waterhouse-Friderichsen syndrome, with bilateral adrenal hemorrhage, peripheral gangrene, deafness associated with meningitis or mastoid osteomyelitis, and aortic insufficiency due to endocarditis [14]. Of the patients who succumb to sepsis, greater than 50 % will die within 48 h of presentation [14]. Although the prognosis was historically dismal, while employing early vaccination and aggressive treatment strategies, recent data suggests that informed patients who seek immediate medical attention have mortality closer to 10 % [14], a drastic improvement from previous data.

Summary

- Minimally invasive splenectomy is safe and has become the gold standard for children today.
- Preoperative imaging is warranted in the setting of massive splenomegaly as adjacent anatomy, especially the splenic vessels, may be severely distorted by the enlarged spleen.
- Most common indications for splenectomy in children are hereditary spherocytosis, immune thrombocytopenia purpura (ITP), and sickle cell disease.
- Anterior and lateral approaches to laparoscopic splenectomy have been described. Steps of the operation include division of the short gastric vessels, division of its ligamentous attachments, ligation of the vascular pedicle, and complete removal of all splenic tissue from the abdomen.
- Children undergoing splenectomy must be immunized for *Haemophilus influenzae*, *Neisseria meningitidis*, and *Streptococcus pneumoniae*, ideally 2 weeks prior to the operation.
- Overwhelming postsplenectomy sepsis (OPSI) is a rare but very dangerous complication after splenectomy, most commonly in children younger than five. OPSI should be considered in any asplenic patient with high fevers and rigors since quick progression to septic shock can occur.

References

1. Rescorla FJ, Engum SA, West KW, et al. Laparoscopic splenectomy has become the gold standard in children. Am Surg. 2002;68:297–302.
2. McClain KL, Mahoney DH, Armsby C. Approach to the child with an enlarged spleen. www.uptodate.com. 10/21/2015.

3. Coran A, Adzick NS, Krummel TM, et al. Chapter 110: the spleen. In: Pediatric surgery, 7th ed. Philadelphia: Elsevier; 2012.
4. Lee J, Moriarty KP, Tashjian DB. Less is more: management of pediatric splenic injury. JAMA Surg. 2012;147(5):437–41.
5. Walsh D. Pediatric laparoscopic splenectomy. SAGES Wiki. www.sages.org/wiki. 11/3/15.
6. Feliciano DV, Bitondo CG, Mattox KL, Rumizek JD, Burch JM, Jordan GL. A four-year experience with splenectomy versus splenorrhaphy. Ann Surg. 1984;201(5):568–73.
7. Velanovich V, Tapper D. Decision analysis in children with blunt splenic trauma: the effects of observation, splenorrhaphy or splenectomy on quality-adjusted life expectancy. J Pediatr Surg. 1993;28(2):179–85.
8. Nakae H, Shimazu T, Miyauchi H, et al. Does splenic preservation treatment (embolization, splenorrhaphy and partial splenectomy) improve immunologic function and long-term prognosis after splenic injury? J Trauma. 2009;67(3):557–64.
9. Al-Salem AH. Indications and complications of splenectomy for children with sickle cell disease. J Pediatr Surg. 2006;41:1909–15.
10. Lesher AP, Kalpatthi R, et al. Outcome of splenectomy in children younger than 4 years with sickle cell disease. J Pediatr Surg. 2009;44:1134–8.
11. Brousse V, Elie C, et al. Acute splenic sequestration crisis in sickle cell disease: cohort study of 190 paediatric patients. Br J Haematol. 2012;156:643–8.
12. Minkes RK, Lagzdin M, et al. Laparoscopic versus open splenectomy in children. J Pediatr Surg. 2000;35(5):699–701.
13. Sinwar PD. Overwhelming post splenectomy infection syndrome—review study. Int J Surg. 2014;12:1314–6.
14. Bridgen ML, Pattullo AL. Prevention and management of overwhelming postsplenectomy infection—an update. Crit Care Med. 1999;27(4):836–42.
15. Moores DC, McKee MA, et al. Pediatric laparoscopic splenectomy. J Pediatr Surg. 1995;30(8):1201–5.
16. Somasundaram SK, Massey L, et al. Laparoscopic splenectomy is emerging 'gold standard' treatment even for massive spleens. Ann R Coll Surg Engl. 2015;97(5):345–8.
17. Corcione F, Pirozzi F, et al. Laparoscopic splenectomy: experience of a single center in a series of 300 cases. Surg Endosc. 2012;26:2870–6.
18. Karadog CA, Erginel B, et al. Impact of spleen size on outcomes in laparoscopic splenectomy in children. Gastroenterol Res Pract. 2015; 1–5. Article ID 603915.
19. Danielson PD, Shaul DB, et al. Technical advances in pediatric laparoscopy have had a beneficial impact on splenectomy. J Pediatr Surg. 2000;35(11):1578–81.
20. de Lagausie P, Bonnard A, et al. Pediatric laparoscopic splenectomy: benefits of the anterior approach. Surg Endosc. 2004;18:80–2.
21. Kathouda N. Chapter 26: laparoscopic splenectomy. The SAGES manual volume 2: advanced laparoscopy and endoscopy, 3rd ed. Springer Science+Business Media; 2012.
22. Wang X, Wang M, Zhang H, Peng B. Laparoscopic partial splenectomy is safe and effective in patients with focal benign splenic lesion. Surg Endosc. 2014;28:3273–8.

23. de la Villeon B, Zarzavadjian Le Bian A, et al. Laparoscopic partial splenectomy: a technical tip. Surg Endosc. 2015;29:94–9.
24. Hery G, Becmeu F, et al. Laparoscopic partial splenectomy: indications and results of a multicenter retrospective study. Surg Endosc. 2008;22:45–9.
25. Hollingsworth C, Rice HE. Hereditary spherocytosis and partial splenectomy in children: review of surgical technique and the role of imaging. Pediatr Radiol. 2010;40:1177–83.
26. Diesen DL, Zimmerman SA, et al. Partial splenectomy for children with congenital hemolytic anemia and massive splenomegaly. J Pediatr Surg. 2008;43:466–72.
27. Rescorla FJ, Breitfeld PP, West KW, et al. A case controlled comparison of open and laparoscopic splenectomy in children. Surgery. 1998;124(4):670–6.
28. Pasternack MS, Weller PF, Thorner AR. Prevention of sepsis in the asplenic patient. www.uptodate.com. 10/21/15.

45. Laparoscopic Adrenalectomy in Children

Craig A. Wengler, Heather R. Nolan, and Joshua Glenn

Introduction

Pediatric surgeons are seeing adrenal disease with increased frequency. The objective of adrenal surgery is to completely resect the tumor, resulting in removal of the malignancy and normalization of endocrine function [1]. Surgical approach is based on likely pathology of the adrenal mass, presence of bilateral masses, and the surgeon's preference. Laparoscopic adrenal resection provides an attractive alternative to the open approach in children.

Laparoscopic adrenalectomy for pediatric patients has only recently been described, and the small body habitus of patients makes this surgery more technically challenging [2]. Although normally benign in the pediatric population, pheochromocytomas and neuroblastomas are seen with physiologic changes. Neuroblastomas are often large and infiltrative, making laparoscopic removal more difficult. Nevertheless, laparoscopic adrenalectomies have been successfully performed in the pediatric population with benefits of shorter hospitalization and rapid resumption of diet, as well as improved cost efficacy [3, 4]. In adults, laparoscopic adrenalectomy has proven to result in less blood loss and decreased need for transfusion, fewer wound complications, and decreased postoperative pain [5]. Most adrenal lesions are small and benign, making laparoscopic surgery both feasible and the appropriate operative choice. Relative contraindications include patients with malignancies that involve lymph nodes, highly vascular pheochromocytomas, and large tumors.

D.S. Walsh et al. (eds.), *The SAGES Manual of Pediatric Minimally Invasive Surgery*, DOI 10.1007/978-3-319-43642-5_45

History

The first anatomic description of the adrenals came in 1563, but it was not until 1805 when the adrenal gland was subdivided into the medulla and the cortex [6]. Later, early animal experimentation uncovered a substance derived from the adrenal medulla that elevated blood pressure. This was subsequently named epinephrine in 1897. Surgical innovation followed with the first surgical removal of adrenal glands performed in Switzerland and the United States by Roux and Charles Mayo, respectively [6]. As more information was uncovered regarding the functional capacity of the adrenals, several disorders were identified and subsequently named after those that first described them. Of these, most notable are Addison who characterized adrenal insufficiency, Cushing who described patients with excess cortisol, and Conn who identified aldosterone and the syndrome resulting from its excess.

Surgical Anatomy

The paired adrenal glands sit superior to the kidneys bilaterally. Located in the retroperitoneum, the typical adrenal gland is roughly 5 cm at greatest length when fully grown. By adulthood, the adrenal gland weighs typically 4–5 g, while at birth the gland weighs just 1 g [7]. Each adrenal gland is supplied by three main arterial beds: superior, middle, and inferior (Fig. 45.1). The superior adrenal arteries arise from the inferior phrenic artery, and the inferior adrenal arteries arise from the renal artery. The middle adrenal arteries are direct branches off the aorta.

The venous drainage of the adrenal gland is less complex with a single vessel draining the entire gland [7]. The course of the vein varies based on laterality with the right adrenal vein draining directly into the inferior vena cava and the left adrenal vein connecting to the IVC by way of the inferior phrenic vein to the left renal vein.

The adrenal gland is grossly divided into the medulla and the cortex. The cortex is largely comprised of lipids giving it a yellow color. The cortex makes up the exterior portion of the gland and accounts for the large majority of the gland's volume. It is subdivided into three zones: the zona glomerulosa, the zona fasciculata, and the zona reticularis. The zona reticularis reaches its final maturity late in childhood. The zona glomerulosa produces mineralocorticoid (aldosterone, 11-doxycorticosterone). The zona fasciculata and the zona reticularis produce glucocorticoids (cortisol) and the adrenal androgens (didehydroepiandrosterone

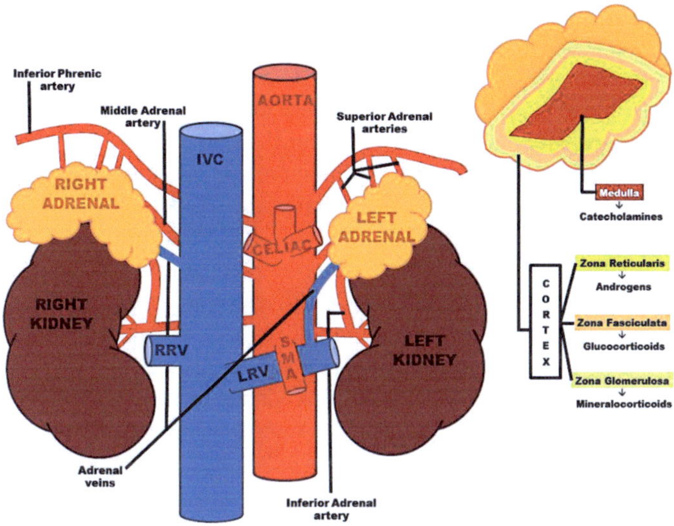

Fig. 45.1. Adrenal anatomy. Note the variances in left- and right-sided venous drainage.

(DHEA), androstenedione, testosterone, estrogen). The medulla comprises a smaller area, only 10–20 % of the total gland. Its cells are derived from neural crest cells and secrete the catecholamines norepinephrine and epinephrine [8].

The lymphatics are divided into two plexuses, one in the medulla and one just under the capsule [1]. The left adrenal lymphatics drain to the nodes near the left renal artery, while the right adrenal lymphatics drain to the periaortic lymph nodes. Innervation to the adrenal gland is primarily composed of splanchnic nerves to the medulla, while the cortex lacks any identifiable innervations.

Indications/Selection of Patients

Almost all adrenal tumors are treated with surgical removal [9]. Congenital adrenal hyperplasia is the only primary hyperfunctioning disorder for which medical therapy is indicated over surgical excision. Bilateral adrenal hyperplasia is much less responsive to surgery than its unilateral counterpart, and selective venous catheterization is used to predict response to surgery. Bilateral hyperplasia is managed medically with spironolactone, and unilateral hyperplasia is treated surgically with unilateral adrenalectomy.

Pheochromocytomas are initially treated with alpha-blockers to manage blood pressure prior to surgical intervention, while definitive treatment requires removal of the adrenal gland [10]. In the pediatric patient, extensive adrenocortical carcinoma is often resected en bloc along with lymph nodes, while minimally invasive techniques predominate for less extensive disease [7].

For adrenal incidentalomas, surgery is the treatment of choice if the mass is enlarging or functioning. In adults, resection is typically indicated for masses greater than 5 cm, but in the pediatric population, some surgeons advocate resection without regard to size. The pediatric population is also unique in that more than 90 % of adrenal masses are neuroblastomas [7]. In neuroblastoma, treatment is resection, although initially unresectable tumors may become resectable following chemotherapy.

Methods

The main techniques for laparoscopic adrenalectomy are the lateral transabdominal and the posterior retroperitoneal approach [5]. Left adrenalectomy and right adrenalectomy are two distinct procedures.

Transabdominal Lateral Approach

The transabdominal lateral approach is more commonly used in the pediatric population. It is performed with patient in the lateral decubitus position with the operative side up allowing gravity to assist in exposure of the adrenal glands. Prior to placing the patient on their side, the stomach and bladder are decompressed with an orogastric tube and Foley catheters. A kidney rest is placed in the lumbar area, and the bed is flexed at the level of the iliac crest to maximally open the space between it and the costal margin for trocar insertion. The bed is placed in a slight reverse Trendelenburg position. The superior arm is supported on pillows on top and the opposite arm is secured to arm board. An axillary roll is placed and all bony prominences are protected. Next, the bean bag is firmed and the patient is secured, again ensuring appropriated padding of all pressure points. The skin is then prepped and draped in the standard fashion with enough skin exposed to allow open laparotomy if necessary.

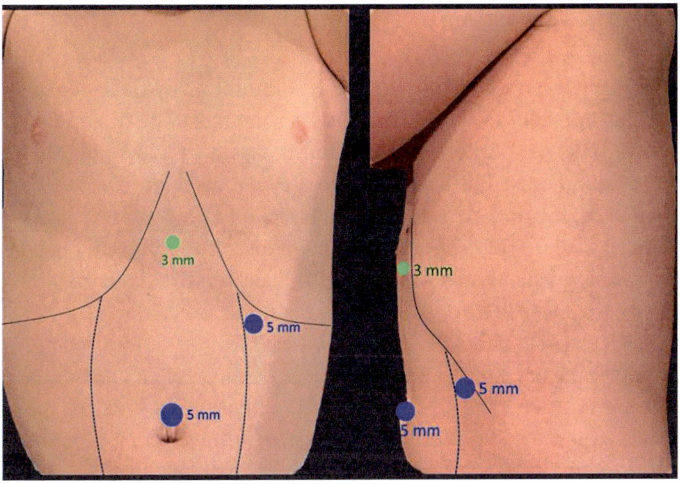

Fig. 45.2. Laparoscopic port placement for left sided adrenalectomy. Anterior and lateral views are shown.

Three to four trocars are placed in a subcostal position on the side of the adrenal gland to be extracted, starting with a 5-mm umbilical port placed under direct vision. The carbon dioxide (CO_2) insufflation begins at a low flow rate with maintenance of intra-abdominal pressure of 10 12 mmHg. A 30° camera should be used, if available. Under direct vision, a 3-mm or 5-mm port should be placed in the upper midline, close to the xiphoid process (Fig. 45.2). A third port (5-mm) should be placed laterally, close to the costal margin. An additional accessory port is often used on the right for either liver retraction or improved exposure.

It has also been described by Cameron et al. to use a 10- or 12-mm incision into the flank at the midclavicular line, two fingerbreadths below the left costal margin [5]. Dissection is carried down to the fascia, which is elevated between two Kocher clamps, and the peritoneal cavity is entered with a Veress needle. After a successful leak test, the peritoneal cavity is insufflated and a 10- or 12-mm trocar is placed at the Veress site. The 10-mm cannula is used in order to remove the specimen through the cannula or the incision. A specimen bag is necessary due to the potential of malignancy. Working ports (5-mm or 3-mm) are placed in a fashion to triangulate the lesion with as much distance between ports as possible depending on the patient's size. Often, the peritoneal attachments to the colon must be divided in order to place the most posterior cannula.

Right Adrenalectomy

In a right adrenalectomy, exposure is improved by dividing the right triangular ligament of the liver, including the most lateral and posterior attachments to the peritoneum. The fourth trocar should be placed in the epigastrium and used as a retractor to elevate the right lobe of the liver. During mobilization of the right hepatic lobe, always recognize the proximity of the inferior vena cava. Laparoscopic ultrasound can assist with this, as well as identifying the borders of the liver, kidney, and major vessels to allow for safe and expeditious dissection.

The retroperitoneum is then incised along the inferior vena cava allowing exposure to the adrenal gland and its vessels. The medial border of the inferior vena cava is carefully exposed, looking for the right adrenal vein at the superior medial border of the adrenal, remembering that this vein is typically broad and short and enters the vena cava slightly posteriorly [5]. Three clips should be used, with distal-most clip at the edge of the vena cava. Clipping the vein first is especially important in cases of pheochromocytomas.

Once the right adrenal vein has been clipped and divided, dissection continues with use of monopolar hook electrocautery to mobilize the medial portion of the adrenal gland. By dissecting from medial to lateral and inferior to superior, the superior pole of the kidney can be used as a dissection plane through the Gerota fascia, and the dissection can progress in a direction away from any anatomic danger areas (inferior vena cava and renal vein) [5]. Visible vessels, including the inferior phrenic vessel which is commonly seen at the superior and lateral border of the gland, are clipped. Before specimen extraction, the operative field is inspected for hemostasis. The adrenal gland is then placed within a bag and extracted without morcellation.

Left Adrenalectomy

Division of the lienocolic ligament up to the level of the gastric fundus improves exposure of the left adrenal gland by allowing the spleen to fall medially, pulling the tail of the pancreas with it. The left colon is also mobilized medially. Laparoscopic ultrasound can be used to verify the borders of the adrenal, kidney, and pancreas. It is important to note that the dissection plane should be relatively avascular and that it is relatively easy to mistake the tail of the pancreas for the adrenal gland.

With small tumors, first dissect the inferior and medial aspect of the adrenal remaining close to the gland until the vein is ligated with endoscopic clips. A right-angle dissector facilitates this exposure. It is important to remember that on the left, this should be done early in the operation after locating it entering the renal vein. Afterward, the gland is then carefully dissected free from the diaphragmatic attachments superiorly, the kidney on its inferior and lateral aspects, and medially from the midline structures. The inferior phrenic artery is frequently encountered along the superior edge of the adrenal and should be sought and ligated with clips and divided [5]. The dissection and extraction then occur in a similar fashion. For large tumors, early identification of the vein may be difficult and mobilization of the gland inferiorly and laterally is often helpful.

Prone Retroperitoneal Adrenalectomy

This can be useful in patients with small tumors and those that are likely to have adhesions from previous abdominal operations [11]. Due to the small retroperitoneal working space, however, limitations include large tumors and morbidly obese patients although some studies are challenging these restrictions [12].

The retroperitoneal approach begins by placing the child in a prone position, close to the lateral border of the table on the side of the procedure to allow manipulation of the lateral grasper. The 12th rib, iliac crest, and paravertebral muscles are then marked on the patient [13]. The first incision is made at the lateral border of the laterovertebral muscles, halfway between the 12th rib and the iliac crest [14]. According to Heloury, blunt dissection is performed until the retroperitoneal space outside the Gerota fascia is reached. Working space is then created by insertion and distension of a homemade balloon. Heloury uses a finger glove attached to a nasogastric tube [14]. A 5-mm port is inserted and secured with an external stitch. Insufflation is connected and maintained at a pressure between 8 and 12 mmHg. The second port (3- or 5-mm) is placed at the tip of the 12th rib and the third port (5-mm) is between the two previously inserted ports. Once inside, the landmarks and dissection are similar to a lateral transperitoneal approach. The specimen is then extracted via a bag without morcellation.

Single-Site Adrenalectomies

Single-site laparoscopic techniques were devised over 10 years ago. The technique for adrenalectomies was described more recently by Walz et al. in 2010 [15]. The technique can be performed in a variety of methods including a 10-mm laparoscope with a working port, two ports placed in a single incision, or most commonly using a specific device. A case–control study published by Walz et al. demonstrated that single-site cases for their institution had a conversion rate of 14 %, longer operative times, similar instances of complications, and a shorter hospital stay [15]. Shi et al. described similar intraoperative hemodynamic values and estimate blood loss, but also reported that while operative times were longer, in hospital analgesics use was less with single-site procedures [16].

Partial Adrenalectomies

Partial or cortical-sparing adrenalectomies have been described for bilateral tumors, hereditary adrenal tumors, and tumors in a solitary adrenal gland [17]. During these procedures, a portion of a single gland or portion of bilateral glands are extracted. Early reports that incorporate all patients, including adults and children, demonstrate few recurrences and ability to remain corticosteroid independent [18]. Specific operative techniques were previously described by Rogers et al. [19]. Tumors were resected with the help of laparoscopic ultrasound aiding the delineation between normal and involved tissues.

Robotics

Use of the robot in pediatrics remains controversial due to cost, size of the equipment, and relatively longer operative times [20]. However, robotic assistance does provide a magnified three-dimensional view as well as an improved ability to more precisely dissect structures [21]. Rogers et al. in 2008 described their institutions' use of a robotically assisted partial adrenalectomy and extra-adrenal pheochromocytomas resection in a pediatric patient with Von Hippel–Lindau disease [19]. Since this time, robotic equipment has become smaller and single-site robotic surgery has become more prevalent. Further case series are needed in this area.

Postoperative Care

Most patients are ready for discharge on postoperative day number one. However, pheochromocytomas require close monitoring in the intensive care unit, and patients with Cushing syndrome require postoperative stress-dose steroids. Patients with aldosterone-producing adenomas often experience a significant diuresis postoperatively and require close monitoring of their fluid balance and electrolytes [5].

Outcomes

Functional adrenal adenoma resection is associated with a 75 % cure rate and a mortality rate of less than 1 % [7]. Early identification of tumors and younger age (< age 5) improve prognosis. In adrenocortical carcinomas, surgical resection is the only chance for a cure. Untreated carcinomas have a mean survival of less than 3 months, with a worse prognosis involving nonfunctional tumors [7]. Complete excision is required; otherwise mortality is high.

Complications

Laparoscopic adrenalectomy is associated with typical laparoscopic risks, including injury to abdominal structures with trocar and instrument placement. These injuries are even more apparent in the pediatric population where thin pliable abdominal walls are commonplace. Additional concerns related to laparoscopy are complications of insufflation and its cardiopulmonary effects.

Patients who present with Cushing's syndrome are more likely to develop thromboses or infectious processes. Conversely, patients with Cushing's disease who have bilateral adrenalectomies can suffer from Nelson's syndrome in which the pituitary tumor undergoes progressive growth and leads to increased ACTH, visual disturbances, and hyperpigmentation.

In patients with pheochromocytomas, anesthesia induction can elicit hemodynamic instability requiring further medical intervention intraoperatively. Postoperatively, hypotension is a known risk and patients often stay in the hospital longer for management and to ensure stability prior to discharge.

After bilateral adrenalectomy, and less commonly after unilateral adrenalectomy, patients can experience adrenal insufficiency.

Summary

- Laparoscopic adrenalectomy is becoming increasingly more frequent in the pediatric population. With the exception of congenital adrenal hyperplasia, adrenal tumors are treated with surgical excision.
- Anatomical differences exist between left and right adrenal anatomy necessitating variances in procedural technique based on location.
- Minimally invasive surgical techniques include laparoscopic transabdominal lateral approach, laparoscopic prone retroperitoneal adrenalectomy, single-site surgery, partial adrenalectomies, and robotic procedures.
- The most frequently described procedure is the laparoscopic transabdominal lateral approach which is done in the lateral decubitus position utilizing 3–4 trocar sites.
- The prone retroperitoneal approach is best suited for small tumors and patients likely to have adhesions from previous intra-abdominal interventions.
- Single-site operations have similar instances of complications but have shown some promise in improved cosmesis and decreased postoperative narcotic use despite the longer operating times.
- Partial adrenalectomies utilize a laparoscopic ultrasound to guide dissection in an attempt to reduce postoperative corticosteroid use.
- Robotic surgery provides excellent visualization and instrument manipulation but is still controversial due to its associated increase in cost and operative times.
- The ideal method of operative intervention is dependent on surgeon preference, history of previous interventions and/or difficulty of dissection, lesion size and location, and cosmesis.
- A review of the literature reveals strong evidence that minimally invasive surgery has excellent outcomes with complete resection leading to the adoption of the laparoscopic approach to pediatric adrenalectomy as the standard of care.

References

1. Caty MG, Escobar MA. Adrenal tumors. In: Coran AG, editor. Pediatric surgery. Philadelphia: Elsevier Saunders; 2012. p. 557–66.
2. Gagner M, LaCroix A, Bolte E. Laparoscopic adrenalectomy in Cushing's syndrome and pheochromocytoma. N Engl J Med. 1992;327(14):1033.
3. Iwanaka T, Arain M, Ito M, Kawashima H, Matoba K, Imaizumi S. Challenges of laparoscopic resection of abdominal neuroblastoma with lymphadenectomy. A preliminary report. Surg Endosc. 2001;15(5):489–92.
4. Stanford A, Upperman JS, Nguen N, Barksdale E, Wiener ES. Surgical management of open versus laparoscopic adrenalectomy: outcome analysis. J Pediatr Surg. 2002;37(7):1027–9.
5. Cameron J, Cameron A. Current surgical therapy. Philadelphia: Elsevier Saunders; 2011.
6. Brunicardi FC, Andersen DK, Billiar TR, Dunn DL, Hunter JG, Matthews J, et al. Schwartz's principles of surgery. New York: McGraw Hill; 2010.
7. Holcomb GW, Murphy JP. Ashcraft's pediatric surgery. Philadelphia: Saunders Elsevier; 2010.
8. Greenfield LJ, Mulholland MW, Oldham KT, Zelenok GB, Lillemoe KD. Surgery scientific principles and practice. Philadelphia: Lippincott Williams & Wilkins; 2001.
9. Stewart JN, Flageole H, Kavan P. A surgical approach to adrenocortical tumors in children: the mainstay of treatment. J Pediatr Surg. 2004;39(5):759–63.
10. Fiser SM. The absite review. Philadelphia: Lippincott Williams & Wilkins; 2010.
11. Berber E, Tellioglu G, Harvey A, Mitchell J, Milas M, Siperstein A. Comparison of laparoscopic transabdominal lateral versus posterior retroperitoneal adrenalectomy. Surgery. 2009;146(4):621–5.
12. Perrier ND, Kennamer DL, Bao R, Jimenez C, Grubbs EG, Lee JE, et al. Posterior retroperitoneoscopic adrenalectomy: preferred technique for removal of benign tumors and isolated metastases. Ann Surg. 2008;248(4):666–74.
13. Lopez PJ, Pierro A, Curry JI, Mushtaq I. Retroperitoneoscopic adrenalectomy: an early institutional experience. J Pediatr Urol. 2007;3(2):96–9.
14. Heloury Y, Muthucumaru M, Panabokke G, Cheng W, Kimber C, Leclair MD. Minimally invasive adrenalectomy in children. J Pediatr Surg. 2012;47(2):415–21.
15. Walz MK, Groeben H, Alesina PF. Single-access retroperitoneoscopic adrenalectomy (SARA) versus conventional retroperitoneoscopic adrenalectomy (CORA): a case–control study. World J Surg. 2010;34(6):1386–90.
16. Shi TP, Zhang X, Ma X, Li HZ, Zhu J, Wang BJ, et al. Laparoendoscopic single-site retroperitoneoscopic adrenalectomy: a matched-pair comparison with the gold standard. Surg Endosc. 2011;25(7):2117–24.
17. Volkin D, Yerram N, Ahmed F, Lankford D, Baccala A, Gupta GN, et al. Partial adrenalectomy minimizes the need for long-term hormone replacement in pediatric patients with pheochromocytoma and von Hippel–Lindau syndrome. J Pediatr Surg. 2012;47(11):2077–82.

18. Baghai M, Thompson GB, Young WF, Grant CS, Michels VV, van Heerden JA. Pheochromocytomas and paragangliomas in von Hippel–Lindau disease: a role for laparoscopic and cortical-sparing surgery. Arch Surg. 2002;137(6):682–9.
19. Rogers CG, Blatt AM, Miles GE, Linehan WM, Pinto PA. Concurrent robotic partial adrenalectomy and extra-adrenal pheochromocytoma resection in a pediatric patient with von Hippel–Lindau disease. J Endourol. 2008;22(7):1501–3.
20. Brunaud L, Ayav A, Zarnegar R, Rouers A, Klein M, Boissel P, et al. Prospective evaluation of 100 robotic-assisted unilateral adrenalectomies. Surgery. 2008; 144(6):995–1001.
21. Berber E, Mitchell J, Milas M, Siperstein A. Robotic posterior retroperitoneal adrenalectomy: operative technique. Arch Surg. 2010;145(8):781–4.

46. Minimally Invasive Support for Placement of Ventricular Shunts

Celeste Hollands

Introduction

Congenital and acquired hydrocephalus in children frequently requires shunting of cerebrospinal fluid (CSF) from the ventricles to another body cavity such as the peritoneal or pleural cavities, heart, or gallbladder. Ventriculoperitoneal shunts (VPS) are the most common shunts used in children. Traditionally neurosurgeons have placed primary shunts using a minilaparotomy with blind distal catheter insertion. Secondary or redo shunts more frequently involve the pediatric surgeon for repeat access to the peritoneal cavity or placement in an alternate body cavity.

The widespread adoption of pediatric minimally invasive surgery has resulted in the use of laparoscopy in patients with existing VPS as well as neurosurgeons and pediatric surgeons working together to use laparoscopy for insertion of VPS and managing their distal complications [1–20].

Epidemiology of Hydrocephalus and Shunt Failure

Congenital hydrocephalus occurs in about 1/1000 live births in the United States. Acquired hydrocephalus in children results from infection, trauma, tumors, and cranial vault anomalies. Most cases are diagnosed by 2 years of age and are related to congenital conditions like Dandy–Walker malformations, myelomeningocele, or complications of premature birth. After the age of 2 years, the incidence decreases with most cases resulting from tumors or x-linked aqueductal stenosis.

D.S. Walsh et al. (eds.), *The SAGES Manual of Pediatric Minimally Invasive Surgery*, DOI 10.1007/978-3-319-43642-5_46

There is no geographic distribution worldwide and, aside from x-linked hydrocephalus, there is no sex predilection. The prognosis for successful management of hydrocephalus is excellent. It is however the underlying cause that will ultimately determine a child's outcome.

Hydrocephalus is most often treated by surgically inserting a shunt system. This system diverts the flow of CSF from the CNS to another area of the body where it can be absorbed as part of the normal circulatory process. A limited number of individuals can be treated with an endoscopic third ventriculostomy. Ventriculoperitoneal shunts (VPS) are the most frequent choice for surgical treatment of hydrocephalus in children [6, 9, 19].

Shunt catheters are foreign bodies with a one-way valve. Slit-valve, unidirectional-flow shunting devices have largely eliminated shunt failure due to the device. Shunts are at risk for infection and mechanical complications on either the proximal (ventricular) or distal (peritoneal, pleural, atrial, gallbladder) ends. The two main shunt complications in pediatric patients are infection and mechanical failure [21]. Shunt failure within the first year occurs in up to 40 % of children [4, 22] with 70–80 % requiring at least one revision [22]. Distal complications account for up to 72 % of VPS failures [23].

Pathophysiology

Hydrocephalus

Possible causes of hydrocephalus include complications of premature birth such as intraventricular hemorrhage, diseases such as meningitis, tumors, traumatic head injury, or subarachnoid hemorrhage, which block the exit of CSF from the ventricles to the cisterns or eliminate the passageway for CSF into the cisterns.

VPS Complications

Once a patient has a VPS, distal complications occur in 5–47 % of patients and include obstruction of the intraperitoneal catheter, inguinal hernia/hydrocele development, perforation of viscera, vaginal perforation, abdominal wall perforation, preperitoneal malposition, pseudocyst formation, tissue inflammation, bowel obstruction, infection, need to lengthen catheter, and shunt disconnection, fracture, or migration [4, 6, 9–21, 24–27]. Some of these can be seen more frequently in patients with abdominal adhesions, obesity, or scoliosis [5].

Laparoscopy in Patients with VPS

The adoption of laparoscopic surgery raised the concern of whether laparoscopic surgery in the presence of a VPS was safe. The general concern was that increased pressure in the peritoneal cavity could hinder drainage of CSF and might allow carbon dioxide to enter the ventricular system as an air embolus. In vitro assessment of the pressure required to cause shunt failure revealed a pressure of 80 mmHg was needed to disrupt shunts [28]. These disruptions occurred at the seals and diaphragms and did not disrupt the valve. Primary valve failure is rare, but depending on the shunt system used, a rate as high as 10 % may exist though a review of the literature fails to identify any reports of pneumocephalus after laparoscopy [28, 29].

Studies utilizing transcranial Doppler have shown decreased cerebral blood flow with intra-abdominal insufflation pressures of 15 mmHg but not at 10 mmHg [30]. Acute neurologic deterioration has been reported due to obstruction of the distal shunt catheter following laparoscopic jejunostomy which was resolved by a return to operating room and flushing of distal catheter [31].

The presence of a VPS has been shown to have no effect on the outcomes of laparoscopic procedures [32]. Multiple studies have shown no increased risk of shunt infection during laparoscopy for clean and clean-contaminated procedures in patients with VPS [27, 29, 33–36]. Finally, in patients with dirty procedures such as pelvic abscess or perforated appendicitis, the studies in the literature that show no increased shunt complications or infections all temporarily externalized the VPS [34, 37].

Preoperative Evaluation

Hydrocephalus is diagnosed through clinical neurological evaluation and by using cranial imaging techniques such as ultrasonography, CT, MRI, or pressure-monitoring techniques. A physician selects the appropriate diagnostic tool based on an individual's age, clinical presentation, and the presence of known or suspected abnormalities of the brain or spinal cord. Shunt failure or complications will present in much the same way and require a similar preoperative evaluation. The discussion will focus on diagnosing shunt failure and distal complications as these are the patients that will most likely involve the pediatric surgeon during the evaluation phase.

History

The patient with hydrocephalus will typically present with signs and symptoms of increased intracranial pressure. These include: rapid increase in head circumference or an unusually large head size; headache followed by vomiting, nausea, blurred, or double vision; downward deviation (also called sunsetting) of the eyes; problems with balance; poor coordination; gait disturbance; urinary incontinence; slowing or loss of developmental progress; lethargy; drowsiness; irritability; seizures; or other changes in personality or cognition including memory loss.

Patients undergoing evaluation for shunt malfunction or failure may present with symptoms or signs of increased intracranial pressure, infection, or distal obstruction.

Infection may produce symptoms such as a low-grade fever, soreness of the neck or shoulder muscles, meningitis, and redness or tenderness along the shunt tract. Distal complications may present with abdominal pain, distention, or fever.

Exam

The patient may have unusually an large head size, downward deviation of the eyes, gait disturbance, fever, redness or tenderness along the shunt tract, abdominal distention or tenderness, or a tender nonreducible mass at the abdominal catheter insertion site.

Labs

Generally, if infection is suspected, CSF cultures will be obtained.

Imaging

Shunt series and head and abdominal CT are the most common imaging modalities used. In the first 6–12 months of life, the diagnosis of hydrocephalus can often be made with an ultrasound of the brain. After the skull fuses, the diagnosis is best made with MRI or CT. All of these imaging modalities can be used to diagnose worsening hydrocephalus associated with shunt malfunction or failure. A shunt series is most useful to evaluate the course of the shunt looking at position, length, and possible disconnection.

Abdominal ultrasound or abdomen and pelvis CT scan will be useful in the evaluation of distal shunt malfunction. Findings such as abdominal pseudocyst or erosion into abdominal or pelvic viscera are best imaged with these modalities.

Surgical Indications

The most common indications for laparoscopic-assisted shunt surgery in children are the initial placement of VPS in patients who have had prior abdominal surgery, are obese, have distorted anatomy, or have evidence of distal shunt complications. Patients with prior abdominal surgery showed limited impact of prior surgery on subsequent non-shunt-related laparoscopic procedures [38], and in patients with hostile abdomens undergoing laparoscopic-assisted shunt, surgery success rates of up to 85 % avoided the need for ventriculoatrial shunts [39].

Technique

Special Considerations

Appendicitis is relatively rare in conjunction with a VPS, although not unheard of: The incidence of a child with appendicitis having a VPS is 1 in 1000, and the incidence of child with VPS having appendicitis is 1 in 750 [37].

Ventriculogallbladder shunts (VGB) have been used with mixed success in patients where the abdomen is no longer useable [40–44].

A technique to prevent distal obstructions where the distal catheter is passed through the falciform and positioned above the liver with the tip pointed at the hepatic flexure has been described in adults [45].

Anatomy

Sites of prior shunt insertion, abdominal incisions, gastrostomy, or enterostomy should be considered; otherwise there are no specific concerns.

Positioning

The patient is positioned in conjunction with the neurosurgeon, typically supine with the head turned away from the side of the shunt [46, 47]. Patients with significant scoliosis and contractures may require additional attention during positioning.

Instruments/Equipment

- 2.7-, 4-, or 5-mm 30-degree laparoscope.
- 3- or 5-mm general laparoscopic instruments such as bowel grasper, Maryland dissector, or DeBakey grasper as appropriate for age and size.
- 10-Fr peel-away sheath and introducer, groove director, or fragmentable needle for distal catheter insertion.
- One or two trocars, 3- or 5-mm.
- Some surgeons have used an 11-mm operating scope in adults [1].

Steps

Entry into the peritoneal cavity is typically made at the umbilicus by the safest method as determined by prior surgical history, anatomy, indications for surgery, and surgeon's experience. In the patient without significant surgical history, access is typically performed with a Veress needle at the umbilicus. Once position in the peritoneal cavity is confirmed, insufflation pressures should be kept as low as possible to complete the operation.

In operations for placement of a VPS, either primary or replacement, several techniques are available to insert the shunt under direct vision-groove director [9], 10-Fr peel-away sheath introducer via a Seldinger technique [7, 20], or a fragmentable needle [6]. In the case of a peel-away sheath, a finder needle is inserted into the abdomen at the desired location for the VP shunt under laparoscopic vision. A guidewire is passed into the abdomen, the needle is removed, and a 1-cm incision is made with a #11 blade. At this point, the neurosurgeon tunnels the catheter from the head to outside the abdomen. A dilating sheath is placed over the wire, and the catheter is advanced into the abdomen. The size of catheter and dilating sheath is determined by the neurosurgeon. The catheter should be positioned in the pelvis, and typically the rigid sheath is adequate to direct the catheter. If not, a working port can be placed to position the catheter. Alternatively, an operative laparoscope or 5-mm hysteroscope may be used.

If the operation is for management of a distal shunt complication, then the steps will depend on the complication being addressed. A single working port placed directly across from the site of the indwelling shunt on the other side of the abdomen can be used to reposition catheters, remove orphaned shunts, drain pseudocysts, or externalize distal shunts to clear distal obstructions. Two working ports may be needed for adhesiolysis. Placement of the shunt catheter and documentation of patency by observing flow of CSF should be noted prior to termination of the procedure, before and after release of pneumoperitoneum [48].

Pearls/Pitfalls

- Two setups/two teams can be helpful and will minimize traffic for infection.
- Use the lowest insufflation pressure needed and monitor end tidal CO2 to keep between 30 and 35.
- A second working port may be needed for difficult adhesiolysis, and one study showed a third was required in seven of 126 patients [16].

Postoperative Care

Postoperatively, the patient's diet is typically advanced as tolerated. Most patients are admitted to the neurosurgery service, and further care is dictated by the neurosurgery team.

Outcomes

A study of 810 adult and pediatric patients undergoing primary or replacement VPS showed a 20 % risk of shunt failure for both open and laparoscopic-assisted procedures. Infection was the most common reason for shunt failure and was equal in both groups. Failure due to distal obstruction was significantly less likely in the laparoscopic group 5.1 vs. 9.9 % [8].

Patients undergoing laparoscopic-assisted surgery for complications of VPS also were found to have infection (6.6–13 %) and distal failure (9.5 %) as the most common complications resulting in up to a 38 %

Table 46.1. Perioperative outcomes of laparoscopic VPS placement.

	Martin et al. [4]	**Buhligen et al. [15]**	**Handler et al. [16]**
Total *n*	17	29	126
Significant adhesions at initial placement	13	[a]	[a]
Failed due to adhesions	7	2	4
VA shunt	[a]	1	1
V pleural shunt	[a]	[a]	2
Laparotomy	[a]	1	1
Failed peritoneal placement	4	1	3

[a]Data not included in the study

subsequent rate of revision or replacement [1, 4, 16, 20]. Patients with prior abdominal surgery who had significant adhesions were noted to have subsequent shunt failure resulting in alternate shunt sites or laparotomy in several studies [4, 15, 16] (Table 46.1).

Complications

The complications of primary or redo VPS insertion are the same as those discussed under indications for surgery for complications of VPS. Those patients who require shunt revisions have a history of progressive difficulties reaching the abdominal cavity, intra-abdominal adhesions, CSF pseudocyst formation, and difficulty retrieving dislocated catheters [20]. Laparoscopic techniques have not decreased the overall shunt failure rate [45].

Summary

- Laparoscopy is safe and useful in inserting primary and redo VPS and in managing distal complications of VPS.
- Minimize CO2 insufflation to reduce hypercapnia.
- Abdominal surgical history is important in operative planning and may dictate port placement.

References

1. Kirshtein B, Benifla M, Roy-Shapira A, Merkin V, Melamed I, Cohen Z, et al. Laparoscopically guided distal ventriculoperitoneal shunt placement. Surg Laparosc Endosc Percutan Tech. 2004;14(5):276–8.
2. Armbruster C, Blauensteiner J, Ammerer H, Kriwanek S. Laparoscopically assisted implantation of ventriculoperitoneal shunts. J Laparoendosc Surg. 1993;3(2):191–2.
3. Goitein D, Papasavas P, Gagne D, Ferraro D, Wilder B, Caushaj P. Single trocar laparoscopically assisted placement of central nervous system-peritoneal shunts. J Laparoendosc Adv Surg Tech A. 2006;16(1):1–4.
4. Martin K, Baird R, Farmer J, Emil S, Laberge JM, Shaw K, et al. The use of laparoscopy in ventriculoperitoneal shunt revisions. J Pediatr Surg. 2011;46:2146–50.
5. Khosrovi H, Kaufman HH, Hrabovsky E, Bloomfield SM, Prabhu V, el-Kadi HA. Laparoscopic-assisted distal ventriculoperitoneal shunt placement. Surg Neurol. 1998;49:127–35.
6. Schubert F, Fijen BP, Krauss JK. Laparoscopically assisted peritoneal shunt insertion in hydrocephalus: a prospective controlled study. Surg Endosc. 2005;19:1588–91.
7. Argo JL, Yellumahanthi DK, Ballem N, Harriga MR, Fisher 3rd WS, Wesley MM, et al. Laparoscopic versus open approach for implantation of the peritoneal catheter during ventriculoperitoneal shunt placement. Surg Endosc. 2009;23:1449–55.
8. Naftel RP, Argo JL, Shannon CN, Taylor TH, Tubbs RS, Clements RH, et al. Laparoscopic versus open insertion of the peritoneal catheter in ventriculoperitoneal shunt placement: review of 810 consecutive cases. J Neurosurg. 2011;115:151–8.
9. Yu S, Bensard DD, Partrick DA, Petty JK, Karrer FM, Hendrickson RJ. Laparoscopic guidance or revision of ventriculoperitoneal shunts in children. JSLS. 2006;10:122–5.
10. Rodgers BM, Vries JK, Talbert JL. Laparoscopy in the diagnosis and treatment of malfunctioning ventriculo-peritoneal shunts in children. J Pediatr Surg. 1978;13(3):247–53.
11. Acharya R, Ramachandran CS, Singh S. Laparoscopic management of abdominal complications in ventriculoperitoneal shunt surgery. J Laparoendosc Adv Surg Tech. 2001;11(3):167–70.
12. Julian TB, Ribeiro U. Laparoscopic removal of a displaced ventriculoperitoneal shunt. J Laparoendosc Surg. 1995;5(1):55–8.
13. Turner R, Chahlavi A, Rasmussen P, Brody F. Laparoscopic revision of a ventriculoperitoneal shunt. J Laparoendosc Adv Surg Tech A. 2004;14(5):310–2.
14. Oak SN, Parelkar SV, Agarwal P, Gera P, Lahiri K, Charvarkar M. Laparoscopic management of pseudocyst and adhesions as a complication of ventriculoperitoneal shunt placement. Ped Endo Innov Tech. 2003;7(1):51–4.
15. Buhligen U, Grosser K, Rolle U, Grafe G, Brock D. Laparoscopy-assisted abdominal shunt revisions in children with hydrocephalus. Ped Endo Innov Tech. 2000;4(2):133–5.
16. Handler MH, Callahan B. Laparoscopic placement of distal ventriculoperitoneal shunt catheters. J Neurosurg Pediatr. 2008;2:282–5.

17. Kavic SM, Segan RD, Taylor MD, Roth JS. Laparoscopic management of ventriculo-peritoneal and lumboperitoneal shunt complications. JSLS. 2007;11:14–9.
18. Holcomb GW, Smith HP. Laparoscopic and thoracoscopic assistance with CSF shunts in children. J Pediatr Surg. 1995;30(12):1642–3.
19. Esposito C, Porreca A, Gangemi M, Garipoli V, De Pasquale M. The use of laparoscopy in the diagnosis and treatment of abdominal complications of ventriculo-peritoneal shunts in children. Pediatr Surg Int. 1998;13:352–4.
20. Liu DC, Wise MW, Loe WA, Hill CB, Nadell JM. Laparoscopically assisted shunt surgery for children with hydrocephalus. Ped Endo Innov Tech. 2000;4(4):271–6.
21. Roth J, Sagie B, Szold A, Elran H. Laparoscopic versus non-laparoscopic-assisted ventriculoperitoneal shunt placement in adults. A retrospective analysis. Surg Neurol. 2007;68:177–84.
22. Reddy GK, Bollam P, Caldito G. Ventriculoperitoneal shunt surgery and the risk of shunt infection in patients with hydrocephalus: long-term single institution experience. World Neurosurg. 2012;78(1/2):155–63.
23. Kast J, Duong D, Nowzari F, Chadduck WM, Schiff SJ. Time-related patterns of ventricular shunt failure. Childs Nerv Syst. 1994;10(8):524–8.
24. Grosfeld J, Cooney D. Inguinal hernia after ventriculoperitoneal shunt for hydrocephalus. J Pediatr Surg. 1974;9(3):311–5.
25. Potineni LB, Hartin CW, Gemme S, Caty MG, Bass KD. Laparoscopic assessment of a migrated ventriculoperitoneal shunt into an inguinal hernia. J Laparoendosc Adv Surg Tech A. 2012;22(3):301–3.
26. Cuatico W, Vannix D. Laparoscopically guided peritoneal insertion in ventriculoperitoneal shunts. J Laparoendosc Surg. 1995;5(5):309–11.
27. Liu DC, Flattmann GJ, Karam MT, Siegrist BI, Loe Jr WA, Hill CB. Laparoscopic fundoplication in children with previous abdominal surgery. J Pediatr Surg. 2000;35(2):334–7.
28. Neale ML, Falk GL. In vitro assessment of back pressure on ventriculoperitoneal shunt valves. Is laparoscopy safe? Surg Endosc. 1999;13:512–5.
29. Fraser JD, Aguayo P, Sharp SW, Holcomb III GW, Ostlie DJ, St Peter SD. The safety of laparoscopy in pediatric patients with ventriculoperitoneal shunts. J Laparoendosc Adv Surg Tech A. 2009;19(5):675–8.
30. Ravaoherisoa J, Meyer P, Afriat R, Meyer Y, Sauvanet E, Tricot A, et al. Laparoscopic surgery in a patient with ventriculoperitoneal shunt: monitoring of shunt function with transcranial Doppler. Br J Anaesth. 2004;92:434–7.
31. Baskin JJ, Vishteh AG, Wesche DE, Rekate HL, Carrion CA. Ventriculoperitoneal shunt failure as a complication of laparoscopic surgery. JSLS. 1998;2:177–80.
32. Backman T, Berglund Y, Sjovie H, Arnbjornsson E. Complications of video-assisted gastrostomy in children with or without a ventriculoperitoneal shunt. Pediatr Surg Int. 2007;23:665–8.
33. Li G, Dutta S. Perioperative management of ventriculoperitoneal shunts during abdominal surgery. Surg Neurol. 2008;70:492–7.
34. Walker DH, Langer JC. Laparoscopic surgery in children with ventriculoperitoneal shunts. J Pediatr Surg. 2000;35(7):1104–5.

35. Collure DWD, Bumpers HL, Luchette FA, Weaver WL, Hoover EL. Laparoscopic cholecystectomy in patients with ventriculoperitoneal (VP) shunts. Surg Endosc. 1995;9(4):409–10.
36. Bui CJ, Tubbs RS, Pate G, Morgan T, Barnhart DC, Acakpo-Satchivi L, et al. Infections of pediatric cerebrospinal fluid shunts related to fundoplication and gastrostomy. J Neurosurg. 2007;107:365–7.
37. Ein SH, Miller S, Rutka JT. Appendicitis in the child with a ventriculo-peritoneal shunt: a 30-year review. J Pediatr Surg. 2006;41:1255–8.
38. Metzelder ML, Jesch N, Dick A, Keubler J, Petersen C, Ure BM. Impact of prior surgery on the feasibility of laparoscopic surgery for children: a prospective study. Surg Endosc. 2006;20:1733–7.
39. Farach SM, Danielson PD, Chandler NM. Diagnostic laparoscopy for intraabdominal evaluation and ventriculoperitoneal shunt placement in children: a means to avoid ventriculoatrial shunting. J Laparoendosc Adv Surg Tech A. 2015;25(2):151–4.
40. Aldana PR, James HE, Postlethwait RA. Ventriculogallbladder shunts in pediatric patients. J Neurosurg Pediatr. 2008;1:284–7.
41. Ketoff JA, Klein RL, Maukkassa KF. Ventricular cholecystic shunts in children. J Pediatr Surg. 1997;32(2):181–3.
42. Stringel G, Turner M, Crase T. Ventriculo-gallbladder shunts in children. Childs Nerv Syst. 1993;9:331–3.
43. Girotti ME, Singh RR, Rodgers BM. The ventriculo-gallbladder shunt in the treatment of refractory hydrocephalus: a review of the current literature. Am Surg. 2009;75(8):734–7.
44. Lobe TE, Schropp KP, editors. Ventricular-gallbladder shunts in infants. In: Lobe TE, Schropp KP, editors. Pediatric laparoscopy and thoracoscopy. Philadelphia: WB Saunders Company; 1994. p. 148–50.
45. Svoboda SM, Park H, Naff N, Dorai Z, Williams MA, Youssef Y. Preventing distal catheter obstruction in laparoscopic ventriculoperitoneal shunt placement in adults: the “Falciform Technique”. J Laparoendosc Adv Surg Tech A. 2015;25(8):642–5.
46. Bax K(N)MA, van der Zee DC. Laparoscopy and ventriculoperitoneal shunts. In: Bax K(N)MA, Georgeson KE, Rothenberg SS, Valla JS, Yeung CK, editors. Endoscopic surgery in infants and children. Berlin: Springer; 2008. p. 479–83.
47. Saxena AK, Eder HG. Ventriculoperitoneal shunt implantation. In: Saxena AK, Hollwarth ME, editors. Essentials of pediatric endoscopic surgery. Berlin: Springer; 2009. p. 297–301.
48. Lobe TE, Schropp KP, editors. Laparoscopic management of ventriculoperitoneal shunt and Tenkhoff catheter malfunction. In: Lobe TE, Schropp KP, editors. Pediatric laparoscopy and thoracoscopy. Philadelphia: WB Saunders Company; 1994. p. 151–2.

47. Bariatric Surgery in Adolescents

Robert Michael Dorman, J. Hunter Mehaffey, and Carroll M. Harmon

Background

Adolescent bariatric surgery has emerged secondary to the growing epidemic of childhood obesity and its comorbidities [1–3]. Weight loss improves or resolves comorbidities in most cases and is projected to improve cardiovascular risk in adulthood [4, 5]. Patients who fail to lose weight with behavioral interventions may be candidates for a weight loss procedure [6–8]. Weight loss procedures have demonstrated excellent short- and mid-term weight loss, improvement in health-related quality of life, and comorbidity improvement in most trials with perioperative safety comparable to adults [9–13].

The most common procedures include laparoscopic gastric bypass, laparoscopic adjustable gastric banding, and sleeve gastrectomy. Gastric banding has largely fallen by the wayside due to a high incidence of weight loss failures and device complications in the adolescent population, leading to band removal or conversion to gastric bypass or sleeve. While bypass may be the most common procedure at present, sleeve gastrectomy is steadily gaining popularity and may surpass bypass as the initial weight loss procedure of choice for most patients.

D.S. Walsh et al. (eds.), *The SAGES Manual of Pediatric Minimally Invasive Surgery*, DOI 10.1007/978-3-319-43642-5_47

Indications and Contraindications for Weight Loss Procedures

Normal body mass index (BMI) changes dramatically in childhood growth periods. For example, 50th percentile BMI for males at ages 8, 12, and 18 years are about 15, 18, and 22 kg/m^2 (Table 47.1). Therefore, up to 18 years of age, percentages of the 95th percentile BMI for age and sex are used to define obesity classes (Fig. 47.1). These correlate well with adult obesity classes and provide greater stratification of extreme weights than an extrapolated 99th percentile.

Most centers define candidacy for operative intervention as either a BMI of >40 kg/m^2 alone or a BMI of >35 kg/m^2 with major comorbidities. About 3 % of US adolescents meet these criteria. Skeletal and physiologic maturity is widely accepted as a prerequisite to surgery. Age (13 years for girls and 15 years for boys) is often used as a surrogate. Comorbid medical and psychiatric conditions should be well stabilized prior to surgery. A treatment algorithm is shown in Fig. 47.2.

In order to achieve both superior safety and outcomes, there must be commitment to a team approach and close follow-up by both a multidisciplinary weight loss team and the patient and the patient's family. Adolescent candidates for weight loss procedures, in comparison to

Table 47.1 Approximate male BMIs for given percentiles

	8 years	**12 years**	**18 years**
50th percentile[a]	15	18	22
85th percentile[a] (overweight)	18	21	25
95th percentile[a] (obesity)	22	26	30
99th percentile[b] (extreme obesity)	26	32	35
120 % of 95th percentile[c] (severe or class II)	24	29	35
140 % of 95th percentile[c] (class III)	28	34	41

[a]CDC

[b]Barlow SE, Expert C. Expert committee recommendations regarding the prevention, assessment, and treatment of child and adolescent overweight and obesity: summary report. Pediatrics. 2007;120 Suppl 4:S164-92

[c]Kelly AS, Barlow SE, Rao G, Inge TH, Hayman LL, Steinberger J, et al. Severe obesity in children and adolescents: identification, associated health risks, and treatment approaches: a scientific statement from the American Heart Association. Circulation. 2013;128(15):1689–712

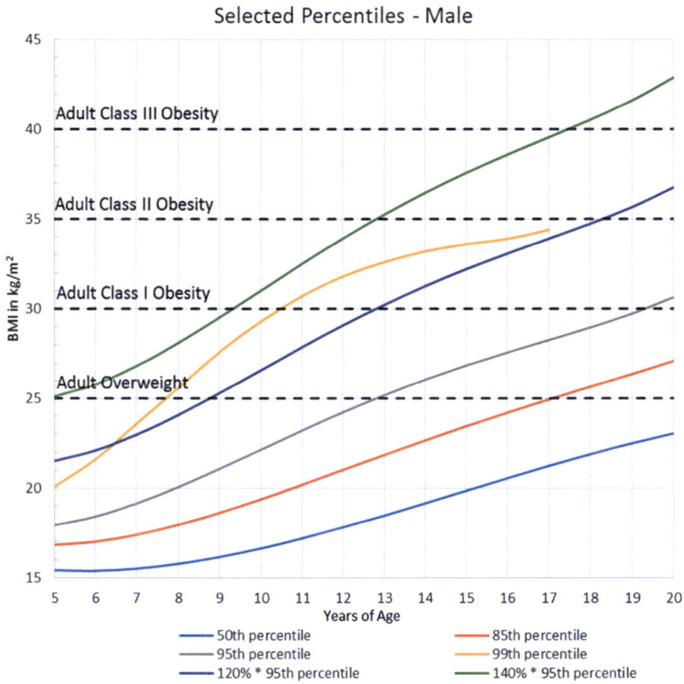

Fig. 47.1. Selected BMI for age percentile curves for male. At approximately age 18, the 85th percentile correlates with adult overweight, 95th percentile with adult class I obesity, 99th or 120 % of 95th percentile with adult class II obesity, and 140 % of 95th percentile with adult class III obesity. Sources—50th, 85th, and 95th percentiles: CDC. 99th percentile: Barlow SE et al. *Pediatrics* 2007.

adults, face the added challenges of psychological immaturity, peer pressure, poor compliance, a propensity for risk-taking behaviors, and possible loss to follow up when beginning college or a career. A 6-month trial of behavioral interventions should be attempted prior to planning an operation, during which compliance and the family and social environment should be evaluated.

Assent of the patient younger than 18 years and a well-informed consent from the parents are necessary. It must be very clear that the family possesses a thorough understanding of risks and realistic expectations of outcomes and the work ahead, and that adequate family and community resources and support are available prior to scheduling an operation.

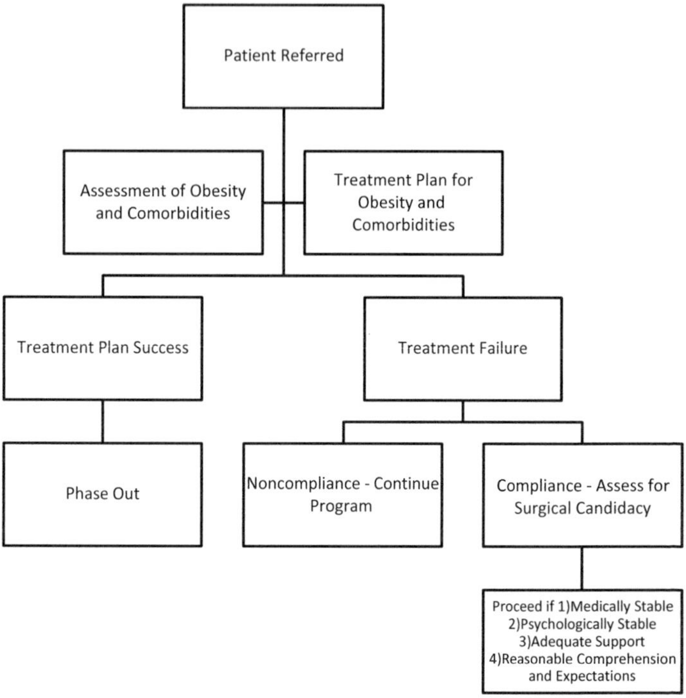

Fig. 47.2. Treatment algorithm for patients referred to a multidisciplinary pediatric obesity clinic.

Patient Positioning and Room Setup

Setup is similar to sleeve gastrectomy and gastric bypass. The patient should be placed in reverse Trendelenburg position in order to visualize the upper abdomen. A footplate is needed to keep the patient from gradually sliding caudally down the table. In all bariatric procedures, padding of all prominences to protect against the skin, vessel, and nerve injury takes on special importance. Even on well-padded surfaces, patients with a BMI upward of 50 are at risk of rhabdomyolysis with a long procedure.

Deep vein thrombosis prophylaxis should consist of pre- and postoperative enoxaparin at a prophylactic dose (e.g., 40 mg subcutaneous for individuals with a BMI $\leq$50 kg/m^2 and 60 mg for individuals with a BMI $\geq$50 kg/m^2) and sequential compression devices placed on both calves prior to induction of anesthesia. Antibiotic prophylaxis against wound infection and covering skin flora are given prior to incision.

The surgeon stands on the right of the patient with the first assistant directly across and both patient arms out. Some surgeons prefer to place both of the patient's legs in stirrups and work alternatively from the right and from between the patient's legs to avoid working at angles.

Trocar Position, Instrumentation, and Technique

Roux-en-Y Gastric Bypass

Roux-en-Y gastric bypass (RYGB) was first reported in 1975 and is the most common procedure performed in adolescents, and nearly all are performed laparoscopically. This is consequently the best-studied procedure in adolescents. RYGB results in a reduced-capacity stomach and diversion of ingested nutrients, as well as removal of parietal cells responsible for the production of ghrelin. A small stomach pouch is created and a Roux limb is brought up at about 50 cm from the ligament of Treitz in order to bypass biliopancreatic secretions and to prevent significant caloric absorption until the common limb is reached (Fig. 47.3). The laparoscopic approach to RYGB is currently the standard in all abdomens without thick adhesions. We begin with construction of the pouch; however the Roux limb can be created first.

Port Placement

- A 12-mm optical-entry trocar is placed in a supraumbilical position slightly left of midline, loaded on a 10-mm zero-angle scope. The abdomen is insufflated to 10 mmHg. A 30-degree 10-mm scope is used for the procedure.
- Under direct visualization, two 5-mm ports are placed, triangulated with the xiphoid on both sides of the abdomen to allow the surgeon to work from any angle and to receive support from a first or second assistant.
- A Nathanson liver retractor is placed through a 5-mm subxiphoid incision made with a 5-mm trocar, the liver is elevated to expose the lesser curvature of the stomach, and the retractor is attached to a fixed post.
- A Tru-Cut biopsy of the liver is taken to test for Non-alcoholic fatty liver disease (NAFLD).

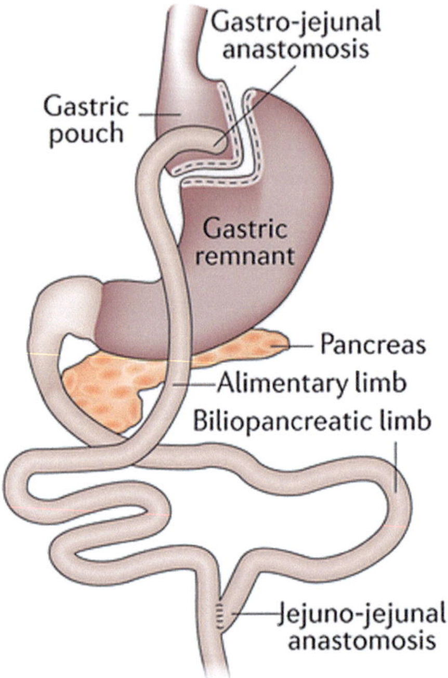

Fig. 47.3. Roux-en-Y gastric bypass surgical anatomy. From Naik RD, Choksi YA, Vaezi MF. Consequences of bariatric surgery on esophageal function in health and disease. Nature Reviews Gastroenterology and Hepatology 2016;13:111–119. Reprinted with permission from Nature Publishing Group.

Pouch Creation

- Gastric pouch creation begins with dissection of the left crus to provide access to the left side of the cardia.
- The hepatogastric ligament is then taken down with an EnSeal® (Ethicon) or Harmonic Ace Shears (Ethicon) about 4 cm down from the gastroesophageal junction (Fig. 47.4).
  - Pitfall—Care is taken to preserve the first two gastric branches of the left gastric artery (to prevent pouch ischemia) and, if present, a replaced left hepatic artery. Be alert for an accessory left hepatic artery as coming partially across one can lead to significant bleeding.

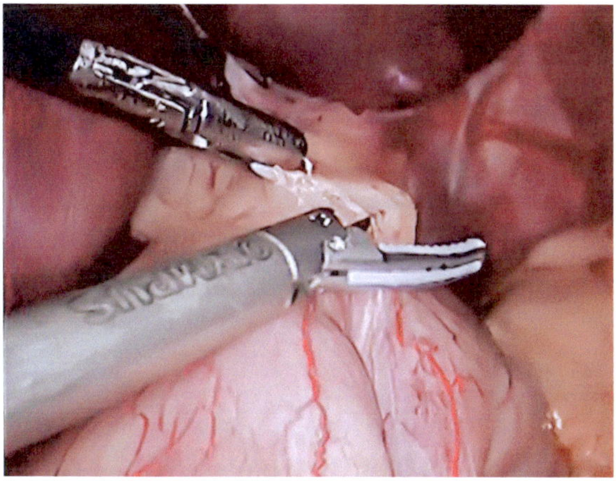

Fig. 47.4. The hepatogastric ligament is carefully opened while evaluating for replaced or accessory left gastric vessels.

- A retrogastric tunnel is bluntly dissected beginning at the lesser curvature, entering the lesser sac, separating the pancreas and other tissues from the back wall of the stomach to allow for stapling, until the dissecting instrument can be seen at the previously created opening in the left phrenoesophageal membrane.
- A 45-mm laparoscopic stapler (with 3.5-mm blue-load staples) is fired horizontally starting at the lesser curve about 4 cm below the GE junction. The horizontal staple line should be approximately 4 cm long.
  - Pearl—This can be measured with an open grasper, which is approximately 2 cm from tip to tip.
- A 32-Fr blunt-end bougie or Ewald tube is placed at the level of the horizontal staple line for sizing of the gastric pouch. The goal is a 30–50-cc pouch, about the size of an egg.
- Subsequent vertical firings complete the pouch. Staple-line bleeding can be controlled with surgical clips.
  - Pitfall—Care is taken to provide clearance from the gastroesophageal junction by angling the final staple load slightly toward the fundus.
  - Pitfall—Care is taken to keep the stomach taut with a grasper and to not let the back wall of the stomach fold so that four layers of the stomach wall are being crossed.

Roux-Limb Creation

- 50 cm of the small bowel is measured distal to the ligament of Treitz with hand-over-hand technique.
  - Pearl—Place a piece of white tape on one grasper 10 cm proximal to the tip to more accurately measure the length of the bowel.
- 100 cm are further measured distally along the jejunum. This distance may vary depending on whether BMI is greater or less than 50 kg/m^2. A white load (3.1-mm staples) is used to divide the jejunum. An absorbable stitch is placed for identification on the end that will be anastomosed to the gastric pouch.
  - Pitfall—Care is taken to rotate the bowel counterclockwise while measuring hand-over-hand to avoid kinking of the mesentery.
  - Pearl—The subsequent jejunojejunostomy can be facilitated by a first suture approximating the mesentery of the biliopancreatic limb and the mesentery of the jejunum where the side-to-side anastomosis is to occur, using a nonabsorbable suture such as Ethibond (Ethicon).
- A side-to-side jejunojejunostomy is created. A jejunostomy is made in the antimesenteric border of each limb with the hot tip of the energy device. The jejunostomy in the biliopancreatic (unmarked) limb is made just proximal to the staple line. A jaw of the stapler is passed through each and a white load is fired.
  - Pearl—Intraluminal bleeding may occur at this staple line. The scope can be passed through the jejunal defect to visualize this prior to closure.
- The resulting jejunal defect is closed with a running 2-0 Vicryl (Ethicon) suture or another white staple load. The resulting mesenteric defect is closed with running or interrupted Ethibond sutures.

Gastrojejunostomy

- The omentum is divided vertically with Harmonic shears in the midline.
- The marked proximal end of the Roux limb is brought up to the gastric pouch between the two divided omental leaves and anterior to the transverse colon.
  - Pitfall—Every effort should be made to ensure stapled anastomoses are not on tension, including division of the mesentery.

- A jejunostomy is made proximal to the staple line in the antimesenteric border of the jejunal Roux limb. A gastrotomy is made in the posterior wall of the pouch near the lesser curve and just proximal to the horizontal staple line.
- The stapler is passed just deep enough to create a 2-cm end-to-side gastrojejunostomy and a white load is fired. The gastrojejunal defect is closed with 2-0 Vicryl suture.
- Alternately, an end-to-end anastomosis stapler with an orally delivered anvil (such as the Covidien OrVil™) may be used. The gastrotomy will be at the junction of the vertical and horizontal staple lines.
- The pseudo-Petersen defect at the jejunal and transverse colonic mesenteries is closed with silk suture.
  - Pitfall—Failure to close mesenteric defects can lead to a high incidence of internal hernia, as demonstrated by Gothberg [14].
- A flexible endoscope is passed into the gastric pouch and past the gastrojejunostomy to ensure patency. The upper abdomen is then filled with saline, and the pouch is gently insufflated to check for air leak at the gastrojejunostomy.

Sleeve Gastrectomy

Sleeve gastrectomy is a chiefly restrictive procedure, although removal of the parietal cells in the fundus may also have a metabolic effect by reducing the production of ghrelin. A stapler is used to tubularize the stomach by placing a bougie of appropriate size within the lesser curvature and amputating the greater curvature and fundus down to about the level of the incisura distally (Fig. 47.5). The advantages of this technique are preservation of the pylorus, which prevents the dumping syndrome prevalent in bypass, reduced malabsorption (although nutritional deficiencies remain a challenge), relative simplicity and shorter operative time versus bypass, and fewer postoperative complications than bypass, as there is only one staple line and no new spaces are created for internal hernia. Although weight loss is slightly less than that after bypass, a sleeve can later be converted to bypass if the malabsorptive component is later necessary or if post-sleeve reflux is refractory. The popularity of sleeve gastrectomy has been increasing, and this may become the standard first-line procedure in adolescents in coming years.

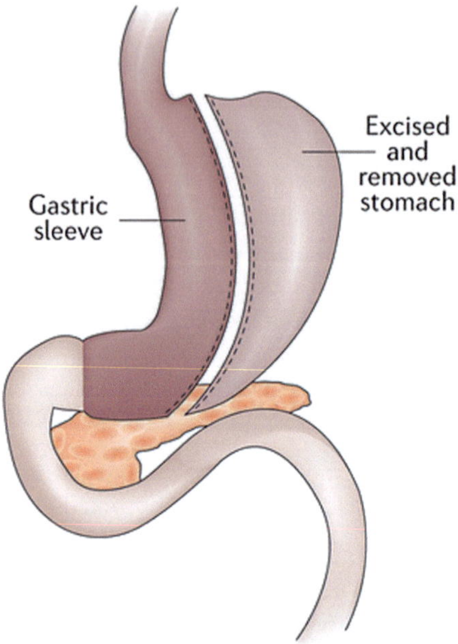

Fig. 47.5. Sleeve gastrectomy surgical anatomy. From Naik RD, Choksi YA, Vaezi MF. Consequences of bariatric surgery on esophageal function in health and disease. Nature Reviews Gastroenterology and Hepatology 2016;13:111–119. Reprinted with permission from Nature Publishing Group.

Port Placement

- A 12-mm optical-entry trocar is placed in the left upper quadrant, loaded on a 10-mm zero-angle scope. The abdomen is insufflated to 10 mmHg. A 30-degree 10-mm scope is used for the procedure.
- Under direct visualization, a 12-mm laparoscopic port is placed in the right upper quadrant and 5-mm ports in right and left lateral subcostal positions.
- A Nathanson liver retractor is placed through a 5-mm subxiphoid incision made with a 5-mm trocar, the liver is elevated to expose the lesser curvature of the stomach, and the retractor is attached to a fixed post.
- A Tru-Cut liver biopsy is taken to test for NAFLD.

Preparation for Gastrectomy

- We begin with dissection of the left crus to provide access to the angle of His.
- The hepatogastric ligament is incised with an EnSeal® (Ethicon) about 4 cm down from the gastroesophageal junction.
  - Pitfall—Care is taken to preserve a replaced left hepatic artery or to come completely across an accessory left hepatic artery.
- If a hiatal hernia is identified, it may be repaired at this time. The incision is extended to incise the phrenoesophageal ligament over the right crus, anterior decussation, and left crus. Herniated abdominal contents are reduced. The distal esophagus is mobilized as necessary to bring the gastroesophageal junction 4 cm below the hiatus without tension, and the hernia is closed anteriorly with interrupted zero-gauge nonabsorbable suture.
  - Pearl—Repair of even small hernias may reduce the incidence of post-sleeve reflux.
  - Pearl—If the esophagus was extensively mobilized for a hiatal hernia repair, we perform a posterior esophagopexy to the median arcuate ligament with a 2-0 silk suture to reduce the likelihood of re-herniation.
- Beginning approximately 5 cm proximal to the pylorus, the greater omentum and gastroepiploic vessels are taken down. These vessels, as well as all of the short gastric vessels, are taken to their full proximal extent.
  - Pearl—The EnSeal has the advantage of not causing bleeding in partially transected vessels as the Harmonic won't do.
  - Pearl—An articulating EnSeal device can significantly aid in following the greater curvature all the way around without changing positions.
  - Pearl—The greater curvature will be removed; therefore it can be closely followed when taking down omentum and vessels in order to avoid injury to the spleen.

Gastrectomy

- A 44-Fr blunt bougie is placed by the anesthesiologist down to the level of the pylorus. A smaller bougie is sometimes used if the stapler will not tightly follow the bougie.

- Due to the thicker gastric muscle at the antrum, the first staple load of the gastrectomy should be a 4.5-mm staple "green load" on an articulating 60-mm gastrointestinal anastomosis (GIA) stapler. Subsequent staple loads should be 3.8-mm "gold loads" then 3.5-mm "blue loads" as the stomach wall becomes somewhat thinner toward the angle of His.
- Retrogastric attachments of the posterior gastric wall to retroperitoneal tissue are bluntly divided along the anticipated path of the stapler, beginning at the greater curvature where gastroepiploic vessels were first taken down and ending at the angle of His.
- The assistant should grasp and laterally retract the posterior wall of the stomach near the greater curvature to ensure no wall of the stomach is folded on itself causing four layers to be included in the staple line. This also prevents the sleeve from twisting as sequential firings take place, resulting in a spiral staple line.
- The stapler is fired at a 30-degree angle to the greater curvature, starting at a point just proximal to where the gastroepiploic vessels were taken down.
- The second firing may need to be at a 45-degree angle to stay parallel to the incisura.
- The remaining stapler firings are adjacent to the bougie with just enough slack given to avoid having the stomach pulled tightly around the bougie and excessive tension on the staple line after firing.
- This is continued until the previously dissected angle of His is crossed.

  – Pitfall—Care is taken to provide clearance from the gastroesophageal junction by angling the final staple load slightly toward the fundus.

- Within a large Endo Catch bag, the amputated greater curvature is then slowly removed from the right upper quadrant port.
- The staple line of the removed portion is inspected for defects. Any areas of concern along the staple line can be imbricated with suture, taking care not to narrow the sleeve excessively. Small bleeding vessels can be controlled with surgical clips.

  – Pitfalls—Bleeding tends to occur where dissection of the gastroepiploics began, and this area should be inspected prior to removal of ports. Sleeve leaks tend to occur proximally, where visualization of the last staple firing is difficult and the esophagus may be crossed.

Postoperative Management

Outcomes

BMI loss after RYGB averages 16.6 kg/m^2 with a preoperative BMI of 49.6 kg/m^2 versus a statistically similar 14.1 kg/m^2 in patients with a preoperative BMI of 48.1 kg/m^2 undergoing sleeve gastrectomy and a statistically lower BMI loss of 11.6 kg/m^2 in patients with a preoperative BMI of 45.8 kg/m^2 undergoing gastric banding [3]. Most weight loss after these operations occurs within 12 months [15]. Mean weight loss of 27 %, and remission of nearly all cases of diabetes, abnormal kidney function, and hypertension, in a mixed procedure prospective cohort, was sustained at 3 years [10]. Other comorbidities, including obstructive sleep apnea, heart failure, polycystic ovarian syndrome, nonalcoholic fatty liver disease, nonalcoholic steatohepatitis, and pseudotumor cerebri have been shown to improve or resolve along with adequate weight loss.

Complications

After RYGB in adolescents, perioperative complications such as anastomotic leakage, bleeding, and conversion to laparotomy occur in 5 % and wound infection in 6 %. Anastomotic leakage and bleeding may present initially only as sustained tachycardia; therefore, the threshold for obtaining an oral and IV contrast-enhanced CT scan in the early postoperative period should be low. Late complications, including obstruction, internal herniation, marginal ulcers, and abdominal wall hernia, occur in 20 % of patients [6]. After sleeve gastrectomy, perioperative complications, including staple line leakage or bleeding, occur in 0.7 %, wound infection occurs in 2 %, and late complications occur in 1 % of patients [7]. Intractable reflux after sleeve gastrectomy may be improved with conversion to gastric bypass. Death in the postoperative period of any weight loss procedure is rarely reported in this population.

Follow-Up Care

Lifelong medical management is imperative. We insist on monthly follow-up visits with the bariatric team in the first year, gradually spacing visits after that to no less than annually in adulthood. Patients that move or go to college should either return to their original program during summer and winter breaks or establish care with a closer bariatric team that includes a surgeon.

Early postoperative diet is a progressive high-protein diet plan that begins with at least 0.5 g/kg of protein broken into 5–6 small meals [5]. Dumping syndrome can occur after RYGB, especially with a high-carbohydrate meal. Most patients reach a weight loss plateau after the first year by which time a sustainable diet plan should be implemented [7].

Routine early blood work includes blood count, chemistry profile, and, if indicated, a nutrition panel. Common nutritional complications include deficiencies in B12, folate, calcium, and thiamine [16]. Menstruating teenagers may require iron supplementation and reliable birth control to prevent a potentially high-risk pregnancy during the dramatic weight loss in the first year. Patients with malabsorptive procedures should be counseled that vitamin supplementation will be especially important should they become pregnant at any future time [17].

Psychological counseling is encouraged to help patients cope with the psychosocial issues and postoperative lifestyle changes, especially in the teenage population. Female patients should be counseled to consider contraception. Weight loss may increase fertility and lead to unexpected pregnancy in the early postoperative period, which may present increased risk to the fetus and mother.

Summary

- Adolescent bariatric surgical patients are a group with significant comorbidities, increased risk of obesity-related disease in adulthood, and increased risk of early death.
- Candidates should be managed in centers with a multidisciplinary team capable of treating adolescents with complications of severe obesity.
- Roux-en-Y gastric bypass and laparoscopic sleeve gastrectomy have been shown to provide excellent short- and mid-term weight loss and amelioration of comorbidities.
- Sleeve gastrectomy has been shown to be safer than bypass although it offers a slightly lesser degree of weight loss.
- Procedures are performed using the same techniques as those used for the adult patient, while pre- and postoperative management and follow-up present unique challenges in adolescents.

References

1. US Department of Health and Human Services. National Institutes of Health. Overweight and obesity statistics. WIN Weight-control information network. 2010. http://win.niddk.nih.gov/statistics/index.htm. Accessed 23 May 2012.
2. Freedman DS, Kahn HS, Mei Z, et al. Relation of body mass index and waist-to-height ratio to cardiovascular disease risk factors in children and adolescents: the Bogalusa Heart Study. Am J Clin Nutr. 2007;86(1):33–40.
3. Singh AS, Mulder C, Twisk JW, van Mechelen W, Chinapaw MJ. Tracking of childhood overweight into adulthood: a systematic review of the literature. Obes Rev. 2008;9(5):474–88.
4. Bibbins-Domingo K, Coxson P, Pletcher MJ, Lightwood J, Goldman L. Adolescent overweight and future adult coronary heart disease. N Engl J Med. 2007;357(23):2371–9.
5. Pories WJ, Mehaffey JH, Staton KM. The surgical treatment of type two diabetes mellitus. Surg Clin North Am. 2011;91(4):821–36. viii.
6. van der Baan-Slootweg O, Benninga MA, Beelen A, et al. Inpatient treatment of children and adolescents with severe obesity in the Netherlands: a randomized clinical trial. JAMA Pediatr. 2014;168(9):807–14.
7. Whitlock EP, O'Connor EA, Williams SB, Beil TL, Lutz KW. Effectiveness of weight management interventions in children: a targeted systematic review for the USPSTF. Pediatrics. 2010;125(2):e396–418.
8. Michalsky M, Reichard K, Inge T, et al. ASMBS pediatric committee best practice guidelines. Surg Obes Relat Dis. 2012;8(1):1–7.
9. Black JA, White B, Viner RM, Simmons RK. Bariatric surgery for obese children and adolescents: a systematic review and meta-analysis. Obes Rev. 2013;14(8):634–44.
10. Inge TH, Courcoulas AP, Jenkins TM, et al. Weight loss and health status 3 years after bariatric surgery in adolescents. N Engl J Med. 2016;374(2):113–23.
11. Inge TH, Zeller MH, Jenkins TM, et al. Perioperative outcomes of adolescents undergoing bariatric surgery: the Teen-Longitudinal Assessment of Bariatric Surgery (Teen-LABS) study. JAMA Pediatr. 2014;168(1):47–53.
12. Kelleher DC, Merrill CT, Cottrell LT, Nadler EP, Burd RS. Recent national trends in the use of adolescent inpatient bariatric surgery: 2000 through 2009. JAMA Pediatr. 2013;167(2):126–32.
13. Varela JE, Hinojosa MW, Nguyen NT. Perioperative outcomes of bariatric surgery in adolescents compared with adults at academic medical centers. Surg Obes Relat Dis. 2007;3(5):537–40. discussion 541–532.
14. Gothberg G, Gronowitz E, Flodmark CE, et al. Laparoscopic Roux-en-Y gastric bypass in adolescents with morbid obesity–surgical aspects and clinical outcome. Semin Pediatr Surg. 2014;23(1):11–6.
15. Mehaffey JH, LaPar DJ, Clement KC, et al. 10-Year outcomes after Roux-en-Y gastric bypass. Ann Surg. 2016;264(1):121–6.
16. Towbin A, Inge TH, Garcia VF, et al. Beriberi after gastric bypass surgery in adolescence. J Pediatr. 2004;145(2):263–7.
17. Bandealy A, Stahl C. Obesity, reproductive health, and bariatric surgery in adolescents and young adults. J Pediatr Adolesc Gynecol. 2012;25(4):277–9.

48. Laparoscopic Management of Pediatric Ovarian Disease

Angela M. Hanna and Jose Alberto Lopez

Introduction

Pediatric ovarian lesions encompass a wide range of clinical pathology including benign cysts, torsion, and benign and malignant tumors (Table 48.1). Management of these lesions has changed over the years. Complete surgical excision remains the standard for most ovarian lesions. Although there may be limitations to minimally invasive management of malignant lesions, it can also have an adjunct role to open procedures such as the ability to assess tumors and examine the peritoneal surface for disease spread [1]. Our ability to treat these lesions in a less invasive manner has grown with advancements in radiographic imaging, the ability to detect biochemical markers, and improved surgical techniques.

Preoperative Evaluation

Physical Exam

Ovarian cysts have a variety of presentations and symptoms. During the neonatal period, they are usually identified prenatally on US as a cystic mass or postnatally with abdominal fullness and presence of a mass. Older patients usually present with abdominal pain and/or fullness that is either acute or chronic. Sometimes the cysts are found on routine physical examination as a mass in the lower abdomen. Torsion usually presents as sudden onset of acute, sharp, or colicky lower abdominal pain (usually the right side) lasting less than 48 h. Nausea and vomiting are usually associated with the pain [2].

D.S. Walsh et al. (eds.), *The SAGES Manual of Pediatric Minimally Invasive Surgery*, DOI 10.1007/978-3-319-43642-5_48

Table 48.1 The different types of ovarian lesions that can be seen

Malignant	Benign
Surface epithelial-stromal tumors	*Follicular cysts*
Mucinous cystadenocarcinoma	Corpus luteum cysts
Serous cystadenocarcinoma	Paraovarian cysts
Adenofibroma	Serous cystadenoma
Adenocarcinoma	Endometriosis
Sex cord-stromal tumors	Gonadoblastomas[a]
Granulosa cell tumors	Torsion[b]
Theca cell tumors	
Fibromas	
Sclerosing stromal tumors	
Sertoli-Leydig cell tumors	
Sex cord tumors with annular tubules	
Steroid cell tumors	
Germ cell tumors	
Dysgerminoma	
Endodermal sinus tumors	
Embryonal carcinomas	
Choriocarcinomas	
Teratomas	
Mixed germ cell tumors	

The italic font describes the class of tumors
[a]Gonadoblastomas can be made up of a mixture of germ cell and sex cord-stromal elements. They can also be malignant
[b]Torsion is not an actual mass of the ovary, but listed as it can present as a mass and is discussed in this chapter

Malignant neoplasms can present with symptoms similar to cysts and torsion. Abdominal enlargement can occur from the mass, ascites, or a combination of both. Pain may be present. If the neoplasm produces hCG, there may be a history of abnormal vaginal bleeding or precocious puberty [3]. Likewise, pregnancy symptoms may present if hCG is produced. A functional lesion may present similar to other ovarian pathology. Acute or chronic pain is usually present, however some present with painless abdominal enlargement. Precocious puberty or virilization (increased muscle strength, acne, hirsutism, frontal hair thinning, deepening of the voice) may occur if androgen production is high [4].

Labs

For benign lesions, laboratory markers can vary and do not directly help in diagnosis. For torsion, the patient may have leukocytosis, elevated lactate, or electrolyte imbalances. Any lesion suspicious for malignancy

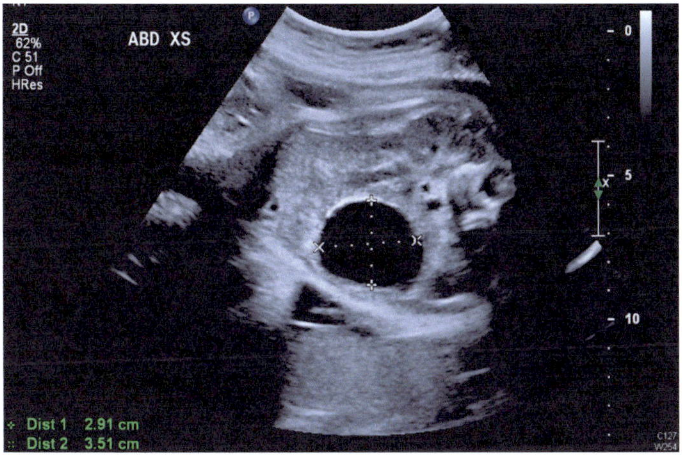

Fig. 48.1. Ultrasound showing a benign simple, right ovarian cyst. Notice the homogeneity and anechoic nature of the cyst. (Courtesy of Robert Weinsheimer, MD, Swedish Medical Center, Seattle, WA).

should have tumor markers evaluated including alpha-fetoprotein, LDH, CA-125, hCG, CEA, LH, FSH, and estrogen levels [5, 6].

Imaging

Ovarian cysts can be diagnosed by ultrasound examination, even in the prenatal population [7]. Although used regularly, ultrasound has some limiting factors: it is operator dependent and can be influenced by patient weight and age (Fig. 48.1). Transvaginal ultrasound is preferred in older patients as it can better visualize adnexal lesions.

If there should be a concern for malignancy or for larger lesions, then evaluation with cross-sectional imaging such as CT or MRI is indicated (Fig. 48.2).

Surgical Indications and Controversies

Ovarian Cyst

For simple, small ovarian cysts, most favor close monitoring. Cysts diagnosed in utero are monitored with serial ultrasounds. These cysts typically regress spontaneously and do not require any intervention. If leading

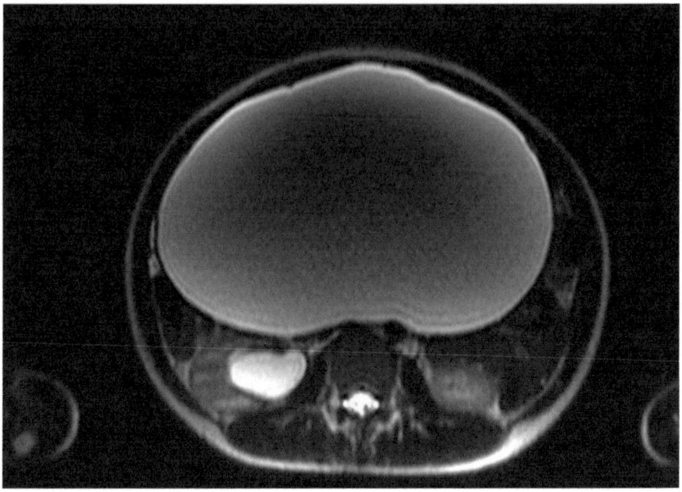

Fig. 48.2. MRI showing a large ovarian benign, simple cyst. Notice the lack of septations and areas of heterogeneity. (Courtesy of Robert Weinsheimer, MD, Swedish Medical Center, Seattle, WA).

to other complications during pregnancy, in utero aspiration is an option but comes with some risk. Postnatally, lesions are followed closely with serial imaging until the cyst has fully resolved or requires intervention. If the cyst grows, is complex, or does not regress, then intervention is warranted. Aspiration of simple cysts greater than 4 or 5 cm is possible; otherwise surgical excision is preferred. Larger cysts are prone to, or may have already undergone, torsion [8].

For simple cysts outside of neonatal populations, usually no intervention is necessary. If they are large or growing, simple aspiration can be performed. If the cysts are >5 cm, complex, or leading to symptoms, then surgical excision is warranted (Fig. 48.3). In every case where malignancy is not suspected or involved, ovarian-sparing excision should be considered.

Ovarian cysts greater than 10 cm, as with large teratomas, can also be challenging to remove. Spillage, domain, and removal of the cyst from the peritoneal cavity are some of the main concerns when developing an operative plan. If imaging shows no concern for malignancy, then laparoscopic techniques can be used [9].

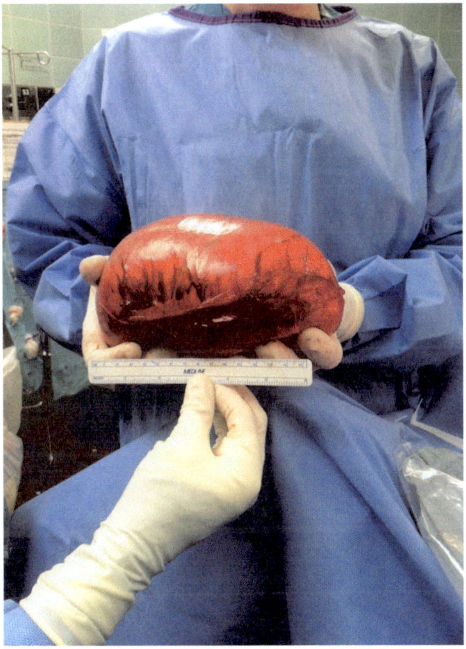

Fig. 48.3. Gross specimen of large ovarian cyst. Note that even benign lesions can grow quite large. (Courtesy of Ian Mitchell, MD, San Antonio, TX).

Ovarian Torsion

Ovarian torsion is considered a surgical emergency in effort to save the ovary. There is an increasing favor to detorse and leave the ovary with postoperative surveillance ultrasounds at designated intervals. This is a departure from the historical management, which consisted of oophorectomy with or without salpingectomy. Commonly a mass or cyst is associated with the torsion, and it can be difficult to interpret where the mass ends and the ovary begins (Fig. 48.4). As a result, it can be difficult to separate the ovary from the mass, and trying to dissect the two free could cause damage to the ovary. In addition, many cysts associated with torsion are functional cysts and can be treated without resection, as they will resolve on their own [10]. An ovary that does not appear viable after detorsion, if left to remain, can be viable in future US surveillance. At follow-up US, if there is a persistent mass, then removal may be warranted and is still a consideration [11].

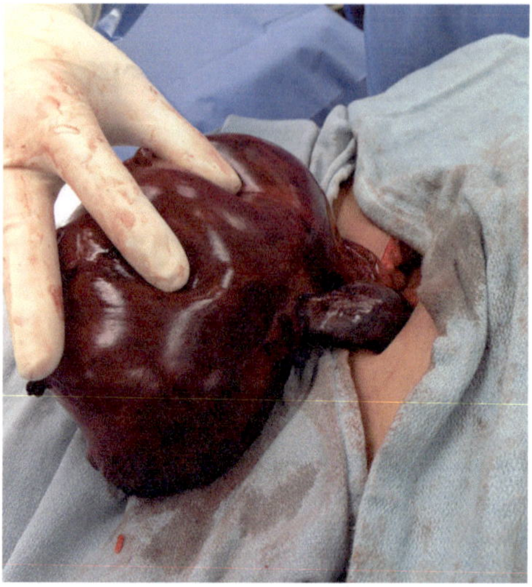

Fig. 48.4. Intraoperative findings of a torsed right ovary and associated large cystic lesion originating from right fallopian tube. (Courtesy of Robert Weinsheimer, MD, Swedish Medical Center, Seattle, WA).

There is no good prospective data to support the use of ovariopexy and its practice appears to be surgeon dependent [12]. Some specific situations may warrant ovariopexy, such as patients undergoing pelvic radiation for a malignancy, bilateral torsion, or recurrent ipsilateral torsion may benefit from a pexy procedure. In addition, pexy may be beneficial if torsion occurs on an ovary with a malformed or excessively long utero-ovarian ligament or in a patient with a single ovary. Clipping the utero-ovarian ligament or infundibulopelvic ligament to the pelvic sidewall or posterior uterus may also serve the same purpose as a pexy.

Teratoma/Malignancy

For malignant lesions, surgical excision is the preferred treatment. This is both diagnostic and therapeutic. In most cases, the extent of the operation depends on intraoperative findings.

Historically, large ovarian tumors over 10 cm in diameter have been removed by laparotomy due to concern for malignancy and risk of spread via rupture or peritoneal seeding. There are arguments that laparoscopy has no role in any lesion over 15 cm, but despite this, laparoscopy is being used more often to approach these lesions [13]. Imaging and tumor markers will aid in determining if the tumor is an appropriate candidate for laparoscopic resection. The goal remains to remove the lesion en bloc without spillage which can upstage the tumor. Spillage rates for ovarian cystectomies can reach upward of 25% during laparoscopy for experienced surgeons [14]. As a result, techniques have been developed to minimize this risk.

Operative Considerations

Anesthesia

It is important to have an anesthesia team familiar with minimally invasive surgery in the pediatric population. General anesthesia should be used in all laparoscopic cases. Prophylactic antibiotics such as cefazolin (first-generation cephalosporin) or some similar antibiotic should be given.

Room Setup

Viewing towers should be optimally arranged to allow the surgeon and assistant to comfortably perform the operation. A screen is placed at the patient's feet. The surgeon will be on the patient's left side facing the feet and assistant will be on the opposite side holding the camera. The scrub nurse will be next to the surgeon. The anesthesiologist is at the head of the bed.

Positioning

The patient is in supine position, with padding on bony prominences. The patient is placed as far down the bed as possible, so the distal part of the surgical bed does not get in the way of towers or viewing monitors. The arms are tucked on both sides to allow for more operating freedom. A Foley catheter is placed to keep the bladder from interfering in the operative field. Trendelenburg position will help with visualization of the pelvic organs.

Laparoscopic Settings

The insufflation setting is based on the patient's age and surgeon's preference. An intraperitoneal pressure of 15 mmHg is usually tolerated by most healthy pediatric patients who weigh more than 5 kg. Intraperitoneal pressures of more than 20 mmHg can lead to decreased venous return and ventilator issues. If the patient is less than 5 kg, an intraperitoneal pressure of 8–12 mmHg is used.

Instrumentation

Standard laparoscopic instruments of appropriate size, either 3- or 5-mm, are sufficient for laparoscopic ovarian procedures. Devices such as monopolar cautery hook or scissors, a sealing device, or ultrasonic energy device can be chosen based on surgeon preference. A 3-mm or 5-mm 30-degree scope is optimal for visualization. Use of blunt graspers will avoid injury to the ovary or surrounding structures. In neonates and smaller patients, 3-mm trocars, instruments, and camera may be used. There is a 3-mm sealing device that is available that is helpful in the neonatal population. If a stapling device will be used, it is possible to use a 5-mm stapler, but otherwise consider which 5-mm port may be upsized to a 12-mm port to allow this if necessary. There are both 5-mm and 10-mm endoscopic specimen bags which can be used.

Trocar Site Placement

The types of trocars used are based on surgeon preference. There are 3- or 5-mm trocars available. The abdominal wall in this population is thin and much more compliant than adults and is an important consideration when placing trocars. Local anesthetic should be used at all trocar sites. A cutdown technique can be used to place the initial trocar in the umbilicus, or a Veress needle with dilatable expandable trocars can be used safely. Once the peritoneal cavity is accessed, additional trocars can be placed under direct vision in a triangulated position to optimize working conditions. The location of the lesion will dictate where the trocars are placed, and with pelvic neoplasms, the trocars sites will usually be mid abdomen or cephalad to the umbilicus.

Surgical Procedure and Technique

Ovarian Cyst

After induction of general anesthesia, an umbilical trocar is placed. A 5-mm camera is placed into the abdomen and additional 3- or 5-mm working ports are placed under direct vision in the RLQ and LLQ. Next, Trendelenburg position aids in visualization and domain with moving bowel out of the pelvis. A four-quadrant exploration should be undertaken to examine and identify any pathology outside of the pelvis. If ascites is present and malignancy is suspected, then a sample should be sent for cytology.

In order to avoid injury to pelvic organs, blunt retraction with a closed grasper is favored over grasping tissue. Suction of the fimbria should be avoided, as this tissue can bleed with excessive suction. Both sides of the pelvis should be examined. Blunt retraction of the uterus toward the anterior abdominal wall will help with visualization of the fallopian tubes and ovaries. In smaller patients, this can be accomplished by passing a suture transabdominally into the uterus and back out to the abdominal wall externally before tightening. This can lift the uterus out of the operating domain.

The lesion must be thoroughly examined and its borders identified. If it is a simple cyst conducive to aspiration, this can be done under direct vision with an aspiration needle. Once decompressed, the opening created from aspiration can be cauterized to obtain hemostasis. To prevent recurrence, marsupialization of the cyst wall can be done. A portion of the cyst wall can be excised with scissors, cautery, or bipolar sealer and the specimen sent to pathology. Any surface of the cyst that remains on the ovary should be cauterized well, as the edges tend to bleed.

If performing a cystectomy, the stripping enucleation technique can be employed to spare the ovary. Aspiration can be done first to help with visualization. The plane between the cyst wall and ovary is identified, and the cyst wall is carefully stripped away [15]. Electrocautery or bipolar sealer can be used for hemostasis as the cyst wall can be oozy. Once the specimen is resected, it can be removed through a trocar or placed into an endobag and removed via trocar or the umbilical incision [16].

If the cyst cannot be separated from the ovary or adjacent tissue, then an oophorectomy or salpingo-oophorectomy may need to be performed. This procedure is discussed later in this chapter.

Ovarian Torsion

Port placement and patient positioning are the same as described above for ovarian cyst. The same tenets apply manipulation of uterus and adnexal structures. The lesion must be thoroughly examined and its borders identified. Blunt retractors are used to detorse the ovary and ensure the vascular pedicle is no longer twisted. Ovarian preservation is preferred, so leaving an ovary that appears necrotic or may have an associated mass is acceptable at the time of detorsion (Fig. 48.5).

If there is a cystic component to be aspirated, an aspiration needle can be passed either transabdominally or through a port. The fluid should be sent for cytology.

If a pexy is to be performed, an absorbable suture or clip is used to pexy the utero-ovarian ligament to the pelvic sidewall or posterior uterus.

Ovarian Teratoma/Tumor

The initial approach for ovarian teratoma or solid tumor is the same as described above. The lesion should be evaluated intraoperatively to determine if ovarian-sparing resection is indicated and possible. If the

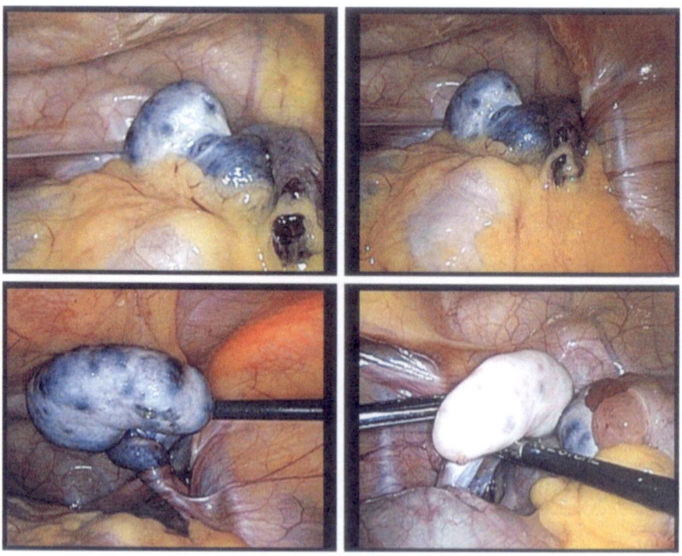

Fig. 48.5. Intraoperative findings of right ovarian torsion and normal left ovary. (Courtesy of Ian Mitchell, MD, San Antonio, TX).

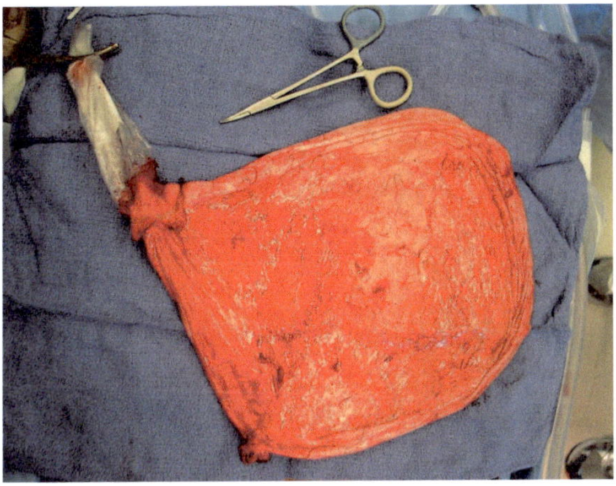

Fig. 48.6. Specimen of large serous cystadenoma. Also seen is the sterile bag technique where the bag is used to minimize spillage from aspiration. (Courtesy of Ian Mitchell, MD, San Antonio, TX).

lesion appears to be benign and ovarian-sparing resection is considered, the lesion should be carefully dissected free from the ovarian tissue [17]. If it appears to invade surrounding tissue and/or is consistent with malignancy, the lesion should be resected en bloc.

If there is a cystic component to a benign-appearing lesion, this can be decompressed prior to removal to minimize risk of rupture and allow for easier removal [18]. The controversy is if the lesion ends up having a malignancy on pathology. To minimize potential risk of spread, a trocar site can be enlarged and the lesion is brought to the incision. A sterile plastic bag is glued (using ethyl-2-cyanoacrylate adhesive) to the surface of the lesion to cover the exposed portion and incision (Fig. 48.6). The wall of the lesion is then accessed with an aspiration needle through the inside of the bag, thus creating a pocket where any spillage will be collected and not allowed to fall into the peritoneal cavity [19]. The contents are collected with suction and a sample sent for cytology.

To proceed with salpingo-oophorectomy, the round ligament on the affected side is identified and transected. Bipolar sealing device capability is ideal, but this can also be accomplished by ligation with a laparoscopic loop suture or with a laparoscopic stapling device. The posterior leaf of the broad ligament is opened with blunt dissection and cautery, and the infundibulopelvic ligament is identified and transected. It is important to identify the ureter during this step. A blunt grasper is used to make a defect in the broad ligament just inferior to where the ovarian

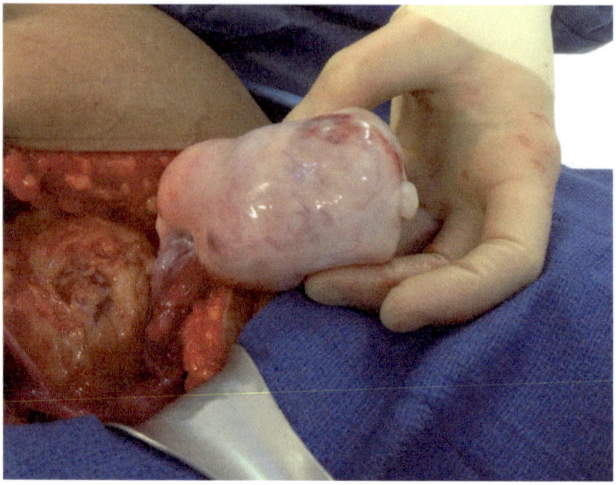

Fig. 48.7. Mature teratoma specimen. (Courtesy of Angela Hanna, MD, Seattle, WA).

ligament attaches to the ovary. This window is used to transect the fallopian tube, mesosalpinx, and ovarian ligament using a laparoscopic loop suture or a stapling device. The broad ligament defect should be closed with absorbable suture.

If there is a distinct capsule that separates the lesion from the fallopian tube, then the fallopian tube may be preserved and transection of the round ligament is usually unnecessary. The ovarian ligament is identified and transected, and the ovary is separated from the surrounding tissue with cautery or bipolar sealing device. Once resected, the specimen should be removed from the peritoneal cavity in a sterile bag, if possible. The bag can be removed through a trocar or through the trocar incision. For larger lesions, an incision may have to be enlarged to facilitate removal (Fig. 48.7).

Closure

Once the procedure is complete, hemostasis should be achieved and the trocars removed under direct vision. All carbon dioxide insufflation should be allowed to escape prior to closing fascial incisions. The fascia should be closed, if feasible, at any port sites that are visible or at least over 10-mm with absorbable suture and the skin approximated with an absorbable suture. Dressing is based on surgeon preference.

Conversion to Open

If at any point it is deemed unsafe to proceed laparoscopically, then conversion to open is necessary. In this instance, it is important to pay close attention to the incision to be made. The specific size of the lesion is important in deciding how large to make the incision to ensure removing the specimen as a whole to minimize the risk of spread throughout the peritoneal cavity.

Postoperative Care

Most postoperative patients will remain inpatient for a day or two. If there was significant pelvic dissection during the procedure, then a Foley catheter can remain in place on the day of operation. It should be removed as early as possible and the patient should void independently before discharge. Postoperative antibiotics are not usually needed. Diet is advanced as tolerated, either on the night of the operation or on postoperative day 1. Pain control is achieved via IV analgesic and converted to oral analgesic once the patient is tolerating a full liquid diet. Activity is not restricted and postoperative ambulation encouraged.

Pearls/Pitfalls

Pearls

- Make sure there is adequate distance between ports. Avoid placing ports too close together or too low.
- It may be necessary to add an extra port for retraction. If so, use the smallest size possible.
- If there appears to be spread of disease, or more disease than originally thought, then tissue or fluid sample should be obtained to restage. Resection at that point may not be indicated.

Pitfalls

- Be sure to avoid adjacent organ injury while using cautery.
- Avoid breaking the capsule of a tumor. Rupture or spillage of a tumor can upstage the patient. If the lesion is too large, consider enlarging the incision or converting to an open approach

Complications

- Bleeding – One may attempt to manage this nonoperatively, but if there is hemodynamic instability, do not hesitate to perform exploration. Type and cross if this is a suspicion.
- Infection/abscess – If small, this may be treated with IV antibiotics. However, percutaneous drainage may be needed if large in size or antibiotics alone are not working.
- Adjacent organ injury – Could present as fevers, hemorrhage, or signs of infection. Keep this possibility in mind when not progressing as usual postoperatively. May need exploration if organ injury is suspected.
- Port-site hernia – Uncommon given small port sizes, but if diagnosed, will need operative repair.

Outcomes

Overall, laparoscopy in the pediatric population has shown favorable results. Despite a small population of patients, Mayer et al. proved laparoscopic excision of pediatric cysts has comparable results to an open approach [9]. They also noted a clear cosmetic advantage using minimally invasive methods compared to open procedures. Michelotti et al. demonstrated a 15-year trend toward minimally invasive procedures for surgical management of ovarian disease in infants, children, and adolescents [20, 21]. Patients who had surgery using minimally invasive techniques had shorter hospital stays, less operative blood loss, and shorter operative times than an open procedure.

Recent publications on management of ovarian torsion suggest ovarian preservation is possible [22–24]. If ovarian detorsion alone is performed, postoperative monitoring with ultrasound is recommended to evaluate the viability of the ovary [25].

Rothenberg et al. demonstrated benefits of minimally invasive surgery in infants less than 5 kg [26]. They performed several common surgical procedures and established that these procedures were safe, effective, and had less operative and hospitalization time than respective open counterparts. MIS for many types of malignancies is being used with greater frequency and has been shown to be safe and effective in the pediatric population [27].

Summary

- There are many types of ovarian lesions, and operative treatment can vary based on pathology.
- The goal of surgery for this population is to adequately resect the lesion in a safe and effective manner.
- Laparoscopic approach to management of pediatric ovarian disease is gaining popularity, with supportive growing evidence of its many benefits.
- Future fertility is an important factor when planning surgical intervention.
- Ovarian-sparing resection is preferred when possible and if pathology allows.
- If the lesion is malignant, salpingo-oophorectomy or oophorectomy is the treatment of choice as the entire lesion needs to be resected in its entirety, but in many cases, this can be accomplished laparoscopically.
- As we incorporate these techniques in modern practices, the techniques will continue to improve and should become the standard of care for the pediatric population.

References

1. Ehrlich PF, Teitelbaum DH, Hirschl RB, Rescorla F. Excision of large cystic ovarian tumors: combining minimal invasive surgery techniques and cancer surgery—the best of both worlds. J Pediatr Surg. 2007;42(5):890–3.
2. Poonai N, Poonai C, Lim R, Lynch T. Pediatric ovarian torsion: case series and review of the literature. Can J Surg. 2013;56(2):103–8.
3. Schultz KA, Sencer SF, Messinger Y, Neglia JP, Steiner ME. Pediatric ovarian tumors: a review of 67 cases. Pediatr Blood Cancer. 2005;44(2):167–73.
4. Spinelli C, Giacomo MD, Cei M, Mucci N. Functional ovarian lesions in children and adolescents: when to remove them. Gynecol Endocrinol. 2009;25(5):294–8.
5. Papic JC, Finnell SM, Slaven JE, Billmire DF, Rescorla FJ, Leys CM. Predictors of ovarian malignancy in children: overcoming clinical barriers of ovarian preservation. J Pediatr Surg. 2014;49(1):144–7.
6. Argawal P, Argawal P, Bagdi R, Balagopal S, Ramasundaram M, Paramaswamy B. Ovarian preservation in children for adenexal pathology, current trends in laparoscopic management and our experience. J Indian Assoc Pediatr Surg. 2014; 19(2):65–9.
7. Bryant AE, Laufer MR. Fetal ovarian cysts: incidence, diagnosis and management. J Reprod Med. 2004;49(5):329–37.

8. Alrabeeah A, Galliani CA, Giacomantonio M, Heifetz SA, Lau H. Neonatal ovarian torsion: report of three cases and review of the literature. Pediatr Pathol. 1988;8(2):143–9.
9. Mayer JP, Bettolli M, Kolberg-Schwerdt A, Lempe M, Schlesinger F, Hayek I, Schaarschmidt K. Laparoscopic approach to ovarian mass in children and adolescents: already a standard in therapy. J Laparoendosc Adv Surg Tech A. 2009;19(1):111–5.
10. Oelsner G, Bider D, Goldenberg M, et al. Long-term follow-up of the twisted ischemic adnexa managed by detorsion. Fertil Steril. 1993;60:976–9.
11. Oltmann SC, Fischer A, Barber R, Huang R, Hicks B, Garcia N. Pediatric ovarian malignancy presenting as ovarian torsion: incidence and relevance. J Pediatr Surg. 2010;45(1):135–9.
12. Spinelli C, Buti I, Pucci V, Liserre J, Nencini L, Alberti E, Alessandra M, Piccolo R, Messineo A. Adnexal torsion in children and adolescents, new trends to conservative surgical approach: our experience and review of literature. Gynecol Endocrinol. 2013;29(1):54–8.
13. Long-Yun Y, Jing-Jing W, Da-Ren L, Guo-Ping D, Li-Ping C. Management of giant ovarian teratoma: a case series and review of the literature. Oncol Lett. 2012;4(4):672–6.
14. Milad M, Olsen E. Factors that increase the risk of leakage during surgical removal of benign cystic teratomas. Hum Reprod. 1999;14(9):2264–7.
15. Canis M, Rabischong B, Houlle C, Botchorishvili R, Jardon K, Safi A, Wattiez A, Mage G, Pouly JL, Bruhat MA. Laparoscopic management of adnexal masses: a gold standard? Curr Opin Obstet Gynecol. 2002;14:423–8.
16. Grabowski A, Korlacki W, Pasierbek M. Laparoscopy in elective and emergency management of ovarian pathology in children and adolescents. Wideochir Inne Tech Maloinwazyjne. 2014;9(2):164–9.
17. Özcan R, Kuruoğlu S, Dervişoğlu S, Eliçevik M, Emir H, Büyükünal C. Ovary-sparing surgery for teratomas in children. Pediatr Surg Int. 2013;29(3):233–7.
18. Salem H, et al. Laparoscopic excision of large ovarian cysts. J Obstet Gynaecol Res. 2002;28(6):290–4.
19. Shozu M, Segawa T, Sumitani H, Inoue M. Leak-proof puncture of ovarian cysts: instant mounting of plastic bag using cyanoacrylate adhesive. Obstet Gynecol. 2001;97(6):1007–10.
20. Michelotti B, Segura BJ, Sau I, Perez-Bertolez S, Prince JM, Kane TD. Surgical management of ovarian disease in infants, children, and adolescents: a 15-year review. J Laparoendosc Adv Surg Tech A. 2010;20(3):261–4.
21. Tseng D, Curran TJ, Silen ML. Minimally invasive management of the prenatally torsed ovarian cyst. J Pediatr Surg. 2002;37:1467–9.
22. Eng-Lunt J. Appelbaum H, Avarello J. Pediatric and adolescent ovarian torsion. ACEP News. 2011; December.
23. Anders J, Powell E. Urgency of evaluation and outcome of acute ovarian torsion in pediatric patients. Arch Pediatr Adolesc Med. 2005;159(6):532–5.
24. Parelkar SV, Mundada D, Sanghvi BV, Joshi PB, Oak SN, Kapadnis SP, Shetty S, Athawale H, Multani P. Should the ovary always be conserved in torsion? A tertiary care institute experience. J Pediatr Surg. 2014;49(3):465–8.

25. Aziz D, Davis V, Allen L, Langer JC. Ovarian torsion in children: is oophorectomy necessary? J Pediatr Surg. 2004;39(5):750–3.
26. Rothenberg SS, Chang JH, Bealer JF. Experience with minimally invasive surgery in infants. Am J Surg. 1998;176:654–8.
27. Spurbeck WW, Davidoff AM, Lobe TE, Rao BN, Schropp KP, Shochat SJ. Minimally invasive surgery in pediatric cancer patients. Ann Surg Oncol. 2004;11(3):340–3.

49. Laparoscopic Management of Testicular Disorders: Cryptorchidism and Varicocele

Armando Rosales, Gavin A. Falk, and Cathy A. Burnweit

Cryptorchidism

Introduction

Cryptorchidism or undescended testes (UDT) is the failure of one or both testes to descend from the pararenal embryological origin to the base of the scrotum. It is one of the most common congenital abnormalities found in newborn males and affects mainly preterm males [1]. It may be located in a non-palpable, intra-abdominal position or may be palpable in an intracanalicular, suprascrotal, or ectopic position. If uncorrected, boys with UDT are at a higher risk of infertility and malignancy [2–5]. It is therefore important to identify these patients early and ensure follow-up so that orchiopexy can be performed in a timely manner if spontaneous descent does not occur.

Epidemiology

The incidence of cryptorchidism is 4–5 % for full-term boys and as high as 30 % in premature boys [1, 6], of which 10 % are bilateral [6]. At 1 year of age, the incidence reduces to as low as 0.8 % [7]. Children with cryptorchidism have a higher risk for malignancy (seminoma) in the ipsilateral testis with a 10–30 fold increased risk [4], as well as increased risk of malignancy in the contralateral testis [8]. This increase in malignancy may be decreased if children undergo an orchiopexy before they reach puberty [9].

D.S. Walsh et al. (eds.), *The SAGES Manual of Pediatric Minimally Invasive Surgery*, DOI 10.1007/978-3-319-43642-5_49

Pathophysiology

It is unclear if cryptorchidism is secondary to an innate testicular defect or if there is direct impairment of the descent mechanism. Genetic and environmental factors have been reported for both congenital and acquired nonsyndromic cryptorchidism. Barthold et al. [10] reported that reduced breastfeeding and increase in soy formula feeding are potential risk factors for acquired cryptorchidism, as hormonally active components of breast milk and soy formula could influence the establishment of normal testis position in the first months of life, leading to apparent ascent of testes in childhood.

Male Sexual Development

The development and descent of testes are dependent on the interaction of multiple chemical and mechanical factors. In humans, gonadal differentiation begins during 6th week of gestation when bipotential gonadal tissue starts undergoing feminization or masculinization. In males, the SRY gene on the Y chromosome produces testes differentiating factor (TDF) that induces the bipotential gonadal tissue to become testes. Sertoli cells in the testes secrete anti-Mullerian hormone that leads to involution of the paramesonephric (Mullerian) duct, which would otherwise result in female internal reproductive structures. Leydig cells in the testes produce testosterone that stimulates the mesonephric (Wolffian) duct to become male internal genitalia. Testosterone is converted to dihydrotestosterone (DHT) that leads to development of external male genitalia.

Testicular descent is required to lower the temperature of the testes by 2–3 °C below body temperature in order for spermatogenesis to occur. Testicular descent is subdivided into the transabdominal migration of testes and the transinguinal descent into scrotum.

Definitions and Classification

A testis is defined as *undescended* if the distance between the top of the pubic crest and the middle of the testes is less than 4 cm in mature boys or less than 2.5 cm in premature boys [7]. They may remain in the abdominal cavity or they may be palpable in the inguinal canal (intracanalicular) or just outside the external ring (suprascrotal) [11]. Testes which in early childhood are located in a scrotal position but then ascend are called *acquired undescended testes* [12–14]. A *retractile testis* represents a normal variant of testicular position; it is not found in the lower part of the scrotum, as the testes is pulled cephalad by the cremasteric muscle, but can be manipulated without pain into the scrotum and remains in place after release [15]. An *absent testis* may be due to agenesis or atrophy secondary to intrauterine vascular compromise, also known as the "vanishing testis syndrome" or testicular regression syndrome [16].

Diagnosis

The diagnosis is mainly by physical exam. In the case of an impalpable testis, it is important to examine the perineum, the base of the penis, and the high thigh, all rare but described positions of ectopic gonads. Imaging, such as ultrasound (US), can aid in the localization, though imaging studies have yield low sensitivity and specificity.

Medical Management

Spontaneous testicular descent usually is completed by 6 months of age [17], and by 1 year of age, the incidence decreases to 0.8 %, possibly secondary to decreasing testosterone levels starting 3–4 months postnatally [7]. Therefore, it is acceptable to observe patients, particularly preterm patients, for up to 6 months of age.

Surgical Management

History

The main challenge of surgical repair is tension-free placement of the testes in the scrotum while avoiding damage to the testicular vessels and atrophy of the testicle. In 1959, Fowler and Stephens described a technique for high UDTs; this technique divides the foreshortened testicular artery, allowing the mobilization of the testis to the scrotum [18]. This was later modified in 1984 by Ransley et al. who described a two-stage technique. First, a preliminary vessel ligation is performed, allowing development of collateral vessels; 6–8 weeks later, the testis is placed in the scrotum [19].

Diagnostic laparoscopy for UDT was first introduced by Cortesi in 1976 and is currently the gold standard for the diagnosis of a non-palpable testis [20]. The laparoscopic approach for cryptorchidism was first described in 1994 [21] and has replaced the combined inguinal/retroperitoneal open approach.

Examination

A UDT may be situated along its normal route of descent or in an ectopic position. Therefore, the role of the physician is to differentiate between palpable or non-palpable and uni- or bilaterally UDT, which will help determine the treatment algorithm [22]. Assessment of UDT may be difficult in an awake and uncooperative child or in an obese child with a large suprapubic fat pad. Also, distinguishing between a testis and thickened gubernaculum can be challenging, perhaps requiring additional examination in a follow-up visit. The baby is positioned supine in a relaxed environment, and each side is assessed with the index finger sliding from above the inguinal area to block off the external ring. If the testis is identified, it should be grasped by the opposite hand and pulled gently down to the scrotum. Once in the scrotum, it is released. If the gonad stays in the scrotum, the diagnosis of retractile testicle is made, and no surgical procedure is warranted. Should there be any question regarding retractile versus cryptorchid testis, a reevaluation can be scheduled. A non-palpable testis could represent testicular agenesis/dysgenesis, an intra-abdominal UDT, or atrophy from antecedent torsion, the distinctions between them made at laparoscopy. A helpful clinical finding is that in the presence of testicular atrophy, the contralateral testis is often hypertrophied [23].

Laboratory Tests

Laboratory tests are not routinely performed. In older boys, semen analysis can be performed to establish a baseline and subsequently during follow-up to assess sperm quality and motility after surgery. In cases where there is bilateral non-palpable UDT, a human chorionic gonadotropin (HCG) simulation test is helpful to determine if there is any functioning testicular tissue [1]. On occasion, full descent will be noted after HCG, allowing the clinician to arrive at the diagnosis of retractile testes. While the testicles will recede as the hormonal stimulation dissipates, the condition will correct itself at puberty.

Imaging

Imaging modalities such as US, computed tomography, and magnetic resonance have been used, although these have low sensitivity and specificity in localizing UDT [2, 3]. Even if no intra-abdominal testes are identified with imaging, their presence is not excluded in an intra-abdominal location [2, 3]. Laparoscopic evaluation is still advised, so many clinicians choose to skip imaging altogether in the case of impalpable testicles.

Surgical Indications

Testicles above the scrotum at 6 months of age are unlikely to descend spontaneously, and surgery should be considered [4, 5]. The appropriate age of orchiopexy has decreased with time; initially orchiopexy was delayed until 5 years of age [1], though others recommended it before 2 years of age [6]. Current recommendations deem that orchiopexy should be performed by age 1 year, as dysplastic changes in the gonad begin to show up at that time, although no improvement in testicular function has been reported.

The indications for surgery are non-palpable abdominal testis, high-canalicular testes, bilateral cryptorchidism, abdominal wall defects, polyorchidism, splenogonadal fusion, and transverse testicular ectopia [7, 24]. A laparoscopic approach may be contraindicated in the presence of extensive prior retroperitoneal or abdominal surgery, prior peritonitis, abdominal wall infection, large hernia, cardiopulmonary disease, or coagulopathy [7].

Anatomy

The testis is a paired organ surrounded by the tunica albuginea and subdivided into numerous lobules by fibrous septa. The seminiferous lobules open into the rete testis, where they join the efferent duct and epididymis, which drains to the vas deferens. The vas courses through the inguinal canal; the seminal vesicles join to form the ejaculatory duct, which opens before the prosthetic urethra. Arterial supply is via the spermatic, vas deferential, and external cremasteric arteries. Venous drainage is through pampiniform plexus, which drains into the internal spermatic vein; the right then joins the IVC, and the left drains directly into the renal vein. Testicular lymphatics drain into the retroperitoneal lymph nodes, the right into the interaortocaval area, and the left into the para-aortic area.

Special Considerations

The operative management of a high intra-abdominal testis can be challenging due to the presence of a short spermatic cord that limits testis mobility and precludes a tension-free orchiopexy. The surgeon must be familiar with various techniques to help determine which option is best for each patient.

Laparoscopic Orchiopexy

Preparation

The patient is catheterized to empty the urinary bladder and then prepped from xiphoid to mid thighs.

Positioning

The patient is positioned supine, and the surgeon will stand on the side opposite the patient's undescended testicle, e.g., on the right side of the table for left cryptorchidism. After port placement, the table should be rolled so the side of cryptorchidism is elevated, allowing easier visualization of the retroperitoneum.

Instruments

- 15-Blade scalpel
- 5-mm 30-degree laparoscope
- Three 5-mm ports
- DeBakey forceps
- Maryland and nontraumatic graspers
- 5-mm clip applier

Steps

- After abdominal access is obtained through the umbilicus, a 5-mm port is placed, and pneumoperitoneum established.
- Inspect the abdomen and abort if the vas and vessels are seen leaving the abdomen at the internal ring. A conventional groin exploration is indicated in this eventuality.
- Look for the vas deferens at its origin and follow it toward the testicle.

- Add two 5-mm working ports on the side of the abdomen contralateral to the affected gonad, lateral to the umbilicus on the side of the table where the surgeon is standing.
- Assess, based on the position of the testicle near to or far away from the internal ring, the probability of getting the testicle well placed and tension-free in the scrotum with a single-stage procedure.
- If a two-stage Fowler-Stephens orchiopexy is advisable, perform high endoclipping of the gonadal vessels and terminate the procedure.
- If a one-stage procedure is chosen, carefully place cephalad traction on the testis to confirm that the epididymis and vas deferens do not loop into the inguinal canal, so that these are not injured during the following step.
- Identify and transect the gubernaculum testis to allow complete mobilization.
- Place traction on the peritoneum and divide it medially to the gonadal vessels, over the median umbilical ligament, and then over the bladder.
- Similarly, the peritoneum lateral to the vessels is dissected as high as possible lateral to the psoas edge.
- This should free up the peritoneum over the gonadal vessels; continue dissection to the root of the small bowel mesentery.
- Using a Maryland grasper, push over the pubic bone while inverting the scrotum.
- Identify the external inguinal ring, which is the thinnest area.
- Push the Maryland grasper gently through the anterior abdominal wall.
- Make an incision in the scrotum to create a sub-dartos pouch.
- On the outside of the body, insert a Maryland grasper all the way through a 5-mm trocar, so that the trocar is pushed up against the handle of the instrument.
- Push the Maryland grasper through the scrotal incision into the abdomen through the hole you have made from above and advance the 5-mm trocar through the scrotum into the abdomen.
- Remove the Maryland dissector.
- Introduce a laparoscopic nontraumatic grasper and grasp the testicle, paying attention not to grasp the epididymis or vas deferens and verifying that the vessels are not twisted.
- Pull the testis through the neo-canal into the trocar and withdraw it with the trocar into the scrotum, being careful to gauge the tension on the vascular pedicle.

- Grab the testis using a DeBakey forceps and place anchoring stitches between its capsule and the dartos pouch using 3-0 Prolene.
- Deflate the abdomen and assess the testicle's position.
- If the length is insufficient to pull the testes into the scrotum, consider a Fowler-Stephens orchiopexy; using an endoclip applier, clip and transect the testicular vessels as high as possible, which should give more length, while the gonad draws its blood supply from collaterals derived from the vas.
- Reinsufflate the abdomen and assess for hemostasis.
- Deflate the abdomen, remove trocars, and close port sites and scrotal skin overlying the testicle.

Pearls/Pitfalls

- The peritoneum around the internal ring of the inguinal canal will allow the development of collateral blood supply to the testis [25]. During the second-stage dissection of the medial aspect of the peritoneum at the level of the internal ring, it is important to preserve the cremasteric artery, as this will contribute to the development of testicular blood supply [26]. If ligation of the vessels in the spermatic cord is necessary to gain length, high ligation preserves the collateral vessels between the testicular and deferential arteries [25].
- If the testicle is so high that a Fowler-Stephens procedure seems inevitable, high division of the testicular pedicle before any peritoneal dissection with return to do the orchiopexy in a few months often allows the collaterals the best chance to develop via the artery of the vas and the cremasters.
- If the *vas deferens* ends blindly, with no testicle at its end, the gonad must still be sought by identifying the distal end of the testicular artery, usually very high in the abdomen. This gonad can be simply resected to remove the risk of malignant degeneration in a testicle which will have no spermatogenic function.

Complications

- Testicular atrophy, if it occurs, is usually evident 6 months after the procedure, although it can be delayed until a year postoperatively.
- Recurrent cryptorchidism may be secondary to insufficient mobilization or inadequate testicular fixation [23, 27]; it can be corrected with a second-stage orchiopexy, performed at least 6 months after the initial procedure [7].

- Bladder injury is minimized by routine urinary catheter placement. This complication should be suspected when hematuria is present postoperatively. The injury is identified with cystoscopy and should be managed with laparoscopic repair and catheter drainage [7].
- Vascular injury to the femoral vessels can occur during the passage of the trocar and testicle through the neo-canal. This can be avoided by ensuring adequate dissection between tissues.
- Avulsion of the testicular vessels could potentially occur, mandating that careful attention be given to traction on the vessels as the testicle is pulled into the scrotum.

Postoperative Care

Laparoscopic orchiopexy is performed as an outpatient procedure. Parents are instructed to limit lifting heavy objects and avoid saddle toys for several weeks [7]; the rest of the postoperative care is similar to inguinal hernia repair.

Follow-Up

The initial follow-up is at 1–2 weeks, 6 months, and 12 months postoperatively. At the last visit, atrophy or high-riding testicles should be evident. It is important to be aware and communicate that the UDT is usually smaller than the other testicle and that this size discrepancy will persist into adulthood [8].

Outcomes

For laparoscopic orchiopexy, the reported incidence for testicular atrophy and recurrent cryptorchidism is between 0 and 35 % [3, 23, 27]. A higher incidence of testicular atrophy has been reported with single-step laparoscopic Fowler-Stephens orchiopexy in comparison to the two-step procedure (3–22 % vs. 0–15 %, respectively) [24]. For this reason, as noted above, it is imperative to make an early decision on the likelihood of a successful one-stage procedure based on the intra-abdominal location of the testicle at laparoscopy. After a two-stage Fowler-Stephens orchiopexy, Esposito et al. [8] reported an 83 % success rate at a 10-year follow-up.

Summary

- Laparoscopy is the gold standard for the diagnosis and management of UDT.
- Pediatric surgeons need to determine if treatment should be performed with one- or two-stage Fowler-Stephens orchiopexy at the initial laparoscopic inspection.
- Serious complications, such as vascular or vesicular injury, can be avoided with attention to detail and meticulous dissection.

Varicocele

Introduction

A varicocele is a collection of abnormally dilated tortuous spermatic veins, which is the most common correctable cause of infertility in males [9]. The reported overall incidence is approximately 13.4 % [10]. Multiple surgical procedures such as microsurgical, laparoscopic, and open (Palomo) and endovascular sclerotherapy have been reported. Laparoscopy has gained popularity as the magnification offered allows for a more accurate identification of structures, thereby minimizing recurrence, hydrocele formation, and testicular dystrophy [28].

Kaouk et al. were the first to report their experience of pediatric laparo-endoscopic single-site varicocelectomy. They demonstrated similar recurrence rates and better cosmetic results with decreased postoperative pain and shortened convalescence in comparison to the conventional approach [11, 29]. However, other authors have not shown any difference in results between laparoscopic and open varicocelectomy [12, 13]. A number of authors have investigated the effectiveness of laparoscopic varicocelectomy in adolescents and analyzed the impact of internal spermatic artery preservation versus ligation on surgical outcomes. Artery preservation demonstrated a higher recurrence rate and offered no advantage in testicular catch-up growth rate than those who underwent artery ligation [14, 15].

Epidemiology

The reported incidence of varicocele in children and adolescents is 10–15 % [12]; 37 % of all infertile men and 81 % of men with secondary infertility have varicocele [10]. Overall 4–15 % of adolescents have a grade 2–3 varicocele [16]. There is a much higher incidence on the left side (70–100 %). The right is rarely affected with an incidence of 0–9 % or bilaterally in 0–23 % [22].

Pathophysiology

The dilatation of the pampiniform plexus at the upper pole of the testicle can be associated with dilated intratesticular veins. Dilation of the renal-spermatic or iliac-deferential venous plexus leads to venous insufficiency, which creates backflow toward the testicle [17]. Testicular atrophy has been thought to be due to abnormal testicular development secondary to varicocele, though reports exist of the testicle size catching up if it is left alone [16, 18, 19]. The increase in venous pressure is mainly due to the above anatomical variances, though it can also be secondary to renal vein obstruction by abdominal or retroperitoneal tumors, retroperitoneal fibrosis, or liver cirrhosis secondary to portal hypertension [22].

Diagnosis

The majority of varicoceles are asymptomatic, and most patients present with painless scrotal swelling. A small number complain of pain or discomfort [22], and because of age of the population, infertility is not generally recognized [7].

Classification

Dubin and Amelar [30] classified clinical varicocele as grade I, small size/only palpable during Valsalva maneuver; grade II, medium size/palpable at rest; and grade III, large size/visible at rest. Hirsh et al. [20] classified varicocele according to the degree of reflux identified by color Doppler US: grade I, reflux induced by Valsalva maneuver with pattern 1 (only very little reflux at the beginning of the Valsalva) or pattern 2 (reflux during the full length of the Valsalva); grade II, intermittent spontaneous venous reflux; and grade III, continuous spontaneous venous reflux.

Medical Management

Transvenous varicocele embolization has been described as an effective and safe nonsurgical approach for varicocele. This is accomplished by catherization of the internal spermatic veins followed by occlusion with either a sclerosant-like sodium tetradecyl sulfate or solid embolic devices with either stainless steel or platinum coils [21].

Surgical Management

There is no gold standard approach for the treatment of varicocele, and accepted approaches include laparoscopy, retroperitoneoscopy, and open surgery. Recent reports have shown that laparoscopy varicocelectomy is a safe and effective approach [12, 31]. The conventional laparoscopic approach is through three ports. In 2007, single-incision laparoscopic surgery was introduced [11, 32].

Examination

Physical examination should be performed in both a supine and standing positions. Varicocele has been described as a "bag of worms" during palpation [22]. It is important to assess testicular consistency and testicle size. If needed, either a Prader or disk orchiodometer should be used to compare and properly document sizes, and growth should be followed in 12-month intervals [33].

Laboratory Test

Semen analysis can give an indication of the level of impaired testicular function, though it does not predict infertility [34].

Imaging

US can be of assistance in identifying a varicocele and for the measurement of testicular volumes [22]. The use of color flow Doppler aids in the identification of reflux flow in the pampiniform plexus [35].

Abdominal ultrasonography or computer tomography should be considered in older patients who present with right-sided varicoceles or a varicocele that does not reduce when supine [36].

Surgical Indications

Surgical correction may be offered for persistent or progressive left-sided testicular hypotrophy, abnormal sperm count, sperm dysmotility, grade increase, pain, or patient's choice.

Contraindications

History of extensive retroperitoneal and abdominal surgery, prior peritonitis, abdominal wall infection, the presence of large hernia, cardiopulmonary disease, and coagulopathy may be contraindications. Laparoscopy can be used to performed varicocelectomy, though its use is limited if the patient has undergone prior groin surgery.

Anatomy

The inguinal canal is a short and oblique passage through the lower abdominal wall that runs medially from the internal inguinal ring to the external inguinal ring; the canal is formed by portions of the external oblique, internal oblique, and transversus abdominis tissues. The spermatic cord runs through the inguinal canal and has three layers of fascia (the external spermatic, the cremasteric, and the internal spermatic), three arteries (artery to the vas and the testicular and cremasteric arteries), three veins (the pampiniform plexus, the cremasteric vein, and the vein of the vas), and three nerves (genitofemoral, sympathetic, and the ilioinguinal nerves).

There are significant anatomical differences between the spermatic veins. The right drains into the IVC obliquely, and the left spermatic vein drains into the left renal vein at a right angle. Also, the left spermatic vein inserts higher than that of the right spermatic vein, thereby generating greater pressures, and in the presence of defective valves, resulting more frequently in varicoceles [22].

Laparoscopic Varicocelectomy

Preparation

The patient should void prior to the procedure, or if the bladder is full, a Foley catheter placement is undertaken. The patient should be prepped from xiphoid to upper thighs including the penis and scrotum.

Positioning

The patient is placed supine in a Trendelenburg position, and the table will be rolled affected side up to more easily expose the retroperitoneum. The surgeon will stand on the side opposite the varicocele, hence most often on the right side of the patient.

Instruments

- 15-Blade scalpel
- Three 5-mm laparoscopic ports
- 5-mm clip applier
- Laparoscopic scissors

Steps

- Obtain abdominal access safely through the umbilicus, placing a 5-mm trocar and establishing pneumoperitoneum.
- Place two more ports, one midway between pubis and umbilicus and the second on the affected side at the umbilical level, lateral to the rectus muscle.
- Identify the gonadal vessels and make an incision in the peritoneum lateral to the gonadal vessels.
- Elevate the peritoneum to allow pneumodissection.
- Incise the peritoneum medial to the iliac vessels.
- Identify the largest vessel and isolate it from the adventitia, preserving the lymphatics.
- Once the veins are isolated, clip and transect the vessels.
- Deflate the abdomen and assess for hemostasis.

Pearls/Pitfalls

The magnification provided with the laparoscope helps in identifying the structures, facilitating proper ligation of the veins. Careful inspection before dissection will assist in locating the artery, which often goes into prolonged spasm, making identification difficult once the dissection starts.

Outcomes

Varicocelectomy is clearly associated with a significant improvement in semen parameters, including sperm concentration, total progressive motility, and morphology [9].

Complications

- Hydrocele is the most common complication if the artery and lymphatics are transected, with an incidence of 25–43 % [37]. It usually presents between 6 and 36 months postoperatively. The majority will resolve with conservative management, and only the persistent or bothersome hydroceles require either sclerosis or hydrocelectomy [7].
- Recurrence or persistent varicocele occurs in 4–5 % [12, 13, 38], usually with preservation of the artery and lymphatics, as part of the venous plexus can accidently be missed [7].
- Genitofemoral nerve injury has been reported in 0–4 %, presenting as numbness or paresthesia. This is managed conservatively with resolution of symptoms seen within 6–9 months [7].
- Testicle atrophy usually occurs if the patient has undergone previous inguinal surgery that compromised the testicular blood supply. If the patient has undergone surgery, careful attention needs to be given to preserve the artery [7].

Postoperative Care

Avoid heavy lifting and saddle toys for a few weeks.

Follow-Up

This is similar to orchiopexy; the patient is seen at 1–2 weeks, 6 months, and 12 months. During these appointments, testicular size is monitored with physical exam, and if needed, a scrotal US can be performed.

Outcomes

The rate of persistent or recurrent varicocele for artery-sparing varicocelectomy has been reported between 3.6 and 37.5 % [39]. Similar results have been reported in comparison to the open Palomo technique, where 63–93 % catch-up on their testicular growth [40, 41].

Summary

- Varicocele is usually asymptomatic.
- Indications for surgery are pain, abnormal semen analysis, and left testicular hypotrophy.
- Multiple modalities for varicocelectomy have been described. The surgeon should select the approach in which he/she feels comfortable performing.
- Most common complication is hydrocele.

References

1. MacKinnon AE. The undescended testis. Indian J Pediatr. 2005;72(5):429–32.
2. Desireddi NV, Liu DB, Maizels M, Rigsby C, Casey JT, Cheng EY. Magnetic resonance arteriography/venography is not accurate to structure management of the impalpable testis. J Urol. 2008;180(4 Suppl):1805–8. discussion 1808–9.
3. Samadi AA, Palmer LS, Franco I. Laparoscopic orchiopexy: report of 203 cases with review of diagnosis, operative technique, and lessons learned. J Endourol. 2003;17(6):365–8.
4. Heyns CF. The gubernaculum during testicular descent in the human fetus. J Anat. 1987;153:93–112.
5. Wenzler DL, Bloom DA, Park JM. What is the rate of spontaneous testicular descent in infants with cryptorchidism? J Urol. 2004;171(2 Pt 1):849–51.
6. Castillo-Ortiz J, Muñiz-Colon L, Escudero K, Perez-Brayfield M. Laparoscopy in the surgical management of the non-palpable testis. Front Pediatr. 2014;2:28.

7. Fine RG, Franco I. Laparoscopic orchiopexy and varicocelectomy: is there really an advantage? Urol Clin North Am. 2015;42(1):19–29.
8. Esposito C, Vallone G, Savanelli A, Settimi A. Long-term outcome of laparoscopic Fowler-Stephens orchiopexy in boys with intra-abdominal testis. J Urol. 2009;181(4):1851–6.
9. Baazeem A, Belzile E, Ciampi A, Dohle G, Jarvi K, Salonia A, et al. Varicocele and male factor infertility treatment: a new meta-analysis and review of the role of varicocele repair. Eur Urol. 2011;60(4):796–808.
10. Barthold JS, Hossain J, Olivant-Fisher A, Reilly A, Figueroa TE, Banihani A, Hagerty J, Gonzalez R, Noh PH, Manson JM (2012) Altered infant feeding patterns in boys with acquired nonsyndromic cryptorchidism. Birth Defects Res A Clin Mol Teratol 94:900–907.
11. Kaouk JH, Autorino R, Kim FJ, Han DH, Lee SW, Yinghao S, et al. Laparoendoscopic single-site surgery in urology: worldwide multi-institutional analysis of 1076 cases. Eur Urol. 2011;60(5):998–1005.
12. Borruto FA, Impellizzeri P, Antonuccio P, Finocchiaro A, Scalfari G, Arena F, et al. Laparoscopic vs open varicocelectomy in children and adolescents: review of the recent literature and meta-analysis. J Pediatr Surg. 2010;45(12):2464–9.
13. Barroso U, Andrade DM, Novaes H, Netto JMB, Andrade J. Surgical treatment of varicocele in children with open and laparoscopic Palomo technique: a systematic review of the literature. J Urol. 2009;181(6):2724–8.
14. Fast AM, Deibert CM, Van Batavia JP, Nees SN, Glassberg KI. Adolescent varicocelectomy: does artery sparing influence recurrence rate and/or catch-up growth? Andrology. 2014;2(2):159–64.
15. Kim KS, Lee C, Song SH, Cho SJ, Park S, Moon KH, et al. Impact of internal spermatic artery preservation during laparoscopic varicocelectomy on recurrence and the catch-up growth rate in adolescents. J Pediatr Urol. 2014;10(3):435–40.
16. Niedzielski J, Paduch D, Raczynski P. Assessment of adolescent varicocele. Pediatr Surg Int. 1997;12(5–6):410–3.
17. Dobanovacki D. Varicocele in adolescents. Med Pregl. 2010;63(11–12):741–6.
18. Zampieri N, Cervellione RM. Varicocele in adolescents: a 6-year longitudinal and follow-up observational study. J Urol. 2008;180(4 Suppl):1653–6. discussion 1656.
19. Rais A, Zarka S, Derazne E, Tzur D, Calderon-Margalit R, Davidovitch N, et al. Varicocoele among 1 300 000 Israeli adolescent males: time trends and association with body mass index. Andrology. 2013;1(5):663–9.
20. Hirsh AV, Cameron KM, Tyler JP, Simpson J, Pryor JP. The Doppler assessment of varicoceles and internal spermatic vein reflux in infertile men. Br J Urol. 1980;52(1):50–6.
21. Dewire DM, Thomas AJ, Falk RM, Geisinger MA, Lammert GK. Clinical outcome and cost comparison of percutaneous embolization and surgical ligation of varicocele. J Androl. 1994;15(Suppl):38S–42.
22. Mohammed A, Chinegwundoh F. Testicular varicocele: an overview. Urol Int. 2009;82(4):373–9.
23. Baker LA, Docimo SG, Surer I, Peters C, Cisek L, Diamond DA, et al. A multi-institutional analysis of laparoscopic orchidopexy. BJU Int. 2001;87(6):484–9.

24. Wein AJ, Kavoussi LR, Partin AW, Peters CA. Campbell-Walsh urology. Philadelphia: Elsevier Health Sciences; 2015. p. 1.
25. Koff SA, Sethi PS. Treatment of high undescended testes by low spermatic vessel ligation: an alternative to the Fowler-Stephens technique. J Urol. 1996;156(2 Pt 2): 799–803. discussion 803.
26. Sampaio FJ, Favorito LA, Freitas MA, Damião R, Gouveia E. Arterial supply of the human fetal testis during its migration. J Urol. 1999;161(5):1603–5.
27. Chang B, Palmer LS, Franco I. Laparoscopic orchidopexy: a review of a large clinical series. BJU Int. 2001;87(6):490–3.
28. Kocvara R, Dvorácek J, Sedlácek J, Díte Z, Novák K. Lymphatic sparing laparoscopic varicocelectomy: a microsurgical repair. J Urol. 2005;173(5):1751–4.
29. Kaouk JH, Palmer JS. Single-port laparoscopic surgery: initial experience in children for varicocelectomy. BJU Int. 2008;102(1):97–9.
30. Dubin L, Amelar RD. Varicocele size and results of varicocelectomy in selected subfertile men with varicocele. Fertil Steril. 1970;21(8):606–9.
31. Méndez-Gallart R, Bautista-Casasnovas A, Estevez-Martínez E, Varela-Cives R. Laparoscopic Palomo varicocele surgery: lessons learned after 10 years' follow up of 156 consecutive pediatric patients. J Pediatr Urol. 2009;5(2):126–31.
32. Autorino R, Cadeddu JA, Desai MM, Gettman M, Gill IS, Kavoussi LR, et al. Laparoendoscopic single-site and natural orifice transluminal endoscopic surgery in urology: a critical analysis of the literature. Eur Urol. 2011;59(1):26–45.
33. Cayan S, Akbay E, Bozlu M, Doruk E, Yildiz A, Acar D, et al. Diagnosis of pediatric varicoceles by physical examination and ultrasonography and measurement of the testicular volume: using the prader orchidometer versus ultrasonography. Urol Int. 2002;69(4):293–6.
34. Cayan S, Woodhouse CRJ. The treatment of adolescents presenting with a varicocele. BJU Int. 2007;100(4):744–7.
35. Sakamoto H, Saito K, Shichizyo T, Ishikawa K, Igarashi A, Yoshida H. Color Doppler ultrasonography as a routine clinical examination in male infertility. Int J Urol. 2006;13(8):1073–8.
36. Beddy P, Geoghegan T, Browne RF, Torreggiani WC. Testicular varicoceles. Clin Radiol. 2005;60(12):1248–55.
37. Rizkala E, Fishman A, Gitlin J, Zelkovic P, Franco I. Long term outcomes of lymphatic sparing laparoscopic varicocelectomy. J Pediatr Urol. 2013;9(4):458–63.
38. Cayan S, Shavakhabov S, Kadioğlu A. Treatment of palpable varicocele in infertile men: a meta-analysis to define the best technique. J Androl. 2009;30(1):33–40.
39. Lee SW, Lee JY, Kim KH, Ha U-S. Laparoendoscopic single-site surgery versus conventional laparoscopic varicocele ligation in men with palpable varicocele: a randomized, clinical study. Surg Endosc. 2012;26(4):1056–62.
40. Poon SA, Kozakowski KA, Decastro GJ, Gjertson CK, Glassberg KI. Adolescent varicocelectomy: postoperative catch-up growth is not secondary to lymphatic ligation. J Pediatr Urol. 2009;5(1):37–41.
41. Muensterer OJ. Genitofemoral nerve injury after laparoscopic varicocelectomy in adolescents. J Urol. 2008;180(5):2155–7. discussion 2157–8.

50. Laparoscopic Resection of Renal Masses

Neel Parekh and Curtis J. Clark

Background

Laparoscopy in pediatric urology has been utilized since the 1970s and has evolved at a rapid pace [1]. Historically, Ehlrich, Kyle, and colleagues initially described laparoscopic nephrectomies for infants and children in the early 1990s, specifically in the setting of multicystic dysplastic kidneys (MCDK) [2, 3]. Advances in technology have made this technique more feasible in the pediatric population and a critical component of surgeon education. The surgeon should have a clear understanding of the indications, renal physiology, tools, and techniques before utilizing laparoscopic surgery.

Laparoscopic resection is an attractive alternative to open surgery given the possibility of superior visualization, the ability to perform fine dissection in limited spaces (such as the retroperitoneum), improved cosmesis, limited analgesic use, and reduced postoperative morbidity [4, 5]. Additionally, as surgical experience and training advance, the disadvantages generally attributed to pediatric laparoscopy, including technical difficulty and longer operative time, are gradually being overcome.

Indications

Renal malignancy accounts for 6–7 % of all childhood tumors [6]. Surgeons are encouraged to manage and treat these conditions using a multidisciplinary approach. It is essential to develop an understanding of the pathophysiology and associated conditions of pediatric renal tumors.

Wilms' tumor (also called nephroblastoma) is the most common pediatric renal malignancy, and surgery is a mainstay of its management.

D.S. Walsh et al. (eds.), *The SAGES Manual of Pediatric Minimally Invasive Surgery*, DOI 10.1007/978-3-319-43642-5_50

Table 50.1. Renal lesions of childhood.

Benign	Malignant
Angiomyolipoma	Wilms' tumor (unilateral or bilateral)
Renal pseudotumor	Clear cell tumor
Metanephric adenoma	Renal cell carcinoma
Multicystic nephroma	Mesoblastic nephroma
Reninoma	Rhabdoid tumor
Ossifying renal tumor of infancy	Multilocular cystic nephroma

Surgical principles established by The National Wilms' Tumor Study Group include understanding key aspects of childhood cancer, surgical expertise in removal without rupture of the tumor, and the ability to intraoperatively stage the patient through assessment of the peritoneum and thorough lymph node sampling [7].

Minimally invasive surgery has been used in Wilms' tumor with success [8]. However, the principles noted above must not be compromised, including removal of the specimen intact and without rupture, which necessitates a larger incision for extraction. As such, MIS should only be considered in appropriately selected patients with small tumors and by those with expertise in laparoscopy to ensure complete excision, intact removal, and lymph node sampling equivalent to that with open surgery.

Refer to Table 50.1 for a list of renal lesions encountered in childhood.

Anesthetic Considerations

Laparoscopy is generally well tolerated by children; however, several anatomic and physiologic differences exist in comparison to adults (see Chap. 1).

Neonates and infants exhibit reduced ventricular compliance, possess a short trachea, and incur increased intra-abdominal pressure resulting in a decrease in functional residual capacity. Hypoxia or visceral stimulation can potentially elicit bradycardia as well [9].

Laparoscopic renal surgery in children can be performed by both retroperitoneal and transperitoneal approaches. The retroperitoneal approach may lead to increased CO_2 absorption and elevated pulmonary artery pressure. These effects are primarily seen in children with central nervous system and/or cardiorespiratory dysfunction [9, 10].

Laparoscopic Radical Nephrectomy

Transperitoneal Approach

Patient Positioning

One must take into consideration patient body habitus, size/location of the renal lesion, and exposure needs when deciding on patient positioning (Fig. 50.1). Positioning can vary from supine to partial flank to full flank. Most cases can be completed in the supine position with a bump placed under the side of the lesion.

In order to increase operative space, the bed may be flexed and/or kidney rest elevated to help widen the angle between the lower ribs and pelvic brim. This may be less beneficial in the younger population due to limited body habitus.

Proper padding of boney sites and soft tissues to ensure patient safety is imperative. The patient is strapped with sturdy cloth tape to allow stability and safety with bed movement.

Port Placement

We find the most predictable point of entry into the peritoneal cavity to be through the umbilical region using an open or Veress needle technique (Fig. 50.2). Either a 5-mm or 10-mm laparoscopic trocar is placed with a 0° scope within the port to allow for direct visualization during entry when using the Veress needle.

Insufflation is started at a pressure of 12 mmHg or less dependent on the age and weight of the patient, with incremental flow of 1–3 L/min. If necessary, higher pressure (up to 15 mmHg) can be used for port placement, after which the pressure should be decreased to the lowest pressure that maintains good visualization.

Two accessory ports are then placed under direct observation after anesthetizing the skin. One working port is placed along the ipsilateral rectus border. The third port can be placed in the midline below the xiphoid. When necessary, an additional port to allow for liver or splenic retraction can be placed subxiphoid as well. Alternatively the original subxiphoid port can be used for retraction and an additional port placed inferiorly based on the anatomy.

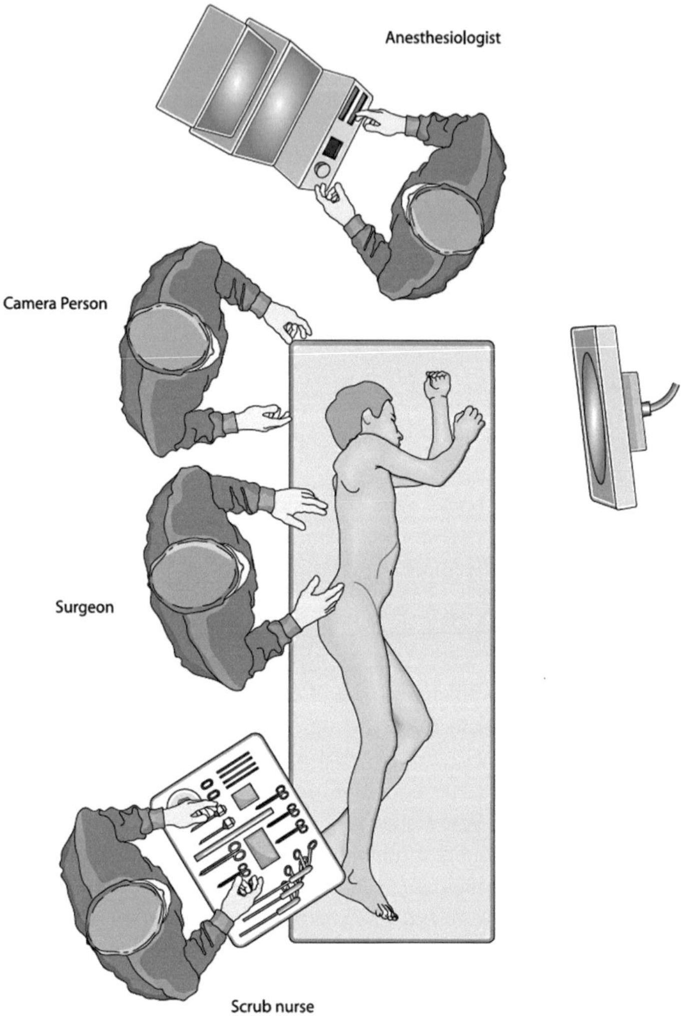

Fig. 50.1. Patient positioning for Laparoscopic Nephrectomy. From Valla JS. Basic Technique: Retroperitoneoscopic Approach in the Lateral Position. In: Endoscopic Surgery in Infants and Children. Bax KMA, et al., eds. 2008:633–638. Reprinted with permission from Springer.

Colon Mobilization

We begin with mobilization of the colon overlying the kidney while maintaining the lateral renal attachments.

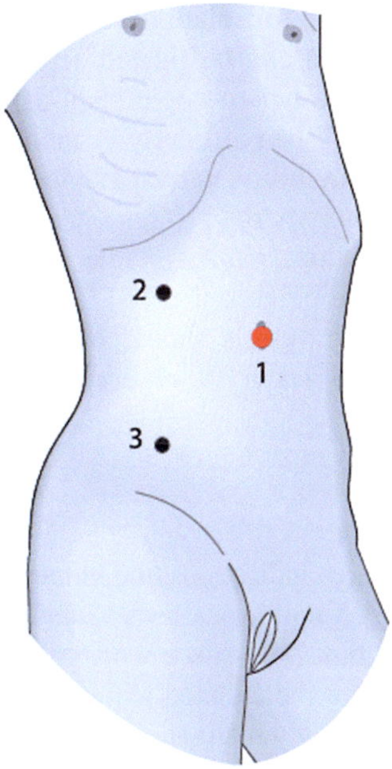

Fig. 50.2. Trocar placement for LN. From Shenoy MU. Total Nephrectomy: Transperitoneal Approach. In: Endoscopic Surgery in Infants and Children. Bax KMA, et al., eds. 2008:639–642. Reprinted with permission from Springer.

The colon is dissected along the white line of Toldt from the splenic flexure on the left or hepatic flexure on the right. Dissection can be performed using harmonic scalpel, cold scissors, or cautery.

Once the ureter is identified as it courses over the psoas muscle, it is followed cephalad to the renal hilum and can be used for retraction. All effort is made to keep Gerota's fascia intact when removing a possible malignant lesion.

Renal Hilum

The ureter and gonadal vein are secured and divided. The hilum should be carefully dissected using gentle technique. Dissection can be performed using a variety of devices. The author's preference is to initially use harmonic scalpel for gross dissection, followed by hook electrocautery for fine dissection using a suction/irrigator with hook attachment. The latter device allows for precise dissection and suction without repeatedly changing instruments.

Efforts should be made to isolate the artery first and vein second. Once isolated, the vessels can be ligated separately with clips. If a 12-mm port is in place, a laparoscopic stapling device with vascular staple load can be used. When difficulty is encountered separating the artery and vein, the entire hilum can be stapled as one, provided adequate visualization. It is important to remember that one can staple or clip across staples, but one cannot staple across previously placed clips.

Secondary renal hilar vessels should be identified and controlled appropriately, with care taken to observe for and control adrenal branches.

Specimen Removal

In the setting of benign indications, the kidney can be extracted from the umbilical region. A 5-mm lens allows visualization through a working port during extraction. The specimen can be divided into smaller pieces laparoscopically or morcellated within a specimen retrieval bag.

If the specimen is possibly malignant or too large for morcellation, a retrieval bag can be deployed and the specimen removed through a Pfannenstiel incision or extension of a port site(s).

Complications

The smaller working space in pediatric patients yields an increased risk of abdominal organ or vascular injury during laparoscopic surgery. Although rare, injury occurring during placement of the initial trocar is a likely cause [11]. Injuries detected intraoperatively should be addressed and repaired. Laparoscopic experience has been found to be the strongest predictor of complication rate during laparoscopic urologic procedures [12].

Retroperitoneal Approach

This approach is preferred by many surgeons due to its convenient access to the renal hilum. The limited retroperitoneal fat in many children can further enhance this advantage. Due to unfamiliar anatomy, fewer landmarks, and limited space, this approach can be technically challenging and is best reserved for experienced laparoscopic surgeons or those who have specific training in its use. Retroperitoneal techniques can be performed in either the lateral or prone position. Both approaches have been reported to have similar outcomes and complication rates [13].

Lateral Approach

We place the patient in the flank position and flex the bed to aid in widening the operative field (Fig. 50.3). The patient is safely secured and pressure points are appropriately padded.

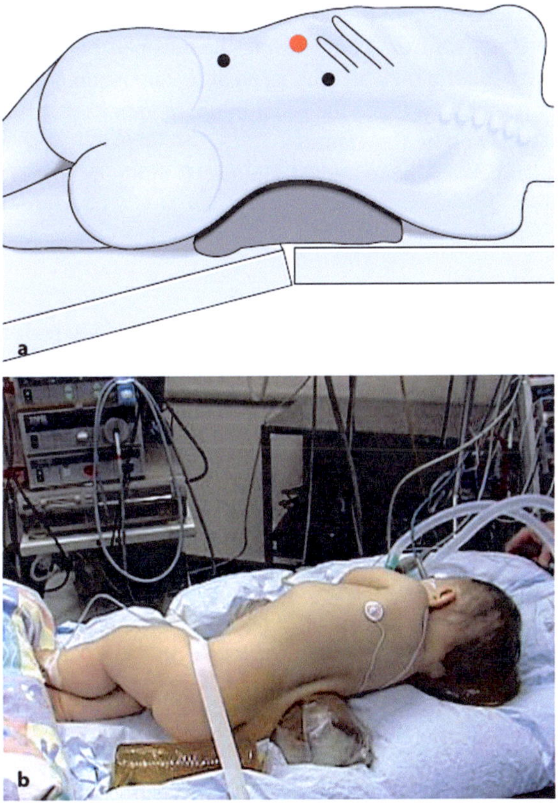

Fig. 50.3. Positioning for lateral retroperitoneal approach. (**a**) Older child, (**b**) baby. From Valla JS. Total Nephrectomy: Lateral Retroperitoneoscopic Approach. In: Endoscopic Surgery in Infants and Children. Bax KMA, et al., eds. 2008:643–649. Reprinted with permission from Springer.

Access is obtained with an incision approximately 1 cm off the tip of the 12th rib. The muscles layers are dissected and peritoneum avoided. The retroperitoneal space can be developed with commercial balloons or using a red rubber catheter and the finger of a glove [14].

Once access to the retroperitoneal space is obtained, a blunt 5-mm or 10-mm trocar is placed to further develop the retroperitoneal space using careful dissection and insufflation. Insufflation should be set to less than 12 mmHg. Two 5-mm trocars are placed under direct visualization anterior to the paraspinous muscles and superior to the anterior superior iliac spine in the anterior axillary line. It is important to avoid transperitoneal port placement. Should peritoneal insufflation occur, a fine angiocatheter can be placed through the abdominal wall as a "vent" to prevent the insufflated abdomen from compressing the retroperitoneum.

The psoas muscle may be used as an anatomic landmark to approach the kidney posteriorly. Once the renal hilum is identified, the artery can be ligated followed by the vein.

The specimen can be extracted via the 10-mm port site as discussed previously.

Prone Approach

The patient must be positioned between chest and hip pads to prevent abdominal compression on the operative table. The initial incision is made at the costovertebral angle, lateral to the paraspinous muscles. Blunt dissection is carried down just lateral to the quadratus lumborum to enter the retroperitoneum. A 10-mm port is placed and pneumoperitoneum further develops the retroperitoneal cavity. Two additional 5-mm ports are placed, one in the posterior midaxillary line approximately 2 cm above the iliac crest and the other at the tip of the 12th rib (Fig. 50.4). The psoas muscle is anteriorly placed in the prone position and therefore is difficult to use as anatomic landmark in the prone position. Similar to the flank technique, dissection and specimen extraction are performed as stated above.

Hand-Assisted Approach

Hand-assisted laparoscopy allows increased tactile sensation, improved depth perception and simple specimen removal and may increase the ease of the operation, particularly for those with less laparoscopic experience.

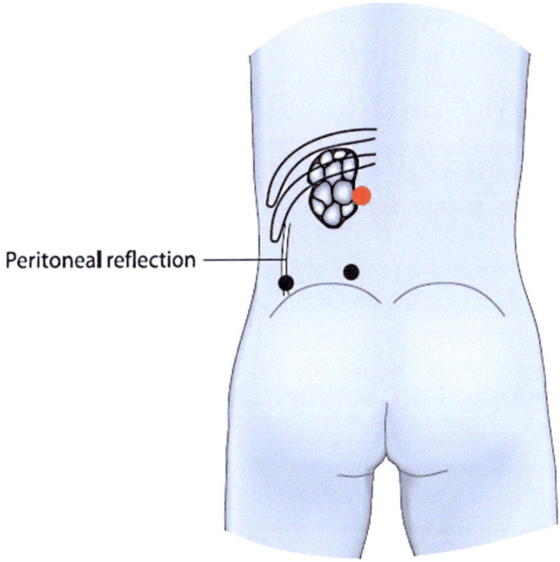

Fig. 50.4. Trocar placement for prone retroperitoneal approach. From Peters CA. Total Nephrectomy: Prone Retroperitoneoscopic Approach. In: Endoscopic Surgery in Infants and Children. Bax KMA, et al., eds. 2008:651–657. Reprinted with permission from Springer.

An incision must be made to accommodate the surgeon's hand. Hand-assisted laparoscopy can be beneficial in cases in which pure laparoscopic resection may prove to be difficult (i.e., prior surgery, infection, etc.). Furthermore, pure laparoscopic surgery may be converted to hand-assisted by extending a trocar site, which can be useful to obtain vascular control or repair an injury in an emergent setting. This technique can be employed for the same indications as transperitoneal or retroperitoneal nephrectomy. Hand assistance is particularly helpful during pediatric living donor nephrectomy where a large incision is required for extraction.

Patient Positioning and Trocar Placement

- Patients are positioned in a similar fashion as for pure laparoscopic nephrectomy.

- The initial incision is for the hand port and will obtain access into the peritoneal cavity
- Pneumoperitoneum is initiated, and subsequent trocar placement is performed under direct visualization using the 30° lens through the hand port.
- Air leak may occur; therefore a variety of devices have been developed to stabilize pneumoperitoneum by providing a seal against the abdominal wall.
- Surgery proceeds as previously described, with the specimen easily removed intact via the hand port.

Laparoscopic Partial Nephrectomy

Background

In the pediatric population, laparoscopic partial nephrectomy (LPN) or heminephrectomy is most commonly utilized to remove a nonfunctioning upper or lower pole resulting from duplication anomalies. Laparoscopic partial nephrectomy in the setting of malignancy is less common; however in select patients, it is an effective approach [14].

When compared to open partial nephrectomy, the laparoscopic technique has been shown to provide a shorter hospital stay, reduced pain medication requirements, and improved cosmesis. However, operating time and costs may be increased [15, 16].

Transperitoneal LPN for Possible Malignant Lesions

This approach allows for a larger working space, and the initial portion is performed similarly to radical nephrectomy, although additional ports may be needed to assist with vascular control or visualization.

Once the colon is mobilized and ureter identified, the hilar vessels are isolated.

At this point intraoperative ultrasonography may be used to confirm the characteristics of the renal mass (location, depth, etc.).

Gerota's fascia is entered and the renal capsule surrounding the tumor is scored with cautery.

Unless the lesion is very exophytic, the renal hilum is then clamped using laparoscopic bulldog clamps. Cold shears are then used to excise the tumor completely. All efforts should be made to minimize warm ischemia time, historically with a goal of less than 30 min.

Hemostasis is critical at this point in the procedure. Options include direct suturing of vessels, hemostatic agents, and bolstering devices. The author's preference is for laparoscopic suturing over a bolster with the addition of hemostatic agent.

In certain situations, the tumor size and location may require entry into the collecting system in order to obtain negative surgical margins. Many surgeons suture the collecting system closed with absorbable suture, although low leak rates have also been seen without formal closure [17]. Many surgeons find that robotic assistance provides a large advantage for intracorporeal suturing. A ureteral stent may be placed based on surgeon preference. A drain should be left near the kidney postoperatively in case of urine leak.

Retroperitoneal LPN

The retroperitoneal approach is technically challenging, but may be an advantage for posteriorly located upper pole tumors. Furthermore, vascular anatomy, prior transperitoneal surgery, and obesity may be additional factors which prompt one to consider a retroperitoneal approach. Most often this approach is used for nonfunctioning renal segments.

The approach for a potentially malignant lesion is similar to the above.

For nonfunctioning segments, the dysplastic kidney can usually be visually identified and excised with cautery, harmonic scalpel, or other devices. Care should be taken to avoid resecting functioning kidney. The base of the resection is often cauterized, and hemostatic agents may be applied if there is concern about the risk of bleeding.

Complications

During any minimally invasive kidney operation, it is essential to identify and be able to manage intraoperative complications. One should never hesitate to add additional ports to aid with suction, hemostasis, or visualization. Further, one should always be prepared to convert to an open procedure if necessary. The following complications can occur:

- Pressure- and nerve-related complications with improper patient positioning.
- Vascular, bowel, or adjacent organ injury.
- Gas embolism.
- Major vascular injury, particularly at the hilum or, retroperitoneal hematoma.
- Ureteral or renal pelvis avulsion may yield ureteral strictures or urinoma.

Summary

- Laparoscopy is a critical component of surgeon education and a key component of the management of pediatric renal masses.
- Maintaining an awareness of the evolving technology and techniques available is fundamental to optimizing patient care.
- The surgeon should have an understanding of the transperitoneal, retroperitoneal, or hand-assisted laparoscopic approaches and consider their role in various clinical scenarios.
- The ability to identify and manage perioperative complications is essential.
- Furthering ones understanding of these conditions and practices will remain a critical part of caring for pediatric patients moving forward.

References

1. Gans SL, Berci G. Advances in endoscopy of infants and children. J Pediatr Surg. 1971;6:199.
2. Ehrlich RM, Gershman A, Mee S, et al. Laparoscopic nephrectomy in a child: expanding horizons for laparoscopy in pediatric urology. J Endourol. 1992;6(6):463–5.
3. Koyle MA, Woo HH, Kavoussi LR. Laparoscopic nephrectomy in the first year of life. J Pediatr Surg. 1993;28(5):693–5.
4. Fahlenkamp D, Rassweiler J, Fornara P, Frede T, Loening SA. Complications of laparoscopic procedures in urology: experience with 2,407 procedures at 4 German centers. J Urol. 1999;162:765.
5. Romao RL, Weber B, Gerstle JT. Comparison between laparoscopic and open radical nephrectomy for the treatment of primary renal tumors in children: single-center experience over a 5-year period. J Pediatr Urol. 2014;10:488–94.
6. Howlader N, Noone AM, Krapcho M, et al., 2013, editors. SEER cancer statistics review, 1975–2010. Bethesda: National Cancer Institute. Available at: http://seer.cancer.gov/csr/1975_2010/. Accessed 3 July 2015.

7. D'Angio GJ, Evans AE, Breslow N, Beckwith B, Bishop H, Feigl P, et al. The treatment of Wilms' tumor: results of the national Wilms' tumor study. Cancer. 1976;38:633e46.
8. Warman S, Godzinski J, Tinteren H, Heij H, et al. Minimally invasive nephrectomy for Wilms tumors in children. J Pediatr Surg. 2014;49:1544–8.
9. Kalfa N, Allal H, Raux O, Lopez M, Forgues D, Guibal MP, Picaud JC, Galifer RB. Tolerance of laparoscopy and thoracoscopy in neonates. Pediatrics. 2005;116(6):e785–91.
10. Bhardwaj N. Retroperitoneal versus transperitoneal approach for nephrectomy in children: anesthetic implications. J Anaesthesiol Clin Pharmacol. 2015;31(1):25–6.
11. Sweeney DD, Smaldone MC, Docimo SG. Minimally invasive surgery for urologic disease in children. Nat Clin Pract Urol. 2007;4:26–38.
12. Peters CA. Laparoscopy in pediatric urology. Curr Opin Urol. 2004;14:67–73.
13. Kim C, McKay K, Docimo SG. Laparoscopic nephrectomy in children: systemic review of transperitoneal and retroperitoneal approaches. Urology. 2009;73:280–4.
14. Cook A, Lorenzo AJ, Salle JL, et al. Pediatric renal cell carcinoma; single institution 25-year case series and initial experience with partial nephrectomy. J Urol. 2006;175(4):1456–60.
15. Piaggio L, Franc-Guimond J, Figueroa TE, et al. Comparison of laparoscopic and open partial nephrectomy for duplication anomalies in children. J Urol. 2006;175(6):2269–73.
16. Robinson BC, Snow BW, Carthwright PC, et al. Comparison of laparoscopic versus open partial nephrectomy in a pediatric series. J Urol. 2003;169:638–40.
17. Bylund JR, Clark CJ, Crispen PL, et al. Hand-assisted laparoscopic partial nephrectomy without formal collecting system closure: perioperative outcomes in 104 consecutive patients. J Endourol. 2011;25(12):1853–7.

51. Minimally Invasive Management of Urinary Reflux

Charlotte Wu and Hans G. Pohl

Introduction

Vesicoureteral reflux (VUR) is the retrograde flow of urine from the bladder to the upper urinary tract through a defective ureterovesical junction (UVJ). Primary reflux is considered to occur as a congenital defect, not associated with any form of bladder pathology resulting in increased intravesical pressure. By contrast, secondary reflux occurs when high bladder pressures, such as in the context of neurological dysfunction or bladder outlet obstruction, overwhelm a normally functioning UVJ. This difference between primary and secondary reflux becomes less distinct when one considers that many children (mostly girls) who are found to have primary VUR in the context of a UTI evaluation also have inherent bladder dysfunction.

Reflux has been described as uncommon among the general pediatric population with an estimated prevalence of less than 1 % [1]. This figure is now thought to be an underestimation. True data on the prevalence of VUR has been difficult to gather as the diagnosis is made almost exclusively in select patients who trigger a workup, such as those with prenatal hydronephrosis, UTI, or family history of VUR. No large population studies have been performed [2]. Also, the natural history of VUR is such that it tends to resolve with time; therefore, prevalence of the condition depends largely on age.

VUR is significantly more common among children presenting with febrile UTI with an incidence in this group estimated at 30–70 %. In one meta-analysis, the prevalence of reflux was estimated to be 30 % for children with UTI and 17 % without infection [3]. Factoring in the epidemiology of UTIs in children, boys and girls tend to present with reflux at different ages. In the neonatal period, UTIs are more common

D.S. Walsh et al. (eds.), *The SAGES Manual of Pediatric Minimally Invasive Surgery*, DOI 10.1007/978-3-319-43642-5_51

in uncircumcised boys, and VUR is more commonly diagnosed in boys in the neonatal age group [4]. In school-age children, the incidence of UTIs and VUR is higher in girls. VUR is 5–6 times more common in girls than boys after 1 year of age. VUR is also tenfold more common in Caucasians than in African Americans, with fair-skinned, red-haired children being most affected [5]. There is a genetic component, though the exact method of inheritance remains unknown. Reports have suggested a predilection for younger siblings to be affected [6].

While reflux is not typically harmful in the absence of bacterial contamination or high bladder pressures, children with reflux and bacteriuria are at a much higher risk for pyelonephritis. It is important to note that in most cases reflux is not a cause of UTI, but rather facilitates bacterial ascent in the urinary tract. Some, however, do regard very high-grade VUR as possibly increasing the risk for UTI based on urinary stasis: the high volume of urine ascending into the upper urinary tract drains back into the bladder as retained residual urine. While this hypothesis seems logical, the degree to which this residual contributes to the risk for UTI is unproven. Repeat episodes of pyelonephritis have been linked to acquired renal scarring, hypertension, renal dysplasia, and progressive renal failure. Reflux nephropathy is the cause of end-stage renal failure in an estimated 3–25 % of children [7]. These all highlight the importance of diagnosis and treatment in the affected pediatric population.

Preoperative Evaluation

History

Children with VUR commonly present with febrile UTI. Parents may report fussiness, lethargy, poor feeding, and fevers. Older children may report dysuria or flank pain. In some instances, there may be episodic unexplained febrile illnesses without a history of documented UTIs. In this patient population, there have been reports of mistakenly treating the child for other conditions such as otitis media, highlighting the importance of urinalysis and culture in the workup for all children with unexplained fever.

As prenatal screening sonography is now routine, hydronephrosis is often detected in utero. About 10–15 % of prenatal hydronephrosis cases are later diagnosed as reflux [8]. If the hydronephrosis is confirmed after birth, it is standard of care to begin suppressive antibiotics until additional workup can be completed.

Urinary reflux often occurs in children with other urologic anomalies, such as in the context of reflux into the lower pole moiety of a duplicated collecting system, ureterocele, or reflux into an ectopic upper pole ureter located at the bladder neck or urethra. Secondary VUR is found in children with a history of posterior urethral valves, bladder exstrophy, prune belly syndrome, or neurogenic bladder [9, 10]. These conditions are associated with bladder dysfunction that may perpetuate primary reflux or cause secondary reflux. Children with behavioral dysfunctional bladder emptying can have similar consequences if the condition is not addressed [11].

Grading

A universal grading system for urinary reflux exists to prognosticate the course of disease at varying degrees of severity. There are five grades of classification, and these depict the appearance of the ureter, renal pelvis, and calyces as seen on voiding cystourethrogram (VCUG). Grade 1, the least severe, is the reflux of urine into a non-dilated ureter. This is followed by grade 2, reflux into the pelvis and calyces without dilatation; grade 3, mild to moderate dilatation of the ureter, renal pelvis, and calyces with minimal blunting of the fornices; and grade 4, moderate ureteral tortuosity and dilatation of the pelvis and calyces. The most severe is grade 5, gross dilatation of the ureter, pelvis, and calyces, loss of papillary impressions, and ureteral tortuosity. Generally, low-grade reflux (grades 1–2) tends to resolve spontaneously with time provided intact function of the lower urinary tract dynamics. Grade 3 reflux resolves in approximately 50 % of cases [12]. High-grade reflux infrequently resolves spontaneously with reported 9–25 % of grade 4–5 cases resolving [13] (Fig. 51.1).

Exam

The child with reflux typically has a normal physical exam. Symptomatic patients have an exam concerning for cystitis or pyelonephritis. This includes lethargy or fussiness, abdominal tenderness, costovertebral angle, or suprapubic tenderness. The urine may be foul-smelling. The child often has a fever or, in rarer instances, high blood pressure if renal damage is present from long-standing disease.

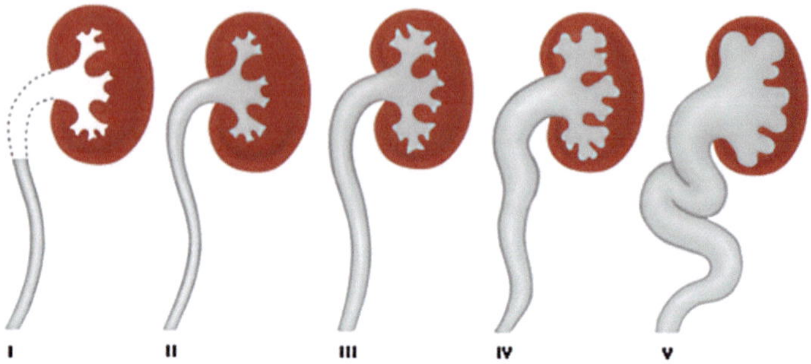

Fig. 51.1. International classification of vesicoureteral reflux (VUR). From Tullus K. Vesicoureteric reflux in children. Lancet. 2015;385(9965):371–9. Reprinted with permission from Elsevier Limited.

Labs

Basic chemistry panel may reveal elevated creatinine or electrolyte abnormalities from chronic renal failure in severe cases. Complete blood count may reveal leukocytosis if an infection is present. Urinalysis demonstrates the presence of leukocytes and/or nitrites with microscopic evaluation revealing urine WBC, RBC, or bacteria. Urine culture should be obtained and may confirm infection.

Imaging

The gold standard diagnostic study for VUR is a voiding cystourethrogram (VCUG). After urethral catheterization, the bladder is passively filled with contrast agent. Fluoroscopy is used to assess for reflux during the filling phase and during the voiding phase when there is active bladder contraction. Several cycles of filling and voiding are sometimes needed to make the diagnosis as VUR may not occur with every void [14]. It is customary to delay obtaining a VCUG until the patient has had at least several days of antibiotics and is no longer febrile, for the simple reason that performing an invasive test on an acutely ill child serves only to further suffering. Typically, the VCUG is performed 1–2 weeks later [15] following recovery from the acute illness. The drawback to this method is that it can miss the diagnosis in individuals with transient VUR that might only manifest during UTI. In these children VUR may not be present in the uninfected bladder, but in the setting of cystitis, inflammation and edema can compromise the borderline valve mechanism at the UVJ. These children may have repeat episodes of pyelonephritis but test negative for reflux on VCUG during uninfected periods. Only then is VCUG during active infection considered.

Radionucleotide cystogram allows for imaging and detection of reflux without the need for urethral catheterization and additionally only requires 1 % the radiation exposure delivered by VCUG [16]. Contrast, usually Technetium Tc99, enters the bladder indirectly by renal excretion and is detected on scintigraphic gamma camera imaging. This study is prone to false-positive results due to contrast not originating from the bladder and misreading of contrast remaining in the ureter or renal pelvis as a sign of reflux. It also is a poor modality for grading the degree of reflux and particularly in diagnosing lower grades of reflux. Given its higher sensitivity as compared with contrast cystography, radionucleotide cystography is most useful to rule out presence of VUR and therefore is most commonly used in children with known history of reflux for follow-up and identification of reflux resolution.

Renal-bladder sonogram is excellent for the initial detection and grading of hydronephrosis. Hydroureteronephrosis in a child with an infection often suggests VUR though is nondiagnostic. Given that ultrasound is a benign testing modality in children, it is the test of choice for initial evaluation of the pediatric patient with symptomatic UTI but should not be considered a proxy for VCUG as it is rarely positive [17]. Renal sonography is also used by some during the follow-up of VUR patients to assess renal growth. In very experienced hands, abnormalities in corticomedullary differentiation and/or renal size are suggestive of renal dysplasia and long-standing reflux.

Nuclear renal scintigraphy is the gold standard for imaging functioning renal parenchyma and renal scar detection. The study is performed by using 99 m Tc-labeled DMSA, which is taken up only by functioning renal cortical tissue (proximal tubules). Renal cortical abnormalities are visualized on DMSA scans as areas of photopenia, and acute pyelonephritis (APN) is distinguished from renal scars based on the persistence of the renal contour or its absence suggesting the loss of cortical volume (scar). Thus, it is useful both in the diagnosis of APN and for long-term assessment of renal cortex health. In fact, DMSA scintigraphy has been found to be more accurate than sonography for the detection of APN [18].

Other Tests

Urodynamic evaluation allows for assessment of bladder functional status, including emptying characteristics. It is particularly valuable for the detection of whether the bladder outlet is functioning properly or whether there is presence of higher resistance during voiding which could lead to abnormally high bladder voiding pressure. These conditions may worsen existing urinary reflux or delay spontaneous resolution.

Surgical Indications

Both medical and surgical managements are geared toward reducing infections and preventing renal cortical scarring. Once reflux is diagnosed, patients are continued on daily low-dose prophylactic antibiotics with regular follow-up and imaging until the reflux resolves or is corrected surgically. Common practice has been to allow all grades of reflux ample time to resolve spontaneously while on suppressive antibiotics, with the understanding that this approach is less successful in high-grade reflux. Some have advocated immediate surgical repair when the likelihood of resolution is slight, such as with bilateral grade IV reflux or unilateral grade V reflux, but this author prefers to observe all children initially. Children with secondary reflux should first be offered a management strategy that includes addressing bladder overactivity with anticholinergics, constipation with laxatives or fiber supplements, and poor emptying with timed voiding or catheterization, as appropriate.

Surgical intervention is typically warranted after medical management has been unsuccessful. In children with recurrent pyelonephritis on antibiotic prophylaxis, including those with breakthrough infections with resistant organisms, medical noncompliance or intolerance, or persistence of reflux with renal scarring, surgical correction is usually advised. Decision to operate will also be dependent in certain circumstances on the sex of the child. As the prime age of post-pyelonephritic renal scarring occurs in children up to age 5, asymptomatic low-grade VUR has less clinical significance in the older child [19]. In boys older than 5 years who have persistent VUR though no prior UTIs on antibiotic prophylaxis, antibiotics may be discontinued, and the child may not need future formal follow-up. In girls, surgical intervention may be recommended to prevent complications associated with APN during future pregnancies, although that recommendation should be tempered by the child's history of UTI and grade of VUR [20, 21]. Ultimately the decision to proceed to surgery and the type of surgical intervention to be undertaken will depend on many factors including the psychosocial needs of the child and family [22].

Technique: Laparoscopic and Robotic Surgery for Vesicoureteral Reflux

Extravesical Ureteral Reimplantation

Special Considerations

Laparoscopic and robotic-assisted laparoscopic surgery has been popularized in recent years with the primary goal of reducing perioperative morbidity associated with surgery while maintaining success rates. Laparoscopic correction of VUR using the Lich-Gregoir extravesical technique, the most commonly performed procedure for laparoscopic correction of reflux, was initially reported in 2000 [23]. With this technique, the bladder is approached from the retroperitoneum, and the distal ureter is dissected from the detrusor, leaving the ureteral orifice intact. Dissection of the detrusor is then carried out cephalad from the ureteral orifice to create a new submucosal tunnel. The ureter is positioned in the new tunnel, and the detrusor is re-approximated over the ureter. The technique has a steep learning curve. Another downside is potentially exposing the child to longer operative times [24, 25].

This same laparoscopic surgery is now done using robotic assistance, called robotic-assisted laparoscopic extravesical ureteral reimplantation (RALUR) using the da Vinci® Surgical System [26]. The robotic surgical system has facilitated performance of laparoscopic surgery and has risen in popularity among pediatric urologists for its ease in dissection and intracorporeal suturing.

Anatomy

The distal ureter passes through a submucosal tunnel in the bladder wall prior to its entry into the bladder lumen at the trigone. With bladder filling, this portion of the ureter stretches, thins, and is compressed against the detrusor back wall, preventing reflux of urine into the upper tracts. Inadequate length of the intramural distal ureter or inadequacy of the detrusor back wall leads to an incompetent valve mechanism. This has been the basis for all surgical interventions performed for surgical correction of VUR. In healthy, non-refluxing ureters, the tunnel length to ureteral diameter is 5:1. For success in definitive reflux correction surgery, the minimum tunnel length to ureteral diameter ratio should be at least 3:1.

Positioning

The patient is placed supine with the lower extremities abducted and frog-legged. Rolls are placed under the bilateral knees to offset the pressure from external rotation of the hips. Older children may be placed in lithotomy. The abdomen, pelvis, and perineum are prepped. Often, a cystoscopy is first performed and bilateral ureteral stents placed. A Foley catheter is left in place. The patient is then repositioned to Trendelenburg for the duration of the surgery.

Instruments

- Laparoscopic [23]:
  - 5-mm trocar
  - 3-mm working port x2
  - 5-mm working port
  - 5- to 3-mm reducer seal
  - 3- or 5-mm 0-degree laparoscope (or 30-degree)
  - 3-mm curved scissors
  - 3-mm tapered curved jaw dissectors x2
  - 5-mm Babcock forceps, ratcheted
  - 3-mm Allis grasper, ratcheted
  - 3- to 5-mm lap needle driver
  - Synthetic absorbable suture on a tapered needle
- Robotic [24]:
  - da Vinci® Surgical System
  - 8.5-mm robotic port
  - 5-mm robotic ports x2
  - Hook electrocautery
  - Maryland grasper
  - Hot scissors

- Needle driver
- 4-0 Prolene® (polypropylene, Ethicon) suture
- PDS® (polydioxanone, Ethicon) suture
- 5-0 Monocryl® (poliglecaprone, Ethicon) suture

Steps

A 5-mm, 0-degree laparoscope is inserted through the umbilicus and pneumoperitoneum is achieved. Traditionally, three working ports have been placed under direct vision along the line of a Pfannenstiel incision at the middle and two ends. The middle port is usually 5-mm and the two end ports 3-mm (Fig. 51.2). The ureter is identified at the pelvic brim and followed down to the distal aspect. The overlying peritoneum is incised. The ureter is identified and grasped with Babcock forceps and freed from the surrounding tissue. Ureteral stents, if placed previously,

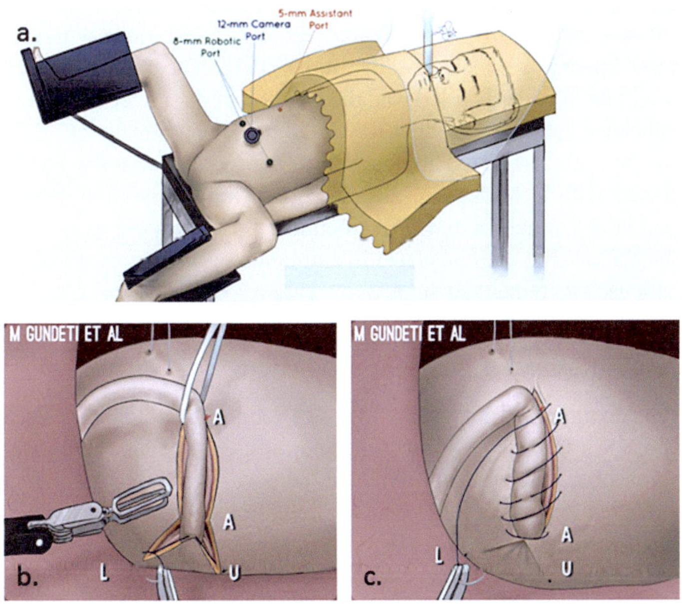

Fig. 51.2. (**a**) Patient positioning for RALUR (not shown is robot docking between the legs). (**b** and **c**) Creation of detrusorrhaphy with closure. From Gundeti MS et al. Robot-assisted laparoscopic extravesical ureteral reimplantation: technique modifications contribute to optimized outcomes. Eur Urol. 2016. Epub ahead of print. Reprinted with permission from Elsevier Limited.

would be removed at this point. A vessel loop or Diamond-Fox retractor can then be passed around the ureter.

Next, the submucosal tunnel is developed. The direction of the tunnel is marked using electrocautery. A traction suture using 4-0 Prolene® is placed at the proximal end of the detrusor tunnel using a straight needle, and the needle is passed back externally through the abdominal wall. This suture can be manipulated externally to achieve the desired tension and elevation of the bladder. The incision of the tunnel is then performed in a proximal to distal manner. This dissection is carried down to but not violating the detrusor mucosa, using scissors rather than cautery to prevent injury to bladder innervation. Detrusor flaps are then created along this plane and elevated for a distance of approximately 4–5 cm. The ureter is placed in the tunnel, and a 5-0 Monocryl® suture is placed at the most proximal end and the detrusor is then closed (detrusorrhaphy) from distal to proximal starting at the ureteral orifice. A recent modification to this technique by Gundeti et al. includes a U-stitch of 5-0 PDS® incorporating the detrusor muscle and ureteral adventitia at the apex of the tunnel, followed by a continuous running suture, incorporating the ureteral adventitia in every other throw [27]. The traction suture is released, the bladder is filled, and the position of the ureter is reassessed. A catheter is left in the bladder for 12–24 h postoperatively.

In the robotic-assisted approach, the endoscope port at the umbilicus is placed with a 30-degree 12-mm scope. The two working ports are placed at the midclavicular line; in children <3 years old, placement is slightly above the umbilicus and in children 3 or older at the level of the umbilicus. The remainder steps in the surgery are the same.

Pearls/Pitfalls

The extravesical approach does not require cystotomy or ureteral anastomosis, thereby eliminating morbidity associated with these. Laparoscopic extravesical reimplant surgery, compared to the open extravesical approach, additionally allows for decreased hospital stay, reduced incisional pain, improved cosmesis, and decreased use of postoperative narcotics. Another benefit of the extravesical approach is that the child's anatomy remains favorable for endoscopic instrumentation later in life should the child need ureteroscopy for stones or other indications.

While many studies have demonstrated feasibility and safety of the laparoscopic approach, the drawback of this approach continues to be long operative times and a steep learning curve [25]. Some challenges worth highlighting are difficulty with exposure of the ureter, trauma to the ureter, and difficulty developing the extravesical tunnel. Laparoscopic ureteral reimplantation, despite high success rates, failed to become widely adopted given the technical challenges [24] and did not show significantly decreased morbidity compared to the open technique [25, 28]. With the addition of the robotic-assisted technology, first described in 2004, there has been improved visualization and suturing techniques over the purely laparoscopic approach.

Another notable pitfall is postoperative urinary retention [24, 29]. In one study, there were no reported cases of postoperative urinary retention in a group of 41 patients, attributed to improved visualization and preservation of the neurovascular bundle lateral to the ureteral hiatus using the robotic-assisted technique [29]. Despite this, other studies have reported difficulty identifying these nerves [24] and that even as the nerves are identified and preserved, the incidence of retention was unchanged [30].

Additional reports both critical and supportive of widespread use of RALUR have acknowledged increased operative times, and subsequently increased cost, versus the open approach. Peters et al. reported that for bilateral ureteral reimplantation, the average time for the open approach was 210 min versus 262 min for RALUR. There has been, however, no finding of significant increased operative times when comparing robotic unilateral reimplantation to robotic bilateral reimplantation.

Postoperative Care (Extravesical)

Most children are kept in the hospital for one night after the surgery. Diet is started right away and advanced as tolerated. Intravenous fluids are kept on until the child demonstrates ability to tolerate oral intake sufficiently. The Foley catheter is removed the day after surgery and the child discharged once voiding spontaneously with a post void residual that is no more than half of the voided volume. The child then follows up in 1 month with an ultrasound.

In experienced hands, the robotic technique has offered similar success rates (reportedly 77–100 %) as the open technique [27]. In one study the success rate of RALUR (as defined by resolution of reflux) was 97.6 % [29], and in one single-surgeon study comparing RALUR to open intravesical ureteral reimplant, the success rate was 97 % versus 100 %, respectively [24]. Two separate reports, one by Schomburg et al. [31] and another by Casale et al. [29], even suggested postoperative VCUG could be avoided given the high success rates in their experience, though other reports by skilled surgeons warned against adopting this approach until a larger series is available to confirm success rates similar to the open technique [24, 25].

As it currently stands, there is insufficient evidence to suggest that RALUR is at a point where it is clearly a superior option to the open technique. Some experts have suggested it may be particularly advantageous in bilateral cases and in cases of older children who would benefit most from the improved pain control [25, 31].

Intravesical Ureteral Reimplantation

Special Considerations

Another minimally invasive technique for VUR correction is endoscopic intravesical (or "transvesical") ureteral reimplantation. The approach was first described in 2005 using standard laparoscopic instruments and combines laparoscopic and endoscopic techniques. A robotic-assisted approach was described the same year by Peters and Woo [32]. This approach is unique in that it does not require transperitoneal access, relying instead on carbon dioxide insufflation of the bladder or pneumovesicum. It has been supported for its potential to reduce postoperative bladder spasms, reduced incisional pain, improved cosmesis, and earlier postoperative catheter removal compared to the standard open ureteral reimplantation technique. The major components of this surgery are dissection of the ureter, creation of the submucosal tunnel, and ureteral neocystostomy similar to open Cohen cross trigonal reimplantation. Robotic assistance has facilitated the delicate dissection and suturing required for this procedure and has improved overall efficiency.

Positioning

The patient is placed supine with the lower extremities abducted and frog-legged or in dorsal lithotomy.

Instruments

- Laparoscopic [33]:
  - 0- or a 30-degree lens cystoscope
  - 4-0 Prolene® suture

- No. 1 monofilament suture (traction suture)
- 5-mm step port x1
- 3- to 5-mm working ports x2
- 5-mm 30-degree lens endoscope
- 4-Fr to 6-Fr catheter
- Hook electrocautery
- Endoscopic scissors
- Endoscopic blunt and fine graspers
- 3-0, 5-0, 6-0 Monocryl® suture
- 5-0 PDS® suture

- Robotic [32]:
  - da Vinci® Surgical System
  - 12-mm 0-degree telescope
  - Hook cautery
  - DeBakey forceps
  - Round-tip scissors
  - Fine-point needle driver
  - 12-mm VersaStep radially expanding cannula
  - 5–10-mm InStep radially expanding sheath
  - 5-mm laparoscopic grasper

Steps

Cystoscopy is first performed and the bladder filled with saline. A traction suture is placed percutaneously to the bladder dome under vision. This serves as an anchor so that the bladder does not pull away when the camera port is placed. A 5-mm port is inserted under cystoscopic guidance, a 5-mm 30-degree lens endoscope is inserted into the port site, and a Foley catheter is placed to decompress the bladder. Carbon dioxide pneumovesicum is established to 10 mmHg pressure, and the Foley catheter is clamped. Two additional 3-mm working ports are placed on either side of the bladder under vesicoscopic guidance.

Next, a 5-Fr feeding tube catheter is inserted into the ureter and secured with a 4-0 Prolene® suture similar to that of the Cohen open procedure. Hook electrocautery is used to incise circumferentially around the ureteral orifice for ureteral mobilization, and 3-mm endoscopic scissors are used to develop the plane of dissection and to mobilize the ureter 2.5–3.0 cm to the extravesical space. The muscular defect in the ureteral hiatus was repaired using 5-0 PDS®.

The submucosal tunnel is then created similar to that in the open Cohen procedure. Hook cautery is used to make an incision at the site of the new ureteral orifice just above the site of the contralateral ureteral orifice across the back wall of the bladder. The submucosal tunnel is developed from the site of the ipsilateral ureteral orifice to the site of the new orifice. The feeding tube is used to pull the ureter through the tunnel. Ureteroneocystostomy was then performed under vesicoscopic guidance with intracorporeal suturing using interrupted 5-0 or 6-0 Monocryl® sutures. Port sites were then closed with 3-0 absorbable sutures. A Foley catheter was left in place for bladder drainage for 24–48 h postoperatively.

Pearls/Pitfalls

This technique essentially allows the open Cohen cross trigonal ureteral reimplantation technique to be performed using minimally invasive techniques. The large open bladder incision and forceful retraction, however, can both be avoided, and this likely has contributed to the significantly lower incidence of postoperative bladder spasms observed with this technique. Superior intravesical vision and excellent ergonomics have also been described owing to the ease of pneumovesicum and drainage of any fluid or blood out of the working space through the gravity-dependent Foley catheter [33, 34].

Despite its advantages, this procedure proves to be extremely challenging technically, even for experienced laparoscopic surgeons. The most difficult steps are dissection of the intramural ureter and intravesical suturing. Fortunately, these challenges have been offset substantially with increased use of robotic-assisted technology.

Finally, a pitfall for both the laparoscopic and robotic-assisted transvesical approaches is the small working space of the bladder, particularly in very young children. In the study by Kutikov et al. of 32 patients, a larger proportion of complications or failures occurred in patients age 2 years or younger with bladder capacity less than 130 ml [34]. For this reason, and with consideration of more recent data, a minimum bladder capacity of 200 ml and a minimum age of 4 years have been recommended [35].

Postoperative Care (Intravesical)

Postoperative course is similar to that for extravesical RALUR except that on postoperative day one, a VCUG is typically performed to rule out a bladder leak. If negative, the Foley catheter can be removed [35]. Recovery is similar to that of other minimally invasive surgery in pediatric urology.

With regard to outcomes and surgical success, Yeung described reflux resolution in 15 of 16 patients [33], and Peters described five in six patients [32]. In a larger series by Jayanthi and Patel of 103 patients, a 94% success rate was described [36], and later Valla and colleagues reported 95% success rate in 72 vesicoscopic reimplants [37]. The patterns seem to indicate that this approach, similar to extravesical RALUR, is associated with a shorter hospital stay and decreased use of postoperative analgesics; however, it may be associated with more bladder leaks and a success rate that approaches, but does not yet equal, that of the open technique.

Technique: Endoscopic Antireflux Surgery

Special Considerations

Despite the near assurance of success for the open gold standard approach, endoscopic antireflux surgery has emerged as a popular alternative given its relative ease and low morbidity. The endoscopic surgery refers to the periureteral injection of a bulking agent, which acts to support the intramural ureter in its antireflux mechanism.

Anatomy

For endoscopic antireflux surgery, the key is familiarity with normal bladder anatomy from a cystoscopic viewpoint. The bilateral ureteral orifices should both be identifiable at the trigone. Additional note should be made for identification of anatomic anomalies such as additional ureteral orifices, ureteroceles, ectopic ureter, and bladder diverticulum, which may hinder the operation.

Positioning

For endoscopic treatment of vesicoureteral reflux, the ureteral orifice is approached from the urethra cystoscopically. The patient is placed in dorsal lithotomy.

Instruments

A standard 0- or 30-degree lens cystoscope and a 3.7-Fr to 5-Fr flexible needle are all that is needed for the endoscopic procedure. In the USA, only Deflux® (dextranomer/hyaluronic acid copolymer, Salix Pharmaceuticals, Inc.) is approved for use as the injectable bulking agent. Other products used around the world include bovine collagen, Macroplastique® (polydimethylsiloxane, Cogentix Medical), and coaptite.

Steps

A cystoscopy is first performed and the bladder should be cleared of any inflammatory changes. The needle is placed through the scope and visualized with the bevel up. The mucosa is then injected 2–3 mm distal to the UVJ, advancing the needle in the submucosal plane for a distance 4–5 mm. An alternative, also widely accepted approach particularly for higher-grade reflux, is to insert the needle directly inside the ureter to increase the length of the intramural portion. Injection should result in the formation of a mound, which may become apparent after injecting 0.1–0.2 ml if the needle is appropriately positioned. The mound should take on a "volcano" appearance, and the ureteral orifice should sit just on top of it [38]. Injection is carried out until the ureteral orifice appears crescent or slit shaped. Injection should occur slowly, and the needle should be kept in position after injection for 1 min to prevent leaking of material from the injection site. The bladder is emptied and lidocaine gel is placed in the urethra. After the procedure, the patient is brought to the recovery room for a brief period and is discharged home the same day.

Pearls/Pitfalls

Historically, a concern for this procedure was particle migration to distant sites, erosion, lack of durability of the injection material, or severe allergic reactions. Deflux®, which has been FDA approved in the USA since 2001 does not migrate, does not cause anaphylaxis, has not been shown to cause obstruction, and is biodegradable [7, 39].

The procedure takes approximately 15 min, including anesthesia time, and requires no skin cuts. Procedure-related complications are extremely rare. There is minimal postoperative pain and there is no associated hospital stay. After one or more injections, endoscopic surgery has the potential to eliminate the need for, and therefore further morbidity of, repeat VCUGs and daily prophylactic antibiotics. In some cases, it can also eliminate the need for ureteral reimplantation. Given its ease and minimal risk of morbidity, endoscopic surgery has been advocated as a first-line therapy following reflux diagnosis by some pediatric urologists [39, 40].

The argument against the widespread use of endoscopic surgery as first line treatment is overtreatment. In light of the natural history of spontaneous resolution, not all cases of reflux are clinically significant to warrant surgical intervention. The indications for correction of reflux should remain unchanged despite the technologic advances available for its correction.

Postoperative Care (Endoscopic Deflux®)

Endoscopic Deflux® injection has been shown to be safe, simple, and effective in the treatment of vesicoureteral reflux. Success rates of endoscopic Deflux® injection are lower than for open surgery, with reported 74 % success rate after one injection and 85 % with one or more injections. The approach is generally more successful in patients with lower-grade reflux. For grade IV reflux, the reported success rate is 63 % after first injection and for grade V, 51 % [41]. Also, lower success rates have been reported for endoscopic correction of VUR in children with bladder and bowel dysfunction [42].

In general, the child is maintained on antibiotics for 3 months. At that time, they follow up with a repeat ultrasound and VCUG. If reflux is persistent, a repeat injection is considered 6 months after the initial injection. Definitive surgery is recommended if there is still no resolution.

Experts have additionally questioned the stability of Deflux® with time, warning of late failure that disproportionately affects those with higher-grade reflux. For this reason, longer follow-ups (>1 year from the time of injection) have been advocated [43], particularly for patients with higher-grade reflux who would be at greater risk of renal damage when endoscopic treatment is not durable [44].

Summary

- The minimally invasive techniques used for correction of VUR are:
  - Laparoscopic or robotic-assisted laparoscopic extravesical ureteral reimplantation

- Laparoscopic or robotic-assisted laparoscopic intravesical ureteral reimplantation
- Endoscopic surgery with Deflux® injection

- Robotic-assisted laparoscopic extravesical ureteral reimplantation (RALUR) is the most commonly performed minimally invasive surgery to permanently correct reflux and, in experienced hands, produces success rates approaching that of the standard open technique. The major drawbacks to this surgery are increased operative time and postoperative urinary retention. Advantages commonly seen are shortened length of hospitalization, improved cosmesis, and decreased postoperative need for analgesics. The procedure has been shown to be safe and efficient though there is insufficient evidence to suggest that RALUR is at a point where it is clearly a superior option to the open technique.
- Laparoscopic or robotic-assisted intravesical ureteral reimplantation uniquely utilizes vesicoscopic technology and pneumovesicum, avoiding the need for transperitoneal access. An advantage of this procedure is that it achieves a Cohen cross trigonal ureteral reimplantation surgery using minimally invasive technique and without the need for a large cystotomy or forceful bladder retraction. It is associated with lower incidence of postoperative bladder spasms, shorter hospital stay, early Foley removal, and decreased postoperative need for analgesics. The major drawback is the technical challenge of the surgery, particularly in smaller bladders, and is therefore recommended primarily for patients over age 4 years with minimum bladder capacity of 200 cc. This procedure is feasible and safe though has been associated with increased incidence of bladder leak, and success rates approach but do not reach that of the open technique.
- Endoscopic surgery with Deflux® injection is the quickest, simplest approach. It is associated with low morbidity and rare procedural-related complications. The most significant drawback is that, while effective, it pales in success rate for VUR resolution (51–85 %) when compared to the gold standard open technique (97–100 %). It is not thought to be a definitive VUR correction surgery, though occasionally one or more Deflux® injections may promote VUR resolution and prevent the need for definitive surgery.
- The choice in surgical approach must be individualized for each patient with regard to the age of the child, the severity of the child's condition, and the family's preferences. These must be balanced with consideration of the surgeon's experiences and outcomes. In light of

the natural history of reflux and its tendency to spontaneously resolve, not all cases require surgical intervention. Technologic advancement and increasing ease of intervention should not change the indications for intervention.

References

1. Arant Jr BS. Vesicoureteric reflux and renal injury. Am J Kidney Dis. 1991;17(5): 491–511.
2. Williams G, Fletcher JT, Alexander SI, Craig JC. Vesicoureteral reflux. J Am Soc Nephrol. 2008;19(5):847–62.
3. Sargent MA. What is the normal prevalence of vesicoureteral reflux? Pediatr Radiol. 2000;30(9):587–93.
4. Majd M, Rushton HG, Jantausch B, Wiedermann BL. Relationship among vesicoureteral reflux, P-fimbriated Escherichia coli, and acute pyelonephritis in children with febrile urinary tract infection. J Pediatr. 1991;119(4):578–85.
5. Chand DH, Rhoades T, Poe SA, Kraus S, Strife CF. Incidence and severity of vesicoureteral reflux in children related to age, gender, race and diagnosis. J Urol. 2003;170(4 Pt 2):1548–50.
6. Connolly LP, Treves ST, Connolly SA, Zurakowski D, Share JC, Bar-Sever Z, et al. Vesicoureteral reflux in children: incidence and severity in siblings. J Urol. 1997;157(6):2287–90.
7. Puri P, Chertin B, Velayudham M, Dass L, Colhoun E. Treatment of vesicoureteral reflux by endoscopic injection of dextranomer/hyaluronic Acid copolymer: preliminary results. J Urol. 2003;170(4 Pt 2):1541–4. discussion 4.
8. Herndon CD, McKenna PH, Kolon TF, Gonzales ET, Baker LA, Docimo SG. A multicenter outcomes analysis of patients with neonatal reflux presenting with prenatal hydronephrosis. J Urol. 1999;162(3 Pt 2):1203–8.
9. Priti K, Rao KL, Menon P, Singh N, Mittal BR, Bhattacharya A, et al. Posterior urethral valves: incidence and progress of vesicoureteric reflux after primary fulguration. Pediatr Surg Int. 2004;20(2):136–9.
10. Morioka A, Miyano T, Ando K, Yamataka T, Lane GJ. Management of vesicoureteral reflux secondary to neurogenic bladder. Pediatr Surg Int. 1998;13(8):584–6.
11. Koff SA, Wagner TT, Jayanthi VR. The relationship among dysfunctional elimination syndromes, primary vesicoureteral reflux and urinary tract infections in children. J Urol. 1998;160(3 Pt 2):1019–22.
12. McLorie GA, McKenna PH, Jumper BM, Churchill BM, Gilmour RF, Khoury AE. High grade vesicoureteral reflux: analysis of observational therapy. J Urol. 1990;144(2 Pt 2):537–40. discussion 45.
13. Weiss R, Tamminen-Mobius T, Koskimies O, Olbing H, Smellie JM, Hirche H, et al. Characteristics at entry of children with severe primary vesicoureteral reflux recruited for a multicenter, international therapeutic trial comparing medical and surgical management. The International Reflux Study in Children. J Urol. 1992;148(5 Pt 2):1644–9.

14. Papadopoulou F, Efremidis SC, Oiconomou A, Badouraki M, Panteleli M, Papachristou F, et al. Cyclic voiding cystourethrography: is vesicoureteral reflux missed with standard voiding cystourethrography? Eur Radiol. 2002;12(3):666–70.
15. Craig JC, Knight JF, Sureshkumar P, Lam A, Onikul E, Roy LP. Vesicoureteric reflux and timing of micturating cystourethrography after urinary tract infection. Arch Dis Child. 1997;76(3):275–7.
16. Diamond DA, Kleinman PK, Spevak M, Nimkin K, Belanger P, Karellas A. The tailored low dose fluoroscopic voiding cystogram for familial reflux screening. J Urol. 1996;155(2):681–2.
17. Hoberman A, Charron M, Hickey RW, Baskin M, Kearney DH, Wald ER. Imaging studies after a first febrile urinary tract infection in young children. N Engl J Med. 2003;348(3):195–202.
18. Majd M, Nussbaum Blask AR, Markle BM, Shalaby-Rana E, Pohl HG, Park JS, et al. Acute pyelonephritis: comparison of diagnosis with 99mTc-DMSA, SPECT, spiral CT, MR imaging, and power Doppler US in an experimental pig model. Radiology. 2001;218(1):101–8.
19. Olbing H, Smellie JM, Jodal U, Lax H. New renal scars in children with severe VUR: a 10-year study of randomized treatment. Pediatr Nephrol. 2003;18(11): 1128–31.
20. Bukowski TP, Betrus GG, Aquilina JW, Perlmutter AD. Urinary tract infections and pregnancy in women who underwent antireflux surgery in childhood. J Urol. 1998;159(4):1286–9.
21. Hollowell JG. Outcome of pregnancy in women with a history of vesico-ureteric reflux. BJU Int. 2008;102(7):780–4.
22. Ogan K, Pohl HG, Carlson D, Belman AB, Rushton HG. Parental preferences in the management of vesicoureteral reflux. J Urol. 2001;166(1):240–3.
23. Lakshmanan Y, Fung LC. Laparoscopic extravesicular ureteral reimplantation for vesicoureteral reflux: recent technical advances. J Endourol. 2000;14(7):589–93. Discussion 93–4.
24. Smith RP, Oliver JL, Peters CA. Pediatric robotic extravesical ureteral reimplantation: comparison with open surgery. J Urol. 2011;185(5):1876–81.
25. Grimsby GM, Dwyer ME, Jacobs MA, Ost MC, Schneck FX, Cannon GM, et al. Multi-institutional review of outcomes of robot-assisted laparoscopic extravesical ureteral reimplantation. J Urol. 2015;193 Suppl 5:1791–5.
26. Peters CA. Robotically assisted surgery in pediatric urology. Urol Clin North Am. 2004;31(4):743–52.
27. Gundeti MS, Boysen WR, Shah A. Robot-assisted laparoscopic extravesical ureteral reimplantation: technique modifications contribute to optimized outcomes. Eur Urol. 2016.
28. Riquelme M, Lopez M, Landa S, Mejia F, Aranda A, Rodarte-Shade M, et al. Laparoscopic extravesical ureteral reimplantation (LEVUR): a multicenter experience with 95 cases. Eur J Pediatr Surg. 2013;23(2):143–7.
29. Casale P, Patel RP, Kolon TF. Nerve sparing robotic extravesical ureteral reimplantation. J Urol. 2008;179(5):1987–9. Discussion 90.

30. Dangle PP, Razmaria AA, Towle VL, Frim DM, Gundeti MS. Is pelvic plexus nerve documentation feasible during robotic assisted laparoscopic ureteral reimplantation with extravesical approach? J Pediatr Urol. 2013;9(4):442–7.
31. Schomburg JL, Haberman K, Willihnganz-Lawson KH, Shukla AR. Robot-assisted laparoscopic ureteral reimplantation: a single surgeon comparison to open surgery. J Pediatr Urol. 2014;10(5):875–9.
32. Peters CA, Woo R. Intravesical robotically assisted bilateral ureteral reimplantation. J Endourol. 2005;19(6):618–21. Discussion 21–2.
33. Yeung CK, Sihoe JD, Borzi PA. Endoscopic cross-trigonal ureteral reimplantation under carbon dioxide bladder insufflation: a novel technique. J Endourol. 2005;19(3):295–9.
34. Kutikov A, Guzzo TJ, Canter DJ, Casale P. Initial experience with laparoscopic transvesical ureteral reimplantation at the Children's Hospital of Philadelphia. J Urol. 2006;176(5):2222–5. Discussion 5–6.
35. Weiss DA, Shukla AR. The robotic-assisted ureteral reimplantation: the evolution to a new standard. Urol Clin North Am. 2015;42(1):99–109.
36. Jayanthi V, Patel A. Vesicoscopic ureteral reimplantation: a minimally invasive technique for the definitive repair of vesicoureteral reflux. Adv Urol. 2008;973616.
37. Valla JS, Steyaert H, Griffin SJ, Lauron J, Fragoso AC, Arnaud P, et al. Transvesicoscopic Cohen ureteric reimplantation for vesicoureteral reflux in children: a single-centre 5-year experience. J Pediatr Urol. 2009;5(6):466–71.
38. Lavelle MT, Conlin MJ, Skoog SJ. Subureteral injection of Deflux for correction of reflux: analysis of factors predicting success. Urology. 2005;65(3):564–7.
39. Lackgren G, Wahlin N, Skoldenberg E, Stenberg A. Long-term followup of children treated with dextranomer/hyaluronic acid copolymer for vesicoureteral reflux. J Urol. 2001;166(5):1887–92.
40. Puri P, Pirker M, Mohanan N, Dawrant M, Dass L, Colhoun E. Subureteral dextranomer/hyaluronic acid injection as first line treatment in the management of high grade vesicoureteral reflux. J Urol. 2006;176(4 Pt 2):1856–9. Discussion 9–60.
41. Elder JS, Diaz M, Caldamone AA, Cendron M, Greenfield S, Hurwitz R, et al. Endoscopic therapy for vesicoureteral reflux: a meta-analysis. I. Reflux resolution and urinary tract infection. J Urol. 2006;175(2):716–22.
42. Peters CA, Skoog SJ, Arant Jr BS, Copp HL, Elder JS, Hudson RG, et al. Summary of the AUA guideline on management of primary vesicoureteral reflux in children. J Urol. 2010;184(3):1134–44.
43. Lee EK, Gatti JM, Demarco RT, Murphy JP. Long-term followup of dextranomer/hyaluronic acid injection for vesicoureteral reflux: late failure warrants continued followup. J Urol. 2009;181(4):1869–74. Discussion 74–5.
44. Sedberry-Ross S, Rice DC, Pohl HG, Belman AB, Majd M, Rushton HG. Febrile urinary tract infections in children with an early negative voiding cystourethrogram after treatment of vesicoureteral reflux with dextranomer/hyaluronic acid. J Urol. 2008;180 Suppl 4:1605–9. Discussion 10.

52. Laparoscopic Approaches to Peritoneal Dialysis Access

Ruchi Amin and Danielle S. Walsh

Introduction

Peritoneal dialysis (PD) is the preferred long-term dialysis modality in the pediatric population [1]. The benefits of PD include a lower incidence of serious complications, improved cost-effectiveness, lack of routine blood access, and improved independence, including the ability to attend school. Peritoneal dialysis is also preferentially used in this population, as it is often difficult to achieve adequate flow rates with hemodialysis, especially in smaller children. In 1959, Richard Ruben was the first to describe the use of peritoneal dialysis for a patient with chronic renal failure [2]. In 1968, Henry Tenckhoff described the placement of an indwelling peritoneal catheter via open surgical technique [3, 4]. This technique has since been modified to allow for catheter placement via open surgical technique using a minilaparotomy incision, percutaneous Seldinger technique, and laparoscopy. The routine use of laparoscopy for PD catheter placement has been described since the early 1990s. Laparoscopic catheter placement is of particular interest as it allows for direct visualization of the peritoneal cavity. This allows the surgeon to perform simultaneous adhesiolysis, omentectomy, and any other indicated procedure, such as inguinal hernia repair, gastrostomy tube placement, or kidney biopsy [5].

Preoperative Evaluation

A thorough history should be taken on every patient considered for PD to ensure they meet criteria for catheter placement. Almost any child with a need for dialysis can be considered for initiation of PD, including

D.S. Walsh et al. (eds.), *The SAGES Manual of Pediatric Minimally Invasive Surgery*, DOI 10.1007/978-3-319-43642-5_52

for fluid removal in neonates requiring ECMO after cardiac surgery [6]. It is also the preferred method of dialysis in older children with bleeding diathesis, labile diabetes mellitus, needle anxiety, active lifestyle, and those with a high likelihood for renal transplantation in the near future [7]. Contraindications include severe inflammatory bowel disease/active colitis, recurrent peritonitis, active abdominal skin/soft tissue infection, and poor social support [7, 8]. It is also important to note that catheter placement may be more challenging in patients that are obese and have had prior abdominal surgeries and in patients with preexisting ostomy, intra-abdominal graft/shunts, or intraperitoneal feeding access when discussing the operative details with these patients [9]. Preoperative risk stratification should be performed to address the risks associated with the use of general anesthesia. In patients who are unable to tolerate a general anesthetic, open or percutaneous methods of catheter placement under local anesthetic and/or sedation are recommended.

A preoperative physical exam is important to ascertain if there are hernias present, as these should be repaired at the time of catheter placement. The catheter exit site should be marked prior to surgery, preferably with the patient sitting, standing, and lying down (as appropriate for age), in order to decrease the risk of postoperative cuff extrusion [10]. The catheter is tunneled inferiorly in the subcutaneous tissue to an exit site location in the lateral abdominal wall to reduce the risk of catheter-associated infection [9]. This site should be placed away from the belt line, diapers, and stomas. Presternal exit sites have been described for children and adults with stomas, incontinence, obesity, or other body habitus concerns [11, 12]. As constipation is a known cause of catheter dysfunction, a preoperative enema, though rarely given, may be of some utility in high-risk patients. A single dose of first- or second-generation cephalosporin should be given intravenously prior to surgery; routine usage of vancomycin is discouraged due to concern for the development of vancomycin-resistant enterococcus [10]. Preoperative showering or bathing with antiseptic soap may also help to reduce postoperative infection.

Technique

Laparoscopic PD catheter insertion is performed with the patient in supine position. Peritoneal access for port placement is obtained by insufflating at the umbilicus using a Veress needle. Standard use of 30-degree, 0-degree, and 3-, 5-, and 10-mm laparoscopes has all been described. Generally, two ports are placed, with one in the paramedian

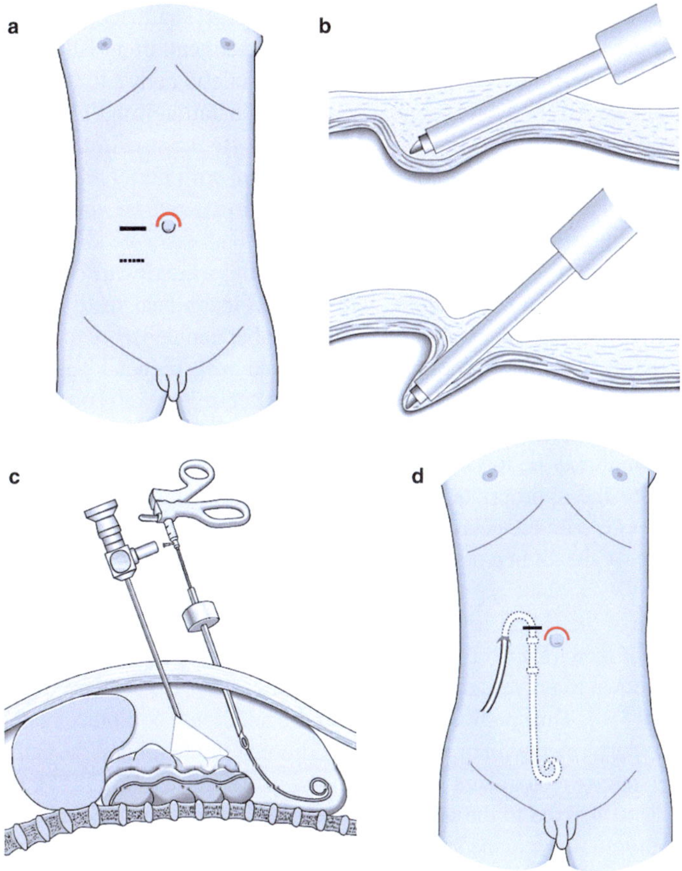

Fig. 52.1. Two-cannula insertion technique. (**a**) Localization of the skin incisions. *Dashed line* shows the entrance of the catheter through the rectus muscle and the peritoneum. (**b**) Creation of the subcutaneous tunnel with a trocar. (**c**) The end of the catheter is pulled out together with the cannula through the abdominal wall and subcutaneous tunnel until the inner cuff comes to lie just above the posterior sheath of the rectus abdominis muscle. (**d**) Final position of the catheter. From Emir H. Endoscopic Surgery for Peritoneal Dialysis Catheters in Children. In: Endoscopic Surgery in Infants and Children, Bax KMA et al., eds. 2008. Springer Berlin Heidelberg, Berlin, Heidelberg, pp 485–498. Reprinted with permission.

fascia corresponding to the catheter size (e.g., 8 Fr) and a second port laterally (3–5 mm) for grasping instruments (Fig. 52.1). In patients with prior abdominal surgeries or those who will need additional surgery during catheter placement, a third port can be placed to facilitate additional grasping and dissection. Single-port laparoscopic catheter insertion has also been described, with placement of a 10-mm port through a supraumbilical incision after partial omentectomy and subsequent passage of a peel-away percutaneous catheter through the trocar [13]. The current SAGES recommendations are to use the smallest port available that will allow for adequate visualization, with preference for noncutting ports to allow for faster healing, minimize leak rate, and decrease time to dialysis initiation [9]. The majority of catheters are silicone with either a pigtail or straight body and two cuffs; a single-cuffed catheter may be used in smaller infants with limited abdominal wall, but these catheters have been associated with a higher incidence of peritonitis [14]. Coiled catheters have been associated with reduced pain, better catheter survival, and lower rate of catheter migration compared to straight catheters [15]. However, the coiled catheters are of a fixed length and may be too long for placement in smaller infants.

Once the appropriate catheter is chosen, it is inserted through the larger port, with the deep cuff positioned between the anterior and posterior rectus sheath in a downward and lateral subcutaneous configuration. This involves tunneling the catheter an additional 4–6 cm (depending on the size of the child), toward the midline pelvis, after it is seen above the posterior rectus sheath right before it enters the peritoneal cavity. This has been shown to prevent migration of the catheter tip and decrease leakage of fluid [16]. This method does not require additional port placement and can be performed with or without an additional suture around the catheter at the anterior rectus sheath to further minimize leakage of fluid [17]. If the inner cuff is fixed to the anterior rectus sheath, care should be taken that this suture is not cinched so tight it occludes the catheter. Suture fixation of catheter to the bladder, uterus, or pelvic sidewall has also been described as a method to decrease the risk for catheter tip migration. However, this technique requires additional port placement, may increase difficulty for future catheter removal, and may increase risk for hernia and adhesion development [18].

It is important to ensure that the inner cuff does not extend into the peritoneum. The superficial cuff should be approximately 2 cm from the exit site to decrease the risk of cuff extrusion, which is a known risk factor for exit site infection [14]. Too short a distance will predispose to cuff extrusion, whereas too long a distance leads to formation of deep sinus tract, granulation tissue formation, and increased risk of tunnel infection. The catheter tip should be in the most dependent portion of the pelvis (Fig. 52.2), right above the bladder reflection, and anterior to the rectum in the rectovesical or rectouterine pouch. If the pelvic space is occluded with dense adhesions from a prior surgery or episode of

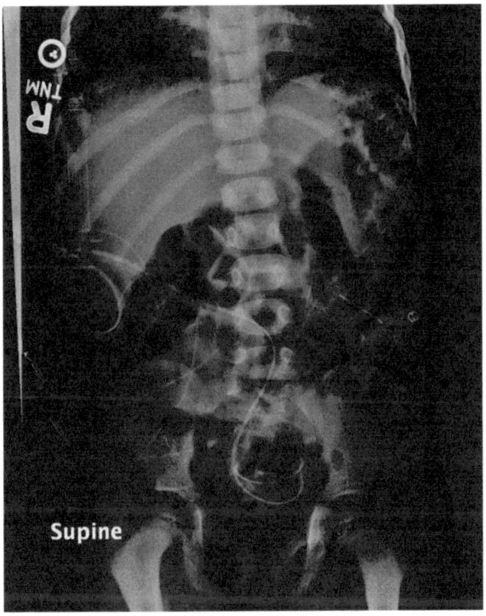

Fig. 52.2. Peritoneal dialysis catheter with pelvic positioning as seen on plain radiograph.

peritonitis, the surgeon may elect to place the catheter over the liver below the right chest wall (Fig. 52.3).

Catheter occlusion due to omental wrapping is more common in children than adults; therefore, routine omentectomy in smaller children and infants is performed. The omentum can be partially removed through the port using electrocautery or ligature. Although omentopexy is preferred to omentectomy in adults [19], the integrity of pediatric omentum poses a technical challenge in regard to suture fixation. Therefore, in smaller children and infants, a formal omentectomy is common. Laparoscopy also allows for repair of inguinal or ventral hernias if present. Comparative trials of open versus laparoscopic hernia repair in PD patients do not exist. However, most experts recommend fixing these defects at the time of surgery [9]. If the child is in need of feeding access, a gastrostomy can be performed with two-point fixation to the fascia using absorbable suture. There is a slightly higher rate of infection in patients with gastrostomy tubes on PD, although independent from timing of gastrostomy placement [9]. Finally, a renal biopsy can also be obtained under direct visualization with the biopsy needle after laparoscopic exposure of the kidney.

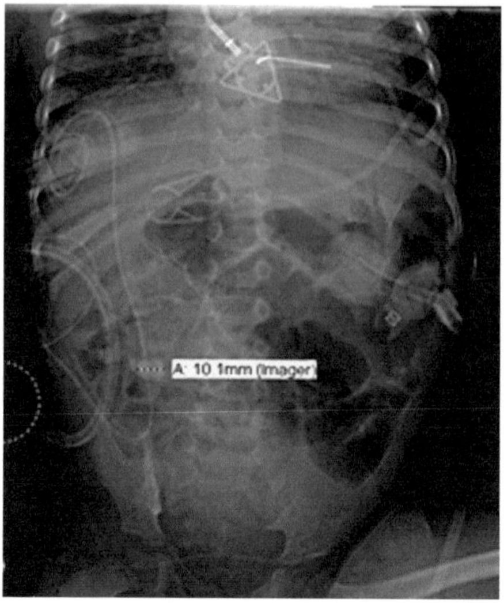

Fig. 52.3. Peritoneal dialysis catheter with suprahepatic position noted on plain radiograph.

After removal of all the instruments and trocars, the fascia at the umbilicus is closed in two layers with an absorbable suture to prevent hernia development. The exit site should be round and small to allow for a snug fit within the surrounding skin. While some surgeons may elect to apply Dermabond (Ethicon Inc., Somerville, NJ, USA) at the exit site, there is clear evidence to suggest that sutures should not be placed at the exit site due to increased risk for bacterial colonization [9]. Fibroblast ingrowth of the Dacron cuff will provide adequate anchorage of the catheter within 2–3 weeks. For patients who require dialysis shortly after catheter implantation, the usage of fibrin glue to the peritoneal cuff suture has been shown to prevent early dialysate leakage; however, this method does not decrease the risk for the development of peritonitis or exit site infection [20]. The fibrin glue is applied around the internal cuff and down the tunnel between the inner and outer cuffs.

The silastic tubing of the catheter is attached to the infusion/drainage system using a titanium connector. This attachment is often prone to mechanical failure from slackening of the tubing, which can lead to eventual disconnection, leaving the patient at risk for bacterial entry with development of peritonitis. As a result, some advocate the use of a "lock-ring" device to further secure this connection [21]. The distal portion of the catheter is attached to a universal male Luer Lock fitting "sealing cap." This cap has a rubber stopper, with a self-sealing injection site for administering medication or drawing peritoneal dialysate samples. Once the dialysis catheter has been assembled, an intraoperative catheter trial using 10 cc/kg of dialysate with 1–2 units of heparin per mL or saline should be performed to ensure adequate inflow and outflow. This instillation and drainage cycle should be continued until the fluid is clear and demonstrates that at least 50 % of the instillate is returned. If at least half the fluid cannot be passively returned in the operating room, the catheter placement should be adjusted.

The catheter should be adequately secured to the abdominal wall to minimize mobility and traction injury. There are commercially available immobilization devices; however, a simple tape or gauze dressing is generally sufficient, as long as the catheter is securely anchored close to the exit site. Some oozing is to be expected; therefore, the exit site is initially dressed with several layers of sterile gauze or an ABD pad. An occlusive dressing should not be used, as these tend to trap fluid, which predisposes the exit site to bacterial growth and subsequent infection [14].

The initial postoperative dressing should not be changed more than once a week during the first 2 weeks, unless there is concern for bleeding or infection [14]. Generally 2 weeks of healing time is given before the initiation of dialysis; however, if early dialysis is necessary, there are no data to suggest a substantial difference in minor versus major leaks in regard to the time of initiation or initial fluid volume [22–24].

Postoperative Care (Outcomes and Complications)

Although there has been vast improvement in catheter quality and surgical technique, the incidence of complications reported in the pediatric population remains relatively high. Basic laparoscopic insertion without using techniques to minimize catheter dysfunction results in similar rates of catheter malfunction as open insertion [25]. Interestingly, advanced laparoscopic PD catheter insertion using lysis of adhesions, catheter fixation with rectus sheath tunneling, and omentopexy has the lowest reported rate of catheter dysfunction in adults, even in patients with prior abdominal surgery. The majority of pediatric studies available have described the use of the omentectomy during both open and laparoscopic catheter insertions; however, none of them have noted a decrease in reoperation for catheter dysfunction [9].

Catheter dysfunction is most often associated with occlusion from thrombosis or with mechanical failure due to kinking, compression, or migration of the catheter. A physical exam should be performed and plain radiographs obtained to rule out constipation. If negative, further studies such as catheterography may be helpful in delineating the underlying etiology. Catheter occlusions secondary to fibrin or blood clot can be managed with tissue plasminogen activator (TPA). Two milligrams of TPA reconstituted in 40 cc of normal saline, and instilled in the catheter for 1 h, resulted in restoration of patency in 57 % of catheters [26]. Another technique described is the use of an endoscopic retrograde cholangiopancreatography cytology brush to manipulate a malfunctioning PD catheter, with subsequent flushing of the catheter with heparinized saline through the injection port to remove any clot or fibrin. The advantage of this method is the ability to also inject contrast through the injection port to confirm the patency of the catheter, while the brush remains within the lumen [27]. If nonoperative treatments such as flushing, thrombolytics, and fluoroscopic manipulation are unsuccessful, then laparoscopy with catheter repositioning may be necessary (Fig. 52.4).

Other complications after PD catheter insertion include bleeding, dialysate leakage, exit site infection, peritonitis, and pain during dialysis. Bleeding generally occurs in 0–5 % patients. This may occur from inferior epigastric injury during insertion through the rectus sheath, intra-abdominally secondary to dissection performed during the omentectomy

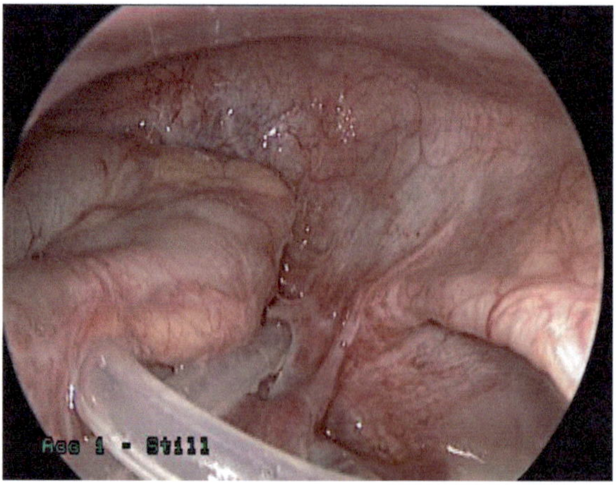

Fig. 52.4. Peritoneal dialysis catheter that was surrounded by dense adhesions requiring laparoscopic revision.

or adhesiolysis, or at the exit site. Angling the insertion site toward the medial border of the rectus, and using nonmetal-bladed trocars or sheaths to insert the catheter through the abdominal wall, may help minimize arterial bleeding [17]. Additionally, limiting the extent and performing careful dissection during adhesiolysis and omentectomy may help minimize intra-abdominal bleeding. Exit site bleeding can be controlled with the application of direct pressure or placement of sutures. Additionally, any coagulopathy should also be identified and corrected to prevent ongoing bleeding.

Leakage of dialysate fluid occurs in 0–12.8 % patients and has been found to be upward of 18 % in infants, secondary to their lack of abdominal wall thickness [1]. This can be treated by transitioning to low-volume or cycled PD initially or with temporary HD for 2–4 weeks if there is a persistent leak. Fibrin glue can be used at the catheter tunnel exit site if leakage is noted within the first 24–48 h and has been shown to decrease the incidence of leak in a randomized prospective study by Sojo et al. in the pediatric population [20].

Uncomplicated exit site infections are initially treated with oral antibiotics for a 2–4-week duration, based upon timing to resolution of symptoms and culture susceptibilities; however, in the pediatric population, these patients will often require surgical salvage. Cuff shaving has been described as an alternative technique for those patients that fail antibiotic therapy—this is performed by shaving off the superficial layer of the subcutaneous cuff and bringing the catheter out at a new exit site. Alternately, the entire subcutaneous tubing can be replaced from above the internal cuff.

Peritonitis has been described in 0–11 % of patients. It is similar in incidence regardless of insertion technique and is managed with intravenous and intraperitoneal antibiotic therapy. Peritonitis should be considered in any child that presents with cloudy peritoneal effluent. Empiric therapy should be initiated in any patient who has an effluent with white blood cell count greater than 100 mm^3 and >50 % of WBC are polymononuclear leukocytes after 2 h of instillation. Empiric therapy should be based upon center-specific antibiotic susceptibility patterns; however, intraperitoneal cefepime monotherapy is suggested as the first-line therapy if available. If unavailable, then a first-generation cephalosporin in combination with ceftazidime or an aminoglycoside can also be used [14]. Catheter removal is suggested in those with persistent infection or with positive fungal cultures. Techniques such as the double-bag system, careful hand-washing habits, treatment of nasal carriage of *Staphylococcus aureus* (intranasal mupirocin twice daily for 5 days), and routine treatment of the exit site with topical mupirocin can lower the rate of peritonitis but not eliminate it [24].

Pain with instillation or drainage of fluid is a rare complication, but can be quite debilitating for patients, especially in the pediatric population. This is best managed with altering the dialysate pH, decreasing the rate of infusion, or performing tidal dialysis with incomplete drainage of PD fluid at the completion of the cycle. If the pain remains refractory to these measures, then the patient may require catheter manipulation, repositioning, or even removal [9].

Summary

- Laparoscopy is an accepted method for peritoneal dialysis catheter placement in the pediatric population.
- A thorough history and physical exam should be performed on each patient; preoperative workup should include proper site marking, assessment for hernia on exam to be repaired at the time of catheter placement, and a first- or second-generation cephalosporin 30 min prior to surgery.
- There is no consensus on port number, size, or placement—the current recommendation is to use the smallest port available that will allow adequate visualization, with a preference for noncutting trocars to allow for faster healing, minimize leak rate, and decrease time to dialysis initiation.
- The silicone-coiled double-cuffed catheter is preferred for PD placement, but there is a role for the straight catheter, especially in smaller infants.
- The catheter should be inserted in a downward and lateral manner in the subcutaneous tissue, with the deep cuff between the anterior and posterior rectus and the superficial cuff approximately 2 cm from the exit site.
- Fibrin glue can be applied around the inner cuff, and in the tunnel between the inner and outer cuff, to prevent early dialysate leakage in patients that will undergo early dialysis.
- Lysis of adhesions, interval suture fixation of the catheter, rectus sheath tunneling, and partial omentectomy or omentopexy have all been described as additional techniques to minimize catheter dysfunction.
- Basic laparoscopic catheter insertion without the abovementioned techniques results in similar dysfunction rates compared to open surgical

PD catheter insertion; however, in adults, advanced laparoscopic PD catheter placement with lysis of adhesions, catheter fixation with rectus sheath tunneling, and omentopexy has been shown to have the lowest rate of catheter dysfunction.

- Complications after PD catheter placement included catheter occlusion and malposition, bleeding, dialysate leakage, exit site infection, peritonitis, and pain with instillation.

References

1. Phan J, Stanford S, Zaritsky JJ, DeUgarte DA. Risk factors for morbidity and mortality in pediatric patients with peritoneal dialysis catheters. J Pediatr Surg. 2013;48:197–202.
2. Drukker W. History of peritoneal dialysis. In: Maher JF. editors. Replacement of Renal Function by Dialysis. 3rd ed. Dordrecht: Kluwer; 1987: p. 475–515.
3. Tenckhoff H, Schechter H. A bacteriologically safe peritoneal access device. Trans Am Soc Artif Intern Organs. 1968;14:181–7.
4. Tenckhoff H, Curtis FK. Experience with maintenance peritoneal dialysis in the home. Trans Am Soc Artif Intern Organs. 1970;16:90–5.
5. Stringel G, McBride W, Weiss R. Laparoscopic placement of peritoneal dialysis catheters in children. J Pediatr Surg. 2008;43:857–60.
6. Sasser WC, Robert SM, Askenazi DJ, et al. Peritoneal dialysis: an alternative modality of fluid removal in neonates requiring extracorporeal membrane oxygenation after cardiac surgery. J Extra Corpor Technol. 2014;46(2):157–61.
7. Shetty A, Oreopoulos G. Peritoneal dialysis: its indications and contraindications. Dial Transplant. 2000;29(2):71–7.
8. Foundation NK. K/DPQI clinical practice guidelines for peritoneal dialysis adequacy: update 2000. Am J Kidney Dis. 2001;37:S65–136.
9. Haggerty S, Roth S, Walsh D, Stefanidis D, Price R, Fanelli RD, Penner T, Richardson W. SAGES guidelines committee. Guidelines for laparoscopic peritoneal dialysis access surgery. Surg Endosc. 2014;28(11):3016–45.
10. Crabtree JH. Construction and use of stencils in planning for peritoneal dialysis catheter implantation. Perit Dial Int. 2003;23:395–8.
11. Crabtree JH, Fishman A. Laparoscopic implantation of swan neck presternal peritoneal dialysis catheters. J Laparoendosc Adv Surg Tech A. 2003;13:131–7.
12. Chadha V, Jones LL, Ramirez ZD, Warady BA. Chest wall peritoneal dialysis catheter placement in infants with a colostomy. Adv Perit Dial. 2000;16:318–20.
13. Milliken I, Fitzpatrick M, Subramaniam R. Single-port laparoscopic insertion of peritoneal dialysis catheters in children. J Pediatr Urol. 2006;2(4):308–11.
14. Warady BA, Bakkaloglu S, Newland J, Cantwell M, Verrina E, Neu A, Chadha V, Yap HK, Schaefer F. Consensus guidelines for the prevention and treatment of catheter-related infections and peritonitis in pediatric patients receiving peritoneal dialysis: 2012 update. Perit Dial Int. 2012;32(2):S32–86.

15. Harvey E. Peritoneal access in children. Perit Dial Int. 2001;21(3):S218–22.
16. Flanigan M, Gokal R. Peritoneal catheters and exit-site practices toward optimum peritoneal access: a review of current developments. Perit Dial Int. 2005;25:132–9.
17. Attaluri V, Lebeis C, Brethauer S, Rosenblatt S. Advanced laparoscopic techniques significantly improve function of peritoneal dialysis catheters. J Am Coll Surg. 2010;211:699–704.
18. Frost JH, Bagul A. A brief recap of tips and surgical manoeuvres to enhance optimal outcome of surgically placed peritoneal dialysis catheters. Int J Nephrol. 2012;2012:1–7.
19. Haggerty SP, Zeni TM, Carder M, Frantzides CT. Laparoscopic peritoneal dialysis catheter insertion using a Quinton percutaneous insertion kit. JSLS. 2007;11:208–14.
20. Sojo ET, Grosman MD, Monteverde ML, Bailez MM, Delgado N. Fibrin glue is useful in preventing early dialysate leakage in children on chronic peritoneal dialysis. Perit Dial Int. 2004;24:186–90.
21. Hudson S, Mackie R, Stewart WK. Lock-ring for Tenckhoff catheter/titanium adaptor junction. Uremia Invest. 1985–1986;9(1):69–71.
22. Ghaffari A. Urgent-start peritoneal dialysis: a quality improvement report. Am J Kidney Dis. 2012;59:400–8.
23. Song JH, Kim GA, Lee SW, Kim MJ. Clinical outcomes of immediate full-volume exchange one year after peritoneal catheter implantation for CAPD. Perit Dial Int. 2000;20:194–9.
24. Rahim KA, Seidel K, McDonald RA. Risk factors for catheter—related complications in pediatric peritoneal dialysis. Pediatr Nephrol. 2004;19:1021–8.
25. Xie H, Zhang W, Cheng J, He Q. Laparoscopic versus open catheter placement in peritoneal dialysis patients: a systematic review and meta-analysis. BMC Nephrol. 2012;13:69.
26. Shea M, Hmiel SP, Beck AM. Use of tissue plasminogen activator for thrombolysis in occluded peritoneal dialysis catheters in children. Adv Perit Dial Conf Perit Dial. 2001;17:249–52.
27. Hummeida MA, Eltahir JMA, Ali HM, Khalid SE, Mobarak AI, Modawi MHA, Abu-Aisha H. Successful management of an obstructed Tenckhoff catheter using an endoscopic retrograde cholangiopancreatography (ERCP) cytology brush. Perit Dial Int. 2010;30(4):482–4.

Index

D.S. Walsh et al. (eds.), *The SAGES Manual of Pediatric Minimally Invasive Surgery*, DOI 10.1007/978-3-319-43642-5

H

U

V

MIX
Papier aus verantwortungsvollen Quellen
Paper from responsible sources
FSC® C105338

If you have any concerns about our products,
you can contact us on
ProductSafety@springernature.com

In case Publisher is established outside the EU,
the EU authorized representative is:
Springer Nature Customer Service Center GmbH
Europaplatz 3, 69115 Heidelberg, Germany

Printed by Libri Plureos GmbH
in Hamburg, Germany